Anesthesiology Keywords Review

SECOND EDITION

ASSOCIATE SPECIAL EDITORS

From the Department of Anesthesiology

Yale University School of Medicine

New Haven, Connecticut

Special Editors For Cardiac Anesthesia Topics
Benjamin Sherman, M.D. - Assistant Professor
Qingbing Zhu, M.D., Ph.D. - Assistant Professor

Special Editors For Critical Care Medicine Topics
Ala S. Haddadin, M.D. - Assistant Professor
Hossam Tatawy, M.D. - Assistant Professor

Special Editor For Neuroanesthesia Topics
Ramachandran Ramani, M.D. - Associate Professor

Special Editor For Obstetric Anesthesia Topics
Lars E. Helgeson, M.D. - Assistant Professor

Special Editor For Pediatric Anesthesia and Endocrine Topics
Mamatha Punjala, M.D. - Assistant Professor

Special Editors For Regional Anesthesia and Pain Topics
Thomas M. Halaszynski, M.D., DMD - Associate Professor
Jodi Sherman, M.D. - Assistant Professor

Special Editor For Statistics and Anesthesia Machine/Equipment Topics
Raj K. Modak, M.D. - Assistant Professor

Special Editors For Thoracic Anesthesia Topics
Shamsuddin Akhtar, M.D. - Associate Professor
Veronica Matei, M.D. - Assistant Professor

Anesthesiology Keywords Review

SECOND EDITION

Edited By

Raj K. Modak, MD
Assistant Professor
Yale University
Department of Anesthesiology
New Haven, Connecticut

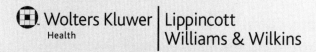 Wolters Kluwer | Lippincott
Health | Williams & Wilkins

Philadelphia • Baltimore • New York • London
Buenos Aires • Hong Kong • Sydney • Tokyo

Acquisitions Editor: Brian Brown
Product Manager: Nicole T. Dernoski
Marketing Manager: Lisa Lawrence
Vendor Manager: Alicia Jackson
Senior Manufacturing Manager: Benjamin Rivera
Design Coordinator: Teresa Mallon
Compositor: S4Carlisle

Printed in the United States

Library of Congress Cataloging-in-Publication Data

Anesthesiology keywords review / edited by Raj K. Modak. — 2nd ed.
    p. ; cm.
  Includes bibliographical references and index.
  ISBN 978-1-4511-2119-3 (alk. paper)
  I. Modak, Raj K.
  [DNLM: 1. Anesthesia—methods—Handbooks. 2. Anesthesiology—methods—Handbooks. 3. Anesthetics—Handbooks. 4. Terminology as Topic—Handbooks. WO 231]

  617.9'6—dc23

                                                                2012043589

Care has been taken to confirm the accuracy of the information presented and to describe generally accepted practices. However, the authors, editors, and publisher are not responsible for errors or omissions or for any consequences from application of the information in this book and make no warranty, expressed or implied, with respect to the currency, completeness, or accuracy of the contents of the publication. Application of this information in a particular situation remains the professional responsibility of the practitioner.

The authors, editors, and publisher have exerted every effort to ensure that drug selection and dosage set forth in this text are in accordance with current recommendations and practice at the time of publication. However, in view of ongoing research, changes in government regulations, and the constant flow of information relating to drug therapy and drug reactions, the reader is urged to check the package insert for each drug for any change in indications and dosage and for added warnings and precautions. This is particularly important when the recommended agent is a new or infrequently employed drug.

Some drugs and medical devices presented in this publication have Food and Drug Administration (FDA) clearance for limited use in restricted research settings. It is the responsibility of the health care provider to ascertain the FDA status of each drug or device planned for use in their clinical practice.

To purchase additional copies of this book, call our customer service department at (800) 638-3030 or fax orders to (301) 223-2320. International customers should call (301) 223-2300.

Visit Lippincott Williams & Wilkins on the Internet: at LWW.com. Lippincott Williams & Wilkins customer service representatives are available from 8:30 am to 6 pm, EST.

10 9 8 7 6 5 4 3 2 1

I dedicate this book to my loving wifey, Marybeth

Draft Editors/Reviewers

Caroline Al Haddadin, M.D.
Stephanie Cheng, M.D.
Mary DiMiceli, M.D.
Jorge A. Galvez, M.D.
Nehal Gatha, M.D., MBA
Shaun Gruenbaum, M.D.
Ashley Kelley, M.D.
Archer K. Martin, M.D.

Kellie A. Park, M.D., Ph.D.
Bijal Patel, M.D.
Roberto Rappa, M.D.
Margaret J. Rose, M.D.
Neil Sinha, M.D.
Anjali B. Vira, M.D.
Suzana M. Zorca, M.D.

Contributors

Tomalika Ahsan-Paik, MD *
Caroline Al Haddadin, MD *
Gregory E. Albert, MD *
Brooke Albright, MD *
Sharif Al-Ruzzeh, MD, Ph.D. *
Emilio G. Andrade, MD *
Michael Archambault, MD—Pediatric Anesthesia Fellow *
Trevor M. Banack, MD *
Holly Barth, MD *
Christina A. Biello, D.O.—Pediatric Anesthesia *
Meredith A. Brown, MD *
Lisbeysi Calo, MD *
Stephanie Cheng, MD *
Anna L. Clebone, MD *
Terrence Coffey, MD *
Frederick Conlin, MD *
Milaurise Cortes, MD *
Nicholas M. Dalesio, MD *
Tiffany Denepitiya-Balicki, MD *
Mary DiMiceli, MD *
Glenn M. Dizon, MD *
Jennifer E. Dominguez, MD, MHS *
Alexey Dyachkov, MD *
Juan J. Egas, MD *
Jammie Ferrara, MD *
Samantha A. Franco, MD-Pediatric Anesthesia *
Dan B. Froicu, MD *
Xing Fu, MD *
Thomas B. Gallen, MD, MPH **
Jorge A. Galvez, MD *
Johnny Garriga, MD *
Nehal Gatha, MD, MBA *
Zhaodi Gong, MD, Ph.D. *
Shaun Gruenbaum, MD *

Gabriel Jacobs, MD *
Ervin A. Jakab, MD *
Rongjie Jiang, MBBS *
Ashley Kelley, MD *
Jinlei Li, MD, Ph.D. *
Christina N. Mack, MD *
Adnan Malik, MD *
Jordan R. Martin, MD *
Archer K. Martin, MD *
Veronica A. Matei, MD—Cardiac Anesthesia Fellow *
Dallen D. Mill, MD *
Amit Mirchandani, MD *
Tori M. Myslajek, MD *
Harika R. Nagavelli, MD *
Donald L. Neirink, MD *
Soumya Nyshadham, MD *
Adrianna D. Oprea, MD *
Kellie A. Park, MD, Ph.D. *
Bijal Patel, MD *
Tara L. Paulose, MD *
Gabriel Pitta, MD *
Roberto Rappa, MD *
Kristin L. Richards, MD *
Margaret J. Rose, MD *
Hyacinth L. Ruiter, MD *
Marianne A. Saleeb, MD *
Svetlana Sapozhnikova, MD *
Christian C. Scheps, MD *
Robert B. Schonberger, MD, M.A. *
James H. Shull, Jr., MD *
Neil Sinha, MD *
Garth C. Skoropowski, MD *
Kimberly A. Slininger, MD *
Dmitri Souzdalnitski, MD *
Kevan C. Stanton, MD *
Jonathan Tidwell, MD *

Alexander A. Timchenko, MD *
Michael Tom, MD *
Margo Vallee, MD—Pediatric Anesthesia
Fellow *
Francis vanWisse, MD *
Anjali B. Vira, MD *
K. Karisa Walker, MD *

Ira Whitten, MD *
Jeffrey S. Widelitz, MD *
Chi H. Wong, D.O. *
Laurie Yonemoto, MD *
Martha Zegarra, MD *
Suzana M. Zorca, MD *

 * Department of Anesthesiology, Yale University School of Medicine, New Haven,
   Connecticut
** Department of Anesthesiology and Perioperative Medicine, Georgia Health Sciences
   University/Medical College of Georgia, Augusta, GA

Preface

The origins of this project date back to the 1980's when the book was first developed as a tool for residents preparing for both the in-service training exams and the written boards. Over the past several years, the project has evolved to meet the educational needs of our current resident physicians. The first edition was met with great success demonstrated by the many favorable reviews, electronic communications, and sales. It was humbling to know that the project aided so many people in anesthesiology, especially the residents.

One of the most unique aspects of this book, and one that residents have found most useful, is the development of a subject index. Not just one index, but multiple indices reflecting different subspecialties, organ systems, and concepts/groupings. The primary premise of the book is not to consolidate exam related topics, but to allow residents the ability to study these exam-emphasized concepts while on various rotations during their residency. Thus, enabling anesthesia residents the ability to identify what is important from a knowledge perspective, to see these important topics demonstrated in live clinical scenarios, and to discuss these topics and scenarios with faculty while on subspecialty rotations.

The authors of the script were asked to provide relevant discussions regarding each keyword topic. Key points were identified and emphasized. Common references were provided to site concept origins and provide a useful link to the appropriate source. These discussions are very successful in bringing the reader to a useful conclusion regarding the key points. Some keywords were ambiguous by nature resulting in a nebulous discussion and conclusion. This cannot be helped, since we will never truly know what the list makers were inferring in some of the keywords.

To maximize the educational benefit of this project, I expect users to go through the various indices in a systematic fashion and read the topics, especially while on clinical rotation. Once the user finds great knowledge in a single area, they should move on to other topics. However, if the user looks at a topic and is relatively uninformed about that topic or feels that the topic was inadequately covered, they should seek the references provided or find additional sources of information including discussions with instructors. In this way, residents can become the most knowledgeable by first identifying the important concepts, then studying the ones they know the least plus potentially engaging in discussion during rotations with clinical relevance. In addition, the indices list the keywords in a similar fashion to the feedback provided from the anesthesia in-service training exam. Residents should be able to cover the topics they missed easily if they save and use this list.

Although we are calling this a 2nd edition, in reality, this book is a 1st edition because new residents wrote all of the topics. As with the annual project that has been created locally at Yale University, this project represents a living process. Each local edition only covers the list at hand, potentially gaining, losing, or repeating topics from year to year. Residents commonly develop a library of 3–4 editions over their residency to get a comprehensive view of the material. This is supported by old versions continuing to be circulated years after their initial collation. In light of this, it may be fair to point out that the 1st edition may continue to hold some value.

The living process is also supported by the dynamic environment of our science. The final topic results from the resident authors represent exposures to current concepts within our specialty via clinical venues, lectures, journal articles, textbooks, meetings, and faculty, all of which are constantly changing. As such, similar topics may have changed their focus slightly over time as can be seen between two similar topics printed in the different editions.

This edition is more comprehensive as topics have been a summation of more than one recent exam list. Resident authors had a higher level of performance based on peer editor reviews. The resident draft editors contributed more in editing than in the previous edition resulting in an overall better product. There were more attending special editors which allowed better concentration on areas of expertise.

In light of *It's Your Book!,* I wanted to make note of a single resident author, Thomas Gallen (Medical College of Georgia, Augusta), who may have steered the project in a new direction by actively seeking participation. Historically, this project was completed entirely at Yale University with local residents and attendings. Thomas' participation changed this project from being solely a local project to a national endeavor.

There are many people to thank on a large project like this. Ajit Modak, my father and retired anesthesiologist, continued to supply critical input after the last publication. Roberta Hines, the Chairperson of my department, continues as one of the projects greatest supporters. At Wolters Kluwer/Lippincott Williams & Wilkins, I appreciate the patience and support of Editors, Brian Brown and Nicole Dernoski.

My resident authors should be given credit to their participation in this fantastic product. I know it will continue to serve you and so many others well. Please make note of the individual draft editors in the contributor list. This edition would not have been possible without them. The attending special editors gave generously of their time and effort to make the final copy. Many thanks to all of you for making this project successful.

Lastly, I want to thank Marybeth, my wife, to whom I dedicate this book. We have been together since the days of my residency. Together, we delicately balance my workplace and our very busy family, including our 3 children: Chloe, Jacqueline, and Julien. Marybeth has endured my own exam preparations over the years and truly understands the importance of this project.

Raj K. Modak

Contents by Alpha Section Keywords

Contents by Alpha Topic Keywords

ALPHA
TOPIC
KEYWORDS

ALPHA TOPIC KEYWORDS

ALPHA TOPIC KEYWORDS

ALPHA
TOPIC
KEYWORDS

ALPHA TOPIC KEYWORDS

ALPHA
TOPIC
KEYWORDS

ALPHA
TOPIC
KEYWORDS

ALPHA
TOPIC
KEYWORDS

ALPHA
TOPIC
KEYWORDS

ALPHA
TOPIC
KEYWORDS

Letter	Alpha Topic	Keywords	Pages	
	Peri-op	Addison's Disease: Periop Rx	26	– 27
	Peri-op	Renal function: periop preservation	490	
	Peripheral Arterial	Arterial waveform: Periph versus central	61	– 62
	Peripheral Nerves	Peripheral Nerves: Sensory versus motor	443	
	Peripheral TPN	Peripheral TPN: Complications	444	– 445
	PFT	Lung resection outcome: PFTs	314	
	pH buffering	pH Buffering: Bicarbonate	446	
	Pharmacodynamics	Ketamine: Pharmacodynamics	293	– 294
	Pharmacodynamics	Vasodilators: pharmacodynamics	600	– 601
	Pharmacokinetics	Cirrhosis: NMB pharme kinetics	150	– 151
	pharmacokinetics	Uptake of inhaled Anesthetics: V/Q Mismatch	594	– 595
	Pharmacolocy	Milrinone: pharmacology	346	– 348
	Pheochromacytoma	Pheochromocytorna: Hypertension Rx	449	
	Pheochromocytoma	Pheochromocytoma: Dx Markers	447	– 448
	Pheochromocytoma	Pheochromocytoma: pre-op Pre-paration	450	
	pH-stat	Circ arrest: pH-stat implications	148	– 149
	pH-stat	Hypothermia: pH stat management	274	– 275
	Physical Exam	FB Aspiration: Physical Exam	206	– 208
	Physician impairment	Physician impairment: Referral	451	
	Physiology	Smoking cessation: acute physiol	516	– 517
	Physiology CV	Renin-Angiotensin CV physiology	495	– 496
	Physiology of	Denervated Heart: Exercise Physiology	173	– 174
	Physiology, cardiac	Neonatal vs. adult cardiac phys	376	– 377
	Physiology, Cardiovasc	Aging: Cardiovasc physiol	31	– 32
	Physiology, Pulm	Aging: Pulm physiol	33	– 34
	Pierre-Robin	Intubation in Pierre-Robin	291	
	Placenta	Chloroprocaine placental transfer	145	
	Placenta	Placental Transfer: Anticholinergic	453	
	Placenta	Placental Transfer: Local Anesthetics	454	
	Placenta accreta	Placenta accreta: Risk factors	452	
	Plasma	FFP: warfarin reversal	225	– 226
	Plasma	Fresh frozen plasma : Indications	225	– 226
	Plateau Airway Pressure	Peak vs. Plateau Airway Pressure	437	– 438
	Plateau effect	Nalbuphine: Plateau effect mech	371	– 372
	Platelet Function	Hetastarch: platelet function	248	
	Platelet Function	Renal failure: platelet function	487	
	Pneumocephalus	Tension pneumocephalus: Dx	549	– 550
	Pneumonectomy	Hypox during pneumonectomy: Rx	278	– 279
	Pneumothorax	Tension pneumothorax: Dx and Rx	551	
	Poisoning	Organophosphate poisoning Rx	415	
	PONV	PONV after pediatric surgery	455	
	PONV	PONV Prophylaxis	456	
	Positioning	Lithotomy position: Nerve injury	307	– 308
	Positioning	Sitting position: BP measurement	514	– 515
	Post-CPB	LV failure Dx/Rx post-CPB	315	
	Post-CPB	Post-CPB creatinine increase: DDx	457	– 458
	Post-dural puncture	PDP headache: Risk factors	436	
	Post-Op	Carotid sinus stim: post-heart tplt	124	– 125
	Post-Op	Morbid obesity: post-op complications	353	– 355
	Post-Op	Myasthenia gravis: postop management	364	– 365
	Post-Op	PONV after pediatric surgery	455	

ALPHA
TOPIC
KEYWORDS

ALPHA
TOPIC
KEYWORDS

ALPHA TOPIC KEYWORDS

ALPHA TOPIC KEYWORDS

ALPHA
TOPIC
KEYWORDS

Contents by Alpha Rotation Keywords

ALPHA ROTATION KEYWORDS

Rotation	Subtopic	Keywords	Pages	
	Circulation	Venous air embolism	605	– 606
	Circulation	Venous air embolism detection	605	– 606
	Coagulation	Cryoprecipitate: fibrinogen content	172	
	Coagulation	Desmopressin for Von Willebrand	175	– 176
	Coagulation	FFP: warfarin reversal	225	– 226
	Coagulation	Hetastarch: platelet function	248	
	Coagulation	Renal failure: platelet function	487	
	Coagulation	Rx: antithrombin III deficiency	502	
	Congenital	Congenital heart disease: Prostaglandin Rx	158	– 159
	Congenital	Patent ductus arteriosus: Dx	434	– 435
	Congenital	TEF: Other abnormalities	547	– 548
	Congenital Disease	Tetralogy of Fallot Rx	552	– 554
	Congenital Syndrome	Prostaglandin for congenital heart: Dx	481	– 482
	CPB	LV failure Dx/Rx post-CPB	315	
	CPB	Post-CPB creatinine increase: DDx	457	– 458
	Electrolytes	Acute hyperkalemia: Rx	19	– 21
	Electrolytes	Calcium chelation; transfusion	105	
	Electrolytes	Hydrochlorothiazide: Blood chem effect	252	– 253
	Electrolytes	Hypercalcemia: Acute treatment	257	– 258
	Electrolytes	Hyperkalemia Rx	19	– 21
	Electrolytes	Hyperkalemia: drugs causing	266	
	Electrolytes	Hypocalcemia: ECG effects	271	– 272
	Electrolytes	Magnesium complications	316	– 317
	Electrolytes	Renal failure: electrolytes	485	– 486
	Electrolytes	Vasopressin Rx diabetes insipidus	602	– 603
	Electrolytres	Renal insufficiency: hyperkalemia	493	
	Endocrine	Hormonal stress response	251	
	Equipment	Arterial waveform: Periph vs central	61	– 62
	Equipment	AV pacing: Hemodynamic effect	79	– 80
	Equipment	Brachial artery catheter: Cx	94	
	Equipment	Bronchial blocker: Advantages	98	
	Equipment	Bronchopleural fistula: Vent management	99	– 100
	Equipment	Cardiac cycle: ECG	111	– 112
	Equipment	Cardiac pacemaker indications	115	– 116
	Equipment	Central line infections: prevention	132	
	Equipment	ECG leads: P wave detection	184	– 185
	Equipment	Gas laws: temp/pressure changes	229	
	Equipment	Hypocalcemia: ECG effects	271	– 272
	Equipment	IABP: Contraindications	282	– 283
	Equipment	Implantable cardiac defibrillator: interventions	284	
	Equipment	Mediastinoscopy: vascular compression	332	
	Equipment	Pacemaker designation	420	– 421
	Equipment	Pacer lead placement: ECG morph	422	– 423
	Equipment	PEEP: Effect on PAOP	439	
	Equipment	Subarachnoid bleed: ECG effects	535	
	Equipment	Synchronized electrical cardioversion	546	
	Equipment	Ultrasound structures: echogenicity	584	
	Equipment	Ultrasound visualization: IJ compress	585	– 586
	Equipment	Venous air embolism detection	605	– 606
	Fluids	Mannitol osmolarity effects	320	
	Geriatrics	Aging: Cardiovasc physiol	31	– 32

ALPHA
ROTATION
KEYWORDS

Rotation	Subtopic	Keywords	Pages	
	Geriatrics	Aging: Pulm physiol	33	– 34
	Geriatrics	LV Function: Geriatric	31	– 32
	Heart Transplant	Denervated heart: exercise physiology	173	– 174
	Heart Transplant	Heart transplant: autonomic effect	234	– 235
	Heme	Age-related P50	29	– 30
	Heme	Calcium chelation; transfusion	105	
	Heme	CO_2 transport: bicarbonate	88	
	Heme	Cryoprecipitate: fibrinogen content	172	
	Heme	Desmopressin for Von Willebrand	175	– 176
	Heme	Elevated INR: Factor Rx	189	– 190
	Heme	FFP: warfarin reversal	225	– 226
	Heme	Fresh frozen plasma : Indications	225	– 226
	Heme	Hetastarch: platelet function	248	
	Heme	Leukoreduction: Viral transmission	306	
	Heme	O_2 release	400	– 401
	Heme	Renal failure: platelet function	487	
	Heme	Rx: antithrombin 3 deficiency	502	
	Heme	Transfusion mortality: Causes	573	– 574
	ID	Central line infections: prevention	132	
	ID	SBE prophylaxis	504	– 505
	Ischemia	Coronary perfusion pressure	167	
	Ischemia	IABP: Contraindications	282	– 283
	Ischemia	Myocardial ischemia: Acute MR	366	– 367
	Labs	ABG: pulm embolism	9	– 10
	Labs	Elevated INR: Factor Rx	189	– 190
	Labs	Hyperkalemia: drugs causing	266	
	Metabolism	ABG: pulm embolism	9	– 10
	Metabolism	Bicarb admin: CO_2 effect	88	
	Metabolism	Cerebral ischemia: deep hypothermia	137	
	Monitors	Brachial artery catheter: Cx	94	
	Monitors	Constrictive pericarditis: venous waveform	161	– 162
	Monitors	ECG: loose lead effect	183	
	Monitors	Uptake of inhaled anesthetics: V/Q mismatch	594	– 595
	Monitors	Venous air embolism	605	– 606
	Monitors	Ventricular PV loops	613	– 614
	Neuro	Carotid sinus stim: post-heart transplant	124	– 125
	Neuro	Magnesium complications	316	– 317
	Neuro	Mannitol osmolarity effects	320	
	Neuro	Neuraxial anesth: cardiovascular effects	382	– 383
	Neuro	Subarachnoid bleed: ECG effects	535	
	Neuro	Vasopressin Rx diabetes insipidus	602	– 603
	Pediatrics	Congenital heart disease: Prostaglandin Rx	158	– 159
	Pediatrics	Hypothermia: Infant vs toddler	273	
	Pediatrics	Patent ductus arteriosus: Dx	434	– 435
	Pediatrics	TEF: Other abnormalities	547	– 548
	Peri-Op	Renal function: periop preservation	490	
	Pharm	Acute hyperkalemia: Rx	19	– 21
	Pharm	Amiodarone: Hemodynamic effect	40	– 41
	Pharm	Atrial flutter: Pharm Rx	69	– 70
	Pharm	Bicarb admin: CO_2 effect	88	
	Pharm	Calcium chelation; transfusion	105	
	Pharm	Carcinoid crisis: Rx	108	– 109

ALPHA ROTATION KEYWORDS

ALPHA
ROTATION
KEYWORDS

Rotation	Subtopic	Keywords	Pages	
	Pulmonary	PEEP: LV effects	441	
	Regional	Ultrasound structures: echogenicity	584	
	Renal	Mannitol osmolarity effects	320	
	Renal	Post-CPB creatinine increase: DDx	457	– 458
	Renal	Renal failure: CPB surgery	484	
	Renal	Renal failure: electrolytes	485	– 486
	Renal	Renal failure: platelet function	487	
	Renal	Renal function: periop preservation	490	
	Renal	Renal insufficiency: hyperkalemia	493	
	Renal	Renin-angiotensin CV physiology	495	– 496
	Respiratory	ABG: pulm embolism	9	– 10
	Respiratory	Age-related P50	29	– 30
	Respiratory	Bicarb admin: CO_2 effect	88	
	Respiratory	CO_2 transport: bicarbonate	88	
	Respiratory	Factors affecting turbulent flow	203	
	Respiratory	Head down position: hypoxemia	232	
	Respiratory	Inhalational anesthesia: ventilatory effects	288	
	Respiratory	Oxygen delivery index determinants	416	
	Respiratory	SVO_2 physiology	543	
	Respiratory	Tension pneumothorax: Dx and Rx	551	
	Respiratory	Uptake of inhaled anesthetics: V/Q mismatch	594	– 595
	Respiratory	V/Q mismatch - emphysema	618	
	Respiratory	Venous air embolism	605	– 606
	Temperature	Cardiac arrest: Induced hypothermia	110	
	Temperature	Cerebral ischemia: deep hypothermia	137	
	Temperature	Circ arrest: pH-stat implications	148	– 149
	Temperature	Hypothermia: Infant vs toddler	273	
	Temperature	Hypothermia: pH stat management	274	– 275
	Tests	Tension pneumothorax: Dx and Rx	551	
	Transplant	Heart transplant: Autonomic pharmacology	234	– 235
	Uterus	Magnesium complications	316	– 317
	Valves	Aortic insufficiency: Hemodynamic Rx	58	– 60
	Valves	Congenital heart disease: prostaglandin Rx	158	– 159
	Valves	IABP: Contraindications	282	– 283
	Valves	Myocardial ischemia: Acute MR	366	– 367
	Vascular	Bradycardia during carotid surgery	95	– 96
	Vascular	Carotid sinus stim: post-heart transplant	124	– 125
Critical Care	ABG	ABG temp correction: PCO_2	13	
	ABG	ABGs: Resp acid/met alk	14	
	ABG	Compensated resp acidosis: ABG	157	
	ABG	Metabolic alk: Resp compensation	333	
	ABG	pH buffering: Bicarbonate	446	
	ABG	Pyloric stenosis: metab abnormality	483	
	ABG	Saline: Hyperchloremic acidosis	503	
	Airway	Metoclopramide: esoph sphincter tone	341	
	Airway	Metoclopramide: gastric effects	342	– 343
	Airway	Nasal fiberoptic intubation	373	
	ASA	ASA sedation guidelines	63	– 64
	Cadiac	Venous air embolism	605	– 606
	Cardiac	Acute septic shock	22	– 23
	Cardiac	Aging: Cardiovasc physiol	31	– 32

ALPHA
ROTATION
KEYWORDS

ALPHA
ROTATION
KEYWORDS

Rotation	Subtopic	Keywords	Pages	
	GI	Metoclopramide: esoph sphincter tone	341	
	GI	Metoclopramide: gastric effects	342	– 343
	GI	Peripheral TPN: complications	444	– 445
	GI	PONV Prophylaxis	456	
	Heart Transplant	Denervated heart: exercise physiology	173	– 174
	Heart Transplant	Heart transplant: autonomic effect	234	– 235
	Heme	Age-related P50	29	– 30
	Heme	Calcium chelation; transfusion	105	
	Heme	CO_2 transport: bicarbonate	88	
	Heme	Cryoprecipitate: fibrinogen content	172	
	Heme	Desmopressin for Von Willebrand	175	– 176
	Heme	Elevated INR: Factor Rx	189	– 190
	Heme	Factor VIII concentrate: indications	202	
	Heme	FFP: warfarin reversal	225	– 226
	Heme	Fresh frozen plasma : Indications	225	– 226
	Heme	Hemolysis: bilirubin levels	239	
	Heme	Hetastarch: platelet function	248	
	Heme	Leukoreduction: Viral transmission	306	
	Heme	Local anes: Methemoglobinernia	309	– 310
	Heme	Maximum ABL calculation	327	
	Heme	Methemoglobinemia: Treatment	337	– 338
	Heme	O_2 release	400	
	Heme	pH buffering: Bicarbonate	446	
	Heme	Renal failure: platelet function	487	
	Heme	Rx: antithrombin III deficiency	502	
	Heme	TRALI: Treatment	570	– 571
	Heme	Transfusion mortality: Causes	573	– 574
	ID	Acute septic shock	22	– 23
	ID	Central line infections: prevention	132	
	ID	Clostridium tetani infection	154	– 155
	ID	Hepatitis B: Needlestick Rx	242	– 243
	ID	Leukoreduction: Viral transmission	306	
	ID	Septic Shock: Vasopressin rx	507	– 508
	Labor	Pre-term labor: treatment	478	– 479
	Labs	ABG: pulm embolism	9	– 10
	Labs	ABG: salicylate toxicity	11	– 12
	Labs	ABG:COPD	3	
	Labs	Air embolism: Dx	605	– 606
	Labs	Anes techniques: suspected MH	48	
	Labs	CO poisoning: clinical features	163	– 164
	Labs	Hemolysis: bilirubin levels	239	
	Labs	Hepatic dysfunction: Dx	240	– 241
	Labs	Hepatic synthetic capacity: Dx	244	– 245
	Labs	Hyperglycemia: complications	263	
	Labs	Hyperkalemia: drugs causing	266	
	Labs	Pheochromocytoma: Dx markers	447	– 448
	Labs	Postoperative ATN: DDx	463	– 464
	LAbs	Preeclampsia: Lab abnormalities	465	
	Labs	Propofol infusion syndrome: Dx	480	
	Labs	Renal insufficiency: Dx	491	– 492
	Labs	SIADH: Lab values	510	– 511
	Labs	SpO_2 effect of methemoglobin	337	– 338

Rotation	Subtopic	Keywords	Pages	
	Liver	Cirrhosis: NMB kinetics	150	– 151
	Liver	Cirrhosis: NMB pharmacokinetics	150	– 151
	Liver	Hemolysis: bilirubin levels	239	
	Liver	Hepatic dysfunction: Dx	240	– 242
	Liver	Hepatic synthesis impairment: Dx	244	– 245
	Liver	Hepatic synthetic capacity: Dx	244	– 245
	Liver	Hepatitis B: Needlestick Rx	242	– 243
	Liver	Postop jaundice DDx	459	– 460
	Metabolic	Anes techniques: suspected MH	48	
	Metabolism	ABG: pulm embolism	9	– 10
	Metabolism	Bicarb admin: CO_2 effect	88	
	Metabolism	Burn management: carbon monoxide toxicity	163	– 164
	Metabolism	Carbon monoxide poisoning: Rx	163	– 164
	Metabolism	Cirrhosis: NMB kinetics	150	– 151
	Metabolism	TPN: metabolic effects	568	– 569
	Metobolism	Brain death pathophysiology	97	
	Monitors	Air embolism: Dx	605	– 606
	Monitors	Anes techniques: suspected MH	48	
	Monitors	Brachial artery catheter: Cx	94	
	Monitors	Bronchospasm: mechanical ventilation Dx	101	
	Monitors	Constrictive pericarditis: venous waveform	161	– 162
	Monitors	ECG: loose lead effect	183	
	Monitors	Fat embolism: Dx	204	– 205
	Monitors	Monitoring for residual NMB	351	– 352
	Monitors	MRI monitoring hazards	358	
	Monitors	Venous air embolism	605	– 606
	Monitors	Ventricular PV loops	613	– 614
	Neuro	Autonomic hypereflexia	73	– 74
	Neuro	Autonomic hyperreflexia: signs	73	
	Neuro	Blood brain barrier: Fluid transfer	90	
	Neuro	Brain death pathophysiology	97	
	Neuro	Carbamazepine toxicity	107	
	Neuro	Cerebral blood flow: Temp effect	136	
	Neuro	Cerebral vasospasm: Rx	138	– 139
	Neuro	CO poisoning: clinical features	163	– 164
	Neuro	Diabetes insipidus intracranial surg.	177	– 178
	Neuro	Glasgow Coma Scale: components	227	– 228
	Neuro	Glasgow coma scale: definition	227	– 228
	Neuro	Increased ICP: Acute rx	286	– 287
	Neuro	Ketamine receptor effects	296	
	Neuro	Lambert-Eaton Syndrome: Physiology	298	
	Neuro	Mannitol osmolarity effects	320	
	Neuro	Mult sclerosis: Exacerbation of Symptoms	359	– 360
	Neuro	Myasthenia gravis : postop management	364	– 365
	Neuro	Myasthenia gravis: postop management	364	– 365
	Neuro	Myasthenia: Musc relax effects	362	– 363
	Neuro	N_2O: CBF and $CMRO_2$	370	
	Neuro	Neuromusc disease: Sux hyperkalemia	386	
	Neuro	Neuromuscular diseases: muscle pain	388	
	Neuro	Paraplegia: Autonomic hyperreflexia	73	– 74
	Neuro	SIADH: Lab values	510	– 511
	Neuro	Subarachnoid bleed: ECG effects	535	

Rotation	Subtopic	Keywords	Pages
	Neuro	Subarachnoid hemorrage: nimodipine	536
	Neuro	Tension pneumocephalus: Dx	549 – 550
	Neuro	Thiopental: $CMRO_2$/CBF relationship	555 – 556
	Neuro	Traumatic brain injury: CPP	575 – 577
	Neuro	Vasopressin Rx diabetes insipidus	602 – 603
	Neuro	Venous air embolism: Diagnosis	605 – 606
	Nutrition	Peripheral TPN: complications	444 – 445
	Nutrition	TPN discontinuation: Hypoglycemia Cx	566 – 567
	Nutrition	TPN discontinuation: hypoglycemia	566 – 567
	Nutrition	TPN: metabolic effects	568 – 569
	Obersity	Metoclopramide: esoph sphincter tone	341
	Obesity	Morbid obesity: post-op complications	353 – 355
	Obesity	Morbid obesity: rapid desaturation	356 – 357
	Obestity	Metoclopramide: gastric effects	342 – 343
	Obstetrics	Oxytocin: Electrolyte effects	419
	Obstetrics	Preeclampsia: Lab abnormalities	465
	Oxygenation	Hypercarbia: Alv gas equation	259 – 260
	PACU	PACU bypass: Rationale	424 – 425
	PACU	PACU Stage I bypass criteria	426 – 428
	Pediatrics	Congen heart Disease: Prostaglandin Rx	158 – 159
	Pediatrics	Hypovolemia signs: Peds	276 – 277
	Pediatrics	Neonatal vs. adult cardiac phys	376 – 377
	Pediatrics	Postop vomiting: Peds vs. adults	461 – 462
	Pediatrics	Pyloric stenosis: metab abnormality	483
	Peri-Op	Renal function: periop preservation	490
	Pharm	ABG: salicylate toxicity	11 – 12
	Pharm	Acetaminophen toxicity	15 – 16
	Pharm	Acute hyperkalemia: Rx	19 – 21
	Pharm	Amiodarone: Hemodynamic effect	40 – 41
	Pharm	Anaphylaxis: Epinephrine Rx	43 – 44
	Pharm	Anes techniques: suspected MH	48
	Pharm	ASA sedation guidelines	63 – 64
	Pharm	Atrial flutter: Pharm Rx	69 – 70
	Pharm	Bicarb admin: CO_2 effect	88
	Pharm	Burn management: carbon monoxide toxicity	163 – 164
	Pharm	Calcium chelation; transfusion	105 –
	Pharm	Carbamazepine toxicity	107 –
	Pharm	Carbon monoxide poisoning: Rx	163 – 164
	Pharm	Cerebral vasospasm: Rx	138 – 139
	Pharm	Cirrhosis: NMB kinetics	150 – 151
	Pharm	Cirrhosis: NMB pharmacokinetics	150 – 151
	Pharm	Clostridium tetani infection	154 – 155
	Pharm	CO poisoning: clinical features	163 – 164
	Pharm	CO poisoning: Dx	163 – 164
	Pharm	CO toxicity: Rx	163 – 164
	Pharm	CO_2 transport: bicarbonate	88
	Pharm	Desmopressin for Von Willebrand	175 – 176
	Pharm	Doxorubicin: Complications	179 – 180
	Pharm	Elevated INR: Factor Rx	189 – 190
	Pharm	Fenoldopam: Renal effects	211
	Pharm	FFP: warfarin reversal	225 – 226
	Pharm	Helium advantage: Small-bore tube	236 – 238

ALPHA ROTATION KEYWORDS

ALPHA
ROTATION
KEYWORDS

Rotation	Subtopic	Keywords	Pages	
	Pharm	Thiopental: $CMRO_2$/CBF relationship	555	– 556
	Pharm	Time constant definition	561	– 562
	Pharm	Vasodilator pharmacodynamics	600	– 601
	Pharm	Vasodilators: renal blood flow	600	– 601
	Pharm	Vasopressin Rx diabetes insipidus	602	– 603
	Pharm	Vasopressors: risk of myocardial ischemia	604	
	Post-Op	Morbid obesity: post-op complications	353	– 355
	Post-Op	Myasthenia gravis : postop management	364	– 365
	Pulmonary	Aging: Pulm physiol	33	– 34
	Pulmonary	Bronchopleural fistula: Vent management	99	– 100
	Pulmonary	CO poisoning: Dx	163	– 164
	Pulmonary	CO toxicity: Rx	163	– 164
	Pulmonary	FRC: definition	221	– 222
	Pulmonary	FRC: Vent settings effects	223	– 224
	Pulmonary	Hyperbaric chamber: MAC effect	254	
	Pulmonary	Hypercarbia: Alv gas equation	259	– 260
	Pulmonary	Low VT ventilation: Protect effect	610	– 611
	Pulmonary	Lung protect vent: Pressure goal	313	
	Pulmonary	Mediastinal tumor: Airway obstr	330	– 331
	Pulmonary	Metabolic alk: Resp compensation	333	
	Pulmonary	O_2 release	400	– 401
	Pulmonary	PEEP: Lung volume effect	440	
	Pulmonary	Smoking cessation resp physiol	516	– 517
	Pulmonary	TRALI: Treatment	570	– 571
	Pulmonary	VE /$PaCO_2$ relationship: Hypoxia	615	– 616
	Pulmonary	Work of breathing: Neonate vs adult	623	
	Renal	Abdominal compartment syndrome: Dx	1	– 2
	Renal	Ketorolac: Renal dysfunction	297	
	Renal	Ketorolac: renal function	297	
	Renal	Mannitol osmolarity effects	320	
	Renal	Post-CPB creatinine increase: DDx	457	– 458
	Renal	Postoperative ATN: DDx	463	– 464
	Renal	Preop renal failure predictors	470	
	Renal	Prerenal oliguria: Dx	475	
	Renal	Renal failure: CPB surgery	484	
	Renal	Renal failure: electrolytes	485	– 486
	Renal	Renal failure: platelet function	487	
	Renal	Renal failure: relaxants	488	– 489
	Renal	Renal function: periop preservation	490	
	Renal	Renal insufficiency: Dx	491	– 492
	Renal	Renal insufficiency: hyperkalemia	493	
	Renal	Renal replacement Rx selection	494	
	Renal	Renin-angiotensin CV physiology	495	– 496
	Respiratory	ABG: pulm embolism	9	– 10
	Respiratory	ABG: salicylate toxicity	11	– 12
	Respiratory	ABG:COPD	3	
	Respiratory	Age-related P50	29	– 30
	Respiratory	Air embolism: Dx	605	– 606
	Respiratory	Bicarb admin: CO_2 effect	88	
	Respiratory	Bronchospasm: mechanical ventilation Dx	101	
	Respiratory	CO_2 transport: bicarbonate	88	
	Respiratory	Factors affecting turbulent flow	203	

ALPHA ROTATION KEYWORDS

ALPHA ROTATION KEYWORDS

ALPHA
ROTATION
KEYWORDS

Rotation	Subtopic	Keywords	Pages	
	Equipment	Unilateral blindness: etiology	588	– 589
	Equipment	Upper extrem tourn pain prevention	592	– 593
	Equipment	Vaporizer output calculation	598	– 599
	Equipment	Ventilator disconnect: Detection	612	
	Equipment	Wall O_2 failure: Signs	619	– 620
	Eye	Anes management: penetrating eye injury	45	– 46
	Eye	Oculocardiac reflex management	406	
	Eye	Unilateral blindness: etiology	588	– 589
	Fetus	Pregnancy: non-OB surg. risks	467	
	Fluids	Intravascular: extracellular volume ratio	289	– 290
	Fluids	Prerenal oliguria: Dx	475	
	GI	Abdominal compartment syndrome: Dx	1	– 2
	GI	ABG: morbid obesity and vomiting	4	– 5
	GI	Bowel distention	92	– 93
	GI	Chronic opioids: side effects	146	– 147
	GI	Compartment syndrome: Dx	1	– 2
	GI	H_2 blockers: Onset time	230	
	GI	Metoclopramide: esoph sphincter tone	341	
	GI	Metoclopramide: gastric effects	342	– 343
	GI	Myotonic dyst: Aspiration risk	369	
	GI	Peripheral TPN: complications	444	– 445
	GI	PONV after pediatric surgery	455	
	GI	PONV Prophylaxis	456	
	GI	Postop vomiting: Peds vs. adults	461	– 462
	GI	Pregnancy GE reflux mechanism	469	
	Heme	Age-related P50	29	– 30
	Heme	Anaphylaxis: Epinephrine Rx	43	– 44
	Heme	Calcium chelation; transfusion	105	
	Heme	CO_2 transport: bicarbonate	88	
	Heme	Elevated INR: Factor Rx	189	– 190
	Heme	Factor VIII concentrate: indications	202	
	Heme	FFP: warfarin reversal	225	– 226
	Heme	Hemolysis: bilirubin levels	239	
	Heme	Hetastarch: platelet function	248	
	Heme	Latex allergy: Foods	305	
	Heme	Leukoreduction: Viral transmission	306	
	Heme	Maximum ABL calculation	327	– 328
	Heme	Renal failure: platelet function	487	
	ID	Acute septic shock	22	– 23
	ID	Clostridium tetani infection	154	– 155
	ID	Hepatitis B: Needlestick Rx	242	– 243
	ID	Leukoreduction: Viral transmission	306	
	ID	SBE prophylaxis	504	– 505
	Labs	ABG: morbid obesity and vomiting	4	– 5
	Labs	ABG:COPD	3	
	Labs	Anes techniques: suspected MH	48	
	Labs	CO poisoning: clinical features	163	– 164
	Labs	Hemolysis: bilirubin levels	239	
	Labs	Hepatic dysfunction: Dx	240	– 241
	Labs	Hepatic synthetic capacity: Dx	244	– 245
	Labs	Hyperglycemia: complications	263	
	Labs	Hyperkalemia: drugs causing	266	

ALPHA ROTATION KEYWORDS

ALPHA ROTATION KEYWORDS

Rotation	Subtopic	Keywords	Pages	
	Labs	Pheochromocytoma: Dx markers	447	– 448
	Labs	Post-op jaundice DDx	459	– 460
	Labs	Renal insufficiency: Dx	491	– 492
	Labs	SpO$_2$ effect of methemoglobin	337	– 338
	Liver	Acetaminophen toxicity	15	– 16
	Liver	Cirrhosis: NMB kinetics	150	– 151
	Liver	Cirrhosis: NMB pharmacokinetics	150	– 151
	Liver	Hemolysis: bilirubin levels	239	
	Liver	Hepatic dysfunction: Dx	240	– 241
	Liver	Hepatic synthesis impairment: Dx	244	– 245
	Liver	Hepatic synthetic capacity: Dx	244	– 245
	Liver	Hepatitis B: Needlestick Rx	242	– 243
	Liver	Post-op jaundice DDx	459	– 460
	Metabolic	Anes techniques: suspected MH	48	
	Metabolism	Bupivacaine toxicity Rx	103	– 104
	Metabolism	Burn management: carbon monoxide toxicity	163	– 164
	Metabolism	Carbon monoxide poisoning: Rx	163	– 164
	Metabolism	Cirrhosis: NMB kinetics	150	– 151
	Metabolism	TPN: metabolic effects	568	– 569
	Monitors	Anes techniques: suspected MH	48	
	Monitors	Brachial artery catheter: Cx	94	
	Monitors	Bronchospasm: mechanical ventilation Dx	101	
	Monitors	Fat embolism: Dx	204	– 205
	Monitors	Monitoring for residual NMB	351	– 352
	Monitors	MRI monitoring hazards	358	
	Monitors	Venous air embolism	605	– 606
	Neuro	Advanced mult scler: anesthetic drugs	28	
	Neuro	Autonomic hyperreflexia	73	– 74
	Neuro	Autonomic hyperreflexia: signs	73	– 74
	Neuro	Cervical fracture: Intub techniques	141	– 142
	Neuro	Chronic opioids: side effects	146	– 147
	Neuro	CO poisoning: clinical features	163	– 164
	Neuro	Evoked potentials: Anes effects	197	– 199
	Neuro	Glasgow Coma Scale: components	227	– 228
	Neuro	Glasgow coma scale: definition	227	– 228
	Neuro	Ketamine receptor effects	296	
	Neuro	Lambert Eaton Syndrome: Physiol	298	
	Neuro	Magnesium complications	316	– 317
	Neuro	Mult sclerosis: Exacerbation of Symptom	359	– 360
	Neuro	Multiple sclerosis exacerbation	361	
	Neuro	Myasthenia gravis : postop management	364	– 365
	Neuro	Myasthenia gravis: postop management	364	– 365
	Neuro	Myasthenia: Musc relax effects	362	– 363
	Neuro	Myotonic dyst: Aspiration risk	369	
	Neuro	Nerve AP termination mechanism	378	– 379
	Neuro	Neuromusc disease: Sux hyperkalemia	386	
	Neuro	NMB drug interactions	393	– 394
	Neuro	Paraplegia: Autonomic hyperreflexia	73	– 74
	Neuro	Preoperative anxiolysis in children	472	– 474
	Neuro	Traumatic brain injury: CPP	575	– 577
	Nutrition	Latex allergy: Foods	305	
	Nutrition	Peripheral TPN: complications	444	– 445

Rotation	Subtopic	Keywords	Pages	
	Nutrition	TPN discontinuation Cx	566	– 567
	Nutrition	TPN discontinuation: hypoglycemia	566	– 567
	Nutrition	TPN: metabolic effects	568	– 569
	Obersity	Metoclopramide: esoph sphincter tone	341	
	Obesity	ABG: morbid obesity and vomiting	4	– 5
	Obesity	Morbid obesity: Hypoxemia physiol	356	– 357
	Obesity	Morbid obesity: post-op complications	353	– 355
	Obesity	Morbid obesity: rapid desaturation	356	– 357
	Obesity	Obesity: airway evalvation	402	– 403
	Obesity	Turnescent liposuction complications	581	
	Obestity	Metoclopramide: gastric effects	342	– 343
	Obseity	Obstructive sleep apnea: Dx	404	– 405
	Obstetrics	Asthma: Postpartum hemorrhage Rx	65	– 66
	Obstetrics	Pregnancy GE reflux mechanism	469	
	Other	Anesthesiologists: substance abuse and fentanyl	53	– 54
	Other	Automated vs. paper anesthesia records	71	– 72
	Other	Ethics: Speaker disclosure	195	– 196
	Other	Lithotomy position: Nerve injury	307	– 308
	Other	Physician impairment: Referral	451	
	Other	Root cause anal: Essential elements	499	– 501
	Pain	Spinal stenosis: Dx	525	– 526
	Pain	Upper extrern tourn pain prevention	592	– 593
	Perfusion	ABG: morbid obesity and vomiting	4	– 5
	Peri-Op	Renal function: periop preservation	490	
	Pharm	Acetaminophen toxicity	15	– 16
	Pharm	Acute hyperkalemia: Rx	19	– 21
	Pharm	Addison's disease: Periop Rx	26	– 27
	Pharm	Advanced mult scler: anesthetic drugs	28	
	Pharm	Anaphylaxis: Epinephrine Rx	43	– 44
	Pharm	Anes management: penetrating eye injury	45	– 46
	Pharm	Anes techniques: suspected MH	48	
	Pharm	Anes uptake: Right-to-left shunt	49	– 50
	Pharm	Anes uptake: Solubility coeff	51	
	Pharm	Anesthesiologists: substance abuse	53	– 54
	Pharm	ASA sedation guidelines	63	– 64
	Pharm	Bupivacaine toxicity Rx	103	– 104
	Pharm	Burn management: carbon monoxide toxicity	163	– 164
	Pharm	Calcium chelation; transfusion	105	
	Pharm	Carbon monoxide poisoning: Rx	163	– 164
	Pharm	Chronic opioids: side effects	146	– 147
	Pharm	Cirrhosis: NMB kinetics	150	– 151
	Pharm	Cirrhosis: NMB pharmacokinetics	150	– 151
	Pharm	Clostridium tetani infection	154	– 155
	Pharm	CO poisoning: clinical features	163	– 164
	Pharm	CO_2 absorbers: volatile anes toxicity	156	
	Pharm	CO_2 transport: bicarbonate	88	
	Pharm	Doxorubicin: Complications	179	– 180
	Pharm	Epiglottitis: inhalation induction	193	– 194
	Pharm	FFP: warfarin reversal	225	– 226
	Pharm	H_2 blockers: Onset time	230	
	Pharm	Herbals: garlic	246	– 247
	Pharm	Hetastarch: platelet function	248	

ALPHA
ROTATION
KEYWORDS

Rotation	Subtopic	Keywords	Pages	
	Pharm	Hydrochlorothiazide: Blood chem effect	252	– 253
	Pharm	Hyperglycemia: complications	263	
	Pharm	Hyperglycemia: Preop Rx	264	– 265
	Pharm	Hyperkalemia Rx	267	– 268
	Pharm	Hyperkalemia: drugs causing	266	
	Pharm	Inhalation anesth: Resp effects	288	
	Pharm	Inhalational anesthesia: ventilatory effects	288	
	Pharm	Ketamine receptor effects	296	
	Pharm	Ketamine: Pharmacodynamics	293	– 294
	Pharm	Local anesthetic: Trans neurol Sx	311	
	Pharm	Magnesium complications	316	– 317
	Pharm	Management: acute heart failure	17	– 18
	Pharm	MAO inhibitor: meperidine toxicity	321	
	Pharm	Metformin: contrast dye interaction	334	
	Pharm	Metoclopramide: esoph sphincter tone	341	
	Pharm	Metoclopramide: gastric effects	342	– 343
	Pharm	Midazolam: Bioavail vs. route	344	– 345
	Pharm	Monitoring for residual NMB	351	– 352
	Pharm	Multiple sclerosis exacerbation	361	
	Pharm	Myasthenia gravis: postop management	364	– 365
	Pharm	Myasthenia: Musc relax effects	362	– 363
	Pharm	Nerve AP termination mechanism	378	– 379
	Pharm	Neuromusc disease: Sux hyperkalemia	386	
	Pharm	Neuromuscular block: vecuronium	387	
	Pharm	NMB drug interactions	393	– 394
	Pharm	NMB reversal: Assessment	395	– 397
	Pharm	NMB: volatile agent interaction	392	
	Pharm	Oral clonidine: MAC effect	412	
	Pharm	Pheochromocytoma: Dx markers	447	– 448
	Pharm	Pheochromocytoma: pre-op preparation	450	
	Pharm	Pheochromocytorma: hypertension Rx	449	
	Pharm	PONV after pediatric surgery	455	
	Pharm	PONV Prophylaxis	456	
	Pharm	Preoperative anxiolysis in children	472	– 474
	Pharm	Renal failure: relaxants	488	– 489
	Pharm	Renal insufficiency: hyperkalemia	493	
	Pharm	SBE prophylaxis	504	– 505
	Pharm	SpO_2 effect of methemoglobin	337	– 338
	Pharm	Steroid prophylaxis indications	533	
	Pharm	Succinylcholine and bradycardia	538	
	Pharm	Succinylcholine: Normal K increase	537	
	Pharm	Surgical stim: Effect on MAC	541	– 542
	Pharm	Time constant definition	561	– 562
	Pharm	Transdermal fentanyl indications	572	
	Pharm	Tumescent liposuction: lidocaine dose	580	
	Positioning	Head down position: hypoxemia	232	
	Post-Op	Morbid obesity: post-op complications	353	– 355
	Post-Op	Myasthenia gravis : postop management	364	– 365
	Post-Op	Myasthenia gravis: postop management	364	– 365
	Pre-Op	Smoking cessation: resp physiol	516	– 517
	Pulmonary	Air trapping:Ventilator management	35	– 36
	Pulmonary	Asthma: Postpartum hemorrhage Rx	65	– 66

Rotation	Subtopic	Keywords	Pages	
	Pulmonary	Bronchospasm triggers: ETT	102	
	Pulmonary	Carcinoid crisis: Rx	108	– 109
	Pulmonary	Inhalation anesth: Resp effects	288	
	Pulmonary	Morbid obesity: Hypoxemia physiol	356	– 357
	Pulmonary	Neg pressure pulm edema: Physiol	374	
	Reanl	Preop renal failure predictors	470	
	Regional	Spinal stenosis: Dx	525	– 526
	Renal	Abdominal compartment syndrome: Dx	1	– 2
	Renal	Postoperative ATN: DDx	463	– 464
	Renal	Pre-renal oliguria: Dx	475	
	Renal	Renal failure: electrolytes	485	– 486
	Renal	Renal failure: platelet function	487	
	Renal	Renal failure: relaxants	488	– 489
	Renal	Renal function: periop preservation	490	
	Renal	Renal insufficiency: Dx	491	– 492
	Renal	Renal insufficiency: hyperkalemia	493	
	Renal	Renal replacement Rx selection	494	
	Renal	Robotic prostatectomy: contraindications	498	
	Renal	TURP syndrome: Rx	582	– 583
	Respiratory	ABG: morbid obesity and vomiting	4	– 5
	Respiratory	ABG:COPD	3	
	Respiratory	Age-related P50	29	– 30
	Respiratory	Bronchospasm: mechanical ventilation Dx	101	
	Respiratory	Chronic opioids: side effects	146	– 147
	Respiratory	CO_2 transport: bicarbonate	88	
	Respiratory	FB aspiration: physical exam	206	– 208
	Respiratory	Head down position: hypoxemia	232	
	Respiratory	Hypercarbia: O_2 release to tissues	261	– 262
	Respiratory	Hypoxemia: Ventilator management	280	– 281
	Respiratory	Inhalational anesthesia: ventilatory effects	288	
	Respiratory	Laparoscopy: increased $PaCO_2$	299	
	Respiratory	Morbid obesity: rapid desaturation	356	– 357
	Respiratory	Obstructive sleep apnea: Dx	404	– 405
	Respiratory	Smoking cessation: resp physiol	516	– 517
	Respiratory	SpO_2 effect of methemoglobin	337	– 338
	Respiratory	Venous air embolism	605	– 606
	Skeletalmuscular	Advanced mult scler: anesthetic drugs	28	
	Skeletalmuscular	Atlantoaxial instability: causes	67	– 68
	Skeletalmuscular	Abdominal Compartment syndrome: Dx	1	– 2
	Skeletalmuscular	Multiple sclerosis exacerbation	359	– 360
	Skeletalmuscular	Myasthenia gravis: postop management	364	– 365
	Skeletalmuscular	Rheumatoid arthr complications	497	
	Sketetalmuscular	Anes techniques: suspected MH	48	
	Spine	Autonomic hyperreflexia	73	– 74
	Spine	Autonomic hyperreflexia: signs	73	– 74
	Statistics	Categorical data: Chi square	127	
	Statistics	Paired vs. unpaired t-test	431	– 432
	Statistics	Power analysis: Study design	527	– 528
	Statistics	Preop testing: Bayes, theorem	471	
	Statistics	SE vs. SD calculation	506	
	Statistics	Statistical anal: power	527	– 528
	Statistics	Statistics: median	529	

ALPHA
ROTATION
KEYWORDS

Rotation	Subtopic	Keywords	Pages	
	Statistics	Stats: ANOVA indications	530	
	Temperature	Malig hypertherm: Assoc disorders	318	
	Tests	Abdominal Compartment syndrome: Dx	1	– 2
	Uterus	Magnesium complications	316	– 317
	Uterus	Pregnancy: non-OB surg. risks	467	
	Vascular	Acute septic shock	22	– 23
	Ventilator	Air trapping:Ventilator management	35	– 36
	Ventilator	Ventilator disconnect: Detection	612	
Neuro	Airway	Atlantoaxial instability: causes	67	– 68
	Assesment	Glasgow Coma Scale: components	227	– 228
	Assesment	Spinal stenosis: Dx	525	– 526
	Bleed	Subarachnoid bleed: ECG effects	535	
	Brain Injury	Closed claims: Brain damage	152	– 153
	Brain Injury	Traumatic brain injury: CPP	575	– 577
	Cardiac	Venous Air embolism Dx	605	– 606
	Cardiac	Autonomic hypereflexia	73	– 74
	Cardiac	Autonomic hyperreflexia: signs	73	– 74
	Cardiac	Autonomic innervation: upper extremity	75	– 76
	Cardiac	Autonomic neurotransmitters	77	– 78
	Cardiac	Bradycardia: Carotid Surgery and Carotid Stent	95	– 96
	Cardiac	Carotid sinus stim: post-heart tplt	124	– 125
	Cardiac	ECT: side effects	186	
	Cardiac	Oculocardiac reflex management	406	
	Cardiac	Subarachnoid bleed: ECG effects	535	
	Cardiac	Vasopressin Rx: Diabetes Insipidus	602	– 603
	Circulation	Cerebral blood flow: Temp effect	136	
	Circulation	Cerebral vasospasm: Rx	138	– 139
	Circulation	Oculocardiac reflex management	406	
	Circulation	Traumatic brain injury: CPP	575	– 577
	Circulation	Venous Air Embolism: Diagnosis	605	– 606
	Complications	Spinal anes complic: MRI indications	518	– 519
	Complications	Venous Air Embolism: Diagnosis	605	– 606
	Drug Interactions	MAO inhibitor: meperidine toxicity	321	
	Drug Interactions	NMB: volatile agent interaction	392	
	ECT	Anesthesia for ECT: lidocaine effect	52	
	ECT	ECT: side effects	186	
	Electrolytes	Diabetes insipidus intracranial surg.	177	– 178
	Electrolytes	Electrolyte homeostasis: hormones	187	– 188
	Electrolytes	SIADH: Lab values	510	– 511
	Electrolytes	Vasopressin Rx diabetes insipidus	602	– 603
	Endocrine	Diabetes insipidus intracranial surg.	177	– 178
	Endocrine	Electrolyte homeostasis: hormones	187	– 188
	Endocrine	Hormonal stress response	251	
	Equipment	Evoked potentials: Anes effects	197	– 199
	Equipment	MRI monitoring hazards	358	
	Equipment	Multiple sclerosis: exacerbation	359	– 360
	Equipment	Sitting position: BP measurement	514	– 515
	Equipment	Spinal anes complic: MRI indications	518	– 519
	Equipment	Spinal cord stim: Reprogramming	522	
	Equipment	Unilateral blindness: etiology	588	– 589
	Eye	Oculocardiac reflex management	406	
	Eye	Unilateral blindness: etiology	588	– 589

ALPHA
ROTATION
KEYWORDS

ALPHA
ROTATION
KEYWORDS

Rotation	Subtopic	Keywords	Pages	
	GI	Metoclopramide: esoph sphincter tone	341	
	GI	Metoclopramide: gastric effects	342	
	GI	Pregnancy GE reflux mechanism	469	
	Heme	Asthma: Postpartum hemorrhage Rx	65	– 66
	Heme	Pregnancy: Hematologic changes	466	
	Labor	Preterm labor: treatment	478	– 479
	Labor	Side effects of tocolytics	512	– 513
	Labs	ABG in pregnancy	8	
	Labs	ABG: morbid obesity and vomiting	4	– 5
	Labs	Amniotic fluid embolus: Dx	42	
	Labs	Fetal blood gas values	212	
	Metabolism	Chloroprocaine metabolism	143	– 144
	Metabolism	Chloroprocaine placental transfer	145	
	MGMT	Anes techniques: first stage labor	47	
	MGMT	Cervical cerclage: Anes management	140	
	Monitors	Amniotic fluid embolus: Dx	42	
	Monitors	Dx of uterine rupture	596	– 597
	Neuro	Magnesium complications	316	– 317
	Neuro	Neuraxial anesth: cardiovascular effects	382	– 383
	Newborn	Meconium: Tracheal suctioning	329	
	Newborn	Neonatal bradycardia: Rx	375	
	Obesity	Metoclopramide: esoph sphincter tone	341	
	Obesity	ABG: morbid obesity and vomiting	4	
	Obestity	Metoclopramide: gastric effects	342	– 343
	Perfusion	ABG in pregnancy	8	
	Perfusion	ABG: morbid obesity and vomiting	4	– 5
	Pharm	Chloroprocaine metabolism	143	
	Pharm	Chloroprocaine placental transfer	145	
	Pharm	Epidural anesthetics: respiratory effects	191	– 192
	Pharm	Epidural test dose: Sx	192	– 268
	Pharm	Hypermagnesemia Rx	267	– 268
	Pharm	Magnesium complications	316	– 317
	Pharm	Methods: uterine relaxation	339	– 340
	Pharm	Metoclopramide: esoph sphincter tone	341	
	Pharm	Metoclopramide: gastric effects	342	– 343
	Pharm	Neuraxial anesth: cardiovascular effects	382	– 383
	Pharm	Nitroglycerin: Uterine relax	389	– 389
	Pharm	Oxytocin: Electrolyte effects	419	
	Pharm	Placental transfer: anticholinergic	453	
	Pharm	Placental transfer: local anesthetics	454	
	Pharm	Pregnancy: SVT Rx	468	
	Pharm	Preterm labor: treatment	478	– 479
	Pharm	Side effects of tocolytics	512	
	Placenta	Chloroprocaine placental transfer	145	
	Placenta	O_2 delivery to fetus in labor	417	– 418
	Placenta	Placenta accreta: Risk factors	452	
	Placenta	Placental transfer: anticholinergic	453	
	Placenta	Placental transfer: local anesthetics	454	
	Pregnancy	Preeclampsia: Lab abnormalities	465	
	Pregnancy	Pregnancy GE reflux mechanism	469	
	Pregnancy	Pregnancy: Hematologic changes	466	
	Pulmonary	Asthma: Postpartum hemorrhage Rx	65	– 66

ALPHA ROTATION KEYWORDS

ALPHA
ROTATION
KEYWORDS

ALPHA
ROTATION
KEYWORDS

Rotation	Subtopic	Keywords	Pages	
	Newborn	Beta thalassemia: Newborn	86	– 87
	Newborn	Neonatal bradycardia: Rx	375	
	Newborn	Neonatal vs. adult cardiac phys	376	– 377
	Newborn	Work of breathing: Neonate vs adult	623	
	Parents	Parental presence: Indications	433	
	Pediatrics	Caudal anesthesia	128	– 129
	Pharm	Anes techniques: suspected MH	48	
	Pharm	Congenital heart disease: prostaglandin Rx	158	– 159
	Pharm	Congenital long QT: management	160	
	Pharm	Epiglottitis: Anes Mgt and Inhal Induction	193	– 194
	Pharm	Helium advantage: Small-bore tube	236	– 238
	Pharm	Midazolam: Bioavail versus route	344	– 345
	Pharm	PONV after pediatric surgery	455	
	Pharm	PONV Prophylaxis	456	
	Pharm	Preoperative anxiolysis in children	472	– 474
	Pharm	Prostaglandin for congenital heart: Cx	481	– 482
	Placenta	O_2 delivery to fetus in labor	417	– 418
	Pulmonary	Bronchospasm triggers: ETT	102	– 103
	Pulmonary	Helium advantage: Small-bore tube	236	– 238
	Pulmonary	Mapleson D: Rebreathing	322	– 323
	Pulmonary	Meconium: Tracheal suctioning	329	
	Pulmonary	Work of breathing: Neonate vs. adult	623	
	Regional	Caudal anesthesia	128	– 129
	Regional	Dural sac: Caudal extent	181	– 182
	Respiratory	FB aspiration: physical exam	206	– 208
	Respiratory	Fetal blood gas values	212	
	Sketetalmuscular	Anes techniques: suspected MH	48	
	Temperature	Hypothermia: Infant vs. toddler	273	
	Ventilator	Helium advantage: Small-bore tube	236	– 238
Regional	Airway	Airway anesthesia: anatomy	37	
	Airway	Superior laryng n anatomy	539	– 540
	Anatomy	Airway anesthesia: anatomy	37	
	Anatomy	Axillary block: Median n rescue block	83	– 85
	Anatomy	Dural sac: Caudal extent	181	– 182
	Anatomy	Femoral nerve block anatomy	209	– 210
	Anatomy	Lumbar nerve roots: Innervation	312	
	Anatomy	Superior laryng n anatomy	539	– 540
	Anatomy	Total knee repl: Reg anes techniques	563	– 565
	Block	Axillary block limitations	83	– 85
	Block	Axillary block: complications	81	– 82
	Block	Axillary block: Median n rescue block	83	– 85
	Block	Celiac plexus block: Side effects	130	– 131
	Block	Celiac plexus block: complications	130	– 131
	Block	Nerve block landmarks	380	– 381
	Block	Stellate ganglion block: effects	531	– 532
	Block	Upper extrem nerve blocks: indications	590	– 591
	Blocks	Total knee repl: Reg anes techniques	563	– 565
	Cardiac	Autonomic innervation: upper extremity	75	– 76
	Cardiac	Epidural test dose: Symptom	192	
	Cardiac	Neuraxial anesth: cardiovascular effects	382	– 383
	Cardiac	Oculocardiac reflex management	406	
	Cardiac	Spinal hypotension Rx	523	– 524

ALPHA
ROTATION
KEYWORDS

ALPHA ROTATION KEYWORDS

Rotation	Subtopic	Keywords	Pages	
	Pharm	Pain management: rib fracture	429	– 430
	Pharm	Peripheral nerves: sensory versus motor	443	
	Pharm	Placental transfer: local anesthetics	454	
	Pharm	Stellate ganglion block: effects	531	– 532
	Pharm	Trigeminal neuralgia: Rx	578	
	Pharm	Trigger point injection indications	579	
	Pharm	Tumescent liposuction: lidocaine dose	580	
	Placenta	Chloroprocaine placental transfer	145	
	Placenta	Placental transfer: local anesthetics	454	
	Reflexes	Paraplegia: Autonomic hyperreflexia	73	– 74
	Regional	Caudal anesthesia	128	– 129
	Regional	Epidural test dose: Symptom	192	
	Regional	Ultrasound structures: echogenicity	584	
	Respiratory	Epidural anesthetics: respiratory effects	191	
	Skeletalmuscular	Advanced multiple scler: anesthetic drugs	28	
	Skeletalmuscular	Multiple sclerosis exacerbation	361	
	Skeletalmuscular	Pain management: rib fracture	429	– 430
	Spinal	Spinal anes spread: Factors	520	– 521
	Spinal	Spinal hypotension Rx	523	– 524
	Spinal Injury	Paraplegia: Autonomic hyperreflexia	73	– 74
	Tests	CRPS I: Early sx and diagnosis	170	– 171
	Tests	Sympathetic block indications	544	– 545
	Uterus	Dx of uterine rupture	596	– 597
Statistics	Statistics	Categorical data: Chi-square	127	
	Statistics	Power analysis: Study design	527	– 528
	Statistics	Preop testing: Bayes' theorem	471	
	Statistics	SE vs. SD calculation	506	
	Statistics	Stats: ANOVA indications	530	
Thoracic	ABG	ABGs: Resp acid/met alk	14	
	ABG	Compensated resp acidosis: ABG	157	
	ABG	Hypercarbia: Alv gas equation	259	– 260
	ABG	Metabolic alk: Resp compensation	333	
	Airway	Bronchial blocker: Advantages	98	
	Airway	FB aspiration: physical exam	206	– 208
	Airway	Mediastinal tumor: Airway obstr	330	– 331
	Airway	Negative Pressure Pulmonary Edema: Physiology	374	
	Airway	Obstructive sleep apnea: Dx	404	– 405
	Cardiac	Factors affecting turbulent flow	203	
	Cardiac	NO hemodynamic effect	398	– 399
	Cardiac	PEEP: LV effects	441	
	Circulation	Calculation pulmonary vs systemic vasc resistance	106	
	Circulation	Haldane effect	231	
	Circulation	Hypercarbia: O_2 release to tissues	261	– 262
	Circulation	Mediastinoscopy: vascular compression	332	
	Circulation	SVO_2 physiology	543	
	Circulation	Tension pneumothorax: Dx and Rx	551	
	Circulation	Uptake of inhaled anesthetics: V/Q mismatch	594	– 595
	Circulation	V/Q mismatch — emphysema	618	
	Electrolytes	Metabolic alk: Resp compensation	333	
	Equipment	Bronchospasm: mechanical ventilation Dx	101	
	Equipment	Gas laws: temp/pressure changes	229	
	Equipment	Hypoxemia: Ventilator management	280	– 281

ALPHA ROTATION KEYWORDS

ALPHA
ROTATION
KEYWORDS

Rotation	Subtopic	Keywords	Pages	
	Respiratory	PEEP to treat hypoxia	442	
	Respiratory	Shunt: effect of increased FiO_2	509	
	Respiratory	Smoking cessation: acute physiol	516	– 517
	Respiratory	SVO_2 physiology	543	
	Respiratory	Tension pneumothorax: Dx and Rx	551	
	Respiratory	Uptake of inhaled anesthetics: V/Q mismatch	594	– 595
	Respiratory	V/Q mismatch — emphysema	618	
	Respiratory	Ventilator: low tidal volume	610	– 614
	Smoking	Smoking cessation resp physiology	516	– 517
	Tests	Lung resection outcome: PFTs	314	
	Tests	Tension pneumothorax: Dx and Rx	551	
	Tumor	Mediastinal tumor: Airway obstr	330	– 331
	Ventilator	Bronchopleural fistula: Vent management	99	– 100
	Ventilator	FRC: Vent settings effects	223	– 224
	Ventilator	Low VT ventilation: Protect effect	610	– 611
	Ventilator	Lung protect vent: Pressure goal	313	
	Ventilator	PEEP: Lung volume effect	440	
	Ventilator	Pressure vs. volume vent: ICU	476	– 477
	Ventilator	Vent modes: Pressure waveform	607	– 609
	Ventilator	Work of breathing: Neonate vs adult	623	
Vascular	Aorta	Aortic crossclamp: CV complications	55	– 57
	Cardiac	Bradycardia during carotid surgery	95	– 96
	Cardiac	Carotid sinus stim: post-heart transplant	124	– 125
	Carotid	Bilat carotid endart: Physiology	89	
	Carotid	Carotid stent: Bradycard Prevention	126	
	Carotid	Carotid stent: Bradycardia cause	126	
	Circulation	Mediastinoscopy: vascular compression	332	
	Coagulation	Cryoprecipitate: fibrinogen content	172	
	Coagulation	Desmopressin for Von Willebrand	175	– 176
	Equipment	Central line infections: prevention	132	
	Equipment	Mediastinoscopy: vascular compression	332	
	Heme	Cryoprecipitate: fibrinogen content	172	
	Heme	Desmopressin for Von Willebrand	175	– 176
	ID	Central line infections: prevention	132	
	Liver	Cirrhosis: NMB kinetics	150	– 151
	Metabolism	Bicarb admin: CO_2 effect	88	
	Metabolism	Cirrhosis: NMB kinetics	150	– 151
	Neuro	Carotid endarterec: CNS monitoring	123	
	Neuro	Carotid sinus stim: post-heart tplt	124	– 125
	Neuro	Cerebral aneurysm clipping: anes management	133	– 135
	Pharm	Bicarb admin: CO_2 effect	88	
	Pharm	Cerebral aneurysm clipping: anes management	133	– 135
	Pharm	Cirrhosis: NMB kinetics	150	– 151
	Pharm	Desmopressin for Von Willebrand	175	– 176
	Respiratory	Bicarb admin: CO_2 effect	88	
	Vascular	Bradycardia during carotid surgery	95	– 96
	Vascular	Carotid body: hypoxic drive	122	
	Vascular	Carotid endarterec: CNS monitoring	123	
	Vascular	Carotid sinus stim: post-heart tplt	124	– 125
	Vascular	Cerebral aneurysm clipping: anes management	133	– 135

ALPHA ROTATION KEYWORDS

Abdominal Compartment Syndrome: Dx

Generic, Clinical Sciences: Anesthesia
Procedures, Methods, Techniques

Tomalika Ahsan-Paik and Dmitri Souzdalnitski

Edited by Ala Haddadin

KEY POINTS

1. Abdominal compartment syndrome can be caused by either primary or secondary factors.
2. The effect involves inadequate organ perfusion to multiple organ systems, including the heart, brain, and lungs.
3. Treatment is multifactorial, involving pharmacological, changes in ventilator management, as well as surgical treatment.

DISCUSSION

Abdominal compartment syndrome is defined as multiorgan dysfunction within and beyond the abdomen resulting from hypertension within the intraabdominal compartment. Intraabdominal pressure can be measured indirectly by instilling 50 mL of normal saline within the bladder and measuring the intravesicle pressure with a Foley catheter. A pressure above 25 mm Hg indicates abdominal compartment syndrome. Conditions such as pregnancy and obesity that increase abdominal wall compliance can be protective. A distended and tense abdomen can raise a red flag and require further investigation and intervention, as abdominal compartment syndrome can often lead to multiple organ failure and death.

Abdominal compartment syndrome can be caused by multiple factors that can be divided into primary and secondary causes (Table 1). Primary causes include major abdominal trauma or surgery. Secondary causes include burn injuries that require profound fluid resuscitation often because of hemorrhage. It often results from profound intraabdominal edema caused by surgical manipulation, massive fluid resuscitation, or shock-induced inflammatory mediators. Trauma patients with fluid resuscitation and emergent surgery who are at higher risk should have a temporary closure for increased abdominal compliance instead of a tight surgical closure.

The effect often involves inadequate organ perfusion, which is not only limited to intraabdominal organs, but can also involve the heart, lungs, and brain. The diaphragm is displaced cephalad, which leads to mechanical compression, V/Q mismatch, atelectasis decreased compliance, and increase work of breathing. Most of these patients require mechanical ventilation, as patients experience shallow, rapid breaths with associated hypoxemia and hypercapnia. The peak airway pressure is elevated along with plateau pressure.

Increased abdominal compartment pressure decreases cardiac output by increasing systemic vascular resistance. Cardiac output is further decreased by elevation of the diaphragm, which decreases ventricular compliance and contractility and therefore venous blood flow. Left ventricular end-diastolic volume index measured with a pulmonary catheter is a better reflection of preload in these patients than pulmonary capillary wedge pressure (PCWP) and central venous pressure (CVP) since they are both falsely elevated. Often these patients do not respond to fluid resuscitation despite their hypovolemic status.

These patients, who are often on mechanical ventilation, should be carefully monitored since mechanical ventilation increases an already high PCWP. When combined with high-volume fluid resuscitation, this can significantly worsen edema and organ perfusion. Elevated abdominal compartment pressure can lead to increased intracranial pressure, where intraabdominal pressure is mediated via CVP to the brain.

Abdominal compartment syndrome can cause bowel ischemia by reducing mesenteric arterial blood flow, which is aggravated by low cardiac output. Direct pressure on the vein leads to edema, ischemia, and mucosal barrier compromise, ultimately leading to multiple organ failure. Hepatic flood blow is also compromised, which results in decreased mitochondrial function and lactate clearance. There can also be decreased renal perfusion secondary to a rise in renal venous pressure, which manifests clinically as oliguria.

Interventions include prompt recognition and immediate paracentesis. Often opening up the abdomen for decompression and relieving intraabdominal tension may be required to allow parenchymal blood flow. If surgical intervention is required, the open abdomen can be covered with a nonadhesive dressing.

To help determine the right timing for intervention, abdominal perfusion pressure (APP) can be measured using the following formula: APP = Mean arterial pressure (MAP) − Intraabdominal blood pressure (IABP). A value of APP <50 mm Hg is associated with poor outcomes such as critical organ dysfunction. Often a neuromuscular blockade is used to relax the abdominal wall.

Table 1. Selected Condition Associated with Abdominal Compartment Syndrome

1. Abdominal trauma
2. Liver transplantation
3. Burns
4. Pancreatitis
5. Bowel obstruction
6. Peritonitis
7. Intraperitoneal hemorrhage
8. Tense ascites

Reproduced with permission from Corbridge T, Wood LDH. Restrictive disease of the respiratory system and abdominal compartment syndrome. In: Hall JB, Schmidt GA, eds. *Principles of Critical Care.* 3rd ed. New York, NY: McGraw-Hill; 2005: 592–593.

SUGGESTED READINGS

Capan L, Miller S. Anesthesia for trauma and burn patients. In: Barash PG, Cullen BF, Stoelting RK, Cahalan M, Stock MC, eds. *Clinical Anesthesia.* 6th ed. Philadelphia, PA: Wolters Kluwer Health/LWW; 2009:922–923.
Corbridge T, Wood LDH. Restrictive disease of the respiratory system and abdominal compartment syndrome. In: Hall JB, Schmidt GA, eds. *Principles of Critical Care.* 3rd ed. New York, NY: McGraw-Hill; 2005:592–593.
Morgan GE, Mikhail MS, Murray MJ. *Clinical Anesthesiology.* 4th ed. New York, NY: McGraw-Hill; 2006:869.

ABG: COPD
Organ-based Clinical: Respiratory

Jammie Ferrara

Edited by Shamsuddin Akhtar

A

KEY POINTS

1. Chronic obstructive pulmonary disease (COPD) is characterized by progressive increased resistance to airflow resulting in gas trapping.
2. Arterial blood gas disturbances in patients with COPD are secondary to hypoventilation and carbon dioxide retention. The primary acid–base disturbance is respiratory acidosis.
3. In chronic bronchitis, chronically elevated levels of CO_2 reset medullary respiratory chemoreceptors, resulting in reduced ventilatory drive.
4. In emphysematous patients, although arterial blood gas values may look essentially normal, these patients often require an increased minute ventilation to maintain a normal $PaCO_2$.

DISCUSSION

COPD includes emphysema, chronic bronchitis, and chronic asthmatic bronchitis. COPD is characterized by gas trapping secondary to increased resistance of small conducting airways. Functionally, it is characterized by irreversible airflow limitation measured during forced expiration, caused by either an increase in the resistance of the small conducting airways, an increase in lung compliance due to emphysematous lung destruction, or both. Gas trapping leads to increased dead space, poor carbon dioxide elimination, and ventilation/perfusion (V/Q) mismatch. The venous admixture from the ventilation perfusion mismatch may also result in hypoxemia. Blood gas disturbances seen in patients with COPD reflect hypoventilation and carbon dioxide retention. COPD is a slowly progressing disease that causes a primary respiratory acidosis with a compensatory metabolic alkalosis. An acute-on-chronic respiratory acidosis can also be seen in COPD patients with acute exacerbations.

In patients with chronic bronchitis, chronically elevated carbon dioxide leads to increased serum bicarbonate concentrations. The elevated level of bicarbonate in the cerebrospinal fluid (CSF) over long periods of time causes the medullary chemoreceptors to "reset" their perceived normal level of CSF bicarbonate. Therefore, these "blue bloaters" often exhibit a poor ventilatory drive in the setting elevate levels of $PaCO_2$.

In patients with emphysema, the major complaint is often an increased work of breathing, as these patients have to increase their minute ventilation in order to maintain a normal $PaCO_2$. Therefore, these "pink puffers" are often thin and visibly dyspneic.

SUGGESTED READINGS

Barash PG, Cullen BF, Stoelting RK, et al, eds. *Clinical Anesthesia*. 6th ed. Philadelphia, PA: Lippincott Williams & Wilkins; 2009:252, 1034.
Longnecker DE, Brown DL, Newman MF, et al, eds. *Anesthesiology*. 1st ed. New York: McGraw-Hill; 2008:137–140, 349.

ABG: Morbid Obesity and Vomiting

Generic, Clinical Sciences: Anesthesia Procedures, Methods, Techniques

Lisbeysi Calo

Edited by Lars Helgeson

1. The arterial blood gas (ABG) is a useful tool to diagnose acid–base imbalances in obese and other surgical patients.
2. Certain predisposing conditions or clinical presentations such as vomiting and hypopnea should alert the anesthesiologist to a possible acid–base imbalance.
3. Decreased chest wall compliance, increased elastic resistance, and decreased functional residual capacity (FRC) are often present in morbidly obese patients.
4. Pathologic obstructive sleep apnea (OSA) occurs in 5% of obese patients and can lead to repeated periods of apnea during sleep. One of the diagnostic criteria for pathologic sleep apnea includes periods of respiratory acidosis.
5. Physiologic abnormalities resulting from OSA include hypoxemia, hypercarbia, and pulmonary and systemic hypertension.
6. The obesity hypoventilation syndrome (OHS, also known as *Pickwickian syndrome*) is characterized by chronically elevated $PaCO_2$, decreased PaO_2, pulmonary hypertension, and body mass index (BMI) ≥ 30 kg per m^2. ABG is the gold standard test to determine daytime hypercarbia.
7. Vomiting results in a loss of acid resulting in metabolic alkalosis.

Respiratory acidosis may be acute or chronic with partial renal compensation. Significant hypercarbia can result from decreased FRC in the obese, which should be corrected by adjusting ventilator setting, specifically by increasing tidal volume, respiratory rate, and use of positive end-expiratory pressure (PEEP). Also useful is changing to pressure control ventilation instead of volume control. A patient with metabolically compensated hypercarbia should not be hyperventilated to keep the pH within normal limits.

Vomiting and nasogastric suctioning can result in metabolic alkalosis, hypokalemia, hypochloremia, and hypovolemia. Although treatment of the cause of the vomiting is necessary, supportive care to correct secondary electrolyte imbalances is also required. This may include intravenous saline infusion to increase the chloride and decrease the serum bicarbonate. Carbonic anhydrase inhibitors such as acetazolamide may be given to increase renal excretion of bicarbonate. Ammonium chloride can be given to increase hydrogen ion concentration. The administration of 0.1 N of hydrochloric acid can correct life-threatening metabolic alkalosis.

Obese patients may have respiratory muscle weakness. Consequently, decreased chest wall pulmonary compliance results in decreased FRC and expiratory reserve volume (ERV). This results in small airway closure, ventilation perfusion mismatch, right-to-left shunt, and arterial hypoxemia. General anesthesia may further worsen this respiratory picture through the reduction of FRC by up to 50% in obese patients (compared with 20% in nonobese persons). Patients with OSA will exhibit the respiratory abnormalities of hypoxemia, hypercarbia, and pulmonary and systemic hypertension and will have respiratory acidosis during periods of sleep.

OHS will ultimately result in cor pulmonale. The main factor affecting patients with OHS is alveolar hypoventilation. These patients are more susceptible to the respiratory depressant effects of anesthetics.

Supine positioning in spontaneously breathing obese patients can decrease the PaO_2 and lead to cardiac arrest. Postoperative ventilation is more likely to be required in obese patients who have coexisting carbon dioxide retention and have undergone prolonged surgery, especially abdominal operations. The semisitting position is often used during the postoperative period to avoid arterial hypoxemia. The maximum decrease in PaO_2 postoperatively usually occurs 2 to 3 days after surgery.

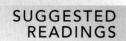

Barash PG, Cullen BF, Stoelting RK, et al, eds. *Clinical Anesthesia*. 6th ed. Philadelphia, PA: Lippincott Williams & Wilkins; 2009:1230–1233.

Hines RL, Marschall K. *Anesthesia and Co-existing Disease*. 5th ed. New York, NY: Churchill Livingstone; 2008:302–306.

Kessler R, Chaouat A, Schinkewitch P, et al. The obesity hypoventilation syndrome revisited: a prospective study of 34 consecutive cases. *Chest*. 2001;120(2):369–376.

Olson AL, Zwillich C. The obesity hypoventilation syndrome. *Am J Med*. 2005;118(9):948.

ABG: Opioid Effect

Pharmacology

Tiffany Denepitiya-Balicki

Edited by Jodi Sherman

1. Opioids are analgesics that work through specific receptors (mu, kappa, delta, and sigma) to decrease pain.
2. Respiratory depression is a well-known side effect resulting from activation of mu-2 receptors.
3. Opioids shift the carbon dioxide (CO_2) response curve to the right, thereby decreasing the respiratory rate until CO_2 accumulates. The resultant arterial blood gas (ABG) will demonstrate an increase in $PaCO_2$ and a decrease in pH.

Opioids are analgesics that work primarily through mu, kappa, delta, and sigma receptors to decrease pain. Respiratory depression is a common consequence of opioid administration. These effects are primarily due to the activation of mu-2 receptors. Opioids cause respiratory depression by increasing the CO_2 apneic threshold in the medulla. The apneic threshold is defined as apnea occurring when CO_2 is at the highest level in the arterial blood. Women appear to be more prone to respiratory depression than men.

Chest wall rigidity is another potential consequence of opioid use in which the chest wall becomes so rigid that ventilation becomes difficult to maintain. The most common agents known to produce this phenomenon are sufentanil, fentanyl, and alfentanil.

Physiologically, opioids change the respiratory pattern at low doses and can decrease tidal volumes at higher doses. Ultimately, under the influence of opioids, the respiratory rate slows, thus allowing CO_2 to gradually accumulate as the CO_2 response curve shifts to the right (Fig .1). Accompanying the change in respiratory rate, hypoxia is often noted. These respiratory changes may be reflected in ABGs analysis. As such, the arterial CO_2 will

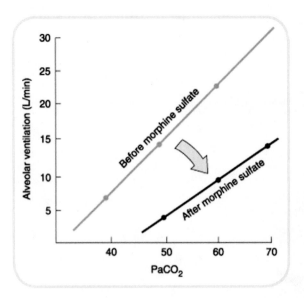

Figure 1. Alveolar ventilation as a function of $PaCO_2$ before and after morphine administration. (From Morgan G, Mikhail M, Murray M. *Clinical Anesthesiology.* 4th ed. New York, NY: McGraw-Hill Medical; 2005:194–195.)

rise and the arterial pH will decrease, reflecting a more acidic environment. Arterial PO_2 decreases as the patient becomes more hypoxic.

SUGGESTED READINGS

Barash PG, Cullen BF, Stoelting RK, et al, eds. *Clinical Anesthesia*. 6th ed. Philadelphia, PA: Lippincott Williams & Wilkins; 2009.

Morgan G, Mikhail M, Murray M. *Clinical Anesthesiology*. 4th ed. New York, NY: McGraw-Hill Medical; 2005:194–195.

Pattinson KTS. Opioids and the control of respiration. *Br J Anaesth*. 2008;100(6):747–758.

ABG in Pregnancy
Subspecialties: Obstetric

Caroline Al Haddadin

Edited by Lars Helgeson

KEY POINTS

1. Pregnancy has major effects on nearly all organ systems including the lungs.
2. Anatomical and hormone shifts are responsible for the pulmonary alterations seen in pregnancy.
3. These pulmonary changes impact the arterial blood gas (ABG), which is partially compensated for by metabolic adjustment.

DISCUSSION

In pregnancy, the diaphragm is mechanically displaced upward as a consequence of the increasing uterine size. The total lung capacity (TLC), however, is not significantly reduced because of the compensatory increased volume of the thoracic cage, particularly the increase of the anteroposterior and transverse diameters of the thoracic cage. During the second half of pregnancy, there is a decrease in the expiratory reserve volume (ERV), residual volume (RV), and the functional reserve capacity (FRC). On the other hand, the inspiratory reserve volume (IRV) and minute ventilation may increase by up to 50% (an increase of 40% in tidal volume and an increase of 15% in respiratory rate). In addition, alveolar ventilation increases by 70% via a progesterone-mediated process. Oxygen consumption increases by 20%.

Arterial CO_2 tension decreases by 10 mm Hg as a result of increased ventilation rate, and arterial oxygen tension increases by 10 mm Hg. The resulting pH becomes slightly alkalotic (7.4 to 7.45). This respiratory alkalosis is compensated metabolically by increased renal bicarbonate excretion.

SUGGESTED READINGS

Barash PG, Cullen BF, Stoelting RK, et al, eds. *Clinical Anesthesia*. 6th ed. Philadelphia, PA: Lippincott Williams & Wilkins; 2009:910.

Prowse CM, Gaensler EA. Respiratory and acid-base changes during pregnancy. *Anesthesiology*. 1965;26(1):381.

ABG: Pulm Embolism

Generic, Clinical Sciences: Anesthesia Procedures, Methods, Techniques

Jennifer Dominguez

Edited by Ala Haddadin

A

KEY POINTS

1. Pulmonary embolism (PE) may be marked by hypocapnia, hypoxemia, and/or a widened Alveolar-arterial oxygen gradient ([A-a] PO_2); however, the arterial blood gas (ABG) may also be normal.
2. PE results in ventilation of underperfused areas of the lung, or alveolar dead space ventilation, which can result in hypocapnia and hypoxemia.
3. The diagnosis of PE cannot be excluded on the basis of a normal ABG or A-a gradient.

DISCUSSION

Although PE produces pathologic changes in gas exchange, the ABG analysis in a patient with PE may be normal. PE can, however, be marked by hypocapnia, hypoxemia, and a widened Alveolar-arterial oxygen gradient ([A-a] PO_2).
Alveolar-Arterial Oxygen Gradient or PO_2 (A-a) Grad.

$$PO_2 \text{ (A-a) Grad} = PO_2 \text{ Alveolar Gas} - PO_2 \text{ Arterial Gas} = PAO_2 - PaO_2.$$
$$PO_2 \text{ Alveolar Gas}(PAO_2) \text{ is derived from the Alveolar Gas Equation (AGE):}$$
$$PAO_2 = FiO_2(PB - PH_2O) - (PACO_2/0.8)$$

Where,

FiO_2 = fraction of inspired oxygen; PB = Pressure Barometic; PH_2O = Pressure Water Vapor at 37°C; $PACO_2$ = Pressure Alveolar CO_2 (most substitute the partial pressure of arterial $CO_2 = PaCO_2$, since they are usually very close in value).
The PO_2 Arterial Gas (PaO_2) is measured by blood gas analysis.

PE results in ventilation of underperfused areas of the lung, or alveolar dead space ventilation. The remaining functional lung must now eliminate the same amount of carbon dioxide. This requires an increase in minute ventilation and usually results in an effective reduction in $PaCO_2$ that may be seen in the ABG. However, if a patient is muscle relaxed and mechanically ventilated, the minute ventilation cannot increase and the $PaCO_2$ will increase. In a normal physiologic state, the end-tidal CO_2 ($EtCO_2$) should approximate the $PaCO_2$, in as much as $PaCO_2$ should approximate $PACO_2$. The creation of alveolar dead space by a PE yields areas of lung in which the $PACO_2$ is nearly zero. The air expired from the alveolar dead space mixes with air from perfused areas of the lungs and results in an overall decrease of the $EtCO_2$. Some have suggested that a fall in $EtCO_2$ is associated with occlusion of greater than 25% of the pulmonary vasculature.

Increased alveolar dead space ventilation, in addition to various other mechanisms, should result in hypoxemia (decreased PaO_2). This high V/Q ratio is also characterized by an increased (A-a) PO_2. However, as described above, if PE produces an increase in minute ventilation, then PaO_2 may be normal or near normal, particularly in patients with no underlying cardiopulmonary disease. There are other mechanisms that also contribute to hypoxia in PE, including intracardiac shunting through a patent foramen ovale with high

A

right-sided heart pressures, intrapulmonary shunting through areas of atelectasis, and a decrease in cardiac output leading to a decrease in the mixed venous oxygen saturation. The Prospective Investigation of Pulmonary Embolism Diagnosis (PIOPED) study looked at a subset of otherwise healthy patients with suspected PE and was unable to distinguish patients with and without confirmed PE on the basis of either (A-a) PO_2 or PaO_2. Another retrospective study of hospitalized patients with PE found that all patients had an elevated (A-a) PO_2, and that PaO_2 was greater than 80 mm Hg in 29% of patients younger than 40 years, compared with only 3% of those older than 40 years.

The diagnosis of acute PE cannot be excluded on the basis of a normal ABG. Although the alveolar-arterial difference is usually elevated, it may occasionally be normal in patients without preexisting cardiopulmonary disease. An elevated $PaCO_2$ (which may be caused by other factors, such as preexisting lung disease or metabolic alkalosis) does not rule out the possibility of acute PE.

SUGGESTED READINGS

Crapo JD, Glassroth J, Karlinsky JB, et al. *Baum's Textbook of Pulmonary Disease.* 7th ed. Philadelphia, PA: Lippincott Williams & Wilkins; 2004:736.

Green RM, Meyer TJ, Dunn M, et al. Pulmonary embolism in younger adults. *Chest.* 1992;101(6):1507–1511.

Hall JB, Schmidt GA, Wood LDH. *Principles of Critical Care.* New York, NY: McGraw-Hill; 2005:347–355.

Hines RL, Marschall K. *Anesthesia and Co-existing Disease.* 5th ed. Philadelphia, PA: Churchill Livingstone; 2008:191–193.

Parrillo JE, Dellinger RP. *Critical Care Medicine.* 3rd ed. St Louis, MO: Mosby Elsevier; 2005:895–904.

Stein PD, Goldhaber SZ, Henry JW. Alveolar-arterial oxygen gradient in the assessment of acute pulmonary embolism. *Chest.* 1995;107(1):139–143.

ABG: Salicylate Toxicity

Subspecialties: Critical Care and Pharmacology

Juan Egas

Edited by Hossam Tantawy

KEY POINTS

1. Salicylate intoxication may produce a wide range of symptoms including tremors, diaphoresis, hyperthermia, nausea, vomiting, hyperventilation, and hearing abnormalities such as hypoacusia and tinnitus.
2. Patients with salicylate intoxication may develop two primary acid–base disorders that may occur together or independently.
3. A hyperventilation syndrome secondary to a direct stimulation of the respiratory center results in respiratory alkalosis. The uncoupling of oxidative phosphorylation and the subsequent inability to effectively produce ATP by the mitochondria may result in a severe anion gap metabolic acidosis.

DISCUSSION

Acetylsalicylic acid (ASA) is a weak acid (pKa 3.5) with antiplatelet and anti-inflammatory properties. In gastric acidic pH, it is largely present in a nonionized form, facilitating absorption by passive diffusion. Despite the changes in the pH from an acidic gastric environment to an alkaline one in the duodenum (with subsequent change from nonionized form to an ionized nonlipid soluble form), most of the ingested ASA will be absorbed in the jejunum because of its large absorptive surface. Salicylate overdose may produce pylorospasm and delayed gastric emptying. In addition, salicylates have the tendency to form concretions (ASA bezoars), which may delay their absorption, reaching peak plasma concentrations more than 4 hours after ingestion. This delayed absorption will allow the use of late therapeutic interventions such as late gastric emptying (up to 4 hours after the ingestion) and repeated doses of activated charcoal.

In normal therapeutic doses, ASA is deacetylated by plasma esterases and eliminated by conjugation. At physiologic pH, salicylates are highly ionized (99%), leading to a low volume of distribution, which increases once metabolic acidosis ensues. During salicylate intoxication, the conjugation pathway becomes rapidly saturated. Unconjugated ASA is excreted by the kidneys. Urinary excretion of unchanged ASA can be enhanced by alkalinization of the urine, increasing its water-soluble fraction. ASA has high water solubility, low molecular weight, with low V_d. Most of the drug will remain in the central compartment, and its elimination can be further enhanced with extra corporeal clearance techniques such as hemodialysis.

Salicylate intoxication may produce a wide range of symptoms including tremors, diaphoresis, hyperthermia, nausea, vomiting, hyperventilation, and hearing abnormalities such as hypoacusia and tinnitus. In addition, salicylate overdose may result in an anion gap metabolic acidosis and, if left untreated, may result in cerebral edema, acute respiratory distress syndrome, kidney failure, hypoprothrombinemia, and/or thrombocytopenia, all of which in conjunction may lead to death.

Patients with salicylate intoxication may develop two primary acid–base disorders that may occur together or independently. A hyperventilation syndrome secondary to a direct

12

stimulation of the respiratory center results in respiratory alkalosis with a secondary loss of bicarbonate in the urine and loss of body's buffering capacity. In addition, the uncoupling of oxidative phosphorylation and the subsequent inability to effectively produce ATP by the mitochondria may result in a severe anion gap metabolic acidosis and hyperthermia.

Collee GG. The management of acute poisoning. *Br J Anaesth.* 1993;70(5):562–573.

Shannon MW, Borron SW, Burns M, et al. *Haddad and Winchester's Clinical Management of Poisoning and Drug Overdose.* 4th ed. Philadelphia, PA: Saunders; 2007:Chapter 48: Salicylates.

SUGGESTED READINGS

ABG Temperature Correction: PCO$_2$
Physics, Monitoring, and Anesthesia Delivery

Sharif Al-Ruzzeh

Edited by Qingbing Zhu

KEY POINTS

1. There is no established evidence that we should routinely correct temperature for arterial blood gas (ABG) results. Most commonly, the noncorrected results at 37° C are used.
2. There is a continuing debate and controversy as to which of the two methods, pH stat or alpha stat, provides better outcomes.
3. Some studies have found better cerebral perfusion and oxygenation, but more cardiac arrhythmias, with the pH-stat method.
4. The current general consensus seems to be that the alpha-stat method is preferred with moderate hypothermia (30° to 32° C), whereas the pH-stat method may be preferred to better maintain cerebral oxygenation with deep hypothermia (below 30° C).

DISCUSSION

Hypothermia and hyperthermia during surgery, especially during cardiopulmonary bypass, induce not only a series of physical and physiologic changes in the blood, but also chemical changes. Cooling the blood down makes it more alkaline, which increases CO$_2$ solubility and consequently lowers PaCO$_2$. In other words, as the body temperature is lowered, the corrected pH will increase and the corrected PaCO$_2$ will decrease. This mechanism is thought to attempt to keep the ratio of $[H^+]/[HCO_3^-]$ at a constant value, which assures continued functioning of enzymes at normal levels. This mechanism has been called alpha-stat regulation. Alpha refers to the protonation state of the α-imidazole side chain of histidine, and allowing the pH to drift with temperature allows the protonation state of histidine to remain "static," hence the name.

It has also been found that animals that have a hibernation cycle will change their ventilation as their metabolism changes, so that as their body temperature drops, the temperature corrected pH and PaCO$_2$ will remain close to normal. As a result, the noncorrected values will show an increased PCO$_2$ and decreased pH measured at 37° C when the body temperature is lower than this, indicating a respiratory acidosis. This mechanism appears to maintain cerebral blood flow and allows better cerebral oxygenation during hypothermia, and has been given the name pH-stat regulation.

The alpha-stat and pH-stat mechanisms have both been studied with induced hypothermia during surgery. Some studies have found better cerebral perfusion and oxygenation, but more cardiac arrhythmias, with the pH-stat method. There is a great debate and controversy in the literature about which method is best to use. The current general consensus seems to be that the alpha-stat method is preferred with moderate hypothermia (30° to 32° C), whereas the pH-stat method may be preferred to better maintain cerebral oxygenation with deep hypothermia (below 30° C). However, this is further complicated by the fact that there is a lack of knowledge about what is "normal" at temperatures other than 37° C.

SUGGESTED READINGS

Granger W. ABG temperature correction: to correct or not to correct; that is the question. *FOCUS: J Respir Care Sleep Med.* 2005;20–23.

Stoelting R, Miller R. *Basics of Anesthesia.* 5th ed. Philadelphia, PA: Churchill Livingstone; 2007:324–325.

ABGs: Resp Acid/Met Alk
Subspecialties: Critical Care

Stephanie Cheng
Edited by Ala Haddadin

KEY POINTS

1. Respiratory acidosis can be the result of several pathophysiologic disease processes.
2. Metabolic alkalosis is the compensatory mechanism for prolonged respiratory acidosis.
3. Acute versus chronic respiratory acidosis results in different compensation estimates in serum bicarbonate and pH.

DISCUSSION

Respiratory acidosis ($PaCO_2 \geq 45$ mm Hg) can be the result of several pathophysiologic disease processes. These processes can be categorized generally as a decrease in CO_2 elimination. The increase in $PaCO_2$ in turn decreases the $HCO_3^-/PaCO_2$ ratio and pH. Hypoventilation can be caused by diseased airways (asthma, chronic obstructive pulmonary disease, sleep apnea, tumors/foreign bodies), central nervous system depression (pharmacologically induced or neurologic deficits), decreased chest wall strength (neuromuscular blocking drugs, neuropathy, myopathy), or lung disease states (pulmonary edema, fibrosis, sarcoid, pneumonia). Increased overall CO_2 can be caused by increased production (maternal hyperthyroidism, hyperthyroidism, high carbohydrate intake), rebreathing, or CO_2 absorption (from laparoscopic surgery). Both mechanisms of increased $PaCO_2$ will lead to increased H^+ ions and thus decreased pH.

Metabolic alkalosis is the compensatory mechanism for prolonged respiratory acidosis. In response to a decreased pH, the kidneys will increase HCO_3^- reabsorption and production. At the same time, there will be an increase in hydrogen ion secretion. If the acidosis continues for days or longer, these mechanisms will increase the body's pH close to normal even in the face of increased $PaCO_2$.

With renal compensation, plasma bicarbonate should rise 3.5 mEq per L for every 10 mm Hg increase in $PaCO_2$.

The change in serum bicarbonate concentration can be estimated with the following guidelines:

1. In an acute respiratory acidosis, HCO_3^- will increase 1 mEq per L for every 10 mm Hg increase in $PaCO_2$.
2. With a chronic respiratory acidosis, HCO_3^- should increase 3.5 mEq per L for every 10 mm Hg increase in $PaCO_2$.

The expected changes in pH with respiratory acidosis can be estimated with the following:

3. In an acute respiratory acidosis: Change in pH $= 0.008 \times (40 - PaCO_2)$.
4. In a chronic respiratory acidosis: Change in pH $= 0.003 \times (40 - PaCO_2)$.

Treatment of severe respiratory acidosis (pH < 7.1) is usually ventilatory support via endotracheal intubation. KCl and/or acetazolamide can be coadministered in efforts to prevent a concomitant metabolic alkalosis that can occur with overventilation. HCO_3^- can also be used for dosing.

SUGGESTED READINGS

Barash PG, Cullen BF, Stoelting RK, et al, eds. *Clinical Anesthesia.* 6th ed. Philadelphia, PA: Lippincott Williams & Wilkins; 2009:290–296.
Miller RD, Stoelting RK. *Basics of Anesthesia.* 5th ed. Philadelphia, PA: Churchill Livingstone; 2007:317–323.

Acetaminophen Toxicity

Pain

Milaurise Cortes

Edited by Jodi Sherman

A

1. Acetaminophen is a nonopioid analgesic and antipyretic.
2. The recommended acetaminophen dose is 10 to 20 mg per kg orally or 20 to 40 mg per kg rectally.
3. Acetaminophen intoxication can result in hepatic failure or renal necrosis.
4. Acetaminophen toxicity can be treated with activated charcoal and N-acetylcysteine (NAC; Mucomyst).
5. Hepatic failure occurs as a result of accumulation of toxic metabolites with depletion of hepatic glutathione levels. These levels are restored with the administration of NAC.

DISCUSSION

Acetaminophen is a nonopioid analgesic that can be administered orally (10 to 20 mg per kg) or rectally as a suppository (20 to 40 mg per kg), the maximum daily dose being 4,000 mg. It is useful for pain management in both children and adults. It works by inhibiting the cyclooxygenase (COX) pathway that potentiates pain. Properties of acetaminophen include analgesic and antipyretic effects, but not anti-inflammatory effects. Physicians will often turn to acetaminophen instead of nonsteroidal anti-inflammatory drugs (NSAIDs) for pain control because even though NSAIDs do carry anti-inflammatory properties, they also have undesirable side effects such as gastrointestinal ulcers and poor platelet function. Acetaminophen, however, is not completely devoid of its own side effects. Given in large quantities, acetaminophen can result in liver toxicity, as well as renal necrosis.

Large doses of acetaminophen can result in fulminant hepatic failure, but even at recommended doses, it can cause liver injury when administered with other medications such as isoniazid or when patients suffer from diseases such as chronic alcoholic cirrhosis. The pathophysiology behind hepatic injury after the administration of large doses of acetaminophen includes depletion of hepatic glutathione, which results in the accumulation of toxic metabolites. To treat acetaminophen toxicity, patients are given NAC (Mucomyst), which prevents hepatic damage by restoring the levels of hepatic glutathione.

Symptoms of excessive acetaminophen ingestion include nausea and vomiting. In order to better estimate potential hepatic damage, it is best to draw acetaminophen levels 4 hours after ingestion for accurate measurements after the medication has been systemically absorbed. This level is applied to an acetaminophen toxicity nomogram to assess the severity of intoxication and assist in therapeutic management (Fig .1). When a patient arrives 2 to 4 hours after ingestion, they can initially be treated with activated charcoal. NAC is given within 8 hours after ingestion, orally or intravenously, if the patient is unable to tolerate the former.

The following are just a few medications that contain acetaminophen, and when taken together, can lead to an unintentional overdose: Alka Seltzer Plus Cold and Sinus, DayQuil, NyQuil, Vicodin, Dimetapp, and Percocet.

16

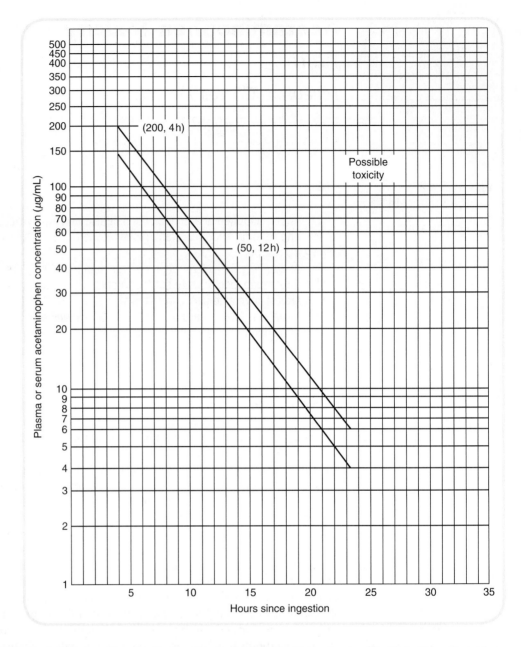

Figure 1. Nomogram for estimating severity of acute acetaminophen poisoning. (Modified with permission from Rumack BH, Matthew H. Acetaminophen poisoning and toxicity. *Pediatrics*. 1975;55:871–876.)

SUGGESTED
READINGS

Barash PG, Cullen BF, Stoelting RK, et al, eds. *Clinical Anesthesia*. 6th ed. Philadelphia, PA: Lippincott Williams & Wilkins; 2009:1486, 1501.
Fleisher GR, Ludwig S, Henretig FM. *Textbook of Pediatric Emergency Medicine*. 5th ed. Philadelphia, PA: Lippincott Williams & Wilkins; 2005:964–965.
Morgan G, Mikhail M, Murray M. *Clinical Anesthesiology*. 4th ed. New York, NY: McGraw-Hill Medical; 2005:369, 394, 1063.

Acute Heart Failure: Management
Organ-based Clinical: Cardiovascular

Christian Scheps

Edited by Qingbing Zhu

1. Acute heart failure can etiologically arise from exacerbation of chronic failure or valvular dysfunction, myocardial infarction, or papillary muscle rupture.
2. Acute heart failure is initially managed by pharmacologic means, including diuretics, inotropes, vasodilators, and exogenous Brain Natriuretic Peptide (BNP).
3. If pharmacologic management fails, mechanical devices such as intraaortic balloon pumps, ventricular assistant devices, and even cardiac transplantation are available options.

Acute heart failure may manifest as a primary heart condition or be the result of an exacerbation in chronic failure. When not related to a chronic condition, acute heart failure can be the consequence of massive myocardial infarction, abrupt onset of valvular dysfunction, or other structural defect such as wall or papillary muscle rupture. Whatever the etiology, low cardiac output along with high ventricular filling pressures and hyper/hypotension ensues. The pathophysiology most closely resembles cardiogenic shock rather than chronic congestive heart failure.

Situations requiring the management of acute heart failure can occur intraoperatively. Acute heart failure is most commonly seen during heart surgery while weaning from cardiopulmonary bypass. Treatment initially focuses on maintaining and/or increasing cardiac output via different pharmacologic interventions. In addition, if the episode is refractory to pharmacologic management, there are mechanical devices that can be implanted for temporary relief of acute failure. Cardiac transplantation is an uncommon option for those episodes that have a bleak and unrecoverable prognosis. Classic pharmacologic therapy centers on diuretics, vasodilators, and inotropes, whereas newer options include calcium sensitizers and exogenous B-type natriuretic peptide.

Loop diuretics such as furosemide are commonly used in initial management and can provide rapid symptomatic relief by reducing the amount of volume overload resulting from a failing pump. In addition, loop diuretics offer benefit by their intrinsic vasodilatory properties, which reduce preload. Targeted vasodilators such as nitroglycerin and nitroprusside are more commonly used for this purpose, however. The effective systemic vasodilation helps the failing heart by lowering left ventricle filling pressure and systemic vascular resistance and by increasing stroke volume.

Depending on the severity of failure, inotropes may be necessary to maintain a viable cardiac output. Inotropes work by improving excitation–contraction coupling by increasing intracellular calcium concentrations via the augmentation of cAMP levels. Inotropes such as milrinone accomplish this by indirectly inhibiting cAMP degradation. Other inotropes such as dobutamine, dopamine, and epinephrine accomplish this by direct beta receptor stimulation. All the inotropes increase the risk of dysrhythmia and can have the deleterious effect of increasing heart rate, myocardial oxygen demand, and oxygen consumption. Thus, short-term use is best.

Newer pharmacologic treatments include calcium sensitizers such as levosimendan, which is widely used in Europe but has not yet been approved for use in the United States. It increases contractility without increasing intracellular calcium levels, and therefore theoretically does not increase the risk of tachycardia, increase in myocardial oxygen demand, and propensity for dysrhythmias that limit the use of other inotropes. Exogenous

B-type natriuretic peptide is an alternative aid as well. It works by promoting arterial, venous, and coronary vasodilation.

If pharmacologic treatment of acute heart failure is not effective, various mechanical devices are available to off-load the work of the failing heart. One such device is the intraaortic balloon pump, which is commonly inserted when the etiology of heart failure is myocardial infarction. This device is inserted percutaneously via the femoral artery and is placed distal to the left subclavian artery. It works by expanding during diastole, which increases diastolic blood pressure and thus increases coronary perfusion pressure and oxygen delivery. During systole, the device deflates and essentially helps pull blood through by negative pressure with improvement in oxygen consumption by decreasing cardiac work.

In addition to balloon pumps, left and right ventricular assist devices have been developed that can be inserted during open heart surgery and percutaneously. These devices work to unload the preload of the heart and distribute the blood distally in the system, thereby decreasing the heart's work. In some circumstances, assist devices can be very effective at allowing the heart to rest acutely. These devices can be explanted once the heart assumes satisfactory function.

SUGGESTED READING

Hines RL, Marschall KE. *Stoelting's Anesthesia and Co-existing Disease.* 5th ed. Philadelphia, PA: Saunders Elsevier; 2008:112–114.

Acute Hyperkalemia: Rx

Pharmacology and Physiology

Mary DiMiceli and Ervin Jakab

Edited by Qingbing Zhu

A

KEY POINTS

1. Hyperkalemia (P_k > 5.5 mEq per L) can be a life-threatening condition caused by excessive intake, inadequate excretion, or extracellular shifts.
2. Hyperkalemia may be manifested by muscle weakness or ECG changes; however, up to 50% of patients may have life-threatening hyperkalemia without any ECG manifestations.
3. Hyperkalemia with ECG changes (tall T waves, lengthening of the PR interval and the QRS duration, heart block, V-Fib) or circulatory compromise, or levels greater than 7.0 mEq per L needs prompt intervention with intravenous (IV) calcium or insulin plus dextrose.
4. Basic understanding of potassium physiology is pertinent in proceeding through treatment for hyperkalemia.
5. Goals of treatment include membrane stabilization/antagonism of potassium on cell membranes, redistribution of potassium intracellularly, and permanent removal from the body achieved by secretion, excretion, or hemodialysis.

DISCUSSION

Electrolyte disturbances, particularly elevated potassium levels, have the potential for some very serious complications. Although hyperkalemia, defined as a plasma potassium level greater than 5.5 mEq per L, may be desired in the local administration of cardioplegia during cardiac surgery with the overall effect to help reduce oxygen consumption and cardiac standstill, it is more often not desirable and can be a life-threatening condition. Hyperkalemia may result from (a) excessive intake, such as that which occurs with massive blood transfusion and cardioplegia, inadequate excretion secondary to renal failure/insufficiency, potassium-sparing diuretics, or angiotensin-converting enzyme (ACE) inhibitors and (b) extracellular shifts that may occur with extensive tissue damage, burns, major trauma, organ transplantation, respiratory or metabolic acidosis, hyperkalemic periodic paralysis, digitalis overdose, malignant hyperthermia, and administration of succinylcholine. Particularly pertinent to the field of anesthesia is hyperkalemia resulting from succinylcholine, since it is known to increase plasma levels by 0.5 mEq per L in normal patients. As anesthesiologists, we must be aware of other circumstances and surgical situations that can predispose a patient to developing hyperkalemia after receiving the depolarizing muscle relaxant. Patients may also have pseudohyperkalemia secondary to red cell hemolysis or thrombocytosis/leukocytosis. Moreover, as discussed in a recent case report, rebound hyperkalemia can ensue after therapeutic barbiturate coma, as barbiturates, particularly thiopental, have been known to cause a transient hypokalemia secondary to an intracellular shift followed by rebound hyperkalemia as potassium shifts extracellularly.

Hyperkalemia is manifested by muscle weakness (>8 mEq per L) and electrocardiographic changes, which can be seen at plasma potassium (P_k) concentrations starting around 6.5 to 7.0 mEq per L. However, having elevated potassium levels does not guarantee clinically evident ECG changes. As a matter of fact, many studies have demonstrated significant hyperkalemia (>7.0 mEq per L) without ECG changes, and other reports only 46% to 55% patients with P_k > 6.0 with ECG changes. Therefore, unless one has a clinical index of suspicion, diagnosing hyperkalemia may actually prove to be difficult and/or otherwise delayed. Hyperkalemia also has the effect of potentiating the effects of neuromuscular blocking agents, and so patients must be monitored very closely intraoperatively.

A

To understand the treatment of hyperkalemia, a basic understanding of the potassium physiology is pertinent, specifically as when applied to cardiac myocytes. Potassium is the dominant intracellular cation, whereas sodium is the dominant extracellular cation. P_k is also mostly determined by renal regulation, with secretion and reabsorption occurring at the distal tubule in the nephron, and a balance is further maintained by insulin, catecholamines, and acid–base equilibrium. The concentration gradient between sodium and potassium, maintained by sodium–potassium ATPase pumps, is what determines a cell membrane's resting membrane potential, which is normally −90 mV. The potassium ion gradient is the most important factor in determining the membrane potential, and as a result when the extracellular concentration increases, the concentration gradient decreases and so does the resting membrane potential (e.g., from −90 to −80 mV). The normal threshold potential is −75 mV; therefore, by making the resting membrane potential less negative (i.e., closer to −75 mV), the cell membrane is more excitable.

These changes are clinically manifested as peaked T waves, prolonged PR interval, and a widened QRS. Phase 1 is due to efflux of potassium ions, which is eventually offset by the influx of calcium, as manifested in phase 2, resulting in a plateau phase. Phase 3 is the result of calcium channels closing and the continued efflux of potassium out of cells leading to cell repolarization. However, with high extracellular levels of potassium, the potassium ion channels have increased conductance across the cell membrane (for unknown reasons), resulting in a higher efflux of ions outward, and thus to a steeper slope in phases 2 and 3, and therefore shortened repolarization time. This is also clinically manifested as ST segment depression and a shortened Q-T interval. With increasing levels of potassium, the sinoatrial (SA) node is increasingly more sensitive and begins to exhibit increased electrical activity without actual atrial depolarization, thus resulting in the loss of P waves. Finally, with worsening levels (>10 mEq per L), the SA node no longer is the focus of depolarization, and the electrical impulse begins in junctional pacemakers, resulting in widened QRS complexes, eventually to the point where the QRS and T wave occur simultaneously, ultimately leading to ventricular fibrillation and asystole.

Accordingly, treatment in the acute setting is directed at minimizing and eliminating the adverse electrophysiologic effects on the myocardium. Additional modes of treatment can then be directed at increasing the flux of potassium ion flow intracellularly and by increasing potassium elimination or renal secretion/excretion. Membrane stabilization is achieved with calcium chloride or calcium gluconate, which acts by reducing the threshold potential of cardiac myocytes. In other words, the normal threshold potential is −75 mV, and with hyperkalemia, the resting membrane potential is less negative (−90 to −80 mV) with resultant increased excitability, but with increased extracellular calcium, the threshold potential is lowered to −60 mV and as a result membrane excitability is decreased along with the potential for arrhythmias. Moreover, with the administration of calcium, the influx of calcium into cells (particularly calcium-dependent cells, such as the SA and atrioventricular nodes) increases the rate of rise of phase 0 in the action potential, therefore counteracting the depressant effects of hyperkalemia as evidenced in a decreased slope of phase 0 (Fig. 1). Calcium gluconate is the preferred solution, as calcium chloride has the untoward side effect of tissue necrosis if it extravasates, and it is administered as 10 to 30 mL of 10% calcium gluconate IV. Hyperkalemia is also worsened by concurrent electrolyte disturbances (hyponatremia, hypocalcemia, acidemia), and so in patients with hyponatremia, the IV administration of hypertonic saline may also aid in reversing ECG changes and membrane stabilization.

One may also try to prevent occurrence of hyperkalemia secondary to excessive intake, which may occur with massive blood transfusion. With prolonged storage of whole blood, the plasma potassium concentration may increase to 30 mEq per L. In one case report, continuous autotransfusion (CAT) devices were used, in which 1 mL of "old" (>4 weeks) blood was washed with 2 mL of normal saline. The unprocessed blood had a potassium level of 39.6 mmol per L, and the final-processed blood using the CATs resulted in a level of 2.3 mmol per L, which was administered intraoperatively to a patient with end-stage kidney disease (ESRD) who ultimately had an uneventful postoperative course. Although there is not much in the literature regarding this method, it is definitely something to consider, especially in trauma patients and patients who will require massive blood transfusions with impaired renal function.

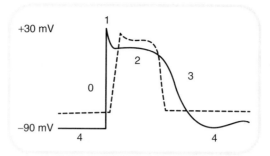

Figure 1. The action potential of a cardiac myocyte. Activation of voltage-gated Na ion channels results in phase 0 of the action potential. The rate of rise of this phase is determined by the membrane potential at the onset of depolarization, which determines the number of sodium channels activated. With hyperkalemia *(dotted line)*, the resting membrane potential is less negative, resulting in less-activated sodium channels and therefore a slower rate in rise correlating with slower conduction through the myocardium and prolonging depolarization. (Reused from Parham WA, Mehdirad AA, Biermann KM, et al. Hyperkalemia revisited. Tex Heart Inst J 2006;33(1):40–47.)

The second goal of therapy, intracellular redistribution of potassium, may be achieved by stimulation of Na-K ATPase pumps typically with an injection of 10 units of regular insulin followed by a bolus of 50% dextrose, thus helping to move potassium inside the cell and sodium out. Catecholamines and beta-agonists have also been shown to help drive potassium intracellularly by the same process. In select patients, particularly those who are significantly acidotic, sodium bicarbonate may be given to help shift potassium inside cells by increasing plasma pH. In patients with an otherwise normal pH, it may not be helpful, as it may have a transient effect with the potential for rebound hyperkalemia. Finally, potassium excretion/secretion may be enhanced by particular medications, although not in the acute setting of severe hyperkalemia. Lasix will help promote elimination of potassium by inhibition of sodium–potassium–chloride transporter in the ascending limb of the loop of Henle in patients with normal renal function. However, in patients with renal insufficiency or failure, cation-exchange resins such as sodium polystyrene sulfonate (Kayexalate) in the oral or rectal form help promote intestinal excretion. Unfortunately, it has a slow onset of effect and has the potential for bowel necrosis, so it is not particularly a favorable medication. Dialysis has also been shown to be an effective method, particularly in renal failure patients, but can result in rebound hyperkalemia in some patients.

SUGGESTED READINGS

Gaba DM, Fish KJ, Howard SK. *Crisis Management in Anesthesiology.* Philadelphia, PA: Churchill Livingstone; 1994:153–155.

Knichwitz G, Zahl M, Van Aken H, et al. Intraoperative washing of long-stored packed red cells using an autotransfusion device prevents hyperkalemia. *Anesth Analg.* 2002;95:324–325.

Morgan GE, Mikhail MS, Murray MJ. *Clinical Anesthesiology.* 4th ed. New York, NY: Lange Medical Books/McGraw Hill; 2006:680–682.

Neil MJ, Dale MC. Hypokalaemia with severe rebound hyperkalemia after therapeutic barbiturate coma. *Anesth Analg.* 2009;108(6):1867–1868.

Weisberg LS. Management of severe hyperkalemia. *Crit Care Med.* 2008;36(12):3246–3251.

Acute Septic Shock
Subspecialties: Critical Care

Gabriel Jacobs
Edited by Hossam Tantawy

KEY POINTS

1. Septic shock is sepsis with hypotension, despite adequate fluid replacement, accompanied by signs of perfusion derangements.
2. The degree of sepsis can be classified by different levels of severity.
3. Treatment of sepsis involves intravenous (IV) antibiotic treatment for infection, maintaining tissue perfusion, and treating any secondary sepsis-induced derangements (acute renal failure [ARF], acute respiratory distress syndrome [ARDS]).

DISCUSSION

Septic shock is a shock in the setting of activation of systemic inflammatory response. Systemic vascular resistance is decreased, and cardiac output is increased; hypotension is present with redistribution of blood flow to different regions resulting in tissue hypoperfusion. Septic shock is associated with infectious processes. The degree of sepsis can be viewed on a scale of different grades of severity.

$$SIRS \rightarrow Sepsis \rightarrow Severe\ sepsis \rightarrow Septic\ shock$$

Systemic inflammatory response syndrome (SIRS) is defined as two or more of the following: core temperature $<36°$ C or $>38°$ C, heart rate >90 beats per minute, tachypnea >20 breaths per minute or a $PaCO_2$ <4.3 kPa, WBC $>12,000$ per mm^3 or $<4,000$ per mm^3 or greater than 10% immature forms.

Sepsis is SIRS in the setting of an infection. Sepsis is termed as being severe when there are signs of end-organ dysfunction. *Septic shock* is a hypermetabolic state in which the body's ability to extract, deliver, and utilize oxygen is impaired secondary to endotoxemia, which can lead to metabolic acidosis and *MODS* (multiorgan dysfunction syndrome). Septic shock is sepsis with hypotension despite adequate fluid replacement and signs of perfusion derangements. Hypotension in the context of septic shock is defined as (a) systolic blood pressure (SBP) <90 mm Hg, (b) mean arterial pressure (MAP) <60 mm Hg, and (c) systemic blood pressure <40 mm Hg of the patient's baseline.

Septic shock is most commonly due to gram-negative rods from the genitourinary tract or the lungs. The hypotension seen in septic shock is due to capillary leak and perhaps increased NO levels. Cardiac depression can also contribute to hypotension. Activation of clotting cascade can contribute to tissue hypoperfusion. The clinical manifestations of septic shock include leukocytosis with a left shift or leukopenia and metabolic acidosis (most commonly lactic acidosis); sometimes a compensatory respiratory alkalosis can also be seen.

The signs of end-organ damage include elevated liver function tests (LFTs) in the setting of liver damage, altered mental status, signs of ARDS or respiratory failure, and elevated renal markers such as an increased creatinine in the setting oliguria and azotemia.

The diagnosis can be made by discovering the nidus of infection with the aid of radiography and cultures of urine, blood, and sputum before the initiation of antibiotic therapy. The treatment includes broad-spectrum IV antibiotics, maintenance of tissue perfusion/oxygenation using oxygen therapy, IV fluid replacement and vasoactive drugs (such as

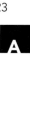

norepinephrine) as needed, and treatment of specific end-organ damage. Activated protein C may be used to counteract sepsis-induced disseminated intravascular coagulation (DIC), and thereby minimize the risk of microvascular thrombus formation.

SUGGESTED READINGS

Barash PG, Cullen BF, Stoelting RK, et al, eds. *Clinical Anesthesia*. 6th ed. Philadelphia, PA: Wolters Kluwer Lippincott Williams & Wilkins; 2009:1453–1455.
Morgan GE Jr, Mikhail MS, Murray MJ. *Lange Clinical Anesthesiology*. 4th ed. New York, NY: Lange Medical Books/McGraw-Hill; 2005:1051–1057.

KEYWORD

SECTION

Addiction: Definition

Generic Clinical Sciences: Anesthesia Procedures, Methods, Techniques

Alexey Dyachkov

Edited by Thomas Halaszynski

KEY POINTS

1. Addiction is a chronic disease.
2. Addiction is defined as a physical or psychological dependence on a substance or activity that is beyond voluntary control.
3. Addiction leads to continuing involvement in dependent behaviors regardless of consequences (often negative) associated with them.
4. Addiction has different definitions in medical and legal societies.

DISCUSSION

Various definitions of the word *addiction* are as follows:

1. *Oxford American Dictionary*: the fact or condition of being addicted to a particular substance, thing, or activity; Origin: late 16th century (denoting a person's inclination or proclivity): from Latin *addictio(n-)*, from *addicere* "assign"
2. *Merriam-Webster*: compulsive need for and use of a habit-forming substance (heroin, nicotine, or alcohol) characterized by tolerance and well-defined physiological symptoms upon withdrawal; *broadly*: persistent compulsive use of a substance known by the user to be harmful

The American Academy of Pain Medicine (AAPM), the American Pain Society (APS), and the American Society of Addiction Medicine (ASAM) issued a consensus document defining physical dependence, tolerance, and addiction as follows:

"***Tolerance*** is a state of adaptation in which exposure to a drug induces changes that result in a diminution of one or more of the drug's effect over time."

"***Physical dependence*** is a state of adaptation that is manifested by a drug class specific withdrawal syndrome that can be produced by abrupt cessation, rapid dose reduction, decreasing blood level of the drug, and/or administration of an antagonist." This term may refer to the use of "regular" medications, for instance, beta-blockers or clonidine.

"***Addiction*** is a primary, chronic, neurobiologic disease, with genetic, psychosocial, and environmental factors influencing its development and manifestations. It is characterized by behaviors that include one or more of the following: impaired control over drug use, compulsive use, continued use despite harm, and craving."

The National Institute on Drug Abuse (NIDA) defines addiction as "a chronic, relapsing disease characterized by compulsive drug seeking and use, despite harmful consequences, and by neurochemical and molecular changes in the brain."

NIDA and the National Institute on Alcohol Abuse and Alcoholism (NIAAA) differentiate dependence and addiction as follows:

"*Physical dependence* refers to adaptations that result in withdrawal symptoms when drugs such as alcohol, heroin, etc. are discontinued. Those are distinct from the adaptations that result in *addiction*, which refers to the loss of control over the intense urges to take the drug *even at the expense of adverse consequences*."

A person moves from misuse to abuse to addiction when craving, drug seeking, and compulsive use dominate his or her life and behavior.

Longnecker D, ed. *Anesthesiology*. New York, NY: McGraw-Hill; 2008:2137–2152.

Savage S, Covington EC, Heit HA, et al. Definitions related to the use of opioids for the treatment of pain, a consensus document from the American Academy of Pain Medicine, the American Pain Society, and the American Society of Addiction Medicine. American Pain Society; 2001.

SUGGESTED READINGS

Addison Disease: Periop Rx
Organ-based Clinical: Endocrine/Metabolic

Johnny Garriga

Edited by Mamatha Punjala

1. Primary adrenal insufficiency (hypoadrenocorticism), also known as Addison disease, is associated with local destruction of all the zones of the adrenal cortex.
2. Addisonian crisis or acute adrenal insufficiency can occur if corticosteroid therapy is discontinued abruptly without a taper or if the corticosteroid dosage is not adequately adjusted for perioperative stresses.
3. The key to the anesthetic management of patients with deficiency is to ensure adequate steroid replacement therapy during the perioperative period.
4. Preoperative preparation includes treatment with an exogenously administered mineralocorticoid, volume status replacement, electrolyte management, and correction of hypotension.
5. There are multiple regimens for perioperative steroid replacement.

Adrenocortical insufficiency can be either primary (adrenal gland dysfunction) or secondary (hypothalamic–pituitary axis dysfunction). The adrenal cortex secretes androgens, mineralocorticoids (i.e., aldosterone), and glucocorticoids (i.e., cortisol). The adrenal medulla secretes catecholamines (i.e., epinephrine, norepinephrine, and dopamine). Cortisol normally increases in response to stressors such as surgery or trauma. In patients who have a disturbance of the hypothalamic–pituitary axis such as resulting from chronic administration (>2 weeks) of a daily equivalent of 5 mg of prednisone in the past 12 months, their body's ability to respond to the stress via a cortisol surge will be inadequate. In this case, an Addisonian crisis could ensue; it is an acute complication of adrenal insufficiency characterized by circulatory collapse, dehydration, nausea, vomiting, hypoglycemia, and hyperkalemia.

Glucocorticoids are essential for life and have multiple physiologic effects. Metabolic actions include enhanced gluconeogenesis and inhibition of peripheral glucose utilization. Glucocorticoids affect vascular and bronchial smooth muscle, allowing them to be responsive to catecholamines. Glucocorticoids cause sodium retention and potassium excretion. Adrenocorticotropic hormone (ACTH) from the anterior pituitary regulates all glucocorticoid secretion. Secretion of ACTH and glucocorticoids exhibits a diurnal rhythm, often increasing plasma levels during stress, and is inhibited by circulating glucocorticoids, as a feedback mechanism.

Normally, the adrenal gland secretes a maximum of 200 mg of cortisol per day. During the perioperative period (extreme stress), the adrenal gland may secrete up to 500 mg per day of cortisol. The level of responsiveness correlates with the duration of the surgery and the degree of the trauma. Therefore, perioperatively, patients with Addison disease require additional corticosteroids to mimic the increased output of the normal adrenal gland during stress. As always, in cases of hemodynamic instability and extreme electrolyte imbalances, rapid administration of intravenous fluids and electrolyte replacement are paramount. In anticipated cases, patients with adrenocortical insufficiency will need additional steroid to cope with the stress. However, what constitutes adequate steroid dose is debatable. The clinical decision is how much steroid to give. Two common regimens are utilized in the perioperative management of patients with Addison disease. The first consists of the administration of 200 to 300 mg per 70 kg of body mass of hydrocortisone in divided doses on the day of surgery. The lower dose is increased depending on the

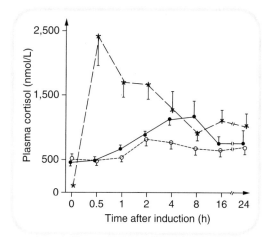

Figure 1. The variation of plasma cortisol concentrations measured in three groups of patients undergoing elective surgery. The first group *(solid circles)* never received corticosteroids. The second group *(open circles)* received preoperative corticosteroids with a normal response to preoperative ACTH (corticotropin) stimulation testing. The third group *(asterisks)* consists of patients who have been receiving long-term corticosteroid therapy. After anesthesia induction, these patients received 25 mg of cortisol intravenously, then a continuous infusion of 100 mg of cortisol for the next 24 hours. Before induction, plasma cortisol levels in this group were lower than in the other two groups; however, after IV administration of cortisol to the third group of patients, plasma concentrations were significantly higher than the two previous groups for the following 2 hours. After this administration, the mean plasma concentrations became similar for all three groups, providing supportive evidence that the key to the anesthetic management of patients with deficiency is to ensure adequate steroid replacement therapy during the perioperative period.

severity and duration of the operation. During the postoperative period, the steroid coverage is tapered to the dose the patient was on previously. The alternative mode of management involves 25 mg of hydrocortisone at the time of anesthesia induction followed by an infusion of 100 mg during the following 24 hours (Fig .1). This has been shown to achieve plasma cortisol levels equal to or higher than those reported in healthy patients undergoing similar elective surgery. One study that used the "low-dose" cortisol replacement regimen found no problems with cardiovascular instability if patients received their usual dose of steroids.

SUGGESTED READINGS

Barash PG, Cullen BF, Stoelting RK, et al, eds. *Clinical Anesthesia*. 6th ed. Philadelphia, PA: Lippincott Williams & Wilkins; 2009:1289–1293.

Marzotti S, Falorni A. Addison's disease. *Autoimmunity*. 2004;37:333–336.

Symreng T, Karlberg BE, Kagedol B, et al. Physiological cortisol substitution of long-term steroid-treated patients undergoing major surgery. *Br J Anaesth*. 1981;53:949.

Advanced Multiple Sclerosis: Anesthetic Drugs

Generic, Clinical Sciences: Anesthesia Procedures, Methods, Techniques

Ervin Jakab

Edited by Ramachandran Ramani

1. The patients should be advised that, although it is controversial, relapse of multiple sclerosis may be precipitated by anesthesia. The discussion should be documented in the preoperative consent.
2. Epidural analgesia, especially in obstetrics, seems to be safe, but higher concentrations of bupivacaine should be avoided.
3. Succinylcholine should be avoided in the setting of paresis/paralysis (hyperkalemia).
4. The response to nondepolarizing muscle relaxants may be influenced by baclofen (increased) and anticonvulsants (decreased).
5. Increases in body temperatures should be avoided (blocked conduction).
6. Volatile anesthetics may have an exaggerated hypotensive effect (autonomic dysfunction).

Perioperative exacerbation of multiple sclerosis may be related to infection, emotional stress, hyperpyrexia, or anesthesia. Although the effect of surgery and anesthesia is controversial, the patient should be advised that a relapse may occur despite a well-managed anesthetic, and the discussion should be documented in the preoperative consent. Both general and regional anesthesia may have unpredictable effects, and they have been reported to exacerbate multiple sclerosis. Elective surgery should be avoided during relapse regardless of the anesthetic technique used.

The mechanism through which spinal anesthesia may precipitate an exacerbation of the disease is not known, but it has been suggested that demyelinated areas of the spinal cord are more sensitive to the effects of the local anesthetic, causing relative neurotoxicity. Higher concentrations of bupivacaine (0.25%) used for epidural analgesia in labor are more likely to cause relapse than lower concentrations, which can be safely used.

Demyelinated fibers are extremely sensitive to increases in body temperatures. Regardless of the anesthetic used, a minimal increase of even 0.5° C may completely block conduction. The effects of nondepolarizing muscle relaxants are influenced by some of the medications used in the treatment of multiple sclerosis: baclofen increases sensitivity because of gamma-aminobutyric acid (GABA) agonist action, whereas anticonvulsants produce resistance to these agents. Succinylcholine could theoretically produce an exaggerated release of potassium, but there are no clinical reports describing this effect. In the setting of paresis or paralysis, succinylcholine should be avoided because of hyperkalemia.

The hypotensive effects of volatile anesthetics may be exaggerated by the autonomic dysfunction present in multiple sclerosis. Patients treated with corticosteroids may require intravenous steroid supplementation.

Barash PG, Cullen BF, Stoelting RK, et al, eds. *Clinical Anesthesia*. 6th ed. Philadelphia, PA: Lippincott Williams & Wilkins; 2009:628–629.

Morgan GE Jr, Mikhail MS, Murray MJ, eds. *Clinical Anesthesiology*. 4th ed. New York, NY: McGraw Hill, Lange Medical Books; 2006:652–653.

Age-related P50

Organ-based Clinical: Respiratory

Rongjie Jiang

Edited by Veronica Matei

A

KEY POINTS

1. The P50 of hemoglobin is defined as the partial pressure of oxygen (PO_2) in blood at which hemoglobin is 50% saturated with oxygen, at 37° C and a pH of 7.4.
2. P50 is the usual method of reporting any shift in the oxygen–hemoglobin dissociation curve.
3. There are three major factors that affect the shift of P50:
   - 2,3-Diphosphoglycerate (DPG)
   - pH
   - Temperature
4. Fetal hemoglobin has a much lower P50 (18 mm Hg) than P50 (27 mm Hg) in adults. Fetal red blood cells have a lower level of 2,3-DPG that may also contribute to this shift.

DISCUSSION

Normal adults have a P50 of 27 mm Hg. The classic oxygen dissociation curve is shown in Figure 1. A low P50 indicates a left shift of the curve, which means an increased affinity of hemoglobin for oxygen. A low 2,3-DPG, increased pH, and lower temperature shift the curve to the left, as does fetal hemoglobin. The right shift is just the opposite.

The lower P50 of fetal hemoglobin (18 mm Hg) makes it easier to bind oxygen from maternal placental circulation. However, it makes releasing oxygen to tissue more difficult.

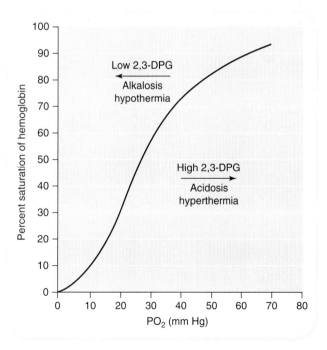

Figure 1. The oxygen dissociation curve. (Reused with permission from Miller RD. Miller's Anesthesia. 7th Edition. Philadelphia, PA: Elsevier, Churchill and Livingstone, 2009: 2663.)

The transition to adult hemoglobin is completed 6 months after birth. The detailed changes are shown in the following table:

Age	Oxygen Consumption (mL/kg/min)	Hemoglobin Concentration (g/dL)	P$_{50}$ (mm Hg)
Term newborn	6.0 ± 1.0	16.5 ± 1.5	18
6 mo	5.0 ± 0.9	11.5 ± 1.0	24
12 mo	5.2 ± 0.9	12.0 ± 0.75	—
2 y	6.4 ± 1.2	12.5 ± 0.5	27
5 y	6.0 ± 1.1	12.5 ± 0.5	—
12 y	3.3 ± 0.6	13.5 ± 1.0	—
Adult	3.4 ± 0.6	14.0 ± 1.0	27

SUGGESTED READINGS

Crone PK. *Pediatric Intensive Care.* Philadelphia, PA: JB Lippincott; 1981. *ASA Refresher Courses in Anesthesiology,* Vol 9.

Miller RD. *Miller's Anesthesia.* 7th ed. Philadelphia, PA: Elsevier, Churchill, and Livingstone; 2009:2663, 1746.

Aging: Cardiovasc Physiol and LV Function

Generic Clinical Sciences: Anesthesia Procedures, Methods, Techniques

A

Laurie Yonemoto and Zhaodi Gong

Edited by Benjamin Sherman

1. As people age, cardiovascular physiology changes in multiple ways, both structurally and functionally.
2. Sympathetic and parasympathetic changes also occur, which affect the cardiovascular system.
3. Left ventricular (LV) hypertrophy can be expected.
4. Diastolic dysfunction can be expected.
5. There is an increase in vascular rigidity and a decrease in vessel compliance.
6. As people get older, there is a decreased maximal attainable heart rate.
7. Patients can develop atrioventricular (AV) conduction defects.
8. Valvular abnormalities, specifically aortic valve calcification, are common.

DISCUSSION

There are many physiologic changes associated with aging that affect each organ system. Some of the most important changes include those involving the cardiovascular system, especially with respect to LV function.

With the normal aging process, there is an overall decrease in the compliance of the central arterial system, veins, and myocardium. The decrease in arterial elasticity is secondary to increased fibrosis of the tunica media, which predisposes patients to systolic hypertension. The myocardium itself also becomes less compliant with age. This decrease in compliance occurs because of ventricular hypertrophy. The LV must work against higher afterload pressures. This ultimately results in impaired relaxation and decreased diastolic filling of the LV, an increased reliance on atrial contraction, and a higher left ventricular end-diastolic pressure (LVEDP). Increased LVEDP leads to an increased vulnerability of congestive heart failure and the development of atrial fibrillation.

With aging, there is increased incidence of atherosclerotic cardiovascular disease and increased incidence of degeneration of cardiac conduction system. Fibrosis of the cardiac conduction system causes damage to the His bundle as it perforates the right fibrous trigone. This can lead to AV conduction defects and various arrhythmias. Fibrosis and calcification of the valves also increases with age. It is not uncommon to find calcification of the aortic valve leading to aortic valve sclerosis or stenosis in the elderly.

Another consequence of aging is a decreased responsiveness of the heart to beta-receptor stimulation. This results in a blunted response to catecholamines and explains the decreased exercise capacity of elderly patients. Maximal attainable heart rate also decreases with aging. Therefore, elderly patients are more dependent on LV end-diastolic volume and preload to maintain adequate cardiac output according to the Frank–Starling relationship (Fig. 1).

A

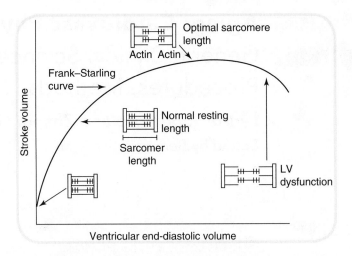

Figure 1. Frank–Starling curve. Increase in ventricular end-diastolic volume results in an increase in stroke volume. (Image: http://www.ncbi.nlm.nih.gov/bookshelf/br.fcgi?book=cardio&part=A709.)

SUGGESTED
READINGS

Barash PG, Cullen BF, Stoelting RK, et al. *Clinical Anesthesia*. 6th ed. Philadelphia, PA: Lippincott Williams & Wilkins; 2009:882–883.

Cheitlin M. Cardiovascular physiology—changes with aging. *Am J Geriatr Cardiol*. 2003;12:9–13.

Folkow B, Svanborg A. Physiology of cardiovascular aging. *Physiol Rev*. 1993;73:725–764.

Goldberger AL, Amaral LAN, Hausdorff JM, et al. Fractal dynamics in physiology: alterations with disease and aging. *Proc Natl Acad Sci U S A*. 2002;99:2466–2472.

Morgan GE, Mikhail MS, Murray MJ. *Clinical Anesthesiology*. 4th ed. New York, NY: McGraw Hill; 2006:952.

Rosenthal R, Zenilman M, Mark K. *Principles and Practice of Geriatric Surgery*. New York, NY: Springer-Verlag Inc; 2001:148–150.

Aging: Pulm Physiol

Generic Clinical Sciences: Anesthesia Procedures, Methods, Techniques

Shaun Gruenbaum

Edited by Shamsuddin Akhtar

KEY POINTS

1. Aging is associated with decreased chest wall compliance, leading to increased residual volume (RV), and increased work of breathing. Functional residual capacity (FRC) remains the same or increases slightly with age.
2. Age-related changes in the lung include dilated alveoli, increases in airspaces, and increased small airway resistance, leading to air trapping and hyperinflation.
3. Diaphragm strength and lung function, including forced expiratory volume in 1 s (FEV1) and diffusing capacity of carbon monoxide (DLCO), decreases with age.
4. Aging is associated with increased pulmonary inflammation.
5. Though adequate gas exchange is maintained throughout life, PaO_2 progressively decreases with aging. Ventilation/perfusion (V/Q) mismatching increases with aging.
6. Elderly are more vulnerable to respiratory failure during high-demand states.

DISCUSSION

Aging is associated with numerous changes in respiratory physiology. The compliance of the chest wall significantly decreases with aging, mostly due to the structural changes in the thoracic rib cage caused by decreased elastance of the connective tissue and calcifications. These changes reduce the ability to expand the lungs during inspiration, and prevent complete emptying of the lungs during expiration leading to increased RV. FRC may increase by 1% to 3% per decade. The reduction in chest wall compliance results in an increased work of breathing. The strength of the diaphragm also reduces with age (by 25%), likely due to muscle atrophy and a reduction in fast twitch fibers. This predisposes older patients to ventilatory failure, when ventilatory demands are increased.

There are age-related anatomical changes in the lung as well. The alveoli dilate and the airspaces enlarge, secondary to either destruction of lung parenchyma or its supporting structures. The small airways close prematurely during normal breathing, which can cause airway resistance, air trapping, and hyperinflation (a phenomenon referred to as "senile emphysema").

Lung function begins to steadily decline after approximately the age of 35 (Fig. 1). Studies demonstrate that both the FEV1 and DLCO decreases with age. Dead space ventilation

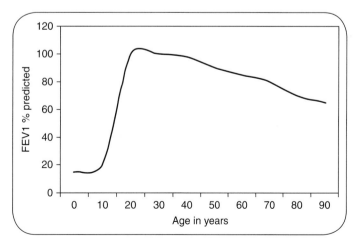

Figure 1. Age-related decline in FEV1 %. (Adapted from Ware JH, Dockery DW, Louis TA, et al. Longitudinal and cross-sectional estimates of pulmonary function decline in never-smoking adults. *Am J Epidemiol.* 1990;132:685–700, with permission.)

A

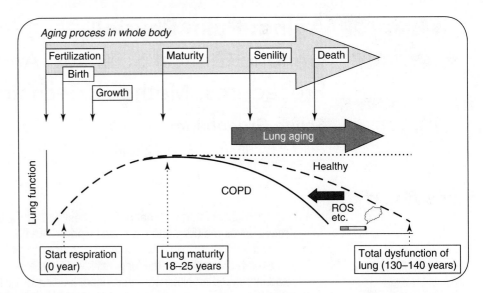

Figure 2. Hypothesis of the development of COPD by accelerated lung injury. (Adapted from Sharma G, Goodwin J. Effect of aging on respiratory system physiology and immunology. *Clin Interv Aging.* 2006;1:253–260, with permission.)

increases by as much as 55%. Aging is associated with increased pulmonary inflammation, and environmental exposure (i.e., to cigarette smoke) may accelerate the decline in lung function. Aging of the lung can accelerate the development of chronic obstructive pulmonary disease (COPD) (Fig. 2).

Complex changes at the alveolar pneumocyte level cause a reduction in arterial oxygen tension with age. It is estimated that the arterial partial pressure of oxygen (PaO_2) decreases by an average rate of 0.35 mm Hg per year. These aforementioned changes are caused by an increased degree of V/Q mismatching and, to a lesser extent, pulmonary shunting. Despite these changes, there is no change in $PaCO_2$. However, the respiratory system reserve decreases with age, and there is decreased sensitivity to hypoxemia and hypercapnia. Thus, the elderly are more vulnerable to respiratory failure during high ventilatory demand states, such as heart failure, pneumonia, and airway obstruction.

SUGGESTED READINGS

Barash PG, Cullen BF, Stoelting RK, eds. *Clinical Anesthesia.* 5th ed. Philadelphia, PA: Lippincott Williams & Wilkins; 2005:238.

Ito K, Barnes PJ. COPD as a disease of accelerated lung aging. *Chest.* 2009;135:173–180.

Sharma G, Goodwin J. Effect of aging on respiratory system physiology and immunology. *Clin Interv Aging.* 2006;1:253–260.

Ware JH, Dockery DW, Louis TA, et al. Longitudinal and cross-sectional estimates of pulmonary function decline in never-smoking adults. *Am J Epidemiol.* 1990;132:685–700.

Air Trapping: Ventilator Mgmt
Organ-based Clinical: Respiratory

Christina Mack

Edited by Shamsuddin Akhtar

A

KEY POINTS

1. Air trapping (aka: auto–positive end-expiratory pressure [PEEP]) can occur in a mechanically ventilated patient when the lungs are not permitted to exhale fully.
2. Auto-PEEP can be identified on the flow–time tracing.
3. Ventilator management includes maneuvers that decrease minute ventilation, increase expiratory time, or application of external PEEP.

DISCUSSION

For a patient who is being mechanically ventilated, PEEP can be generated if there is insufficient time for the lungs to return to their resting state, also known as functional residual capacity (FRC). When this occurs, it is termed "intrinsic PEEP" or "auto-PEEP." When auto-PEEP is generated, the alveolar pressure is higher than the airway opening pressure, which causes air trapping.

Auto-PEEP is commonly seen in patients with dynamic hyperinflation. Conditions such as chronic obstructive pulmonary disease and asthma are the classic examples of this phenomenon. It can also be observed in patients with acute respiratory distress syndrome if high minute ventilation is used on mechanical ventilation.

The causes of auto-PEEP are mostly related to ventilator settings and management. Ventilator-associated factors leading to auto-PEEP are flow limitation, dynamic hyperinflation, high minute ventilation, and short expiratory times. However, high intrabdominal pressure related to patient disease or surgical technique can also lead to generation of intrinsic PEEP by increasing expiratory resistance.

Intrinsic PEEP or auto-PEEP can have many effects on the respiratory and cardiovascular systems. The adverse effects on the respiratory system include the increased risk of barotrauma, increased work of breathing, and impairment of the patients to trigger the ventilator (if the patient is breathing spontaneously). The benefit of intrinsic PEEP, as is the benefit of applied PEEP, is an improvement in oxygenation. The principle adverse effect of intrinsic PEEP on the cardiovascular system is a decrease in venous return, which can lead to a decrease in cardiac output and potential worsening of ventilation/perfusion matching.

On the ventilator, the flow–time tracing can be used to identify auto-PEEP. Typically expiratory flows return to baseline before the next breath is delivered (Fig. 1). Auto-PEEP is identified when the expiratory flow does not return to zero before the next breath is delivered (Fig. 2). An end expiratory maneuver can be used to measure the amount of auto-PEEP. When an end expiratory hold is done, the alveolar, central airway, and ventilator

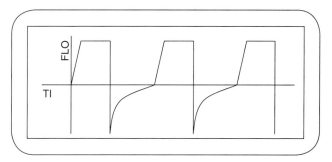

Figure 1. Normal flow–time curve. Exhalation is completed before inspiration is started.

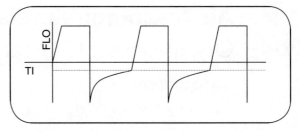

Figure 2. Air trapping on flow–time curve. This waveform displays that inspiration occurs before exhalation of the previous breath is completed. Air-trapping (auto-PEEP) is denoted at the dotted line.

pressures are equilibrated. The pressure read on the manometer during this maneuver is auto-PEEP.

There are several strategies than can be used to decrease auto-PEEP. These include decreasing minute ventilation (decreasing respiratory rate, decreasing tidal volume), decreasing airway resistance (bronchodilators), increasing expiratory time (increasing inspiratory flow rate, changing I:E ratio), and applying external PEEP.

SUGGESTED READINGS

Hall JB, Schmidt GA, Wood LDH, eds. The obstructed patient. *Principles of Critical Care*. 3rd ed. New York, NY: McGraw-Hill; 2005:124–127.

Kacmarek R, Hess D. Mechanical ventilation for the surgical patient. In: Longnecker DE, Brown DL, Newman MF, et al, eds. Anesthesiology. New York: McGraw-Hill; 2008:1852–1873.

Airway Anesthesia: Anatomy

Anatomy

Kellie Park

Edited by Thomas Halaszynski

KEY POINTS

1. The upper airway is separated into the pharynx, hypopharynx, and larynx, which are subsequently separated into various segments.
2. These three segments contain both sensory and motor innervations.
3. Innervation of the airway can be separated into three neural pathways: trigeminal (V), glossopharyngeal (IX), and vagus (X) nerves.
4. These innervations become important for anesthesiologists when anesthetizing for procedures such as awake fiberoptic intubation.

DISCUSSION

The upper airway begins at the nose and mouth; these orifices provide access to the nasopharynx and oropharynx, respectively. The nasopharynx and oropharynx are communicating spaces and are referred together as the pharynx. They are divided partially by the hard and soft palates.

The laryngopharynx, or hypopharynx, is caudal to the pharynx and is the space between the epiglottis proximally and the glottis (vocal cords and intervening space) distally. The larynx is defined by the vocal cords proximally and the cricoid cartilage distally. Finally, the trachea attaches to the larynx at the cricoid cartilage by the cricotracheal ligament. The first ring of the trachea is approximately at the level of the sixth cervical spinous process.

In total, nine cartilages combine to form the larynx. The thyroid cartilage is palpable and forms the prominence commonly referred to as the "Adam's apple." This cartilage protects the vocal cords anteriorly. The cricothyroid membrane spans the space between the thyroid cartilage and the cricoid cartilage. This membrane is subject to penetration during cricothyroidotomy to gain emergency airway access.

Innervation of the upper airway is divided into sensory and motor. In a cranial to caudal direction, sensory innervation to mucosal membranes of the nose is provided by the ophthalmic and maxillary divisions of the trigeminal nerve (V). The maxillary division of the trigeminal nerve provides sensory innervation to the hard and soft palate. Both the trigeminal and the facial (VII) nerves innervate the tongue, whereas the glossopharyngeal nerve (IX) supplies the sensory innervation to the tonsils and part of the soft palate. Branches of the vagus nerve (X) supply sensation to the epiglottis. The superior laryngeal nerve innervates the hypopharynx, whereas the recurrent laryngeal nerve provides sensory innervation to the larynx and trachea. The recurrent laryngeal nerve supplies all motor innervation to the larynx, with the exception of the cricothyroid muscle, which is innervated by the external laryngeal nerve. This anatomy becomes important for topicalization of the airway or airway nerve blockade to block sensory innervation to these areas when performing an awake fiberoptic intubation in patients with a difficult airway. Either of these techniques aims at blocking the sensory innervations as described above.

SUGGESTED READINGS

Barash PG, Cullen BF, Stoelting RK, et al, eds. *Clinical Anesthesia*. 6th ed. Philadelphia, PA: Lippincott Williams & Wilkins; 2009:752.

Stoelting RK, Miller RD, eds. *Basics of Anesthesia*. 5th ed. Philadelphia, PA: Churchill Livingstone; 2007:207.

KEYWORD

SECTION

Airway Assessment: Coexist Disease

Generic Clinical Sciences: Anesthesia
Procedures, Methods, Techniques

Adnan Malik

Edited by Hossam Tantawy

KEY POINTS

1. Airway assessment has many variables for the anesthesiologist to consider, all of which can help predict a difficult airway.
2. Many congenital syndromes are associated with a difficult airway.
3. Several pathologic states are also associated with a difficult airway or can alter airway management; these can be traumatic, infectious, neoplastic, or inflammatory in origin and can range from the common (diabetes mellitus) to more rare causes of airway issues (papillomatosis).

DISCUSSION

Airway assessment is a crucial element of the initial physical examination for an anesthesiologist. Symptoms such as hoarseness, inspiratory stridor, dysphagia, dyspnea, or orthopnea can often be suggestive of disease pathology resulting in a difficulty to ventilate and/or difficulty intubating.

Range of motion can often be restricted in individuals involved in traumas involving cervical spine instability (C-collar). In addition, patients with histories of rheumatoid arthritis have been shown to have atlantooccipital instability, and manipulation of the neck can result in subluxation resulting in spinal cord injury. In patients with severe hand malformations and skin nodules, there is the greatest risk of atlantoaxial subluxation. More commonly, patients with diabetes mellitus also have reduced mobility of the atlantooccipital joint, which can make direct laryngoscopy difficult.

Infectious disease processes can involve the floor of the mouth, tonsils, and pharynx and can result in limited oral aperture as well as facial trauma. Tumors can also limit oral opening, depending on the location and extent of involvement. With neck involvement, there can be compression and/or deviation of the trachea. In more systemic disease processes such as scleroderma, skin tightness and decreased mandibular motion can also result in a small oral aperture. Patients with Down syndrome have not only atlantooccipital instability but also macroglossia, which can further complicate airway management in these patients.

There are other coexisting diseases that are important to airway assessment including: epiglottitis, airway abscesses, croup, foreign bodies in the airway, and laryngeal edema, which direct laryngoscopy can worsen and make visualization of the airway and intubation very difficult. Neoplastic upper or lower airway tumors can also cause airway obstruction and difficult intubation, and these patients also have had radiation to the airway many times, leading to distorted airway anatomy as well as a more rigid neck.

Obesity is one of the most common causes of a difficult airway, secondary to obstruction, especially after induction of anesthesia. Mask ventilation is also made more difficult in these patients because of tissue mass. Ankylosing spondylitis also often leads to fusion of the cervical spine, which can render laryngoscopy and visualization of the airway difficult if not impossible. Other pathologic states that are less thought of and important to airway assessment include papillomatosis, which can cause airway obstruction; sarcoidosis, which can also cause airway obstruction secondary to enlarged lymphoid tissue; hypothyroidism, in which patients often have macroglossia; and abnormal soft tissue, which can make mask ventilation or intubation difficult.

Many congenital anomalies can make for difficult airway managements because of significant craniofacial deformities. These patients often have altered airway anatomy, large tongues, small subglottic diameters, neck rigidity, or difficulty with mouth opening. Such conditions that fall under this category include Treacher Collins syndrome, Goldenhar syndrome, Pierre Robin syndrome, Down syndrome as mentioned above, Turner syndrome, and Klippel–Feil syndrome, in which patients have neck rigidity secondary to cervical vertebral fusion.

SUGGESTED READINGS

Barash PG, Cullen BF, Stoelting RK, et al. *Clinical Anesthesia*. 6th ed. Philadelphia, PA: Lippincott Williams & Wilkins; 2009:570–572.

Dunn PF, Alston TA, Baker KH, et al. *Clinical Anesthesia Procedures of the Massachusetts General Hospital*. Philadelphia, PA: Lippincott Williams & Wilkins; 2007:208–211.

KEYWORD
SECTION

Amiodarone: Hemodynamic Effect

Organ-based Clinical: Cardiovascular

Jordan Martin

Edited by Benjamin Sherman

KEY POINTS

1. Amiodarone is a class III antiarrhythmic that can be used to treat both atrial and ventricular dysrhythmias.
2. Amiodarone works by exerting effects on Na, K, Ca, and alpha- and beta-adrenergic receptors.
3. Amiodarone has multiple potential hemodynamic side effects including:
   - Hypotension
   - Bradycardia
   - Decreased cardiac output.

DISCUSSION

Amiodarone is categorized as a class III antiarrhythmic agent on the basis of its potassium channel blocking properties. This medication also has effects on sodium and calcium channels and blocks alpha- and beta-adrenergic receptors. It can be used to treat a variety of both atrial and ventricular dysrhythmias. As part of the advanced cardiovascular life support (ACLS) algorithm, it is given for ventricular tachycardia or ventricular fibrillation that has not responded to Basic Life Support (BLS), epinephrine, and defibrillation. Amiodarone is also used in ventricular dysrhythmias that are due to Bupivacaine toxicity, such as those following inadvertent intravascular injection during regional anesthesia. It can be useful in the treatment of atrial fibrillation, and is sometimes given preoperatively to patients undergoing pulmonary resection as prophylaxis against atrial fibrillation/flutter in the postoperative period.

Figure 1 depicts the five phases of the cardiac cell action potential with the ion movement associated with each phase (not labeled is phase 0 or the upstroke of the action

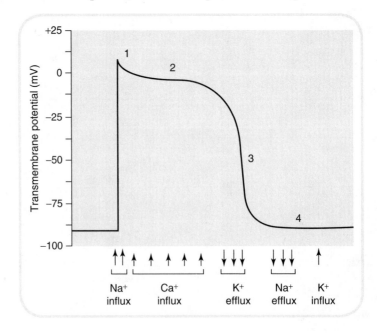

Figure 1. Cardiac action potential. (Reused with permission from Miller RD. *Miller's Anesthesia*. 7th ed. Philadelphia, PA: Elsevier; 2009.)

potential). Although amiodarone affects numerous ion channels and receptors, the mechanism of action for treating dysrhythmias is by a prolongation of the action potential (by prolonging phase 3 of the cardiac action potential—i.e., repolarization) and by increasing the refractory state of the cardiac cells.

This mechanism of action, however, can also lead to conduction abnormalities, QT prolongation, and can even rarely degenerate into Torsades de Pointes. Other hemodynamic side effects include hypotension, bradycardia (especially if infused too rapidly), and a decreased cardiac index. Some studies have shown a bolus of amiodarone causing elevation of right heart pressures, changes in systemic vascular resistance (SVR) and pulmonary vascular resistance (PVR), generally causing severe systemic and coronary vasodilation, and heart failure. Patients who already have depressed cardiac function are more likely to have negative hemodynamic effects with amiodarone boluses. Generally, with slower infusions of amiodarone, these hemodynamic changes can be avoided or decreased.

SUGGESTED READINGS

Barash PG, Cullen BF, Stoelting RK, et al. *Clinical Anesthesia*. 6th ed. Philadelphia, PA: Lippincott Williams & Wilkins; 2009:1149, 1543–1544.

Miller RD. *Miller's Anesthesia*. 7th ed. Philadelphia, PA: Elsevier; 2009.

Toyama T, Hoshizaki H, Yoshimura Y, et al. Combined therapy with carvedilol and amiodarone is more effective in improving cardiac symptoms, function, and sympathetic nerve activity in patients with dilated cardiomyopathy: comparison with carvedilol therapy alone. *J Nucl Cadiol*. 2008;15(1):57–64.

Amniotic Fluid Embolus: Dx
Subspecialties: Obstetrics

Bijal Patel

Edited by Lars Helgeson

1. The exact pathophysiology of amniotic fluid embolus (AFE) is unclear; however, it is believed to be a type of anaphylactoid response to amniotic fluid/fetal tissue.
2. It is considered to be a diagnosis of exclusion, and as such, one must be guided by high clinical suspicion.
3. AFE is characterized by the sudden onset of hypoxia, hemodynamic instability, and coagulopathy.
4. There is a biphasic presentation of symptoms, the first being hemodynamic instability and hypoxia, followed by left ventricular (LV) failure, coagulopathy, and variable elevations of pulmonary artery pressure.
5. Treatment for AFE is supportive by attempting to correct the hypoxia, hemodynamic instability, and coagulopathy.

AFE is an uncommon, but a very serious complication of pregnancy. It can occur at any time during pregnancy (any trimester) and during the postpartum period. It is most common during the immediate peripartum period. The exact pathophysiology of AFE is unclear. It is believed to be a type of anaphylactoid response to amniotic fluid/fetal tissue entering the maternal circulation through rupture of uterine veins or a tear in a placental membrane.

It is important to note that amniotic fluid material found in the pulmonary circulation of a pregnant patient is not considered pathognomonic. It is considered to be a diagnosis of exclusion, and as such, one must be guided by high clinical suspicion. AFE is characterized by the sudden onset of hypoxia, hemodynamic instability, and coagulopathy. Patients have also been reported to present with signs/symptoms such as seizures, dyspnea, pulmonary edema, cardiac arrest, and dysrhythmias. Symptoms are highly variable, as the patient may present with isolated hypoxia or even isolated coagulopathy. Generally, there is a biphasic presentation of symptoms with there first being hemodynamic instability and hypoxia and later LV failure, coagulopathy, and variable elevations of pulmonary artery pressure.

AFE is a diagnosis of exclusion. It is important to consider the differential diagnosis such as pulmonary embolism, disseminated intravascular coagulation (DIC), hypovolemic or septic shock, peripartum cardiomyopathy, myocardial infarction, local anesthetic toxicity, anaphylaxis, uterine rupture, aspiration, placental abruption, eclampsia, and cerebrovascular accident (CVA).

Treatment for AFE is supportive, attempting to correct the hypoxia, hemodynamic instability, and coagulopathy.

Hughes SC, Levinson G, Rosen MA. *Shnider and Levinson's Anesthesia for Obstetrics.* 4th ed. New York, NY: Lippincott Williams & Wilkins; 2001:355–359.

Kumar V, Abbas AK, Fausto N. *Robbins and Cotran Pathologic Basis of Disease.* 7th ed. Philadelphia, PA: Elsevier Saunders; 2005:137.

Stoelting RK, Miller RD. *Basics of Anesthesia.* 5th ed. Philadelphia, PA: Churchill Livingstone Elsevier; 2007:497.

Anaphylaxis: Epinephrine Rx

Pharmacology

Harika Nagavelli

Edited by Hossam Tantawy

1. Anaphylaxis is a life-threatening emergency; understanding the proper treatment protocol is key for a good outcome.
2. Epinephrine is the drug of choice in the treatment of anaphylactic shock.
3. Epinephrine is a catecholamine that affects all the adrenergic receptors.
4. Various infusion rates can target different adrenergic receptors, but the recommended dose for cardiovascular collapse is 1.0 mg of epinephrine.

Anaphylaxis is a life-threatening allergic reaction that leads to clinically significant mortality and morbidity perioperatively. Intravenous (IV) drugs normally trigger allergic reactions within 5 minutes of administration, and therefore having an action plan before any signs of anaphylaxis is of paramount importance for a good outcome. The presentations for allergic reactions have a broad spectrum of signs and symptoms. In particular, anaphylaxis involves an IgE-triggered release of active mediators. This type of reaction is termed type I hypersensitivity and is an immediate reaction. Each mediator released from IgE activation then secondarily triggers various end-organ responses. These responses should cause a knee-jerk reflex for every anesthesiologist, especially after administering the pharmacologic agent to a patient, introducing blood products or volume expanders such as Hextend, or other colloids, or even exposing a patient to an environmental substance such as latex.

On the surface of mast cells and basophils are two IgE antibodies that trigger a cascade-mediator activity within these cells when an antigen/allergen binds the two antibodies. These mediators include histamine, eosinophilic chemotactic factors, and arachidonic acid metabolites such as leukotriene and prostaglandin. An initial sensation of impending doom, unfortunately often masked by anesthetic agents already introduced, is then followed by end-organ responses. These mediator cascades cause effects to the skin, in forms such as urticaria, erythema, and edema. The lungs and upper respiratory system are affected in ways including smooth muscle contraction, bronchospasm, and constriction, and upper airway edema leading to hypoxia and hypercapnia. Finally, cardiovascular collapse may occur as a result of extreme vasodilation. Initially the vasodilation is secondary to the vastly increased capillary permeability, eventually resulting in a decreased venous return, hypotension, and changes in cardiac contractility.

The use of epinephrine has become an established treatment against the life-threatening outcome of anaphylaxis. Epinephrine is classified as a catecholamine along with norepinephrine and dopamine. Naturally produced by the adrenal medulla from norepinephrine via the enzyme phenyethanolamine-*N*-methyltransferase, epinephrine can additionally activate beta-2 receptors responsible for bronchodilation, compared with norepinephrine. Epinephrine produces sympathetic responses by activating all the adrenergic receptors: alpha-1, alpha-2, beta-1, and beta-2. Alpha-1 receptors when activated produce vasoconstriction especially targeting the smooth muscle, and this increases afterload, blood pressure, and peripheral vascular resistance. Only stimulated by epinephrine and dopamine, beta-2 adrenoreceptors are located on smooth muscle and produce bronchodilation. Beta-2 receptors are also thought to inhibit active release of mediators from basophils and mast cells. Finally, beta-1 receptors increase heart rate, conduction, and contractility, and they are the primary and most abundant receptor sites for epinephrine.

Management of Anaphylaxis During General Anesthesia

Initial Therapy

1. Stop administration of antigen.
2. Maintain airway and administer 100% O_2.
3. Discontinue *all* anesthetic agents.
4. Start intravascular volume expansion (2 to 4 L of crystalloid/colloid with hypotension).
5. Give *epinephrine* (5 to 10 μg IV bolus with hypotension, titrate as needed 0.1 to 1.0 mg IV with cardiovascular collapse).

Secondary Treatment

1. Antihistamines (0.5 to 1.0 mg per kg diphenhydramine).
2. Catecholamine infusion (standing doses: epinephrine, 4 to 8 μg per minute; norepinephrine 4 to 8 μg per minute; or isoproterenol, 0.5 to 1 μg per minute as an infusion; titrated to desired effects).
3. Bronchodilators: inhaled albuterol, terbutaline, and/or anticholinergic agents with persistent bronchospasm.
4. Corticosteroids (0.25 to 1 g hydrocortisone; alternatively, 1 to 2 g methylprednisolone).
5. Sodium bicarbonate (0.5 to 1 mEq per kg with persistent hypotension or acidosis).
6. Airway evaluation (before extubation).
7. Vasopressin for refractory shock.

SUGGESTED READINGS

Barash PG. *Clinical Anesthesia.* 6th ed. Philadelphia, PA: Lippincott Williams & Wilkins; 2009:257–260.

Levy JH. *Anaphylactic Reactions in Anesthesia and ICU.* 2nd ed. Stoneham, MA: Butterworth-Heinemann; 1992:162.

Miller RD. *Miller's Anesthesia.* 7th ed. Philadelphia, PA: Elsevier, Churchill Livingstone; 2009:chap 12, 35.

Anes Management: Penetrating Eye Injury

Generic, Clinical Sciences: Anesthesia Procedures, Methods, Techniques

Kristin Richards

Edited by Ramachandran Ramani

KEY POINTS

1. Penetrating injuries need to be dealt with urgently, as there is an increased risk of infection, endophthalmitis, vitreous loss, and retinal detachment.
2. Local anesthetic technique/blocks are usually avoided with open eye injuries.
3. Inhalational agents reduce intraocular pressure (IOP).
4. IV induction agents reduce IOP except ketamine.
5. Nondepolarizing muscle relaxants have no effects on IOP.
6. Succinylcholine can increase IOP.
7. Control ventilation during the procedure, aiming for low to normal end-tidal carbon dioxide.
8. A slight head-up tilt helps reduce IOP.

DISCUSSION

Traumatic eye injuries can be blunt or penetrating. Penetrating injuries are also known as open eye injuries. The incidence of this type of injury is highest in young adult males and children.

There is an increased risk of infection, endophthalmitis, vitreous loss, and retinal detachment with penetrating injuries, and hence these injuries need to be dealt with emergently. The dilemma with emergency eye surgery, as with all emergency surgery, is that the patients may have a full stomach. If the damage to the eye is severe enough that the surgery is not going to improve sight, the surgeon may delay the surgery until the patient has fasted for a number of hours. In this case, these patients are admitted for bed rest and have an eye shield cover the injured eye until they undergo primary closure of the eye wounds.

If the eye is still largely intact and the visual prognosis is good, it needs to be dealt with without delay.

Local anesthetic techniques are usually avoided because they may cause an increase in IOP, which can worsen vitreous loss.

Most intravenous induction agents reduce IOP, thus preventing further damage to the injured eye.

Exception: Ketamine possibly raises IOP, although the literature is conflicting. Most textbooks state that it should be avoided in open eye injuries. If it is necessary to use, it is recommended that it be used in combination with small doses of a benzodiazepine to blunt its excitatory effects.

Nondepolarizing muscle relaxants can be used without adverse effects on the eye, so the choice should be based on other factors.

Succinylcholine increases IOP. The exact mechanism is unclear. The extent of the rise in IOP depends on the other drugs used and the response to laryngoscopy and intubation. Its use in penetrating eye injury anesthesia is controversial.

The increase in IOP associated with succinylcholine presents a dilemma in the case of rapid sequence intubation. The nondepolarizing neuromuscular blocker rocuronium has a rapid onset of action with the duration of 30 to 40 minutes. It can be used, but still does not have as rapid an onset, or as short a duration of action, as succinylcholine.

Once the patient is intubated, it is recommended to ventilate to mild hypocarbia, as this further reduces IOP. A slight head tilt upward can also help to further decrease IOP.

SUGGESTED READINGS

Libonati MM, Leahy JJ, Ellison N. The use of succinylcholine in open eye surgery. *Anaesthesiology*. 1985;62:637.
Miller RD. *Miller's Anesthesia*. 6th ed. Philadelphia, PA: Elsevier, Churchill, Livingstone; 2005.
Wilson A, Soar J. Anaesthesia for emergency eye surgery. *Update Anaesth*. 2000;Issue 11:Article 10.

Anes Techniques: First Stage Labor
Subspecialties: Obstetric Anesthesia

Hyacinth Ruiter

Edited by Lars Helgeson

KEY POINTS

1. Pain during the first stage of labor results from uterine contractions and cervical dilation, which is confined to the T11-T12 dermatomes during the latent phase but also involves the T10-L1 dermatomes during the active phase of labor.
2. The most frequently chosen methods for labor analgesia are systemic medications and regional analgesia.
3. Adverse side effects of systemic opiates include nausea and vomiting, pruritus, urinary retention, allergic reactions, maternal and neonatal dose–related sedation, and respiratory depression.
4. Epidural and spinal analgesia provide excellent pain relief with minimal maternal sedation or respiratory depressant effects and no known direct fetal effects.

DISCUSSION

In the first stage of labor, parturients experience visceral pain resulting from uterine contractions and cervical dilation. The T11-T12 dermatomes are involved during the latent phase. As labor progresses into the active phase, the T10-L1 dermatomes become involved. Several methods of pain relief are available to the laboring patient. By far, the most popular methods are systemic medication and regional analgesia.

Systemic opioids are commonly administered, but careful monitoring should be done to avoid maternal or neonatal respiratory depression. Meperidine is commonly administered systemically. Its major side effects are nausea and vomiting, respiratory depression, and orthostatic hypotension. Other opioids such as fentanyl, alfentanil, and remifentanil are more potent than meperidine, but their short duration of action limits their long-term effectiveness. Longer-acting narcotics such as morphine are sometimes used. Narcotics readily cross the placenta, which frequently leads to neonatal depression at delivery.

Regional techniques, such as epidural or intrathecal blocks either alone or in combination, provide excellent analgesia with minimal respiratory effects on both mother and fetus. Epidural analgesia is commonly used using a low concentration of local anesthetic combined with lipid-soluble opioids. Bupivacaine or ropivacaine are long-acting local anesthetics that provide effective sensory blockade with less motor function blockade. Intrathecal injection produces fast and reliable analgesia lasting 90 to 120 minutes, but has the disadvantage of a potential postdural puncture headache, especially with the need to do repeated injections for prolonged labor. Maternal hypotension resulting from sympathectomy is a common complication that can affect uterine blood flow resulting in fetal distress. Combined spinal/epidural blockade produces rapid onset of analgesia (intrathecal injection) with long duration made possible by a continuous epidural catheter.

Contraindications to regional analgesia include the presence of coagulopathy, sepsis, infection at the site of needle insertion, and hypovolemia. Epidural analgesia blunts the maternal sympathetic response to painful uterine contractions. Therefore, hypotension is a common and potentially serious complication of central neuraxial blockade. Maternal blood pressure should be regularly monitored, every few minutes for approximately 15 to 20 minutes after block placement and routinely thereafter.

SUGGESTED READINGS

Barash PG, Cullen BF, Stoelting RK, et al, eds. *Clinical Anesthesia*. 6th ed. Philadelphia, PA: Lippincott Williams & Wilkins; 2009:1142–1145.

Morgan GE, Mikhail MS, Murray MJ. *Clinical Anesthesiology*. 4th ed. New York, NY: McGraw-Hill; 2006:894–901.

Anes Techniques: Suspected MH
Subspecialties: Pediatrics

Christina Biello

Edited by Mamatha Punjala

KEY POINTS

1. Malignant hyperthermia (MH) is caused by a defect in the ryanodine receptor causing an overwhelming release and altered uptake of calcium from skeletal muscle, leading to sustained muscle contractions and a hypermetabolic state.
2. A nontriggering anesthetic should be used in the management of these cases with the intent of avoiding all inhalational anesthetics and succinylcholine.
3. Avoiding agents that alter temperature regulation or that cause increases in sympathetic tone is important.

DISCUSSION

MH is a genetic disorder of skeletal muscle that causes a hypermetabolic state in the presence of triggering anesthetic agents. Triggering agents during anesthesia include all volatile anesthetics and succinylcholine. An uncontrollable release of calcium from the sarcoplasmic reticulum of skeletal muscle occurs, and a defect in its uptake pathway results is sustained contractions of the skeletal muscle.

When a patient presents with a susceptibility to MH, steps must be taken to ensure that a safe anesthetic is provided to him or her. Succinylcholine should not be in the immediate vicinity of the anesthesia workstation. The vaporizers should be removed from the anesthesia machine. If this is not possible, a method of ensuring that they will not be turned on by accident should be in place, for example, tape across the vaporizer dials. The CO_2 absorbent should be replaced with new soda or baralyme, and the anesthesia circuit should also be removed and replaced with a new one. Finally, the anesthesia machine should be flushed with oxygen at a rate of 10 L per minute for approximately 10 to 12 minutes, depending on the age and manufacturer of the machine. All the above steps help to assure that a minimal amount of the triggering inhalational agents is present.

Because stress can play a role in the initiation of MH, a low stress induction should be planned. EMLA cream and premedication with midazolam 0.5 mg per kg orally can provide anxiolysis before intravenous (IV) placement. After an IV is placed, induction can be performed with Propofol or a barbiturate. Narcotics and nondepolarizing muscle relaxants can be used. Avoid drugs that increase temperature or cause increased sympathetic tone. Avoid phenothiazines and anticholinergics. Atropine can be used if there is a significant risk of bradycardia. Monitoring should include standard ASA monitors, listening to precordial heart sounds, ECG, noninvasive blood pressure monitoring, pulse oximetry, and end-tidal carbon dioxide monitoring. Core temperature should be monitored. Although invasive hemodynamic monitors and urinary catheters are not necessary, they can be helpful in obtaining blood gases and urine myoglobins. The anesthesia machine and circuit can be used to provide mechanical ventilation with oxygen, air, and nitrous oxide, provided the machine has been flushed before being attached to the patient.

SUGGESTED READINGS

Cote C, Lerman J, Todres ID, eds. *A Practice of Anesthesia for Infants and Children.* 4th ed. Philadelphia, PA: Saunders-Elsevier; 2009:847–855.

Etsuro KM, Peter JD, eds. *Smith's Anesthesia for Infants and Children.* 7th ed. Philadelphia, PA: Saunders-Elsevier; 2006:1025.

Anes Uptake: Right-to-left Shunt

Pharmacology

Soumya Nyshadham

Edited by Raj K. Modak

KEY POINTS

1. Right-to-left shunting refers to a situation in which blood from the right heart (mixed venous, desaturated blood) reaches the left heart without being oxygenated in the lungs, resulting in a decrease in the oxygen content of arterial blood delivered to the systemic circulation. Thus, right-to-left shunt results in hypoxemia (as opposed to left-to-right shunt).
2. Uptake of volatile anesthetic agent is determined by three factors: partial pressure difference between venous blood and alveolar gas, anesthetic solubility in blood, and pulmonary blood flow.
3. The rate of rise of alveolar concentrations of volatile anesthetics lags behind the inspired gas concentration due to the uptake of anesthetic agent by the pulmonary circulation during induction. The greater the uptake, the slower the rate of induction.
4. Theoretically, induction with volatile anesthetic agents is slowed by right-to-left shunt because a portion of the blood is not exposed to the inhaled anesthetic in the lungs and returns to the systemic circulation, decreasing the rate of rise in anesthetic concentration.

DISCUSSION

Right-to-left shunting refers to a situation in which blood from the right heart (mixed venous, desaturated blood) reaches the left heart without being oxygenated in the lungs, resulting in a decrease in the oxygen content of arterial blood delivered to the systemic circulation. Thus, right-to-left shunt results in hypoxemia (as opposed to left-to-right shunt). When blood is shunted from the right side of the heart to the left, mixing of deoxygenated right-sided blood with blood from the left heart, the resulting blood is referred to as venous admixture. Venous admixture can be intracardiac or intrapulmonary. Intracardiac shunts most commonly occur because of congenital heart disease, examples of which are ventricular septal defects, atrial septal defects, and tricuspid atresia. Intracardiac shunts can be classified into simple—which are definitive communications between the right and the left heart—and complex—which are caused by shunting that results from ventricular outflow obstruction. Intrapulmonary shunts can be caused by a variety of pulmonary mechanisms, examples of which are pneumonia, endobronchial intubation, and atelectasis. Intrapulmonary shunts can be categorized into absolute shunt, which refers to lung units in which ventilation–perfusion ratio equals zero, and relative shunt, which refers to a low ventilation–perfusion ratio.

Uptake of volatile anesthetic agent is determined by three factors: partial pressure difference between venous blood and alveolar gas, anesthetic solubility in blood, and pulmonary blood flow. Tissue uptake determines the gradient between venous blood and alveolar gas. Anesthetic uptake by tissues depends on blood flow through tissues, the gradient between arterial blood and tissue, and agent solubility in tissue. This gradient must exist in order for pulmonary uptake of anesthetic to occur. Solubility in blood also determines anesthetic uptake. The more soluble an agent, the easier that agent is taken up by the blood. The anesthetic's solubility is determined by its blood/gas coefficient, which is the ratio of the concentrations of the anesthetic gas in these two phases at equilibrium (or equal partial pressures). Finally, pulmonary blood flow determines anesthetic uptake. Theoretically, pulmonary blood flow should equal cardiac output, which is directly proportional to the degree of anesthetic uptake by blood. Hence, as cardiac output increases, so does arterial uptake of anesthetic, slowing the rise in alveolar partial pressure and thus delaying induction. The rate of rise of alveolar concentrations of volatile anesthetics lags behind the inspired gas concentration due to the uptake of anesthetic agent by the pulmonary circulation during induction. The greater the uptake, the slower the rate of induction.

Given the above factors determining volatile anesthetic uptake, induction is slowed by right-to-left shunt because a portion of the blood is not exposed to the inhaled anesthetic in the lungs and returns to the systemic circulation. This dilution effect decreases the rate of rise of anesthetic concentration in the systemic circulation, and induction is prolonged. An example of a right-to-left shunt can be seen in patients with an atrial septal defect. The Fa/Fi ratio difference (using halothane, in this case) in patients with the defect, and hence with the shunt, and those without, can be seen in Figure 1.

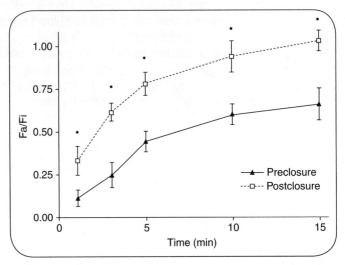

Figure 1. Mean ratio values of arterial to inspired halothane in patients pre- and postclosure of atrial fenestration. (From Huntington JH, Malviya S, Voepel-Lewis T, et al. The effect of a right-to-left intracardiac shunt on the rate of rise of arterial and end-tidal halothane in children. *Anesth Analg*. 1999;88(4):759–762, with permission.)

SUGGESTED READINGS

Dunn PF, Alston TT, Baker KH, et al. *Clinical Anesthesia Procedures of the Massachusetts General Hospital*. 7th ed. Philadelphia, PA: Lippincott Williams & Wilkins; 2007:424.

Huntington JH, Malviya S, Voepel-Lewis T, et al. The effect of a right-to-left intracardiac shunt on the rate of rise of arterial and end-tidal halothane in children. *Anesth Analg*. 1999;88(4):759–762.

Morgan GE, Mikhail MS, Murray MJ. *Clinical Anesthesiology*. 4th ed. Philadelphia, PA: McGraw-Hill Professional; 2006:157–159, 480–482, 555.

Stoelting RK, Miller RD, eds. *Basics of Anesthesia*. 5th ed. Philadelphia, PA: Churchill Livingstone Elsevier; 2007:86, 326.

Anes Uptake: Solubility Coeff
Physics, Monitoring, and Anesthesia Delivery

Tara Paulose
Edited by Raj K. Modak

KEY POINTS

1. The uptake of inhaled anesthetics is affected by their solubility in blood.
2. The solubility coefficient represents a composite number given to a specific inhaled anesthetic, which describes its blood solubility.
3. Agents, which are considered less soluble in blood, tend to have quicker onset as the alveolar concentrations parallel the inspired concentrations at a faster rate.
4. The blood solubility of commonly used inhaled anesthetics in least to greatest order is desflurane, nitrous oxide, sevoflurane, isoflurane, and halothane.

DISCUSSION

The uptake of inhalational anesthetic agents is greatly affected by their solubility in blood. This relationship is defined as the solubility coefficient (or blood–gas partition coefficient), a number derived from various studies that serves as a means of comparison across different agents. The blood–gas coefficient describes the ratio of a specific gas dissolved in blood versus alveolar gas at equilibrium (at the same temperature, pressure, and volume), with respect to their partial pressures (Table 1).

Table 1. Blood/Gas Partition Coefficients of Volatile Anesthetics at 37° C

Agent	Desflurane	Nitrous Oxide	Sevoflurane	Isoflurane	Halothane
Blood/gas coefficient	0.42	0.47	0.65	1.4	2.4

Table excerpted from Morgan GE, Mikhail MS, Murray MJ. *Clinical Anesthesiology*. 4th ed. Philadelphia, PA: McGraw-Hill Medical; 2006:157–160, with permission.

This relationship largely affects the speed of anesthetic induction across the various inhalational agents. As the value of the solubility coefficient increases, this signifies a greater degree of blood solubility and therefore prolonged induction time secondary to slow rise of alveolar partial pressure. The alveolar gas concentration of inhalational agents with lower solubility coefficients, therefore, more rapidly approaches the inspired gas concentration, with respect to more soluble agents.

Of the inhalational agents currently used, desflurane is the least soluble agent, followed by nitrous oxide, sevoflurane, isoflurane, and halothane. The solubility of the agent is inversely proportional to the onset of action.

SUGGESTED READINGS

Barash PG, Cullen BF, Stoelting RK, et al., eds. *Clinical Anesthesia*. 6th ed. Philadelphia, PA: Lippincott Williams & Wilkins; 2009:415–417.
Morgan GE, Mikhail MS, Murray MJ. *Clinical Anesthesiology*. 4th ed. Philadelphia, PA: McGraw-Hill Medical; 2006:157–160.
Stoelting RK, Miller RD, eds. *Basics of Anesthesia*. 5th ed. Philadelphia, PA: Churchill Livingstone Elsevier; 2007:84–86.

KEYWORD

SECTION

Anesthesia for ECT: Lidocaine Effect

Generic, Clinical Sciences: Anesthesia Procedures, Methods, Techniques

Kimberly Slininger

Edited by Ramachandran Ramani

KEY POINTS

1. The use of lidocaine before initiation of seizures during electroconvulsive therapy (ECT) should be avoided because of lidocaine's ability to raise the seizure threshold and potentially shorten seizure duration.
2. Lidocaine is still appropriate to use for the management of postseizure ventricular arrhythmias.

DISCUSSION

Lidocaine is a ubiquitous drug in the world of anesthesiology as a local anesthetic and antiarrhythmic drug. Its side effects and toxicities as a result are well known. Lidocaine has the ability to produce both central nervous system (CNS) stimulation and depression with toxic doses. The concern with the use of lidocaine during ECT is its potential to raise the patient's seizure threshold. Despite seizures being one of lidocaine's CNS toxicities, lidocaine has been used as an alternative therapy for generalized convulsive status epilepticus refractory to conventional therapy. The current recommendation for the administration of anesthesia for ECT is to avoid the use of lidocaine before initiation of seizures. It has also been shown to potentially decrease seizure duration, and as there are studies showing duration of a seizure for ECT is as important as seizure intensity, lidocaine should be avoided. Lidocaine is still clinically appropriate to use for ventricular arrhythmias that occur after seizure.

SUGGESTED READINGS

Albin MS. *Textbook of Neuroanesthesia with Neurosurgical and Neuroscience Perspectives.* New York, NY: McGraw-Hill; 1997:724.

Diprio JT, Talbert RL, Yee GC, et al, eds. *Pharmacotherapy: A Pathophysiologic Approach.* 7th ed. New York, NY: McGraw-Hill; 2008:960–961.

Anesthesiologists: Substance Abuse and Fentanyl

Generic, Clinical Sciences: Anesthesia Procedures, Methods, Techniques

Kevan Stanton and Jonathan Tidwell

Edited by Raj K. Modak

KEY POINTS

1. While the prevalence of substance abuse among anesthesiologists is less than that of physicians in general, anesthesiologists are overrepresented in treatment centers.
2. Substance abuse includes nitrous oxide and the volatile anesthetics as well as intravenous (IV) drugs.
3. Identification of physicians afflicted with substance abuse does not generally occur until late in the disease. Time until detection of abuse is inversely proportional to the potency of the drug abused. Accordingly, fentanyl abuse is not typically detected until 6 to 12 months after the onset of abuse while sufentanyl abuse is typically detected within 1 to 6 months after abuse onset.
4. Job performance is usually last to be affected by substance abuse.
5. Most physicians are able to successfully return to work.

DISCUSSION

Drug addiction is a chronic, relapsing disease. Drug addiction amongst physicians occurs across all specialties. Physicians have a 2.1% annual and 7.9% lifetime prevalence of drug addiction compared with 16% for the general population. However, physicians are five times more likely to use sedatives than illicit substances. Alcohol abuse is also a problem, with physician abuse surpassing that of the general population by the time physicians are in their mid-50s.

In specific regard to anesthesiologists, there is a 1% to 2% prevalence of substance abuse, less than that of physicians in general, though anesthesiologists are overrepresented in treatment centers. The risk of drug-related death and suicide is much higher in anesthesiologists than other physicians. For suicide, the risk is 1.45 times that for internists, and for drug-related death, the risk is 2.79 times that of internists. This substance abuse can include nitrous oxide and volatile anesthetics in addition to IV drugs. Characteristics of anesthesiologists associated with drug addiction include the following:

- Fifty percent are younger than 35 years old, with residents being overrepresented— addiction begins early in the career with curiosity
- Academically accomplished—many are members of Alpha Omega Alpha (AOA)
- Seventy-six percent to 90% use opioids
- Thirty-three percent to 50% are polydrug abusers
- Thirty-three percent have a family history of addictive disorders
- Sixty-five percent are associated with academic departments
- Easy access to potent drugs
- Colleagues are generally last to know

Causes of substance abuse include stress, availability of drugs, and drug potency. Stress is not necessarily a precipitating factor, but can play a role in those with certain preexisting personality traits, family history of substance addiction or abuse, and those with previous recreational drug use. Availability is a factor, not only in that the drugs are immediately

A

available but also in that they are actually given by anesthesiologists, unlike other specialties in which the drug is ordered by the physician but given by someone else. Finally, drug potency also plays a role in substance abuse, leading to addiction. Generally, abuse is more common than addiction among physicians, but the addiction potential of potent opioids is so high that after experimenting, there is enormous risk of becoming chemically dependent.

Identification of those afflicted by substance abuse does not generally occur until late in the disease, and time of detection is inversely proportional to the potency of the drug being abused. The first changes seen in physicians abusing drugs is withdrawal from outside interests followed by increased trouble in their home life. This is followed by the appearance of frequent, unexplained illnesses, personality changes, multiple jobs, and frequent moves. Individuals also seek additional shifts, particularly when they will be alone, such as overnight call. Physical findings such as unexplained trauma to the face (i.e., bruising, abrasions from falling asleep while under the influence) may be one of the few only signs. Job performance is usually last to be affected, which is often why colleagues are last to know.

Perhaps the most important information regarding opioid, particularly fentanyl, use are the clinical manifestations of intoxication and withdrawal. Opioid intoxication typically produces behavioral changes (dysphoria, apathy, psychomotor retardation, euphoria), papillary constriction, drowsiness, slurred speech, and attention impairment. Withdrawal from opioids often produces nausea, myalgia, pupillary dilation, piloerection, sweating, diarrhea, fever, and insomnia. These signs and symptoms can be clues to an opioid addict.

While opioid addiction among anesthesiologists often leads to morbid outcomes, recovery among anesthesiologists addicted to fentanyl is possible. Success seems to depend on several factors, including the motivation of the recovering anesthesiologist and the structure of the recovery program. Many anesthesiologists with drug abuse problems are able to successfully reenter the workplace after documented recovery and treatment, though reentry into the operating room environment remains a topic of much debate.

Help should be sought if substance abuse is suspected. Treatment generally consists of detailed evaluation followed usually by inpatient therapy. Reentry to the workforce is often possible, though it may be difficult being placed into the environment, which lead to the initial drug use. Support is extremely important for physicians recovering from substance abuse. In the long run, most physicians are able to successfully return to work, though some do relapse.

SUGGESTED READINGS

Barash PG, Cullen BF, Stoelting RK, et al, eds. *Clinical Anesthesia*. 6th ed. Philadelphia, PA: Lippincott Williams & Wilkins; 2009:74–77.

Bryson EO, Silverstein JH. Addiction and substance abuse in anesthesiology. *Anesthesiology*. 2008;109(5):905–917.

Miller RD, Eriksson LI, Fleisher LA, et al., eds. *Miller's Anesthesia*. 7th ed. Philadelphia, PA: Churchill Livingstone; 2010:3066–3069.

Aortic Cross-clamp: CV Complications

Organ-based Clinical: Cardiovascular

Karisa Walker

Edited by Qingbing Zhu

KEY POINTS

1. In view of the potential for cardiovascular instability in cases requiring aortic cross-clamping, monitoring may include arterial line placement, transesophageal echocardiography, and/or pulmonary artery catheterization.
2. Cardiovascular consequences of aortic cross-clamping are increased systemic blood pressure above the clamp and potentially left ventricular failure and myocardial ischemia.
3. Infrarenal cross-clamping of the aorta results in less dramatic hemodynamic alteration.
4. Hemodynamic complications associated with aortic cross-clamping are more pronounced in patients with preexisting heart disease.
5. Unclamping of the aorta yields the greatest potential for hemodynamic instability; risk of instability becomes greater with longer cross-clamp time.

DISCUSSION

Cross-clamping of the aorta is done to facilitate surgery on the descending thoracic and abdominal aorta. Significant cardiovascular complications can occur during this procedure because of the redistribution of cardiac output and changes in systemic vascular resistance (SVR) both during the time the clamp is in place and after it has been removed. In view of the potential for these problems, monitoring may consist of arterial line placement, transesophageal echocardiography, and pulmonary artery catheterization, depending on the patient's baseline cardiovascular disease, volume status, and risk of the specific procedure.

Initial changes observed with cross-clamping of the aorta are increases in systemic blood pressure, with mean arterial pressure (MAP) increasing up to 50% above baseline (Table 1). This occurs because of the dramatic, sudden increase in SVR with clamp placement and redistribution of blood volume to vessels proximal to the clamp. Systemic pressure below the level of the clamp is consequently decreased, leading to decreased perfusion of the lower extremities and potentially vital organs, such as the kidneys, depending on clamp location. Effects of clamp placement can be attenuated by lowering the blood pressure before cross-clamp application.

Location of the aortic cross-clamp influences its effect on both afterload and preload. Afterload increase is less pronounced with infrarenal rather than suprarenal placement of the cross-clamp. Placement of the clamp in relation to the splanchnic circulation, however, influences more the redistribution of blood volume such that preload is increased more with supraceliac clamping than in infraceliac clamping because of the high capacitance of the splanchnic vessels.

Particularly in patients with preexisting heart disease, clamp placement may precipitate cardiac ischemia and left ventricular failure. Logically, patients with coronary artery disease and diastolic left ventricular dysfunction are at high risk. These consequences can be prevented and/or treated by reducing afterload (i.e., with nitroprusside) or encouraging coronary artery dilatation and coronary perfusion with nitroglycerin.

Removal of the cross-clamp poses two cardiovascular problems: sudden decrease in afterload and reperfusion of underperfused tissues. Use of short-acting drugs to manipulate afterload is advantageous, so they can be titrated off before clamp removal. Reperfusion of tissues and redistribution of blood volume result in release of humoral factors (prostaglandins, catecholamines, cytokines, complement, activation of the renin–angiotensin system). Effects of these humoral factors increase with longer cross-clamp time. Complications postremoval of cross-clamp may include hypotension (decreased cardiac output from impaired cardiac contractility coupled with shift of blood volume away from the heart), pulmonary edema, metabolic acidosis, and renal failure.

Table 1. Physiologic Changes with Aortic Cross-clamping[a] and Therapeutic Interventions

Hemodynamic Changes
  ↑ Arterial blood pressure above the clamp
  ↓ Arterial blood pressure below the clamp
  ↑ Segmental wall motion abnormalities
  ↑ Left ventricular wall tension
  ↓ Ejection fraction
  ↓ Cardiac output[b]
  ↓ Renal blood flow
  ↑ Pulmonary occlusion pressure
  ↑ Central venous pressure
  ↑ Coronary blood flow
Metabolic Changes
  ↓ Total body oxygen consumption
  ↓ Total body carbon dioxide production
  ↑ Mixed venous oxygen saturation
  ↓ Total body oxygen extraction
  ↑ Epinephrine and norepinephrine
  Respiratory alkalosis[c]
  Metabolic acidosis
Therapeutic Interventions
  Afterload reduction
    Sodium nitroprusside
    Inhaled anesthetics
    Amrinone
    Shunts and aorta-to-femoral bypass
  Preload reduction
    Nitroglycerin
    Controlled phlebotomy
    Atrial-to-femoral bypass
  Renal protection
    Fluid administration
    Distal aortic perfusion techniques
    Selective renal artery perfusion
    Mannitol
    Drugs to augment renal perfusion
  Others
    Hypothermia
    ↓ Minute ventilation
    Sodium bicarbonate

[a]These changes are of greater significance with longer duration of Cross-clamping and with more proximal cross-clamping.
[b]Cardiac output may increase with thoracic cross-clamping.
[c]When ventilatory settings are unchanged from preclamp levels.
From Miller RD, Eriksson LI, Fleisher LA, et al. Miller's Anesthesia. 7th Edition. Philadelphia, PA: Churchill Livingstone, 2009:1997.

Table 2. Factors That May Influence the Magnitude and Direction of Physiologic Changes Occurring with Aortic Cross-clamping

Level of aortic cross-clamp

Species differences

Anesthetic agents and techniques

Use of vasodilator therapy

Use of diverting circulatory support

Degree of periaortic collateralization

Left ventricular function

Status of the coronary circulation

Volume status

Neuroendocrine activation

Duration of aortic cross-clamping

Body temperature

From Miller RD, Eriksson LI, Fleisher LA, et al. Miller's Anesthesia. 7th Edition. Philadelphia, PA: Churchill Livingstone, 2009:1997.

Table 3. Physiologic Changes with Aortic Unclamping[a] and Therapeutic Interventions

Hemodynamic Changes

$\downarrow$ Myocardial contractility

$\downarrow$ Arterial blood pressure

$\uparrow$ Pulmonary artery pressure

$\downarrow$ Central venous pressure

$\downarrow$ Venous return

$\downarrow$ Cardiac output

Metabolic Changes

$\uparrow$ Total body oxygen consumption

$\uparrow$ Lactate

$\downarrow$ Mixed venous oxygen saturation

$\uparrow$ Prostaglandins

$\uparrow$ Activated complement

$\uparrow$ Myocardial depressant factor(s)

$\downarrow$ Temperature

Metabolic Acidosis

Therapeutic Interventions

$\downarrow$ Inhaled anesthetics

$\downarrow$ Vasodilators

$\uparrow$ Fluid administration

$\uparrow$ Vasoconstrictor drugs

Reapply cross-clamp for severe hypotension

Consider mannitol

Consider sodium bicarbonate

[a]These changes are of greater significance with longer duration of cross-clamping and with more proximal cross-clamping.
From Miller RD, Eriksson LI, Fleisher LA, et al. Miller's Anesthesia. 7th Edition. Philadelphia, PA: Churchill Livingstone, 2009:2001.

SUGGESTED READINGS

Barash PG, Cullen BF, Stoelting RK, et al. *Clinical Anesthesia*. 6th ed. Philadelphia, PA: Lippincott Williams & Wilkins; 2009:1123–1126.

Miller RD, Eriksson LI, Fleisher LA, et al. *Miller's Anesthesia*. 7th ed. Philadelphia, PA: Churchill Livingstone; 2009:1997, 2001.

Morgan GE, Mikhail MS, Murray MJ. *Clinical Anesthesiology*. 4th ed. New York, NY: McGraw-Hill; 2006:528–533.

Aortic Insufficiency: Hemodynamic Rx
Organ-based Clinical: Cardiovascular

Suzana Zorca

Edited by Benjamin Sherman

KEY POINTS

1. Aortic insufficiency (AI) is incompetence of the aortic valve that results in regurgitant blood flow into the left ventricle (LV) during diastole.
2. Severe acute AI is associated with a rapidly increasing left ventricular end-diastolic pressure (LVEDP), severe pulmonary edema, compensatory tachycardia, and systemic vasoconstriction.
3. Chronic insufficiency leads to eccentric LV hypertrophy with an increased end-diastolic volume, relatively normal LVEDP, increased stroke volume, and a compensatory relative tachycardia. These chronic adaptations can sometimes restore hemodynamics to near-normal values.
4. Hemodynamic goals for the treatment of AI are as follows:
   a. Maintain high-normal HR.
   b. Reduce afterload to assist forward flow and decrease the regurgitant fraction.
   c. Maintain adequate preload by appropriate fluid administration.

DISCUSSION

Aortic valve incompetence causes regurgitant blood flow into the LV during diastole. This leads to a decreased effective cardiac output for a given stroke volume, and a marked fall in diastolic blood pressure. The resulting widened pulse pressure has a negative effect on coronary artery perfusion.

Common etiologies for chronic AI include disorders that cause dilatation of the aortic root (ascending aortic aneurysms, syphilis, Marfan, Ehlers–Danlos), congenital malformations, subacute bacterial endocarditis, or valvular calcifications impairing valve closure. In contrast, acute AI is a rare condition most often caused by trauma, acute dissecting aneurysms, or acute severe endocarditis.

Symptoms of chronic AI include dyspnea on exertion, orthopnea, paroxysmal nocturnal dyspnea, palpitations, and, less frequently, angina. Exercise tolerance is usually well preserved until late in the disease process. On ECG testing, LV hypertrophy, LV strain, and occasionally signs of ischemia can be seen; the rhythm is usually sinus. In chronic AI, the increased diastolic filling of the LV causes LV dilatation and eccentric hypertrophy (Fig. 1). This acts predominantly to increase LV compliance, thereby avoiding significant increases in LV filling pressure. Cardiac output is preserved despite the regurgitant flow due to profoundly increased stroke volume from the dilated ventricle. In the face of severe valve incompetence, cardiac output can further be augmented by a high-normal heart rate.

As valve incompetence worsens, diastolic pressures continue to fall, leading to progressively lower coronary perfusion pressures. In addition, the geometrically unfavorable LV dimensions and spherical remodeling of eccentric hypertrophy further impair left ventricular ejection fraction. Eccentric dilation causes an increase in wall stress, as predicted by LaPlace's law: $T = PR/2h$, or Wall tension (T) = Pressure difference across the wall (P) × Radius of cylinder (R)/2 × Wall thickness (h). Increased wall stress leads to increased myocardial work and oxygen utilization. Patients may report anginal pain even in the absence of coronary artery disease because of increasing wall stress, falling coronary perfusion, and diminishing ejection fraction (EF). This is, however, much less common than with Aortic Stenosis (AS), where concentric LV hypertrophy causes much higher O_2 demand. Because such severe remodeling and impaired hemodynamics are difficult to reverse, outcomes for valve replacement in chronic AI are better in patients with less advance disease, that is, with normal EF (>55%) and LV diameters less than 55 mm.

In acute AI, aortic and LV end-diastolic pressures equilibrate without any compensatory increase in LV compliance, resulting in highly elevated LVEDP. This generally leads to severe congestive heart failure and worsened contractility, which can precipitate pulmonary edema. Of note, pulmonary capillary wedge pressure (PCWP) may underestimate the true LVEDP under these conditions (Jaffe et al., p. 352). Compensation from tachycardia and peripheral vasoconstriction rapidly ensues. Therapeutic goals for acute AI, therefore, include afterload reduction, inotropic support, and acute valve replacement.

Hemodynamic considerations. The essential goal of hemodynamic therapy is to decrease regurgitant flow and avoid worsening LV wall stress, and therefore lowering afterload, maintaining the compensatory tachycardia, and allowing full stroke volumes (a "full, mildly vasodilated, and modestly tachycardic" heart, Barash et al., p. 1082) are desirable (Table 1). Decreasing afterload with mild vasodilation creates a more favorable pressure gradient that decreases the regurgitant fraction. Arterial vasodilators (nicardipine or nitroprusside) permit increased forward flow. At the time of vasodilation, sufficient volume must be administered to maintain adequate preload. In general, contractility is usually adequate, so inotropes (dopamine vs. epinephrine) may not be needed. Relative tachycardia avoids overdilatation of the LV, decreasing pulmonary congestion, wall stress, and myocardial oxygen requirements. It also serves to decrease the time of diastolic runoff, decrease the regurgitant fraction, maintain diastolic blood pressure, and increase coronary perfusion.

Patients requiring aortic valve replacement with cardiopulmonary bypass (CPB) require special attention in regard to monitoring heart rate, rhythm, and LV filling pressures. Upon the initiation of CPB, AI can cause severe LV distention with subsequent myocardial ischemia and pulmonary edema. This can usually be avoided if the heart maintains a normal sinus rhythm with an adequate heart rate. If the heart fibrillates or severe bradycardia occurs and the LV distends, insertion of an LV vent or aortic cross-clamp may be required to overcome this problem (Jaffe et al., p. 350). Furthermore, myocardial protection with cardioplegia must be given either retrograde through the coronary sinus or directly into

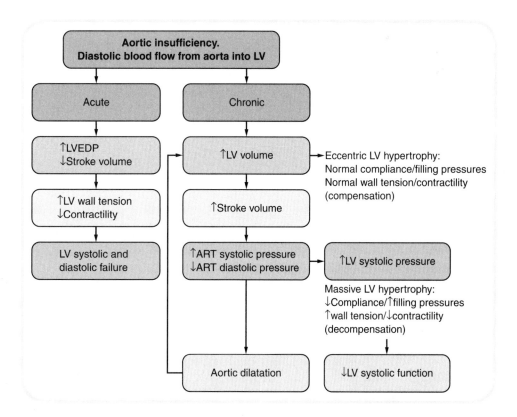

Figure 1. Pathophysiology of AI. ART, arterial.

Table 1. Hemodynamic Goals in AI

Preload	Normal to slightly ↑
Afterload	↓: with anesthetics or vasodilators (to decrease regurgitant fraction)
Contractility	Usually adequate
Rate	↑: reduces ventricular volume and raises diastolic aortic pressure
Rhythm	Usually sinus; not a problem
MVO$_2$	Usually not a problem
CPB	Beware (and observe) for ventricular distention (pre- and post-AXC: regurgitant flow increases if ↓ HR or nonbeating heart)

↑, increase; ↓, decrease; MVO$_2$, myocardial oxygen consumption; CPB, cardiopulmonary bypass; AXC, aortic cross-clamp; HR, heart rate.

From Skubas NJ, Lichtman AD, Sharma A, et al. Anesthesia for cardiac surgery. In: Barash PG, Cullen BF, Stoelting RK, et al, eds. Clinical Anesthesia. 6th edition. Philadelphia, PA: Lippincott Williams & Wilkins, 2009: 1082.

the coronary ostia rather than into the aortic root. Anterograde cardioplegia will not flow through the coronary circulation if LV distention occurs from aortic regurgitation of the solution. Adequate myocardial protection can occur only if the root pressure filled with cardioplegia is higher than the LV cavity pressure (LVEDP), thus promoting forward flow down the pressure gradient.

In summary, patients with AI benefit from high-normal HR, afterload reduction to assist forward flow, and fluid administration to maintain adequate preload. These hemodynamic interventions help maintain cardiac output. After bypass, patients with AI may require inotropic support and careful attention to maintain LV filling (Jaffe et al., pp. 351–352).

SUGGESTED READINGS

Barash PG, Cullen BF, Stoelting RK, et al, eds. *Clinical Anesthesia*. 6th ed. Philadelphia, PA: Lippincott Williams & Wilkins; 2009:1081.

Herrera A. Valvular heart disease. In: Hines RL, Marshall KE, eds. *Stoelting's Anesthesia and Co-Existing Disease*. 5th ed. Philadelphia, PA: Saunders; 2008:38–40.

Jaffe RA, Samuels SI, Schmiesing CA, et al, eds. *Anesthesiologist's Manual of Surgical Procedures*. 4th ed. Philadelphia, PA: Lippincott Williams & Wilkins; 2009:351–352.

Skubas NJ, Lichtman AD, Sharma A, et al. Anesthesia for cardiac surgery. In: Barash PG, Cullen BF, Stoelting RK, et al, eds. *Clinical Anesthesia*. 6th ed. Philadelphia, PA: Lippincott Williams & Wilkins; 2009:1082.

Arterial Waveform: Periph Versus Central

Physics, Monitoring, and Anesthesia Delivery

Caroline Al Haddadin

Edited by Benjamin Sherman

KEY POINTS

1. Although the most often utilized site for intraarterial blood pressure measurement is via cannulation of the radial artery, more central arteries can be utilized if necessary (femoral, axillary, brachial, or aorta).
2. Depending on the location of the measurement, the arterial waveform may differ in appearance.
3. The more peripheral the measurement, the higher the systolic pressures and the lower the diastolic pressures, with equal mean arterial pressures (MAPs) at all sites.
4. Cardiopulmonary bypass (CPB) may alter the waveform morphology, causing higher central systolic pressures and lower peripheral systolic pressures due to peripheral vasodilation and concomitant vasodilator medication administration.

DISCUSSION

Arterial blood pressure is usually measured via cannulation of the radial artery. Arterial waveforms are transmitted through a fluid-filled catheter and tubing, where the wave is measured by a transducer. The accuracy of this measurement is based on positioning of the catheter, the transducer, and the integrity of the fluid column within the tubing.

Although the radial artery is the most common site of blood pressure measurement, arterial blood pressure can be measured anywhere along the arterial system, peripherally or centrally. Depending on the location of measurement, the arterial waveform will appear different (Fig. 1). Peripheral arterial measurements will have a wider pulse pressure than central measurements, with higher systolic and lower diastolic readings. MAP, however, should remain equal at all sites. The dicrotic notch, which represents the transient increase

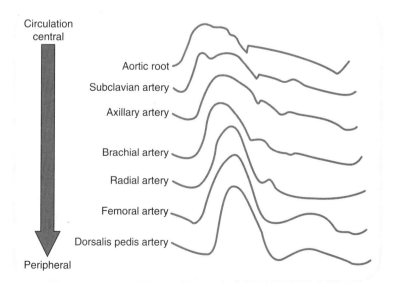

Figure 1. Arterial waveforms central to distal. From Lake CL, Hines RL, Blitt CD, ed. Clinical Monitoring: Practical Applications in Anesthesia and Critical Care Medicine. Philadelphia, PA: WB Saunders, 2001.

A

in pressure corresponding to closure of the aortic valve, also becomes less pronounced, as the measurement is taken farther away from the central arteries toward the periphery.

One exception to this pattern can be found in patients after hypothermic CPB for cardiac surgery. They tend to have higher systolic pressures centrally after CPB because of decreased vascular resistance in the periphery and because of the effects of vasodilating medications such as nitroglycerin and inhaled anesthetics.

SUGGESTED READINGS

Barash PG, Cullen BF, Stoelting RK, et al. *Clinical Anesthesia*. 6th ed. Philadelphia, PA: Lippincott Williams & Wilkins; 2009:702–704.

Lake CL, Hines RL, Blitt CD, ed. *Clinical Monitoring: Practical Applications in Anesthesia and Critical Care Medicine*. Philadelphia, PA: WB Saunders; 2001:182.

Miller RD. *Miller's Anesthesia*. 7th ed. Philadelphia, PA: Elsevier, Churchill, and Livingstone; 2009:308–309.

Morgan GE, Mikhail MS, Murray MJ. *Clinical Anesthesiology*. 4th ed. New York, NY: McGraw-Hill; 2006:119–120.

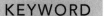
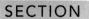

ASA Sedation Guidelines

Generic, Clinical Sciences: Anesthesia
Procedures, Methods, Techniques

Alexander Timchenko

Edited by Jodi Sherman

A

1. The guidelines include recommendations for procedures to be performed in a variety of settings (hospital, clinics, etc.) by practitioners who are not specialists in anesthesiology.
2. The guidelines exclude minimal sedation, general anesthesia, and major conduction anesthesia.
3. The guidelines are applicable to conscious sedation and deep sedation, when the patient is able to make a purposeful response to verbal or tactile stimulation, and both respiratory and cardiovascular function are usually maintained.

DISCUSSION

Definitions of moderate sedation/analgesia (conscious sedation) and deep sedation/analgesia:

	Minimal Sedation (Anxiolysis)	Moderate Sedation/ Analgesia (Conscious Sedation)	Deep Sedation/ Analgesia	General Anesthesia
Responsiveness	Normal response to verbal stimulation	Purposeful response to verbal or tactile stimulation	Purposeful response after repeated or painful stimulation	Unarousable, even with painful stimulus
Airway	Unaffected	No intervention required	Intervention may be required	Intervention often required
Spontaneous ventilation	Unaffected	Adequate	May be inadequate	Frequently inadequate
Cardiovascular function	Unaffected	Usually maintained	Usually maintained	May be impaired

1. Preprocedure patient evaluation and preparation improves clinical efficacy and reduces adverse outcomes. Specific points to be addressed are as follows:

- Abnormalities of the major organ systems
- Previous adverse experience with sedation/analgesia and general anesthesia
- Drug allergies
- Current medications and possible interactions
- Time and nature of the last oral intake
- Preprocedure fasting recommended to decrease adverse outcomes, but there is no significant evidence from the literature
- In emergency situations—when preprocedural fasting is not practical—recommend less sedation or protect the trachea by placing ET tube
- Patients undergoing elective procedures should not eat or drink for a sufficient time to allow for gastric emptying (clear liquids—2 hours, breast milk—4 hours, infant formula, nonhuman milk, light meal—6 hours)
- History of tobacco, alcohol, substance abuse
- Physical examination including airway assessment and laboratory assessment

A

2. Patient monitoring and recording of monitored parameters during sedation:

- This should include pulse oximetry, ECG, and automated noninvasive blood pressure (NIBP).
- Monitoring of ventilator function by observation/auscultation is recommended. Capnography is a reliable method for monitoring respiratory activity and should be considered for deep sedation or if observation/auscultation is not possible. Pulse oximetry is not a substitute for monitoring of respiratory function, but helps in early detection of hypoxemia.
- Vitals are recommended to be monitored every 5 minutes once a stable level of sedation is achieved. NIBP should be measured at 5-minute intervals unless it interferes with procedure (e.g., NIBP stimulation may arouse sedated patient).
- ECG should be used in all patients with deep sedation.
- Patient response monitoring to verbal and tactile stimuli is recommended to prevent drifting into a state of general anesthesia. If verbal response cannot be monitored, ability to give "thumbs up" or other indication of consciousness in response to verbal or tactile stimulation suggests that the patient will be able to control his or her airway. Reflex withdrawal from pain is not considered purposeful (conscious) response and is related to state of general anesthesia.

3. A person other than the practitioner performing the procedure should be available to perform procedural monitoring and should be trained in airway management and resuscitation.
4. Availability of emergency and airway equipment, and a means of positive-pressure ventilation. Defibrillator should be immediately available.
5. The use of supplementary oxygen is recommended. Oxygen can be delivered to all patients unless contraindicated and should be administered to all patients with deep sedation.
6. Maintenance of IV access until the patient is no longer at risk for cardiorespiratory depression. Equipment for IV access should be available throughout the procedure.
7. Medications. Combination of sedatives and analgesics given IV is preferred and should be given incrementally with sufficient time between doses to assess effects. Repeat doses of oral medications are not recommended. Pharmacologic antagonists (e.g., naloxone and flumazenil) and basic resuscitative medications should be immediately available.
8. Postprocedural recovery observation and monitoring until the patients are no longer at risk for cardiorespiratory depression is recommended.

SUGGESTED READINGS

American Society of Anesthesiologists: practice guidelines for sedation and analgesia by non-anesthesiologists. *Anesthesiology.* 2002;96:1004–1017.

American Society of Gastrointestinal Endoscopy: guidelines for conscious sedation and monitoring during gastrointestinal endoscopy. *Gastrointest Endosc.* 2003;58(3):317–322.

American Society of Gastrointestinal Endoscopy: guidelines for the use of deep sedation and anesthesia for GI endoscopy. *Gastrointest Endosc.* 2002;56(5):613–617.

Luginbühl M, Vuilleumier P, Schumacher P, et al. Anesthesia or sedation for gastroenterologic endoscopies. *Curr Opin Anesthesiol.* 2009;22:524–531.

Asthma: Postpartum Hemorrhage Rx
Subspecialties: Obstetric Anesthesia

Lisbeysi Calo

Edited by Lars Helgeson

A

1. Postpartum hemorrhage (PPH) occurs in 4% of patients and is defined as postpartum blood loss exceeding 500 mL. It is associated with prolonged third stage of labor, preeclampsia, multiple gestation, forceps delivery, and mediolateral episiotomy.
2. Prevention of PPH includes oxytocin therapy after delivery of the baby, but before delivery of the placenta, clamping the cord within 20 seconds after delivery, and "controlled" traction of the cord.
3. The treatment of PPH consists of supportive measures (intravenous [IV] fluids, blood transfusion) and identification and management of the cause (i.e., uterine atony and repair of lacerations).
4. Special attention must be paid to asthmatic patients. Medications used to treat uterine atony can cause bronchospasm.

PPH is defined as postpartum blood loss exceeding 500 mL. Up to 4% of patients may experience PPH. It is often associated with a prolonged third stage of labor, preeclampsia, multiple gestation, forceps delivery, and mediolateral episiotomy. Common causes of PPH also include uterine atony, retained placenta, obstetric lacerations, uterine inversion, and use of tocolytic agents.

The management of PPH is first directed at prevention. Active management of stage 3 of labor includes use of oxytocin after delivery of the baby, but before delivery of the placenta, clamping the cord within 20 seconds after delivery, and "controlled" traction of the cord. This approach reduces by 6% to 18% the incidence of significant PPH and the need for maternal blood transfusion.

The treatment of PPH includes supportive treatment and identification and management of the cause (i.e., uterine atony and repair of lacerations). Supportive measures include establishment of venous access and resuscitation with fluid and blood transfusions.

Uterine atony is the most common cause of PPH and is associated with prolonged and augmented labor, uterine overdistention, multiple gestations, and polyhydramnios. When prevention of uterine atony has failed, uterine massage and supportive measures are provided. If necessary, the following medications can be used to help the uterus contract:

- Oxytocin, 20 to 40 units in 1 L at 10 to 15 mL per minute. Can be given intramuscularly (IM) undiluted, if there is no IV access.
- Methylergonovine, 0.2 mg IM or intrauterine repeated every 2 to 4 hours. It is an ergot alkaloid derivative and a vasoconstrictor. Side effects include hypertension (HTN) and bronchospasm.
- Hemabate (Carboprost Tromethamine), 0.25 mg IM every 15 to 90 minutes up to a maximum of eight doses. Hemabate can cause HTN, bronchospasm, and pulmonary edema.
- Misoprostol (PGE1 analog) 600 μg PO or PR if no response to the above measures, unless clear contraindication such as preeclampsia. Advantages over Hemabate are that misoprostol does not elevate blood pressure or cause bronchospasm or pulmonary edema.

These medications should be used with caution in asthmatic patients. Careful preoperative evaluation of the asthmatic patient is important to avoid bronchoconstriction and the need for airway protection if PPH occurs. Asthmatic patients may benefit from inhaler treatment to prevent bronchoconstriction prior to general anesthesia, if bleeding is uncontrolled and emergent laparotomy ± hysterectomy is pursued. Early ligation of the hypogastric arteries may help reduce blood loss and avoid hysterectomy.

SUGGESTED READINGS

Chestnut D, Polley LS, Tsen LC, et al. *Chestnut's Obstetric Anesthesia, Principles and Practice.* 4th ed. Philadelphia, PA: Mosby Elsevier; 2009: 368.

Morgan GE, Mikhail MS, Murray MJ. Clinical anesthesiology. 4th ed. *Obstetric Anesthesia.* New York, NY: McGraw Hill; 2005:912–913.

Khan GQ, John IS, Wani S, et al. Controlled cord traction versus minimal intervention techniques in delivery of the placenta: a randomized controlled trial. *Am J Obstet Gynecol.* 1997;177:770–774.

O'Brien P, El-Refaey H, Gordon A, et al. Rectally administered misoprostol for the treatment of postpartum hemorrhage unresponsive to oxytocin and ergometrine: a descriptive study. *Obstet Gynecol.* 1998;92:212–214.

Rogers J, Wood J, McCandlish R, et al. Active versus expectant management of third stage of labour. *The Hinchingbrooke randomised controlled trial.* Lancet 1998; 351:693-699.

Atlantoaxial Instability: Causes
Organ-based Clinical: Neurologic and Neuromuscular

Ira Whitten

Edited by Ramachandran Ramani

KEY POINTS

1. Atlantoaxial instability (AAI) can complicate airway management.
2. AAI can result from trauma, systemic disease, infection, congenital anomalies, or genetic conditions.
3. Screening for AAI can be achieved by flexion and extension plain radiographs, whereas CT scan and/or MRI can determine the degree of spinal canal involvement.
4. Failure to recognize possible AAI and to take ample precautions can have devastating consequences.

DISCUSSION

AAI is defined as excessive laxity of the ligaments between the C1 and the C2 joint, and this condition can lead to subluxation at the atlantoaxial joint, resulting in devastating neurologic injury. Subluxation at the atlantoaxial joint may force the odontoid process into the spinal canal and result in symptoms ranging from pain and myelopathy in cases of minor cord impingement to complete quadriplegia in cases of severe spinal cord compression (Fig. 1). Atlantoaxial instability can be diagnosed on plain radiograph by measurement of an atlantodens interval space of greater than 3 mm in adults and 5 mm in children.

Commonly encountered etiologies of AAI include blunt trauma, rheumatoid arthritis, ankylosing spondylitis, and Down syndrome, whereas malignancy, dwarfism, Grisel syndrome, Chiari malformation, and congenital cervical spine anomalies are less common causes of this condition. Blunt trauma patients have an incidence of cervical spine injuries of 2% to 4%, with head injuries carrying an associated incidence of cervical injuries on the order of 2% to 10%. Between 50% and 80% of patients with rheumatoid arthritis will have cervical spine involvement during the course of their disease, and this can result in atlantoaxial subluxation or pannus formation, which then results in compression of the spinal cord. Ankylosing spondylitis is also associated with AAI due to inflammatory changes and laxity of the cervical ligaments, and this disorder has an incidence of atlantoaxial subluxation of 21%. AAI is commonly seen in Down syndrome, and the pediatric population has an incidence of 15%. Malignancy can result in cervical instability by direct invasion or metastases, although the cervical spine is rarely a site of metastatic disease. Grisel syndrome is atlantoaxial subluxation due to inflammation or infection of the oropharynx and may occur in the setting of ENT surgery.

AAI is especially important to the anesthesiologist because this condition prevents the practitioner from properly maneuvering the patient's head and neck to achieve alignment of the laryngeal, oral, and pharyngeal axes. Patients with AAI must be dealt with carefully, and may require neck immobilization in a cervical collar and awake fiberoptic intubation for both patient safety and airway management.

A

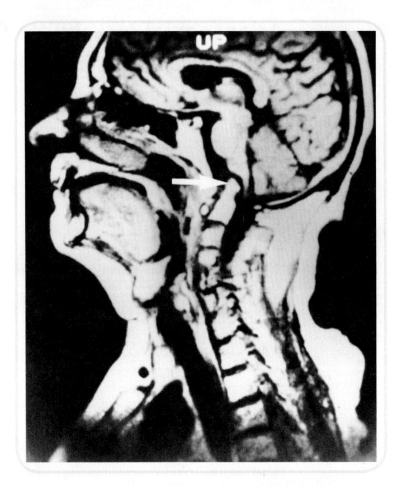

Figure 1. MRI of a patient with advanced rheumatoid arthritis shows invagination of the odontoid process of C2 *(arrow)* through the foramen magnum, compressing the brain stem. Notice the degeneration of C4 and C5, a common problem in rheumatoid arthritis. (From Miller RD, Eriksson LI, Fleisher LA, et al. *Miller's Anesthesia.* 7th ed. Philadelphia: Elsevier, Churchill-Livingstone, 2009: Chapter 70, with permission.)

SUGGESTED
READINGS

Barash PG, Cullen BF, Stoelting RK, eds. *Clinical Anesthesia.* 6th ed. Philadelphia, PA: Lippincott; 2009:636–637, 892.

Canale TS. *Campbell's Operative Orthopaedics.* 11th ed. Philadelphia, PA: Mosby Elsevier; 2007:1150–1155.

Crosby ET. Considerations for airway management for cervical spine surgery in adults. *Anesthesiol Clin.* 2007;25:511–533.

Meleger AL, Krivickas LS. Neck and back pain: musculoskeletal disorders. *Neurol Clin.* 2007;25:419–438.

Miller RD, Eriksson LI, Fleisher LA, et al. *Miller's Anesthesia.* 7th ed. Philadelphia, PA: Elsevier, Churchill and Livingstone; 2009:2409–2420.

Atrial Flutter: Pharm Rx

Organ-based Clinical: Cardiovascular

Tiffany Denepitiya-Balicki

Edited by Qingbing Zhu

KEY POINTS

1. Atrial flutter is a rhythm with an atrial rate of 250 to 350 beats per minute (bpm).
2. The pattern is recognized by the characteristic "saw tooth" pattern of the P wave, also known as flutter waves.
3. Pharmacologic control of the ventricular rate may be achieved with the use of amiodarone, diltiazem, or verapamil if the patient is hemodynamically stable.
4. If the patient is hemodynamically unstable, synchronized cardioversion should be considered.

DISCUSSION

Atrial flutter is a rhythm with an atrial rate of 250 to 350 bpm. Often, however, patients will present in atrial flutter with a 2:1 conduction block, therefore presenting with a heart rate of 150 bpm. This dysrhythmia is often associated with atrial fibrillation or tachycardia.

Diagnosis is based on electrocardiogram analysis, as depicted above. The pattern is recognized by the characteristic "saw tooth" pattern of the P wave, also known as flutter waves (Fig. 1). As stated previously, usually half of the atrial excitation is conducted through the ventricle, resulting in a ventricular rate of 120 to 160 bpm. It is important to realize that atrial fibrillation and atrial flutter may convert back and forth between each another.

If a patient with atrial flutter is hemodynamically unstable, cardioversion is imperative. Approximately 50 J of energy may be enough to convert a patient back into sinus rhythm. For those who are hemodynamically stable, pacemaker is a treatment option. Furthermore, similar to patients with atrial fibrillation, if the patient has been in atrial flutter for more than 48 hours, performing a TEE to rule out clot is important before attempting cardioversion. These patients may benefit from anticoagulation therapy.

Pharmacologic control of the ventricular rate may be achieved with the use of amiodarone, diltiazem, or verapamil. If, however, the ventricle conducts every atrial excitation and a rate of 300 bpm is achieved, a re-entry pathway must be considered and the use of

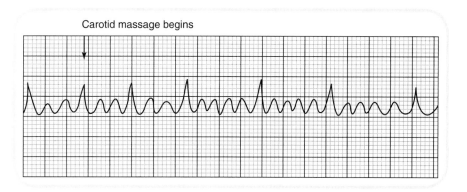

Carotid massage begins

Figure 1. Atrial flutter. (From Barash PG, Cullen BF, Stoelting RK, et al. Clinical Anesthesia. 6th Edition. Philadelphia, PA: Lippincott Williams & Wilkins, 2009: 1580, with permission.)

70

procainamide may be useful. It is important to remember that these agents will control ventricular rate, but will likely not convert the patient to sinus rhythm.

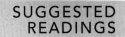

SUGGESTED READINGS

Barash PG, Cullen BF, Stoelting RK, et al. *Clinical Anesthesia*. 6th ed. Philadelphia, PA: Lippincott Williams & Wilkins; 2009:1580.
Hines R, Marschall K. *Anesthesia and Co-Existing Disease*. 5th ed. Philadelphia, PA: Churchill Livingstone; 2008:66–68.

Automated vs. Paper Anesthesia Records
Mathematics, Statistics, Computers

Trevor Banack, Emilio Andrade, and Jennifer Dominguez
Edited by Raj K. Modak

KEY POINTS

1. Research suggests that automated anesthesia information management systems (AIMSs) provide more accurate information regarding intraoperative incidents or deviations from normal physiologic ranges than voluntary reporting by anesthesia providers.
2. Studies have shown that AIMS do not decrease the vigilance of the anesthesia provider, but rather may allow the provider to focus on patient care, instead of manual record keeping.
3. From an anesthesia patient care standpoint, it has been shown that computerized records are more accurate compared with handwritten ones.
4. AIMS provide a centralized database with consistent variables for research purposes, as well as a means of quickly obtaining information about a patient in emergent situations.
5. Rather than increasing malpractice exposure, AIMS may be beneficial in risk management.
6. There can be system errors that can potentially cause inaccurate data collection.

DISCUSSION

AIMS have been adopted by many practices and institutions in recent years. This has been, in part, motivated by pressure from the public and from the government to move toward a fully electronic medical record to facilitate quality monitoring, billing, ease of transmission of records, and to decrease administrative costs. However, the transition from the traditional paper record to an electronic medical record has been slowed by cost, limitations of the commercially available software systems, and implementation. Despite these obstacles, it seems that once in place, AIMS offer many advantages from a patient care standpoint, as well as in mitigating malpractice exposure.

Research suggests that automated AIMS provide more accurate information regarding intraoperative incidents or deviations from normal physiologic ranges than from voluntary reporting by anesthesia providers. They eliminate some of the major problems with manual record keeping, such as averaging of physiologic variables around a trend and omission of abnormal values.

Studies have shown that AIMS do not decrease the vigilance of the anesthesia provider, but rather may allow the provider to focus on patient care, instead of manual record keeping. This becomes especially relevant during labor-intensive portions of the case, traumas, or unexpected intraoperative events when accurate manual charting becomes logistically difficult. AIMS may also improve patient care by facilitating communication between providers through a centralized database that is easy to access during an emergency, or in preparation for a scheduled case. Information about previous intubations or unexpected reactions may be easily found in such a database, compared to the traditional paper record. These data may also be used for research purposes and quality assurance, both of which are ultimately of benefit to patients.

Last, some critics have argued that AIMS may increase malpractice exposure for anesthesia providers. However, research seems to suggest that they may actually help mitigate risk by providing juries with legible, accurate, and complete records. They also provide a "third party" form of documentation that may be considered more favorably by juries, whereas the paper chart is ultimately created by the person who would require it for their defense, should the need arise. However, vigilance by the anesthesia provider and

72

examination of the automated record is still necessary, as errors and omissions are still possible due to system failure.

The major pitfalls for paper anesthesia record keeping are as follows:

- Omission of abnormal values
- Lack of legibility of normal values
- Adjusting abnormal values to within the expected upper or lower physiologic limits
- Averaging of a number of measurements around an abnormal value

The major pitfalls of AIMS are as follows:

- Limited mobility
- Several companies have systems that are not compatible with each other
- System errors can potentially cause inaccurate data collection
- Requires significant time for installation and training

SUGGESTED READINGS

Balust J, Macario A. Can anesthesia information management systems improve quality in the surgical suite? *Curr Opin Anaesthesiol.* 2009;22:215–222.

Barash PG, Cullen BF, Stoelting RK, et al, eds. *Clinical Anesthesia.* 6th ed. Philadelphia, PA: Lippincott Williams & Wilkins; 2009:47–48.

Edsall DW, Deshane P, Giles C, et al. Computerized patient anesthesia records: less time and better quality than manually produced anesthesia records. *J Clin Anesth.* 1993;5:275–283.

Ehrenfeld JM. Anesthesia information management systems—a guide to their successful installation and use. *Anesthesiology News.* September, 2009:1–7.

Feldman JM. Do anesthesia information systems increase malpractice exposure? Results of a survey. *Anesth Analg.* 2004;99(3):840–843.

Lerou JG, Dirksen R, van Daele M, et al. Automated charting of physiologic variables in anesthesia: a quantitative comparison of automated versus handwritten anesthesia records. *J Clin Monit.* 1988;4:37–47.

Sanborn KV, Castro J, Kuroda M, et al. Detection of intraoperative incidents by electronic scanning of computerized anesthesia records: comparison with voluntary reporting. *Anesthesiology.* 1996;85(5):977–987.

Thrush DN. Are automated anesthesia records better? *J Clin Anesth.* 1992;4:386–389.

Weinger MB, Herndon OW, Gaba DM. The effect of electronic record keeping and transesophageal echocardiography on task distribution, workload, and vigilance during cardiac anesthesia. *Anesthesiology.* 1997;87:144–155.

Autonomic Hyperreflexia: Signs and Paraplegia

Organ-based Clinical: Neurologic and Neuromuscular and Generic, Clinical Sciences: Anesthesia Procedures, Methods, Techniques

Kimberly Slininger, Holly Barth, and Meredith Brown

Edited by Ramachandran Ramani

KEY POINTS

1. Patients with spinal cord lesions above the T7 level are at high risk for autonomic hyperreflexia, characterized by a reflex sympathetic discharge in response to a noxious stimulus.
2. Autonomic hyperreflexia typically presents as sudden bradycardia and hypertension.
3. Autonomic hyperreflexia should be treated by first removing the precipitating stimulus, then increasing the anesthetic depth, and finally treating hypertension with direct-acting vasodilators.
4. By blocking the autonomic reflexes in the spinal cord, neuraxial anesthesia is a good alternative to general anesthesia in patients at risk for developing autonomic hyperreflexia.

DISCUSSION

Typically, autonomic hyperreflexia occurs in response to a noxious stimulus in patients with chronic spinal cord lesions above the T7 level. As a result of the spinal cord injury, the central nervous system is unable to modulate the response of the sympathetic nervous system to stimuli. Sixty percent to 70% of patients with spinal cord injuries above T7 may experience vascular tone instability as a result, and reports show approximately a 20% perioperative mortality in patients with spinal cord transection. The triggering stimulus can be proprioceptive, cutaneous, or visceral stimulation (i.e., overdistended bladder or rectum). The result is activation of a spinal cord reflex that fails to be inhibited by the central nervous system. Elevation in blood pressure is sensed by the baroreceptors in the carotid sinus and aorta and thus activates parasympathetic hyperactivity via the vagus nerve that may result in bradycardia, heart block, ventricular ectopy, and reflex vasodilation above the level of the spinal cord injury that is manifested as flushing and sweating. The symptoms of autonomic hyperreflexia reflect the sympathetic discharge below the level of the lesion, causing severe vasoconstriction, which is partly compensated by vasodilatation above the level of the lesion. Stimuli capable of inducing this reflex include bladder distention, rectal stimulation, and surgical stimulation. The incidence is higher in men than in women.

When autonomic hyperreflexia occurs during surgery, the hypertensive changes can lead to increased blood loss, seizures, retinal, cerebral and subarachnoid hemorrhage, stroke, or even death. In addition to hypertension and bradycardia, other commonly observed cardiac changes include heart failure, tachycardia in high cervical spinal cord lesions, and myocardial ischemia.

Induction of general anesthesia in patients with autonomic hyperreflexia must be done with great caution. Too little anesthesia may induce a hypertensive crisis, whereas too much anesthesia may induce profound hypotension. Succinylcholine should be avoided because of its propensity to cause hyperkalemia in paraplegic patients.

When autonomic hyperreflexia occurs, it must be treated immediately to avoid the consequences of hypertensive crisis. The first step is to remove the noxious stimulus, and the anesthetic depth should be immediately deepened. Hypertension should be treated with direct-acting vasodilators. If the patient does not already have a foley catheter in place, one should be placed to ensure that bladder distention is not the cause. The risk of autonomic hyperreflexia persists in the postoperative period, and great care should be taken to prevent it.

Neuraxial anesthesia is a good alternative to general anesthesia in urologic procedures. Spinal anesthesia is particularly effective in preventing autonomic hyperreflexia by blocking the afferent pathways in the spinal cord. Similarly, there is evidence that epidural opioids also block the autonomic reflexes. Because these patients have a sensory deficit below the level of the lesion, however, the level of anesthesia in a neuraxial block is difficult to test.

SUGGESTED READINGS

Barash PG, Cullen BF, Stoelting RK. *Clinical Anesthesia*. 5th ed. Philadelphia, PA: Lippincott Williams & Wilkins; 2009:1052.

Miller RD, Eriksson LI, Fleisher LA, et al. *Miller's Anesthesia*. 7th ed. Philadelphia, PA: Elsevier Churchill Livingston; 2009:1085.

Ruskin KJ, Rosenbaum S. *Anesthesia Emergencies*. 1st ed. New York, NY: Oxford University Press; 2011:144–145.

Autonomic Innervation: Upper Extremity

Anatomy

Anna Clebone

Edited by Jodi Sherman

A

KEY POINTS

1. The autonomic innervation of the upper extremities is exclusively sympathetic, with most preganglionic neurons arising in the intermediolateral column of T3 to T6 spinal segments.
2. Postganglionic neurons join the brachial plexus from the middle cervical and stellate ganglia. Sympathetic innervation to the upper extremity may also exit via the T2 and T3 paravertebral ganglia.
3. The target organs of sympathetic innervations of the upper extremities include blood vessels, hair follicles, and sweat glands. Sympathetically mediated pain can disrupt the normal regulation of these organs.
4. Completely sympathetic denervation of an upper extremity may require blocking the T3 and T4 ganglia in addition to the stellate ganglion.

DISCUSSION

The autonomic nervous system is divided into the sympathetic and parasympathetic systems. The cell bodies of the sympathetic preganglionic neurons reside in the spinal segments from T1 to L2 in the intermediolateral cell column of the spinal cord. The cell bodies of the parasympathetic preganglionic neurons reside in the brain stem as well as the spinal segments from S2 to S4.

The axons of the sympathetic preganglionic neurons exit the spinal column via the ventral roots to paravertebral ganglia (also called sympathetic chain), autonomic ganglia residing adjacent to the vertebrae (Fig. 1). Many of these preganglionic neurons synapse onto the cell bodies of postganglionic neurons within the adjacent ganglia, or travel within the sympathetic chain up or down several spinal levels before synapsing on postganglionic neurons. Some preganglionic axons do pass through the ganglia without synapsing.

The autonomic innervation to the upper extremities is exclusively sympathetic and includes neurons originating primarily in T3 to T6 spinal segments, but also includes those originating in T2 to T8 spinal segments. The preganglionic neurons synapse on postganglionic neurons that include the middle cervical and stellate ganglia and the upper thoracic paravertebral ganglia. From these ganglia, the postganglionic neurons join the nerve roots of the brachial plexus and may also travel along blood vessels. Anatomic variants are common, occurring in more than half the population.

Sympathetic innervations of the upper extremities function primarily to regulate temperature and blood pressure. The target organs of postganglionic neurons are blood vessels, hair follicles, and sweat glands. These specific innervations explain the symptoms characteristic of sympathetically mediated pain syndromes: temperature and color changes of skin, edema, and changes in hair growth along affected areas.

Because of the wide spread of the sympathetic neurons within the sympathetic chain, achieving full sympathetic blockade to the upper extremities can be difficult. Complete sympathetic denervation of an upper extremity may require blocking the T2 and T3 ganglia in addition to the stellate ganglion.

76

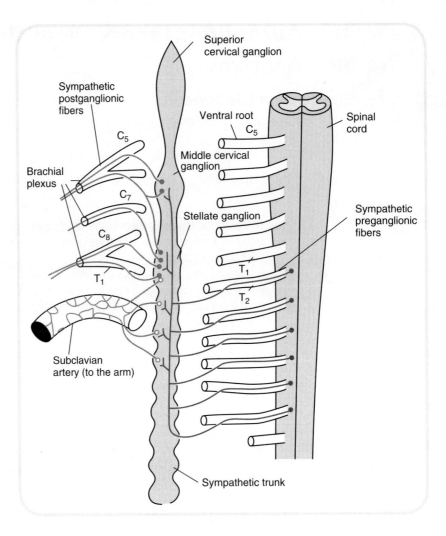

Figure 1. Sympathetic innervation of the upper extremity. The preganglionic fibers come from the upper thoracic segments of the cord and synapse in the ganglia of the sympathetic trunk up to the middle cervical ganglion. The postganglionic fibers follow partly the spinal nerves and partly the subclavian artery to the arm. (From Brodal P. *The Central Nervous System: Structure and Function.* New York, NY: Oxford University Press; 2004: 371–379 with permission.)

SUGGESTED READINGS

Brodal P. *The Central Nervous System: Structure and Function.* New York, NY: Oxford University Press; 2004:371–379.

Fishman SM, Ballantyne JC, Rathmell JP. *Bonica's Management of Pain.* 4th ed. Philadelphia, PA: Lippincott Williams & Wilkins; 2009.

Schiller Y. The anatomy and physiology of the sympathetic innervations to the upper limbs. *Clin Auton Res.* 2003;13(suppl 1):I2–I5.

Autonomic Neurotransmitters

Physiology

Frederick Conlin

Edited by Qingbing Zhu

A

KEY POINTS

1. The autonomic nervous system (ANS) consists of the sympathetic nervous system (SNS) and parasympathetic nervous system (PNS).
2. All preganglionic ANS neurons release acetylcholine (ACh) to activate postganglionic neurons.
3. PNS postganglionic neurons release ACh, activating muscarinic ACh receptors on target organs, causing decreased heart rate, bronchoconstriction, and general gastrointestinal activation.
4. All other SNS postganglionic neurons release norepinephrine onto target organs, whereas activation of the adrenal medulla releases epinephrine and norepinephrine in the bloodstream, causing systemic effects.
5. Four subtypes of adrenergic receptors have different affinities to epinephrine and norepinephrine; therefore, the predominant effect with different infusion rates can be significantly different.

DISCUSSION

The ANS regulates many of the involuntary physiologic activities, enabling the body to adapt to varying conditions and stressors. The ANS comprises the SNS and PNS. The ANS exerts its influence over target organs with only a few neurotransmitters, including ACh, norepinephrine, epinephrine, and dopamine.

All preganglionic ANS neurons release ACh to activate postganglionic neurons. ACh is also released by postganglionic PNS neurons to affect target organs, as well as postganglionic SNS neurons innervating sweat glands. All other SNS postganglionic neurons influence their target organs with the neurotransmitter norepinephrine. Also a member of the SNS, the adrenal medulla is innervated by ACh releasing from preganglionic neurons, and this when activated, releases both norepinephrine and epinephrine into the bloodstream to create a systemic humeral effect on multiple target organs (see Fig. 1).

Acetylcholine: Two types of ACh receptors mediate postsynaptic neuron responses. Nicotinic receptors mediate responses at the neuromuscular junction in the PNS, and are also present in the ganglionic synapses. Muscarinic receptors mediate PNS effect at target organs. Activation of cardiac muscarinic receptors leads to a decrease in myocardial contractility as well as a decrease in heart rate by slowing pacemaker activity and conduction velocity. Activation of smooth muscle muscarinic receptors causes contraction, with the particular effect dependent on the target organ: bronchial constriction, and within the GI tract peristalsis, glandular secretions (but also sphincter relaxation). The effect of ACh on blood vessels is ultimately dilation, via the release of nitric oxide.

Adrenergic receptors: These receptors mediate SNS activity on target organs. Four subtypes of adrenergic receptors mediate the SNS: alpha-1, alpha-2, beta-1, and beta-2. The primary role of alpha-1 receptors is arterial constriction; other actions include hepatic glycogenolysis, piloerection, and uterine contraction. Alpha-2 receptors are presynaptic, and respond to norepinephrine within the synaptic cleft by inhibiting the presynaptic neuron (modulating the effect). Beta-1 receptors respond to activation by increasing the force and rate of cardiac contraction and stimulating lipolysis and the release of insulin and renin. Beta-2 receptor activation leads to bronchodilation and vasodilation of skeletal muscle blood vessels.

Norepinephrine: This neurotransmitter has the strongest affinity to alpha receptors, with very little beta-2 activity. Norepinephrine can selectively influence target organs

78

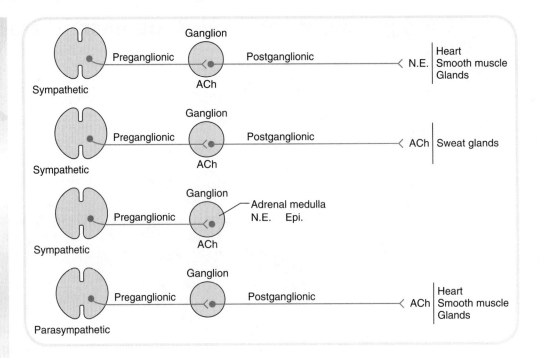

Figure 1. ANS schematic. (From Miller RD, ed. *Miller's Anesthesia*. 7th ed. Philadelphia, PA: Churchill Livingston; 2009:261–304 with permission.)

by postsynaptic activation of target organs or systemically through adrenal release into the bloodstream. Systemically released or infused norepinephrine causes intense arterial vasoconstriction to increase mean arterial pressure and systemic vascular resistance (alpha-1) and increased inotropy (beta-1), although an increase in heart rate is tempered by reflexive bradycardia. Dysrhythmias can also occur secondary to influence on cardiac pacemaker cells and conduction pathways.

Epinephrine: Released by the adrenal medulla on sympathetic stimulation, epinephrine exerts activity at both alpha and beta receptors. Because of differences in receptor subtype affinity, the rate of epinephrine infusion determines the predominant effect. Lower doses of epinephrine stimulate primarily beta-2 receptors, leading to a relaxation of bronchial smooth muscle, as well as dilation of skeletal muscle vasculature, effectively decreasing systemic vascular resistance. Intermediate doses of epinephrine also activate beta-1, causing significantly increased chronotropy and cardiac contractility. At high doses of epinephrine, alpha-1 activation causes intense arterial vasoconstriction, potentially causing severe hypertension. At intermediate and high epinephrine doses, cardiac dysrhythmias commonly occur, as does myocardial ischemia in susceptible patients, because of increased oxygen demand with cardiac artery constriction.

Dopamine: Although a neurotransmitter that does have adrenergic activity, endogenous dopamine within the SNS is primarily a precursor to epinephrine and norepinephrine in postsynaptic neuron terminals. Exogenous dopamine can have variable effects, depending on the infusion rate due to different receptor affinities. The low "renal" dose was previously believed to cause vasodilation of renal and mesenteric arteries via dopamine 1 receptors, a premise no longer considered valid. The intermediate infusion dose promotes beta-1 activity, whereas higher doses activate alpha-1 receptors and lead to vasoconstriction.

Barash PG, Cullen BF, Stoelting RK, eds. *Clinical Anesthesia*. 6th ed. Philadelphia, PA: Lippincott Williams & Wilkins; 2006:275–294.
Miller RD, ed. *Miller's Anesthesia*. 7th ed. Philadelphia, PA: Churchill Livingstone; 2009:261–304.
Stoelting RK, Miller RD. *Basics of Anesthesia*. 5th ed. Philadelphia, PA: Churchill Livingstone; 2007:64–69.

SUGGESTED READINGS

AV Pacing: Hemodynamic Effect
Organ-based Clinical: Cardiovascular

Juan Egas

Edited by Benjamin Sherman

A

KEY POINTS

1. Normal hemodynamics are maintained by an adequate cardiac output (CO) and a normal systemic vascular resistance (SVR) (mean arterial pressure [MAP] = SVR × CO).
2. The main determinants of the CO are the stroke volume and the heart rate.
3. The sinus nodal cells are the pacemakers of the heart because of their high rate of depolarization. AV nodal response is delayed as a result of slow conduction from SA to AV nodal cells, thus allowing the atria to contract prior to the ventricles.
4. Pacemakers emulate the actions of the cardiac conducting system by creating the action potentials, therefore maintaining an adequate CO.
5. In patients with diastolic dysfunction or impaired ventricular filling, atrial contraction may contribute to a substantial portion of the diastolic ventricular filling. In these patients, AV pacing is preferred over ventricular pacing alone.

DISCUSSION

Normal hemodynamics are maintained by an adequate CO and SVR as explained by the formula:

$$MAP = SVR \times CO$$

Changes in either variable can occur under physiologic and/or pathologic conditions with compensatory changes in the other. Compensatory mechanisms are able to maintain an adequate MAP and organ perfusion pressure up to a certain extent; once the compensatory mechanisms have been overwhelmed, a dramatic decrease in perfusion pressure will occur, with end-organ damage. The organs of foremost concern are the heart and brain, followed by the kidneys and lungs.

The main determinants of the CO are the stroke volume and the heart rate. For an adequate pump function, a normal anatomic and physiologic electrical conductive and contractile system is mandatory. Under normal conditions, the initial action potential of the heart originates from sinus node cells. All specialized myocardial cells have the ability to generate action potentials spontaneously (spontaneous diastolic depolarization of phase 4 due to a positive ion inward current), but sinus node cells depolarize at a higher rate, making them the physiologic pacemaker of the heart. Once these cells generate an action potential, it will travel along the myocardial electrical system composed of specialized muscle fibers. Through these fibers, the action potential distributes evenly in a synchronized way between the atrial and the ventricular myocardium. During physiologic conditions, the distribution of the action potential follows a sequential pattern as follows:

SA node (RA and LA) → AV node → Bundle of His and Purkinje fiber system (RV and LV).

Note that there is a physiologic delay in the AV node resulting from slow myocardial conducting fibers, allowing an initial synchronized contraction of the atria, whereas the ventricles are relaxed in the late phase of ventricular diastolic filling. Normal electromechanical physiology can be altered in many pathologic conditions, such as sinus node cells that do not fire at an adequate rate, or the presence of ectopic pacemakers (cells that depolarize faster than the SA node). These abnormal conditions may have a severe effect on the

A

CO, which overwhelms the compensatory mechanisms of the cardiovascular system to maintain an adequate MAP. If CO is not maintained, end-organ damage is the result.

Pacemakers emulate the actions of the cardiac conducting system, creating almost physiologic action potentials allowing for an adequate CO.

Indications for temporary pacing:

1. Rate support for hemodynamically significant or symptomatic bradycardia refractory to positive chronotropic medications.
2. To overdrive and terminate atrial flutter or monomorphic VT.
3. Bridge to implantation of a permanent pacemaker.

Indications for permanent pacing:

1. Symptomatic bradycardia
2. Second degree Mobitz II AV block and third degree AV block
3. Bifascicular block with recurrent third degree block and syncope
4. Acute MI for persistent second and third degree AV block
5. Acute MI survivors with newly acquired left bundle branch block or right bundle branch block with a fascicular block
6. Sinus node dysfunction: sick sinus syndrome, bradycardia–tachycardia syndrome
7. Hypersensitive carotid sinus syndrome

The decision to utilize atrial ventricular pacing versus ventricular pacing alone depends on the patient's comorbidities. Ideally, if possible, atrial ventricular pacing should be utilized because it more closely replicates physiologic conditions. In patients with diastolic dysfunction and reduced ventricular relaxation, the atrial contraction's contribution to the ventricular filling may represent a significant portion of the end-diastolic ventricular volume, and therefore ventricular pacing alone may significantly reduce ventricular volume, and ultimately CO. In addition, the AV interval should be delayed long enough to allow the atrium to empty during contraction.

SUGGESTED READINGS

Hensley FA, Martin DE, Gravlee GP, eds. *A Practical Approach to Cardiac Anesthesia.* 4th ed. Philadelphia, PA: Lippincott Williams & Wilkins; 2008:461–475.
Miller RD, Stoelting RK. *Basics of Anesthesia.* 5th ed. Philadelphia, PA: Churchill Livingstone; 2007:49–51.
Morgan GE, Mikhail MS, Murray MJ. *Clinical Anesthesiology.* 4th ed. New York, NY: McGraw Hill; 2006:415–417.

Axillary Block: Complications

Regional Anesthesia

Nehal Gatha

Edited by Jodi Sherman

KEY POINTS

1. Axillary blocks are well suited for surgical procedures involving the distal humerus, elbow, forearm, wrist, and hand.
2. Incomplete anesthesia/analgesia is the most common complication because of the need for multiple needle redirections.
3. The musculocutaneous nerve exits the plexus early, travels in the coracobrachialis muscle, and is therefore not in immediate proximity to the vasculature. This nerve requires special treatment as it is most commonly missed.
4. Because of the proximity of the nerves to the artery and vein, intravascular injection is a possible but rare complication.
5. Local toxicity due to large volume injections is possible; therefore, maximal doses should be calculated and carefully adhered to.

DISCUSSION

Axillary blocks are well suited for surgical procedures involving the distal humerus, elbow, forearm, wrist, and hand. The brachial plexus travels within a neurovascular bundle that includes the axillary artery and vein, radial nerve, ulnar nerve, median nerve, and musculocutaneous nerve. In the anatomically neutral position, the axillary artery runs at the lateral border of the first rib and continues toward the teres minor muscle; the vein runs parallel and more superficial to the artery; the median nerve lies superior to the artery, with the radial nerve lying posterior, and the ulnar nerve inferior. Fascia envelops these nerves, creating separate compartments. The musculocutaneous nerve exits the plexus early, travels in the coracobrachialis muscle, and is therefore not in immediate proximity to the vasculature. It is important to note that these anatomic relationships vary somewhat with arm positioning and with proximal to distal evaluation, as well as with normal, congenital, or traumatic anatomic variations.

Incomplete anesthesia/analgesia is the most common complication because of the need for multiple needle redirections. Since an axillary block involves nerves that are contained in different fascial planes, one or more nerves may be incompletely anesthetized. Variant nerve distributions or missed nerves may require supplemental anesthetic. The musculocutaneous nerve requires special treatment, as it is most commonly missed.

The intercostobrachial nerve is a lateral cutaneous branch of the second intercostal nerve and does not originate from the brachial plexus. It supplies sensation to the medial arm and axilla. If regional anesthesia is the primary anesthetic and if a tourniquet is used, this nerve should be blocked for optimal patient comfort.

Because of the proximity of the nerves to the artery and vein, intravascular injection is a possible complication. Intravascular injection can lead to seizures, or dysrhythmias, or total cardiovascular collapse. Addition of epinephrine to the local anesthetic, as well as a slow injection with frequent aspiration, provides a safeguard against intravascular injection. There is also a risk of hematoma, which may be higher in the transarterial method to the axillary block. Exceptionally, rare vascular complications include loss of circulation (from vascular injury or vasospasm), thrombus formation, decreased venous drainage, or the formation of a venous wall aneurysm.

As with any regional block, nerve damage is a rare but possible complication of this block. Avoiding injection when there are paresthesias or pressure on injection is advised. Infection is also a rare complication shared with all regional blocks, and procedures should be avoided when there is a local infection, and catheters avoided if systemic infection.

Lastly, local anesthetic toxicity is a possible but serious complication. This is of particular concern with the axillary plexus block, as it requires multiple needle redirections, and possibly supplementation. Maximal doses of local anesthetic should be calculated and carefully adhered to, as large volume injections increase the risk associated with toxicity.

SUGGESTED READINGS

De Jong RH. Axillary block of the brachial plexus. *Anesthesiology.* 1961;22:215–225.

Morgan GE, Mikhail MS, Murray MJ. *Clinical Anesthesiology.* 4th ed. New York, NY: McGraw-Hill; 2006:334–337.

KEYWORD

Axillary Block: Limitations and Median Nerve Rescue Block

SECTION

Regional Anesthesia

Jamie Ferrara and Thomas Gallen

Edited by Jodi Sherman

KEY POINTS

1. Axillary block is one approach to the brachial plexus block and can effectively provide anesthesia or analgesia for surgical procedures of the distal humerus, elbow, forearm, wrist, and hand.
2. An incomplete block is the most common complication of an axillary block.
3. The medial brachial cutaneous nerve and the intercostobrachial nerve are missed with an axillary, and need to be blocked separately if a tourniquet is planned.
4. Single terminal nerves, such as the median nerve, can be blocked individually to supplement an incomplete axillary block.
5. The median nerve blockade is useful for the anterolateral surface of the hand, including digits one through three.
6. The median nerve is preferably blocked at the level of the elbow or at the mid-to-distal aspect of the anterior forearm.

DISCUSSION

Regional anesthesia for the upper extremity can be provided by blocking the brachial plexus with one of four approaches: interscalene, supraclavicular, infraclavicular, and axillary. The axillary approach is effective for surgical procedures of the distal humerus, elbow, forearm, wrist, and hand, and is well suited for patients with pulmonary disease who cannot tolerate the risk of potential phrenic nerve anesthetization. There are several well-described approaches to the axial block, including transarterial, elicitation of paresthesia, ultrasound, and nerve stimulator technique. Understanding the anatomy is critical to achieving successful block and avoiding complications. If only a partial block is obtained, a single nerve may be targeted for anesthesia, for example, the median nerve, rather than repeating the brachial plexus block in its entirety.

The axillary perivascular sheath is formed by the continuation of the prevertebral fascia and contains the brachial plexus as well as the axillary artery and vein. In the anatomical position, the median nerve lies superficially and slightly lateral to the axillary artery, the radial nerve is posterior and slightly medial to the artery, and the ulnar nerve is deep and lateral to the artery. This relationship is commonly encountered, although anatomical variations occur with great frequency, and positioning alters this relationship. Quite consistently, however, the radial nerve is deep to the axillary artery, and so a blind transarterial approach to blocking this nerve is routinely successful.

The musculocutaneous nerve exits the brachial plexus early and travels within the coracobrachialis muscle belly, separately from the main neurovascular bundle. This nerve becomes the lateral antebrachial cutaneous nerve, serving the lateral half of the palmar forearm and the lateral one-third of the dorsal forearm, and is frequently missed if care is not taken.

The axillary block alone does not provide total coverage of the upper extremity. The medial brachial cutaneous nerve innervates the skin of the medial aspect between the axilla and the elbow joint on both the flexor and the extensor aspect of the arm. It leaves the brachial plexus sheath before the axilla, and therefore must be blocked separately. Likewise, the intercostobrachial nerve, which is the lateral cutaneous branch of the T2 intercostal nerve and therefore does not travel in the sheath at all, serves the medial and posterior proximal upper arm. These nerves are usually covered with a separate superficial

84

A

field block from the deltoid prominence to the most inferior aspect of the medial upper arm, and are important to cover if surgical anesthesia is desired and a tourniquet is planned.

Among the advantages to the axillary compared with other approaches to the brachial plexus block named above is the lack of risk of neuraxial anesthesia, phrenic nerve anesthesia, or pneumo/hemothorax. It can provide profound anesthesia or anesthesia for the elbow, forearm, wrist, and hand. Among the disadvantages are insufficient anesthesia for the shoulder and upper arm, and a requirement for abduction of the arm at the shoulder for block placement. One of the most common complications of an axillary block is an incomplete block; therefore, single terminal nerve techniques such as the median nerve block can help "rescue" a failed block.

The median nerve supplies the anterolateral surface of the hand including the thumb through the middle finger. It causes flexion at the metacarpophalangeal joints and extension at the interphalangeal joints of digits two and three. The nerve also innervates the muscles that produce flexion and opposition of the thumb and middle and index fingers, and pronation and flexion of the wrist. Lack of sensory block in this area is an indication for the need of supplemental block.

The brachial artery serves as the main landmark for the median nerve at the level of the elbow. At the antecubital crease, the nerve lies just medial to the brachial artery pulsation, which is approximately 1 cm to the ulnar side of the biceps brachii tendon (Fig. 1). At the level of the wrist, the median nerve lies deep to the flexor retinaculum and in between the palmaris longus tendon and the flexor carpi radialis muscle. The forearm and elbow locations are preferred supplemental block approaches over the wrist location because of the risk of carpal tunnel syndrome exacerbation from injecting a large volume of local anesthetic solution into the limited space of the tunnel.

At the elbow and forearm, nerve stimulation and/or ultrasound imaging can be used to guide the procedure. The optimal nerve stimulation response is flexion and opposition of digits one through three, flexion of the wrist, and pronation of the forearm and usually occurs at 1- to 2-cm depth (see Fig. 2). Under ultrasound, the median nerve is at

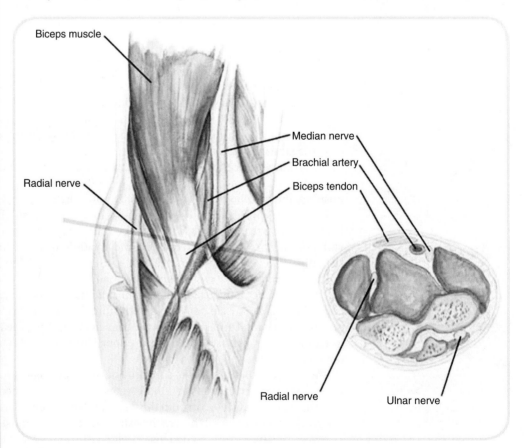

Figure 1. The nerve is medial to the brachial artery.

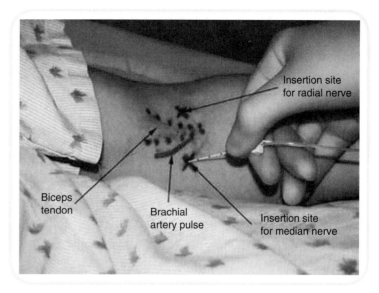

Insertion site
for radial nerve

Biceps
tendon

Brachial
artery pulse

Insertion site
for median nerve

Figure 2. Anterior elbow approach using nerve stimulation. (Courtesy of http://www.arapmi.org/maraa-book-project/Chapt11.pdf.)

approximately 1 to 2 cm depth and medial to the brachial artery and tendon of the biceps brachii muscle. At the level of the elbow and forearm, approximately 5 to 7 mL of local anesthetic should be adequate to block the nerve.

SUGGESTED READINGS

Barash PG, Cullen BF, Stoelting RK, et al, eds. *Clinical Anesthesia*. 6th ed. Philadelphia, PA: Lippincott Williams & Wilkins; 2009:977–979.
Longnecker DE, Brown DL, Newman MF, et al, eds. *Anesthesiology*. New York, NY: McGraw-Hill; 2008:1032–1034.
Morgan GE, Mikhail MS, Murray MJ. *Clinical Anesthesiology*. 4th ed. New York, NY: McGraw-Hill; 2006:334–337.

Beta Thalassemia: Newborn

Organ-based Clinical: Hematologic

Gabriel Jacobs

Edited by Mamatha Punjala

1. Beta thalassemia is a disorder involving defective production of the globin chains on the hemoglobin molecule found on chromosomes 11 and 16.
2. Anemia caused by beta thalassemia is secondary to underhemoglobinized cells (diminished oxygen transport) and/or truncated red blood cell life span.
3. Thalassemia minor is associated with microcytic anemia, which causes modest anemia even though up to 50% of the globin chain production is affected.
4. Thalassemia intermedia symptoms are caused by the anemia itself and by organ dysfunction such as hepatosplenomegaly, cardiomegaly, bone marrow proliferation, and skeletal muscle changes.
5. Thalassemia major can be a life-threatening condition at a very early age, and patients are transfusion dependent. Clinical manifestations usually present between 6 and 9 months, as hemoglobin F production stops and hemoglobin alpha increases.

Beta thalassemia is a disorder that involves the defective production of globin chains of the hemoglobin molecule. The genes for the globin chains are found on chromosomes 11 and 16. In adults, the majority of mature globin molecules consist of two alpha chains and two beta chains that come together to form a tetramer. Thalassemia can be alpha or beta, depending on which chain is defective. Beta thalassemia is most common in Mediterranean countries, Southeast Asia, and areas of Africa. The anemia caused by Beta thalassemia is developed through two mechanisms: underhemoglobinized cells (diminished oxygen transport) and truncated red blood cell life span secondary to excess alpha chains that bind and precipitate, causing membrane damage and cell death. Beta thalassemias can be divided by the severity of clinical symptoms.

Thalassemia Minor
Patients who are heterozygous for either the alpha or the beta mutation can have thalassemia minor. The associated microcytic anemia is modest even though up to 50% of the globin chain production is affected.

Thalassemia Intermedia
In regard to genotype, these patients tend to have beta thalassemia with high levels of hemoglobin F, a combined alpha and beta thalassemia, or a milder form of homozygous beta thalassemia. Clinically, thalassemia intermedia is more severe than thalassemia minor. Symptoms are brought on by the anemia itself and organ dysfunction (hepatosplenomegaly, cardiomegaly, bone marrow proliferation, and skeletal muscle changes).

Thalassemia Major
Thalassemia major can be a life-threatening condition at a very early age. Patients are transfusion dependent. Clinical manifestations of thalassemia major usually present between 6 and 9 months, as hemoglobin F production stops and hemoglobin alpha increases. Transfusion therapy not only helps with correcting the anemia (hemoglobin levels between 3 and 6 g per dL), but also helps ameliorate secondary physiologic derangements brought on

by excess erythropoietin. However, in heavily transfused patients, cardiac disease caused by iron overload and secondary hemochromatosis is a major source of mortality.

Anesthetic Considerations

Anesthetic considerations should be focused on the severity of the anemia and managing any associated organ dysfunction such as congestive heart failure, hepatomegaly, and skeletal muscle damage. Liver failure, endocrinopathies, and right-sided heart failure secondary to associated iron overload should also be considered when making an anesthetic plan. In the setting of a neonatal ICU, citrate toxicity, leukocytosis, transfusion reactions, and platelet sensitization should be kept in mind when transfusing large volumes.

SUGGESTED READINGS

Hines R, Marschall K. *Stoelting's Anesthesia and Co-Existing Disease.* 5th ed. Philadelphia, PA: Saunders; 2008:414–415.

Kumar V. *Robbins and Cotran Pathologic Basis of Disease.* 7th ed. Philadelphia, PA: Elsevier Saunders; 2005:632–634.

Miller RD. *Miller's Anesthesia.* 6th ed. Philadelphia, PA: Elsevier Churchill Livingstone; 2000:2482–2483.

Bicarbonate Admin: CO$_2$ Effect and CO$_2$ Transport

Physiology

Jinlei Li and James Shull

Edited by Ala Haddadin

KEY POINTS

1. The majority of carbon dioxide is transported in the blood in the form of bicarbonate.
2. Bicarbonate is formed from the dissociation of H$_2$CO$_3$ formed in a reaction between carbon dioxide and water in red blood cells.
3. Bicarbonate administration will result in an increase in expired CO$_2$, as well as blood gas CO$_2$ measurements.
4. Bicarbonate administration during resuscitation attempts has not been shown to improve outcomes. Rather, metabolic abnormalities associated with its administration have worsened outcomes.
5. Current clinical recommendations restrict the administration of bicarbonate during resuscitation to patients having significant hyperkalemia, severe metabolic acidosis, or phenobarbital or tricyclic overdose.
6. In select situations, bicarbonate should be administered judiciously, dosed at 1 mEq per kg as needed according to blood pH measurements.

DISCUSSION

Bicarbonate/carbon dioxide is a major buffer system in the body. Carbon dioxide exists in three forms, which include dissolved carbon dioxide, bicarbonate, and carbamino compounds.

Bicarbonate accounts for 85% to 90% of total carbon dioxide in the blood, providing the primary means of transport of CO$_2$ to the lungs for elimination. In tissue capillaries, plasma CO$_2$ enters the erythrocytes and is converted to bicarbonate by carbonic anhydrase. In pulmonary capillaries, bicarbonate is converted back to CO$_2$ by the same enzyme. CO$_2$ is transported across the erythrocyte membrane in exchange for a chloride anion (known as the "chloride shift"), which maintains the electrical gradient. Following administration of bicarbonate, an increased concentration of CO$_2$ will be exhaled during ventilation, resulting in a higher EtCO$_2$ and PaCO$_2$/PvCO$_2$.

Bicarbonate is commonly administered during cardiopulmonary resuscitation (CPR) to supposedly buffer the acidosis arising from CO$_2$ buildup in tissues during asystole and low flow states. However, studies have not shown improved outcomes when bicarbonate was administered during CPR. Rather, bicarbonate administration during resuscitation has been associated with hyperosmolarity, hypernatremia, and metabolic alkalosis, which in turn are associated with poor outcomes.

Current clinical recommendations restrict the administration of bicarbonate during resuscitation to patients having significant hyperkalemia, severe metabolic acidosis, or phenobarbital or tricyclic overdose. In these instances, bicarbonate should be administered judiciously, dosed at 1 mEq per kg as needed according to blood pH measurements.

SUGGESTED READINGS

Barash PG, Cullen BF, Stoelting RK, et al, eds. *Clinical Anesthesia*. 6th ed. Philadelphia, PA: Lippincott Williams & Wilkins; 2009:1513.

Morgan GE, Mikhail MS, Murray MJ, eds. *Clinical Anesthesiology*. 4th ed. New York, NY: McGraw-Hill; 2006:537–570.

Bilat Carotid Endart: Physiology
Physiology

Ervin Jakab

Edited by Shamsuddin Akhtar

1. The carotid bodies are areas of specialized tissue located near the bifurcation of the carotid arteries that contain peripheral chemoreceptors that monitor changes in blood PaO_2 and $PaCO_2$.
2. When PaO_2 drops below 60 mm Hg, the carotid bodies increase their signals to the medullary respiratory center, causing an increase in minute ventilation.
3. Bilateral carotid endarterectomy is associated with the following:
   a. Loss of normal ventilaton responses to acute hypoxia
   b. Loss of arterial pressure responses to acute hypotension
   c. Increased resting partial pressure of arterial carbon dioxide

DISCUSSION

The carotid bodies are areas of specialized tissue located near the bifurcation of the carotid arteries. They are fast-responding monitors of the arterial blood, responding to a fall in blood PaO_2, rise in blood $PaCO_2$ or H^+ ion concentration, or fall in their perfusion rate. CO_2 affects respiratory drive mainly by central mechanisms, but PaO_2 regulation is highly dependent on the carotid body chemoreceptors. When PaO_2 drops below 60 mm Hg, the carotid bodies increase their signals to the medullary respiratory center, causing an increase in minute ventilation. Carotid bodies also serve indirectly as peripheral baroreceptors for blood pressure. As mean arterial pressure drops under 80 mm Hg, the carotid bodies perceive it as a drop in PaO_2 and signal the medullary centers to increase minute ventilation and blood pressure.

Bilateral carotid endarterectomy may abolish compensatory hyperventilation and cause hypoxemia. Also, bilateral carotid body resection may preclude compensatory ventilation when hypoxemia develops. However, it has been reported that, in patients who underwent bilateral carotid body resection for asthma, the ventilatory response to increased $PaCO_2$ was reduced, but hypoventilation did not occur. Because of this, medications that depress respiratory drive should be avoided in the immediate postoperative period.

SUGGESTED READINGS

Barash PG, Cullen BF, Stoelting RK, et al, eds. *Clinical Anesthesia*. 6th ed. Philadelphia, PA: Lippincott Williams & Wilkins; 2009:1117.

Crapo JD, Glassroth J, Karlinsky JB, et al. *Baum's Textbook of Pulmonary Disease*. 7th ed. Philadelphia, PA: Lippincott William & Wilkins; 2004:1272.

Lumb AB. *Nunn's Applied Respiratory Physiology*. 6th ed. Philadelphia, PA: Elsevier; 2005:63.

Miller RD, Eriksson LI, Fleisher LA, et al, eds. *Miller's Anesthesia*. 7th ed. Philadelphia, PA: Churchill Livingstone; 2010:2033.

Blood–Brain Barrier: Fluid Transfer

Physiology

Rongjie Jiang

Edited by Ramachandran Ramani

KEY POINTS

1. The blood–brain barrier is formed by tight junctions that prevent large molecules and most ions from entering the brain.
2. Fluid transfer is mainly determined by the osmolar gradient between plasma and the brain. Both hypertonic saline and mannitol can reduce brain edema by increasing serum osmolality and promoting fluid shift out of the brain.
3. Medications that cross the blood–brain barrier need to meet certain criteria. They need to be small molecules, have a low degree of ionization, need to be unbound from any plasma protein, and have high lipid solubility. The direction of movement is determined by the concentration gradient between plasma and the brain.

DISCUSSION

The presence of the tight junctions in the blood–brain barrier results in a fluid transfer mainly determined by the osmolar gradient. This makes osmotic diuresis possible. When there is no externally administered substance such as mannitol, the serum osmolality is calculated using the following formula:

$$\text{Serum osmolality} = (\text{Serum Na}) \times 2 + \text{Glucose}/18 + \text{BUN}/2.8$$

Because most people have relatively stable glucose and blood urea nitrogen (BUN), the serum sodium concentration becomes the key factor in determination of the serum osmolality.

There is evidence to suggest that the integrity of the blood–brain barrier is not purely anatomical. It is also energy dependent. Ischemia can damage the blood–brain barrier. In the presence of brain edema, the choice of intravenous (IV) fluids becomes critical. The following table shows sodium content and osmolality in commonly used IV fluids. This explains why hypotonic solutions should be avoided when brain edema is concerned and why hypertonic saline and mannitol can be used to reduce brain edema in acute settings.

Fluid	Osmolality (mOsm/kg)	Na$^+$ (mEq/L)
Plasma	289	141
Crystalloid		
0.9% NS	308	154
0.45% NS	154	77
3% NS	1,030	515
Lactated Ringer's	273	130
Plasma-Lyte	295	140
Mannitol (20%)	1,098	0
Colloid		
Hetastarch (6%)	310	154
Albumin (5%)	290	

Any particle that crosses the blood–brain barrier needs to be a small molecule, have a low degree of ionization, be unbound from any plasma protein, and have high lipid solubility. The direction of the movement is determined by the concentration gradient between plasma and the brain. The same rules apply to medications that have CNS effects.

Miller RD. *Miller's Anesthesia.* 7th ed. Philadelphia, PA: Elsevier, Churchill, and Livingstone; 2009:322, 731, 2903.

SUGGESTED READING

Botox: Pain Relief Mechanism
Subspecialties: Pain

Archer Martin

Edited by Thomas Halaszynski

1. Botulinum toxin type A (Botox) is useful in low doses for treatment of many chronic pain conditions including myofascial pain syndrome, fibromyalgia, and hand dystonia.
2. Botulinum toxin in low doses for treatment of pain conditions works primarily through chemical denervation of the muscle. Muscle spasms are primarily responsible for the above syndromes.
3. Botox produces partial chemical denervation of the muscle, resulting in a localized reduction in muscle activity, therefore reducing pain.

In certain conditions, chronic pain may be a result of muscles that are continuously being stressed or continuously and repeatedly contracted. Due to this state of contraction and increased muscle tone, blood flow to the individual muscles may be reduced, allowing byproducts of normal metabolism to remain locally. Secondary to the decreased blood supply along with byproducts of metabolism that are not being diffused away, this may stimulate pain receptors in the distribution effected as the metabolic contaminants accumulate.

Botox blocks neuromuscular transmission by binding to acceptor sites on motor or sympathetic nerve terminals. The Botox enters the nerve terminals and inhibits the release of acetylcholine. This inhibition occurs as the neurotoxin cleaves SNAP-25, which is a protein integral to the successful docking and release of acetylcholine from vesicles situated within nerve endings. When injected intramuscularly, at therapeutic doses, Botox produces partial chemical denervation of the muscle, resulting in a localized reduction in muscle activity. In addition, the muscle may atrophy, axonal sprouting may occur, and extrajunctional acetylcholine receptors may develop. There is also evidence that reinnervation of the muscle may occur, thus slowly reversing muscle denervation produced by Botox.

Botulinum toxin's (type A) mechanism of action is that once it becomes absorbed inside the cell, it acts as a zinc-dependent endoprotease to cleave polypeptides that are vital to exocytosis of cholinergic vesicles. As a result of this process, the nerve can no longer transmit impulses via release of acetylcholine. Therefore, the neuromuscular junction becomes defunct, and the muscles that rely on impulses for contraction are now permitted to rest.

The pain relief attained by the injection of the toxin into the muscles is maintained until the nerve that innervates the muscle is able to form new synaptic contacts, thus restoring the integrity of the neuromuscular junction.

Simpson LL. Botulinum toxin: a deadly poison sheds its negative image. *Ann Intern Med.* 1996;125(7):616–617.
Subin B, Saleemi S, Morgan GA, et al. Treatment of chronic low back pain by local injection of botulinum toxin-A. *Internet Pain Symptom Control Palliat Care.* 2003;2(2).

Bowel Distention

Physiology

Roberto Rappa

Edited by Lars Helgeson

1. Bowel distention is a pathologic state that may be precipitated by a variety of clinical conditions.
2. Use of nitrous oxide is best avoided during abdominal procedures, especially in the setting of bowel obstruction and/or ischemia.
3. Nitrous oxide is approximately 31 times more soluble in blood than is nitrogen and has the ability to readily diffuse into closed gas spaces.
4. The diffusion of nitrous oxide into closed gas spaces continues until it equilibrates with alveolar air.
5. Inhaling a 75% nitrous oxide gas mixture may result in a 4-fold increase in intracavitary volume, whereas inhaling a 50% nitrous oxide mixture may only double a gas-filled space.

Bowel distention is a pathologic state that may be precipitated by a variety of clinical conditions. It is most often seen in the setting of mechanical or functional obstruction of the intestine.

General anesthesia produces a number of physiologic changes in the human body. The degree and extent of those changes are dependent on interpatient variability and the type of anesthetic utilized. Age, medical pathology, and genetic susceptibility all influence the physiologic parameters of anesthetized patients. Use of nitrous oxide is best avoided during abdominal procedures, especially in the setting of bowel obstruction and/or ischemia. To minimize nitrous oxide–induced distention, lower concentrations of nitrous oxide for shorter periods of time can be used.

Nitrous oxide has the ability to readily diffuse into closed gas spaces. A number of closed gas spaces exist within the human body. These spaces can be either absolute or potential and differ by the relative compliance of their surrounding walls. Examples of highly compliant closed gas spaces include the bowel, intrapleural space, and intraperitoneal compartment. These spaces can accommodate large volumes of gas with minimal changes in intracavitary pressures. In contrast, the structures of the middle ear and intraocular space are generally noncompliant. In fact, the diffusion of even small amounts of gas may cause dramatic increases in intracavitary pressure.

The blood–gas partition coefficient is directly responsible for the rate of transfer and subsequent diffusion of gases into closed gas filled spaces. These spaces eventually equilibrate with alveolar air. Nitrogen is the predominant component.

The blood–gas partition coefficient for nitrogen (0.015) is significantly less than that of nitrous oxide (0.468). Nitrous oxide is approximately 31 times more soluble in blood than is nitrogen. Physiologically, this means that nitrous oxide diffuses into closed gas spaces much quicker than nitrogen does. This difference leads to the increased volume and pressure of closed gas spaces with nitrous oxide use.

The diffusion of nitrous oxide into closed gas spaces continues until it equilibrates with alveolar air. As a result, the degree to which nitrous oxide expands closed gas spaces is proportional to its concentration in alveolar air, its duration of administration, and the amount of air already present in the closed gas space. For example, inhaling a 75% nitrous oxide gas mixture may result in a 4-fold increase in intracavitary volume, whereas inhaling a 50% nitrous oxide mixture may only double a gas-filled space.

SUGGESTED READINGS

Barash PG, Cullen BF, Stoelting RK, eds. *Clinical Anesthesia*. 5th ed. Philadelphia, PA: Lippincott Williams & Wilkins; 2006:1053–1071.

Eger EI II. Inhaled anesthetics: uptake and distribution. In: Miller RD, Eriksson LI, Fleisher LA, et al, eds. *Miller's Anesthesia*. 7th ed. Philadelphia, PA: Churchill Livingstone; 2009.

B

Brachial Artery Catheter: Cx
Generic, Clinical Sciences: Anesthesia Procedures, Methods, Techniques

Marianne Saleeb

Edited by Benjamin Sherman

KEY POINTS

- Some of the complications that arise from a brachial artery catheter are as follows:
  - Kinking due to its location in the antecubital fossa
  - Brachial artery obstructions/thrombosis leading to possible ischemia
  - Paresthesias
  - Microembolization
  - Claudication
  - Pseudoaneurysm
  - Hemorrhage

DISCUSSION

Invasive pressure monitoring may be indicated in patients with cardiovascular disease undergoing a high-risk procedure. Most commonly, the radial artery is cannulated; however, if alternative access is required, one may cannulate the brachial artery.

Some advantages of brachial artery catheterization are as follows:

1. Large and easily identifiable in the antecubital fossa
2. Provides less waveform distortion because of its proximity to the aorta

Despite these advantages, some complications may arise. An indwelling catheter may cause limb ischemia because of obstruction from the catheter, although studies have shown that there is a low incidence of permanent ischemic complications. A thrombus may form with or without embolization, and arterial transection may occur leading to hemorrhage or hematoma. All these aforementioned complications may ultimately lead to claudication. Finally, instrumentation of the artery may create a pseudoaneurysm. In view of the many potential complications, it is not common practice to use the brachial artery for invasive monitoring.

SUGGESTED READINGS

Lipchik EO, Sugimoto H. Percutaneous brachial artery catheterization. *Radiology.* 1986;160:842–843.
Moran KT, Halpin DP, Zide RS, et al. Long-term brachial artery catheterization: ischemic complications. *J Vasc Surg.* 1988;8(1):76–78.

Bradycardia: Carotid Surgery and Carotid Stent

Organ-based Clinical: Cardiovascular and Generic, Clinical Sciences: Anesthesia Procedures, Methods, Techniques

Emilio Andrade and Svetlana Sapozhnikova

Edited by Qingbing Zhu

B

1. The carotid sinus baroreceptor resides in the carotid bifurcation.
2. Bradycardia may result from stimulation of the vagal nerve during manipulation of the carotid sinus.
3. Cessation of manipulation and infiltration of local anesthetic restores the hemodynamics.
4. Intraoperative management of bradycardia includes infiltration of the carotid bifurcation with a local anesthetic by a surgeon, cessation of traction on the carotid sinus, and administration of an anticholinergic medication such as atropine.

DISCUSSION

Carotid artery stenosis can be repaired with carotid endarterectomy as well as with endovascular carotid stenting. During carotid surgery, manipulation of the carotid sinus may result in hypotension and bradycardia. Bradycardia and hypotension have been seen in up to 68% of patients undergoing endovascular carotid stenting. Hypovolemia can worsen these symptoms. A decrease in baroreceptor stimulation during carotid artery cross-clamping can result in tachycardia and hypertension.

The carotid sinus baroreceptor is found in the adventitia of the carotid bifurcation. Stimulation of the sinus sends afferent impulses through the glossopharyngeal nerve to the vasomotor center in the medulla (Fig. 1). This causes inhibition of the central sympathetic activity, causing bradycardia and hypotension. Inactivation of the sinus produces a reverse effect.

If bradycardia occurs, ask the surgeon to reduce or release traction on the carotid bifurcation. Administration of an anticholinergic drug, such as atropine, may be necessary for resolution of the bradycardic episode. Some surgeons infiltrate the carotid bifurcation prophylactically with a local anesthetic to avoid the hemodynamic instability; however, caution is advised, as this action may result in both intraoperative and postoperative hypertension.

96

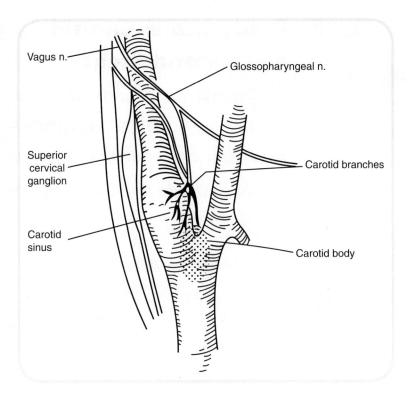

Figure 1. Illustration of carotid sinus and carotid body. The nerve of Hering courses toward the glossopharyngeal nerve. (From Rutherford RB. *Vascular Surgery.* 6th ed. Philadelphia, PA: Elsevier Saunders; 2005:2073–2074, with permission.)

Barash PG, Cullen BF, Stoelting RK, et al, eds. *Clinical Anesthesia.* 6th ed. Philadelphia, PA: Lippincott Williams & Wilkins; 2009:1120–1121.

Jenkins L, Wong D. *Anaesthetic Management of Carotid Endarterectomy.* London, UK: Lloyd-Luke (Medical Books) Ltd.; 1987:136–137, 157.

Longnecker DE, Brown DL, Newman MF, et al. *Anesthesiology.* New York, NY: McGraw-Hill; 2008.

Miller RD, Eriksson LI, Fleisher LA, et al. *Miller's Anesthesia.* 7th ed. Philadelphia, PA: Churchill Livingstone; 2010:2029.

Morgan GE, Michael NS, Murray MJ. *Clinical Anesthesiology.* 4th ed. New York, NY: McGraw-Hill; 2006:629.

Rutherford RB. *Vascular Surgery.* 6th ed. Philadelphia, PA: Elsevier Saunders; 2005:2073–2074.

Yastrebov K. Intraoperative management. *Anesthesiol Clin North Am.* 2004;22(2):276.

Brain Death Pathophysiology
Subspecialties: Critical Care

Neil Sinha

Edited by Ramachandran Ramani

KEY POINTS

1. Brain death is the irreversible cessation of all brain function.
2. The first signs of imminent brain death manifest as the Cushing reflex and are followed by the "autonomic storm."
3. Anaerobic metabolism is increased, as evidenced by hyperglycemia and increased lactate levels in the circulation.

DISCUSSION

Brain death is a legal definition that refers to the irreversible cessation of all cerebral and brain stem function. The clinical criteria for brain death include:

- Coma, defined as the absence of response to any stimulus including movement, withdrawal, grimace, or blinking.
- A negative apnea test: the absence of spontaneous breathing efforts when the patient is disconnected from the ventilator with a $PaCO_2$ greater than 60 or 20 mm Hg above baseline. (This test is typically done last, as it may increase intracranial pressure.)
- Pupils dilated and unresponsive to light.
- The absence of brainstem reflexes including pupillary, oculovestibular, gag, cough (in response to tracheal suction), and corneal reflexes, as well as loss of caloric responses.

Before establishing the diagnosis of brain death, reversible medical conditions, including severe electrolyte or endocrine disorders, severe hypothermia (core temperature ≤32° C), hypotension, drug intoxication, poisoning, or the presence of neuromuscular blocking agents must be ruled out. In patients older than 18 years, confirmatory testing (including cerebral angiography, electroencephalogram, transcranial Doppler ultrasonography, and cerebral scintigraphy) is not necessary, but could be used to confirm the diagnosis.

The pathophysiology of brain death is a complex process, and the changes that occur are a function of time. The first signs of imminent brain death manifest as the bradycardia, with transient hypotension, and an irregular respiratory pattern; this is followed by the "autonomic storm" presenting with tachycardia, hypertension, vasoconstriction, and elevated levels of catecholamines in the plasma (before herniation). Direct cellular injury is a result of a cycle of the absence of blood flow and hypoxia resulting in cerebral acidosis and endothelial swelling of the brain; herniation and aseptic necrosis of the brain follow.

At this point, anaerobic metabolism is increased, as evidenced by hyperglycemia and increased lactate levels in the circulation. These changes maximally affect mitochondria. In addition, there is disruption of the hypothalamic–pituitary axis, resulting in a fall in the levels of antidiuretic hormone, insulin, cortisol, and thyroid hormones. There is also an increased expression of major histocompatibility complex (MHC) antigens, upregulation of cytokines and lymphokines, and an increased expression of cell adhesion molecules.

Microscopically, there is necrosis throughout the nervous tissue, with foci located in the brainstem and the cerebellum. On gross examination, the brain reveals a congested cerebral cortex, generalized swelling, swollen pituitary, and a macerated cerebellum.

SUGGESTED READINGS

Marshall VC. Pathophysiology of brain death: effects on allograft function. *Transplant Proc.* 2001;33(1–2):845–846.

Wijdicks Eelco FM. The diagnosis of brain death. *N Engl J Med.* 2001;344:1215–1221.

Bronchial Blocker: Advantages

Generic Clinical Sciences: Anesthesia Procedures, Methods, Techniques

Ashley Kelley

Edited by Veronica Matei

KEY POINTS

1. Bronchial blockers are an alternative to double-lumen tubes (DLTs) when one-lung ventilation is required or requested for surgery.
2. Bronchial blockers are used with single-lumen endotracheal tubes and may be preferable and easier to place than DLTs in patients with a known or suspected difficult airway.
3. Use of a bronchial blocker negates the need to exchange a DLT for a single-lumen tube at the conclusion of the surgical procedure.

DISCUSSION

Options for lung isolation when one-lung ventilation is required or requested for surgery include DLTs or bronchial blockers. Bronchial blockers are used with single-lumen endotracheal tubes. The choice of a DLT or a bronchial blocker must be tailored to the specific patient and surgical conditions.

In patients with known or suspected difficult airways, the safest option may be to perform an awake fiberoptic intubation with a single-lumen endotracheal tube and subsequently place a bronchial blocker to allow for lung isolation. The relatively larger external diameter and size of a DLT compared with a single-lumen tube may make it harder to place, especially in a patient with a difficult airway. Another advantage of a bronchial blocker used with a single-lumen tube is that the bronchial blocker can be removed through the endotracheal tube at the completion of the surgical procedure, negating the need to exchange a DLT after fluid shifts and airway edema may have occurred.

One disadvantage of using a bronchial blocker is that a relatively high pressure is needed to fully inflate the balloon at the distal tip of the blocker. This pressure may cause the blocker to slip out of the mainstem bronchus and instead obstruct the trachea or allow spillage of contents from one lung to the other. Another disadvantage of a bronchial blocker is that the channel within the blocker that allows the lung to deflate is small compared with the lumen of a DLT, thus making deflation of the desired lung slower.

SUGGESTED READINGS

Barash PG, Cullen BF, Stoelting RK, et al, eds. *Clinical Anesthesia*. 6th ed. Philadelphia, PA: Lippincott Williams & Wilkins; 2009:1048–1051.

Morgan GE, Mikhail MS, Murray MJ. *Clinical Anesthesiology*. 4th ed. New York, NY: McGraw-Hill; 2006:592–594.

Bronchopleural Fistula: Vent Mgmt
Organ-based Clinical: Respiratory

Dallen Mill

Edited by Veronica Matei

1. A bronchopleural fistula (BPF) is a communication between the main or segmental bronchi and the pleural space. Causes of BPF include trauma, iatrogenic insult, alveolar injury from ARDS, or erosion from carcinoma or an inflammatory process.
2. Positive pressure ventilation (PPV) should be avoided whenever possible so as to minimize the risk of developing air leak and tension pneumothoraces and allow for healing of the BPF.
3. Lung separation is indicated for acute, large, or infection-associated BPFs.
4. The lowest minute ventilation and mean intrathoracic pressure tolerated by the patient should be employed when mechanical ventilation is required.
5. High-frequency oscillatory ventilation (HFOV) and high-frequency jet ventilation (HFJV) for management of BPF have been described, but with questionable benefit particularly in patients with underlying lung disease.

DISCUSSION

BPF is an air leak resulting from direct communication between the main or segmental bronchi and the pleural space. The most common causes of BPF include blunt or penetrating chest trauma, iatrogenic insult (e.g., pneumonectomy and barotrauma), alveolar injury associated with acute respiratory distress syndrome (ARDS), and bronchi erosion secondary to carcinoma or inflammatory processes.

Spontaneous respiration is the preferred mode of ventilation in patients with BPFs. When PPV is required, the lowest minute ventilation and mean intrathoracic pressure tolerated by the patient should be employed. The former may require a degree of permissive hypercapnia and the latter, the avoidance of both ventilator administered positive end expiratory pressure (PEEP) and intrinsic PEEP. Peak and plateau airway pressures should be minimized. Table 1 describes additional principles of ventilator management in patients with BPF.

Several risks are associated with the use of PPV in the setting of BPF. Tension pneumothoraces constitute the greatest of these risks and necessitate chest tube placement before initiating mechanical ventilation. PPV can also increase the amount of air leak from the breathing circuit. Compensating for air leak by increasing minute ventilation should be avoided for two reasons: (1) lost volume participates in ventilation and (2) increased minute ventilation leads to increased air leak. Another significant implication of air leak is disruption of healing and thus perpetuation or worsening of the air leak.

In certain settings, lung isolation may be desirable. If the BPF is acute, a double-lumen tube (DLT) may be appropriate, whereas for a chronic process, lung isolation may not be necessary. The size of the air leak also plays a role in endotracheal tube selection, with a larger leak more likely requiring DLT placement. If an infectious process such as an empyema is associated with the BPF, a DLT can minimize the risk of infectious material spilling over into the unaffected lung. If surgical repair of a BPF is indicated, lung isolation can facilitate the procedure.

HFOV and HFJV for management of BPF have been described, but these modalities have fallen out of favor. In principle, these ventilator settings decrease air leak while avoiding barotrauma to the unaffected lung. Although some evidence suggests a benefit in the setting of BPF resulting from surgical procedures, patients with BPF occurring in the setting of underlying lung disease such as ARDS have done poorly with these alternative modalities.

B

Table 1. Principles of Ventilator Management in the Patient with a Bronchopleural Fistula

- Use the lowest number of mechanical breaths that permits acceptable alveolar ventilation (reduce both mean airway pressure and number of high-pressure breaths).
  - Wean the patient completely if possible.
  - Partial ventilatory support may be preferable to total ventilatory support (e.g., pressure-support ventilation).
  - Avoid or correct respiratory alkalosis (to minimize minute ventilation).
  - Unless contraindicated, consider the use of permissive hypercapnia to reduce minute ventilation by allowing $PaCO_2$ to rise.
- Limit effective (returned) tidal volume to <6–8 mL/kg.
- Minimize inspiratory time.
  - Keep inspiration:expiration ratio low (e.g., 1:2).
  - Use high inspiratory flow (e.g., 70–100 L/min).
  - Avoid end-inspiratory pause and inverse ratio ventilation.
  - Use low-compressible-volume ventilator circuit to minimize delivered tidal volume.
- Minimize both dialed-in and endogenous positive end-expiratory pressure.
- Use the least amount of chest tube suction that maintains lung inflation.
- Explore positional differences; avoid placing the patient in positions that exacerbate leak.
- Treat bronchospasm and other causes of expiratory airflow obstruction.
- Consider specific or unconventional measures (e.g., independent lung ventilation and endobronchial measures) if the patient remains unstable or develops clinically harmful, uncorrectable respiratory acidosis despite the above measures.
- Treat the underlying cause of respiratory failure, maintaining nutritional and other support, with the goal of discontinuing mechanical ventilation as soon as possible.

Reproduced from Pierson DJ. Barotrauma and bronchopleural fistula. In: Tobin MJ, ed. *Principles and Practice of Mechanical Ventilation.* 2nd ed. New York, NY: McGraw-Hill; 2006:943–963.

SUGGESTED READINGS

Miller RD, ed. Anesthesia for thoracic surgery. In: *Miller's Anesthesia.* 7th ed. Philadelphia, PA: Elsevier; 2008:1866–1867.

Nicotera SP, Decamp MM. Special situations: air leak after lung volume reduction surgery and in ventilated patients. *Thorac Surg Clin.* 2010;20:427–434.

Pierson DJ. Barotrauma and bronchopleural fistula. In: Tobin MJ, ed. *Principles and Practice of Mechanical Ventilation.* 2nd ed. New York, NY: McGraw-Hill; 2006:943–963.

Tobin MJ. *Principles and Practice of Mechanical Ventilation.* Blacklick, OH: McGraw-Hill Professional Publishing; 2006:958.

Bronchospasm: Mechanical Ventilation Dx

Organ-based Clinical: Respiratory

B

Garth Skoropowski

Edited by Veronica Matei

KEY POINTS

1. Signs of bronchospasm include desaturation, **wheezing**, diminished breath sounds, prolonged expiration, **increased airway pressures**, rising end-tidal CO_2, and reduction in tidal volumes.
2. If a laryngeal mask airway (LMA) is being used, consider aspiration as a cause of bronchospasm.
3. Initial management steps include providing 100% oxygen and deepening anesthesia.
4. When initial treatment of bronchospasm fails, consider pneumothorax or pulmonary edema.

DISCUSSION

Bronchospasm is an important cause of perioperative morbidity that can be a challenge to diagnose. Any patient with a history of asthma, bronchitis, chronic obstructive pulmonary disease, gastroesophageal reflux disease, or heavy smoking is at increased risk for development of bronchospasm.

Although asthma is the most common cause of bronchospasm, there are several disease states that can cause or mimic the signs of bronchospasm. These include anaphylaxis, endobronchial intubation, pneumothorax, mechanical obstruction, right mainstem obstruction, inadequate anesthesia, pulmonary aspiration, pulmonary edema, pulmonary embolism, and an acute asthma attack.

Signs of bronchospasm include desaturation, wheezing, diminished breath sounds, prolonged expiration, increased airway pressures, rising end-tidal CO_2, and reduction in tidal volumes. With anaphylaxis, the above signs may be noted after the development of a rash or hypotension. The initial management of bronchospasm is to provide 100% oxygen, cease stimulation, obtain assistance, and deepen the level of anesthesia.

When performing mask ventilation or using an LMA, aspiration, laryngospasm, and airway obstruction may cause bronchospasm. Administration of muscle relaxants can help differentiate between light anesthesia and bronchospasm. Adding volatile agents may improve bronchospasm, as they can help with smooth muscle relaxation. Potential causes for mechanical obstruction should be ruled out, which can be accomplished with a fiberoptic scope. If bronchospasm is still suspected, treatment with beta-2 agonists followed by corticosteroids can be initiated. If there is still no improvement, then other causes such as pulmonary edema or pneumothorax need to be explored and treated accordingly.

SUGGESTED READINGS

Hepner DL. Sudden bronchospasm on intubation: latex anaphylaxis? *J Clin Anesth.* 2000;12:162–166.

Hines RL, Marshall KE. *Stoelting's Anesthesia and Co-existing Disease.* 5th ed. Philadelphia, PA: Churchill Livingstone; 2008:166–167.

Westhorpe RN, Ludbrook GL, Helps SC. Crisis management during anaesthesia: bronchospasm. *Qual Saf Health Care.* 2005;14:e7.

Bronchospasm Triggers: ETT
Organ-based Clinical: Respiratory

Kellie Park

Edited by Shamsuddin Akhtar

KEY POINTS

1. Bronchospasm occurs commonly in individuals with reactive airways.
2. Endotracheal tube (ETT) placement causes bronchospasm secondary to vagal stimulation.
3. Wheezing may be appreciated with bronchospasm, although in severe cases, no wheezing may be appreciated.
4. The main treatment of bronchospasm is albuterol through the ETT, or, in severe cases, intravenous epinephrine can be used.

DISCUSSION

Bronchospasm occurs most commonly in patients with reactive airway disease, such as in individuals with asthma. These patients are more prone to bronchospasm than normal individuals. There are many causes for increased airway reactivity (neural, humoral, and inflammatory). Parasympathetic stimulation causes bronchospasm, and some patients are predisposed to bronchospasm because they have a hyperreactive airway most likely caused by increased parasympathetic tone. Bronchospasm on placement of an ETT is likely secondary to vagal stimulation. The stimulation of the vagus, which innervates the airway, causes constriction of the bronchioles, via the release of acetylcholine, which stimulates the muscarinic receptors (m_3).

With bronchospasm, airway pressures increase and air trapping occurs. Subsequently, there is an increase in residual volumes. There may be either inspiratory or expiratory wheezes with auscultation. However, if bronchospasm is severe, wheezing may not be appreciated if air movement cannot occur.

Treatment for bronchospasm in the acute setting includes beta-2 agonists, including albuterol, which may be given via the ETT. Epinephrine may also be given in severe cases. Glucocorticoids may have a small effect in the acute setting by decreasing inflammation, but most likely the effects are not fully achieved until hours after administration. Anticholinergics, such as ipratroprium, may also be given through the ETT.

Prevention of bronchospasm is critical. Use of propofol or etomidate is preferred. Ketamine may be used in selected patients because of its propensity to bronchodilate. However, side effects, including lowered seizure threshold and delusions/delirium must be considered. Prior to intubation, administration of intravenous or inhaled lidocaine may reduce the incidence of bronchospasm. Deeping anesthesia with sevoflurane prior to intubation also may be desirable as light anesthesia can lead to bronchospasm. Desflurane is avoided as it is irritating to the airway.

SUGGESTED READINGS

Hurford WE. The bronchospastic patient. *Int Anesthesiol Clin.* 2000;38(1):77–90.

Morgan GE, Mikhail MS, Murray MJ. *Clinical Anesthesiology.* 4th ed. New York, NY: Lange/McGraw-Hill; 2006:573–576.

Stauffer JL, Olson DE, Petty TL. Complications and consequences of endotracheal intubation and tracheotomy. A prospective study of 150 critically ill adult patients. *Am J Med.* 1981;70(1):65–76.

Bupivacaine Toxicity: Rx

Pharmacology

Anjali Vira

Edited by Thomas Halaszynski

Anjali Vira

Edited by Thomas Halaszynski

KEY POINTS

1. Bupivacaine is the most cardiotoxic local anesthetic currently used and may lead to arrhythmias and hemodynamic instability.
2. Bupivacaine toxicity that progresses to cardiac symptoms can prove difficult to treat.
3. The treatment of bupivacaine toxicity is largely supportive, including advanced cardiac life support (ACLS) and mechanical ventilation.
4. An additional new strategy (in addition to no. 2 above) for treatment of bupivacaine toxicity is intravenous administration of a 20% lipid solution.

DISCUSSION

When toxic plasma levels are reached, all local anesthetics may cause central nervous system (CNS) toxicity, initially by producing CNS depression (lower doses) followed by CNS excitation including seizure activity. However, these same local anesthetics are also capable of causing cardiotoxicity. Bupivacaine remains the most cardiotoxic local anesthetic currently used in the United States. When compared with other commonly used local anesthetics, bupivacaine has a very high affinity for cardiac sodium channels and dissociates from them slowly. This phenomenon can lead to cardiac arrhythmias and myocardial depression. Bupivacaine also causes systemic vasodilation, which can quickly lead to hemodynamic instability in the face of a new arrhythmia.

Prevention of bupivacaine toxicity is important as a first step because it is difficult to treat. Aspiration before injection may lower the frequency of inadvertent intravascular injection as well as incremental injection of bolus doses. When using bupivacaine to perform neuraxial anesthesia or a peripheral nerve block, careful monitoring with continuous electrocardiogram, pulse oximetry, and noninvasive blood pressure cuff can aid in early detection of bupivacaine overdose. The maximum dose of bupivacaine that should be used is 3 mg per kg.

When either intravascular injection or an overdose of bupivacaine occurs, treatment is mostly supportive. It is important to ensure satisfactory ventilation and to avoid hypoxia, acidosis, and hypercarbia. If seizures occur, they must be treated quickly because they can exacerbate bupivacaine toxicity by causing hypoxia, hypercarbia, and acidosis. Seizures can be treated with multiple agents including thiopental (50 to 100 mg), propofol (1 mg per kg), and midazolam (2 to 5 mg).

Cardiovascular depression and vasodilation from bupivacaine overdose can lead to hypotension and bradycardia. ACLS should be instituted and continued throughout treatment for, or with, suspected bupivacaine local anesthesia cardiotoxicity. Under the influence of bupivacaine toxicity, an emphasis on adequate ventilation (as discussed above), pharmacologic support of blood pressure (with drugs such as ephedrine), and treatment of ventricular arrhythmias (with drugs such as amiodarone and even with electrical cardioversion) should be entertained. The cardiovascular effects of bupivacaine can be difficult to treat and may require repeated doses of vasoactive and antiarrhythmic drugs; however, resistant dysrhythmias and hypotension may now be treated with a new therapy: 100 cc of 20% lipid emulsion solution (Intralipid). This treatment works in part due to the lipid solubility of bupivacaine. Propofol is not an appropriate lipid solution for this therapy and can actually worsen bupivacaine toxicity by contributing to myocardial depression.

104

B

Local anesthetic systemic toxicity (LAST) and treatment with lipid emulsion therapy (20%):

1. Administer at first signs of LAST, but after airway management.
2. Continue ACLS.
3. Dosing: 1.5 mg per kg of 20% lipid emulsion as a bolus (can be repeated).
4. Infusion after bolus: 0.25 to 0.50 mL/kg/min for at least 10 minutes after circulatory stability.

SUGGESTED READINGS

Barash PG, Cullen BF, Stoelting RK, et al, eds. *Clinical Anesthesia*. 6th ed. Philadelphia, PA: Lippincott Williams & Wilkins; 2009:539–545.
Morgan GE, Mikhail MS, Murray MJ. *Clinical Anesthesiology*. 4th ed. New York, NY: Lange McGraw-Hill; 2006:270–271.

Calcium Chelation: Transfusion
Organ-based Clinical: Hematologic

Laurie Yonemoto

Edited by Qingbing Zhu

KEY POINTS

1. Packed red blood cells (PRBCs) are stored with citrate containing solutions to chelate calcium and prevent premature blood clotting.
2. Citrate is metabolized by the liver into bicarbonate.
3. Neonates, patients with liver dysfunction, or those receiving rapid transfusion may suffer from citrate intoxication or clinically significant hypocalcemia.
4. Signs and symptoms of hypocalcemia include hypotension, prolonged QT interval, widened QRS complexes, flat T waves, and narrow pulse pressures.

DISCUSSION

PRBCs are used to treat anemia with the goal of increasing the oxygen-carrying capacity of blood. PRBCs are prepared by collecting whole blood in bags containing solutions of citrate, phosphate, dextrose, and adenine (CPDA) or citrate, phosphate, and dextrose (CPD). The citrate added to these solutions acts to chelate ionized calcium necessary for clot formation, thus preventing coagulation. Centrifugation then separates the whole blood into components of PRBCs, platelets, cryoprecipitate, and plasma. PRBCs prepared with CPDA have a shelf life of 35 days.

Normally, the citrate in the CPD/CPDA solution is rapidly metabolized by the liver into bicarbonate. It also has the potential to bind to calcium, leading to hypocalcemia. This is usually insignificant because of mobilization of calcium stores from bone and the rapid metabolism of citrate to bicarbonate by the liver. Supplemental calcium may be necessary with rapid administration of PRBCs (volume of transfusion >1 mL per kg) in neonates or in patients with compromised liver function. In these situations, citrate intoxication may occur. The clinical signs and symptoms of citrate intoxication are secondary to hypocalcemia resulting in hypotension, a prolonged QT interval, widened QRS complexes, flat T waves, and narrow pulse pressures.

SUGGESTED READINGS

Barash PG, Cullen BF, Stoelting RK, et al, eds. *Clinical Anesthesia*. 6th ed. Philadelphia, PA: Lippincott Williams & Wilkins; 2009:377–378.
Stoelting RK, Miller RD. *Basics of Anesthesia*. 5th ed. Philadelphia, PA: Elsevier; 2007:359–360.

Calculation: Pulmonary vs. Systemic Vascular Resistance

Organ-based Clinical: Cardiovascular

Martha Zegarra

Edited by Qingbing Zhu

KEY POINTS

1. The basis for the physiologic equation blood pressure (BP) ~ cardiac output (CO) × systemic vascular resistance (SVR) is similar to Ohm's law: $V = I \times R$.
2. SVR or left ventricular afterload can be calculated by SVR = (MAP − CVP)/CO × 80.
3. PVR or right ventricular afterload can be calculated by PVR = (MPAP − PCWP/CO) × 80.

DISCUSSION

The basis for the physiologic equation BP ~ CO × SVR is similar to Ohm's law: $V = I \times R$. Ohm's law states that the pressure in a system is the product of forward flow and resistance to flow in that system, with BP analogous to voltage, CO to current and SVR to resistance.

Rearranging this equation to solve for SVR, we see that SVR, which is commonly equated with left ventricular afterload, can be calculated by dividing BP, or more accurately back pressure (MAP) minus forward pressure (CVP) and then dividing by CO:

$$\text{SVR (dynes} \times \text{seconds per cm}^5) = [(\text{MAP} - \text{CVP})/\text{CO}] \times 80$$

where MAP is mean arterial pressure (mm Hg), CVP is central venous pressure (mm Hg), and CO is cardiac output (L per minute). The constant 80 is added to convert the Wood units to dynes × seconds per cm^5.

In turn, right ventricular afterload is equated clinically with pulmonary vascular resistance (PVR) and can be calculated using the following equation:

$$\text{PVR (dynes} \times \text{seconds per cm}^5) = [(\text{MPAP} - \text{LAP})/\text{CO}] \times 80$$

where MPAP is mean pulmonary arterial pressure, LAP is left atrial pressure (in practice PCWP is substituted as an approximation of LAP), and CO is cardiac output.

SUGGESTED READINGS

Barash PG, Cullen BF, Stoelting RK. *Clinical Anesthesia*. 6th ed. Philadelphia, PA: Lippincott Williams & Wilkins; 2009:165, 706.

Morgan GE, Mikhail MS, Murray MJ. *Clinical Anesthesiology*. 4th ed. New York, NY: Lange Medical Books/McGraw-Hill; 2006:424–425.

Carbamazepine Toxicity
Subspecialities: Pain

Bijal Patel

Edited by Jodi Sherman

1. Carbamazepine is a medication used in the treatment of various disorders such as trigeminal neuralgia, partial and generalized tonic–clonic seizures, and mood disorders.
2. Carbamazepine blocks voltage-gated sodium channels, thereby increasing the time to recovery after cell depolarization.
3. Acute intoxication with carbamazepine may result in stupor, coma, respiratory depression, convulsions, and hyperirritability.
4. Long-term use may result in vertigo, ataxia, blurred vision, diplopia, drowsiness, and water retention leading to hyponatremia and hyposmolality.
5. Severe complications of carbamazepine use include agranulocytosis and aplastic anemia, although the incidence is low.

Carbamazepine is a medication used in the treatment of neurologic disorders such as trigeminal neuralgia, partial and generalized tonic–clonic seizures, and mood disorders. It has a structure similar to tricyclic antidepressants and works through the blockage of voltage-gated sodium channels, thereby increasing the time to recovery after cell depolarization. It also has some antidiuretic effects that may be related to decreased plasma antidiuretic hormone levels. Carbamazepine is broken down into an active metabolite that is subsequently broken down into an inactive form. Several adverse effects are associated with carbamazepine use. With acute intoxication, patients may develop hyperirritability, convulsions, respiratory depression, stupor, or coma. Long-term use may result in vertigo, ataxia, blurred vision, diplopia, and drowsiness. In addition, its long-term use may result in water retention leading to hyponatremia and hyposmolality. Supratherapeutic levels have been found to actually increase seizure activity in some cases. Carbamazepine use may also be associated with agranulocytosis and aplastic anemia, although the incidence is low. A transient leukopenia and thrombocytopenia have been known to occur during initiation of therapy. Other side effects linked to carbamazepine use are nausea, vomiting, a transient transaminitis, and hypersensitivity reactions such as splenomegaly, lymphadenopathy, eosinophilia, and dermatitis.

Finally, there are many drug–drug interactions noted with carbamazepine use. Of note, long-term carbamazepine use may result in decreased sensitivity to neuromuscular blockade with agents such as pancuronium, rocuronium, and vecuronium. In addition, it is known to be an inducer of cytochromes, specifically CYP2C, CYP3A, and UGT, resulting in increased metabolism of certain drugs that are normally broken down by these proteins.

Barash PG, Cullen BF, Stoelting RK, et al, eds. *Clinical Anesthesia.* 6th ed. Philadelphia, PA: Lippincott Williams & Wilkins; 2009:515.
Brunton LL, Lazo JS, Parker KL. *Goodman and Gilman's: The Pharmacological Basis of Therapeutics.* 11th ed. New York, NY: McGraw-Hill; 2006:512–513.

Carcinoid Crisis: Rx
Organ-based Clinical: Endocrine/Metabolic

Kristin Richards

Edited by Mamatha Punjala

1. Treatment of carcinoid crisis is best accomplished with an octreotide infusion; however, if this is unsuccessful, then additional boluses of octreotide may be administered.
2. Carcinoid tumor management includes perioperative blockade of serotonin receptors, special attention to procedures, treatments and drugs that may stimulate release of vasoactive substances from tumor cells, including tumor debulking, hepatic artery embolization, biotherapy, and chemotherapy.
3. Treatments include long-acting somatostatin analogues, anxiolytics to prevent stress-triggered release of serotonin; H1- and H2-blockers to block the effects of histamine; symptomatic therapy (e.g., bronchodilators for wheezing); inhibiting bradykinin with H2-blockers, diphenhydramine, and steroids; and aprotinin (kallikrein inhibitor) to treat hypotension refractory to octreotide.

Carcinoid tumors release vasoactive peptides, which then circulate into the systemic circulation and produce carcinoid syndrome. It occurs in approximately 20% of patients with carcinoid tumors. Clinically, these patients can show signs including cutaneous flushing of the head, neck, and upper thorax; bronchoconstriction; hypotension; hypertension, diarrhea; and carcinoid heart disease. The most effective treatment for carcinoid tumors is complete surgical excision. Biotherapy with interferon and octreotide may reduce tumor bulk and attenuate the release of vasoactive amines.

Management should aim to block histamine and serotonin receptors and to avoid medications that would promote mediator release from tumor cells. For example, opioids and muscle relaxants that release histamine, including succinylcholine, mivacurium, atracurium, and d-tubocurarine, are all medications that can result in mediator release. Epinephrine, norepinephrine, histamine, dopamine, and isoproterenol are also known to provoke carcinoid crises.

Carcinoid crises can be precipitated by physical or chemical factors that can potentially trigger mediator release. Examples include stress, chemotherapy, and succinylcholine-induced fasciculations. All these are possible triggers of mediator release and therefore carcinoid crises.

The most effective treatment of carcinoid crises is octreotide, which is a synthetic octapeptide that mimics the effects of somatostatin. An octreotide infusion starts at a rate of 50 to 100 μg per hour. If more is required, intravenous boluses of 25 to 100 μg can be administered as well. Bradycardia and heart block through an effect on the cardiac conduction system are both potential adverse reactions of bolus doses of octreotide. Aprotinin, a kallikrein inhibitor, may be used for hypotension if there is a refractory response to octreotide.

The majority of the currently available induction agents and muscle relaxants including propofol, etomidate, vecuronium, cis-atracurium, and rocuronium can be used successfully for anesthesia. However, caution is recommended with drugs such as thiopental and succinylcholine that can release histamine. The short-acting synthetic opioids sufentanil, alfentanil, fentanyl, and remifentanil are all acceptable for use.

SUGGESTED READINGS

Barash PB, Cullen BF, Stoelting RK, et al, eds. *Clinical Anesthesia*. 6th ed. Philadelphia, PA: Lippincott Williams & Wilkins; 2009:1227–1228.

Cortinez FLI. Refractory hypotension during carcinoid resection surgery. *Anaesthesia*. 2000;55:505–506.

Dierdorf SF. Carcinoid tumor and carcinoid syndrome. *Curr Opin Anaesthesiol*. 2003;16:343–347.

Dilger JA, Rho EH, Que FG, et al. Octreotide-induced bradycardia and heart block during surgical resection of a carcinoid tumor. *Anesth Analg*. 2004;98:318–320.

Farling PA, Durairaju AK. Remifentanil and anaesthesia for carcinoid syndrome. *Br J Anaesth*. 2004;92:893–895.

C

Cardiac Arrest: Induced Hypothermia
Generic Clinical Sciences: Anesthesia
Procedures, Methods, Techniques

Kimberly Slininger
Edited by Qingbing Zhu

1. Induced hypothermia (32° to 34° C) can improve neurologic outcomes after pulseless ventricular fibrillation (v-fib) or ventricular tachycardia (v-tach) arrest.
2. During cardiac surgery, systemic hypothermia can be given to reduce oxygen requirements and decrease metabolic rate, both serving cardioprotective efforts.
3. The duration of hypothermia should be between 12 and 24 hours.
4. Rewarming should be passive to decrease the risk of releasing accumulated metabolic products into circulation, further myocardial depression, hypotension, and acidosis.

Several studies have shown that induced hypothermia after a v-fib arrest can improve a patient's neurologic outcome. Patients are considered to be eligible for this therapy if they have suffered an out-of-hospital pulseless v-fib or v-tach arrest and remain unresponsive after successful resuscitation. Ideally, induction of hypothermia (goal core temperature of 32° to 34° C) should be initiated within 1 to 2 hours, if patients are intubated and hemodynamically stable after cardiopulmonary resuscitation was started.

Systemic hypothermia is also used for myocardial protection during cardiac surgery. Hypothermia can reduce myocardial oxygen requirements and metabolic rate. It also decreases the release of excitatory neurotransmitter and decreases oxidative phosphorylation. For every 1° C reduction in core body temperature, there is a corresponding 8% decrease in metabolic rate.

Hypothermia can be achieved through active or passive means. Passive hypothermia requires allowing the body to equilibrate with the environment. The speed at which this occurs depends on exposed body surface area and ambient temperature. Most patients during cardiac surgery, however, will require active cooling. This can be done with cooling blankets or other devices designed for this purpose.

The induced hypothermia should last between 12 and 24 hours. Patients should be sedated and receive neuromuscular blocking agents to prevent shivering. Hypothermia can cause metabolic and electrolyte disturbances, which should be monitored. Rewarming of the patient should be allowed to occur passively after the therapeutic duration of hypothermia is over. Passive rewarming decreases the risk of releasing accumulated metabolic products into circulation, further myocardial depression, hypotension, and acidosis.

Barash PG, Cullen BC, Stoelting RK, et al, eds. *Clinical Anesthesia*. 6th ed. Philadelphia, PA: Lippincott Williams & Wilkins; 2009:919, 1089–1090, 1555.

Marino PL. *The ICU Book*. 3rd ed. Philadelphia, PA: Lippincott Williams & Wilkins; 2007:290–291.

Miller RD, Eriksson LI, Fleisher LA, et al, eds. *Miller's Anesthesia*. 7th ed. Philadelphia, PA: Churchill Livingstone Elsevier; 2010:2914.

Cardiac Cycle: ECG

Physiology

Kevan Stanton

Edited by Benjamin Sherman

1. The electrical and mechanical events of the cardiac cycle are closely coupled.
2. Atrial systole occurs from the initiation of the P wave up to the QRS complex.
3. The PR interval represents a delay in the conduction of the electrical impulse through the atrioventricular (AV) node.
4. Ventricular systole begins with the end of the R wave and continues up to the midpoint of the T wave.
5. Ventricular systole consists of three phases—isovolumetric contraction, a rapid ejection, and a reduced ejection.
6. Ventricular diastole also consists of three phases—isovolumetric relaxation, a rapid filling, and a reduced filling.

The cardiac cycle consists of both mechanical and electrical events, repeating itself with every heartbeat. The electrical events, represented on an ECG, and the mechanical events, consisting of chamber filling and ejection, are closely coupled.

The cardiac cycle begins with the initiation of an action potential in the sinoatrial (SA) node, which is propagated throughout both atria, causing atrial contraction and a resultant P wave on the ECG. This atrial systole occurs up to the QRS complex, at which point atrial diastole occurs, along with repolarization of the atria (obscured by the QRS complex). When this signal reaches the AV node, it is further conducted to the ventricles after a delay. This delay is represented on the ECG by the PR interval. After this delay, conduction continues to the His bundle and Purkinje fibers, which results in depolarization of the ventricles, represented on the ECG by the QRS complex. Ventricular systole begins with the end of the R wave on the ECG. The initial phase consists of isovolumetric contraction—the ventricles contract, but sufficient pressure has not been generated to open the pulmonic and aortic valves, resulting in an intraventricular volume that remains unchanged. As the intraventricular pressure builds and overcomes that in the pulmonary artery and aorta, the pulmonic and aortic valves open, respectively. This results initially in a phase of rapid ejection, followed by reduced ejection as the ventricles reach their maximal contractile state.

When the intraventricular pressures fall below those of the pulmonary artery and aorta, the pulmonic and aortic valves close as the ventricles continue to relax, resulting in a phase of isovolumetric relaxation. The beginning of this phase marks the beginning of ventricular diastole and coincides with the peak of the T wave (the T wave representing ventricular repolarization). As the intraventricular pressure falls below that of the intra-atrial pressure, the tricuspid and mitral valves open, resulting in a phase of rapid ventricular filling followed by reduced ventricular filling as the pressure between the atria and the ventricles equilibrates. This cycle then repeats itself with the initiation of SA node depolarization and atrial systole. A summary of these events and their temporal correlation can be seen in Figure 1:

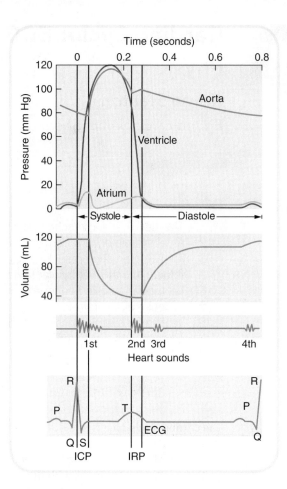

Figure 1. Electrical and mechanical events during the cardiac cycle. (From Barash PG, Cullen BF, Stoelting RK, eds. *Clinical Anesthesia*. 6th ed. Philadelphia, PA: Lippincott Williams & Wilkins; 2009:212.)

SUGGESTED READINGS

Barash PG, Cullen BF, Stoelting RK, eds. *Clinical Anesthesia*. 6th ed. Philadelphia, PA: Lippincott Williams & Wilkins; 2009:211–212.

Boron WF, Boulpaep EL. *Medical Physiology*. 1st ed. Philadelphia, PA: Saunders; 2003:508–519.

Miller RD, Eriksson LI, Fleisher LA, et al, eds. *Miller's Anesthesia*. 7th ed. Philadelphia, PA: Churchill Livingstone; 2010:393–395.

Cardiac Morbidity: Pre-op Factors
Organ-based Clinical: Cardiovascular

Alexander Timchenko

Edited by Benjamin Sherman

c

KEY POINTS

1. Cardiovascular risk factors according to the AHA/ACC guidelines are divided into major, intermediate, and minor predictors of cardiovascular morbidity, including emergency surgery and urgent/elective surgery.
2. Major clinical factors include unstable coronary syndromes, decompensated congestive heart failure (CHF), severe valvular disease, significant arrhythmias, and supraventricular arrhythmias with uncontrolled ventricular rate.
3. Intermediate clinical predictors include mild angina, prior or compensated CHF, previous MI, diabetes, or renal insufficiency with creatinine greater than or equal to 2.0 mg per dL.
4. The revised cardiac risk index is a clinical tool based on a point system to estimate risk of cardiac complications during the perioperative course.

DISCUSSION

Cardiovascular complications account for 25% to 50% of deaths following noncardiac surgery. Perioperative myocardial infarction, pulmonary edema, CHF, arrhythmias, and thromboembolism are most commonly seen in patients with preexisting cardiovascular disease.

Cardiovascular risk factors according to the AHA/ACC guidelines are divided into major, intermediate, and minor predictors of cardiovascular morbidity. The guidelines also describe the following specific situations:

- Emergency surgery—should proceed with surgery with optimal medical management. No risk stratification is performed.
- Urgent/elective surgery with history of coronary revascularization within 5 years—if no recurrent symptoms or signs—proceed with surgery. If recurrent symptoms or signs are present, but stress test or catheterization is favorable—proceed with surgery.
- For all other cases—stratification of risk is performed by clinical predictors (patient factors), surgical risk, and functional capacity as shown below:

Major clinical predictors:

• Unstable coronary syndromes
• Decompensated CHF
• Severe valvular disease
• Significant arrhythmias:
  (a) High-grade AV block
  (b) Symptomatic arrhythmias in the presence of underlying heart disease
  (c) Supraventricular arrhythmias with uncontrolled ventricular rate
	• Consider canceling or delaying surgery
	• Optimize medical management
	• Consider further workup—e.g., cath or cardiology evaluation

Intermediate clinical predictors:

	Functional Capacity <4 METS		Functional Capacity >4 METS	
• Mild angina • Prior or compensated CHF • Prior MI • Diabetes mellitus • Renal insufficiency with creatinine ≥2.0 mg/dL	• Surgical risk: low • Proceed to OR	• Surgical risk: intermediate/high • Noninvasive testing	• Surgical risk: low/intermediate • Proceed to OR	• Surgical risk: high • Noninvasive testing

Minor clinical predictors:

	Functional Capacity <4 METS		Functional Capacity >4 METS
• Advanced age • Rhythm other than sinus • Abnormal ECG (LVH, LBBB, ST-T abnormalities) • Low functional capacity • History of stroke • Uncontrolled systemic HTN	• Surgical risk: low/intermediate • Proceed to OR	• Surgical risk: high • Noninvasive testing	• Any surgical risk • Proceed to OR

At the same time, surgical risk can be divided into:

Low	Intermediate	High
• Endoscopic • Superficial • Breast • Cataract	• Carotid endarterectomy • Intraperitoneal • Intrathoracic • Head and neck • Orthopedic • Prostate	• Emergent surgeries • Major vascular surgeries • Prolonged procedures with extensive fluid shifts or blood loss

There are many clinical tools to estimate risk. The revised cardiac risk index is simple and well validated and provides a reasonable estimate for cardiac complications.

Each of the risk factors below represents 1 point:

- High-risk surgery (intraperitoneal, intrathoracic, suprainguinal vascular)
- History of ischemic heart disease
- History of CHF
- Cerebrovascular disease
- Preoperative insulin use
- Creatinine greater than 2.0 mg per dL

Number of Risk Factors	Risk Class	% Major Cardiac Complications
0	I	0.4
1	II	0.9
2	III	6.6
3 or more	IV	11

Major cardiac complications: MI, pulmonary edema, cardiac arrest, complete heart block.

SUGGESTED READINGS

Fleisher LA, Beckman JA, Brown KA, et al. ACC/AHA 2006 Guideline update on perioperative cardiovascular evaluation.*Circulation.* 2006;113:2662–2674.

Hines RL, Marschall KE, eds. *Anesthesia and Co-existing Disease.* 5th ed. Philadelphia, PA: Saunders Elsevier; 2008:13–16.

Lee TH, Marcantonio ER, Mangione CM, et al. Derivation and prospective validation of a simple index for prediction of cardiac risk of major cardiac surgery. *Circulation.* 1999;100(10):1043–1049.

Cardiac Pacemaker Indications

Organ-based Clinical: Cardiovascular

Ira Whitten

Edited by Qingbing Zhu

KEYWORD

SECTION

C

KEY POINTS

1. Permanent cardiac pacemakers are indicated for a number of arrhythmias, including complete heart block, bifascicular/trifascicular block, sinus node dysfunction, cardiomyopathies, and class III/IV heart failure.
2. The ACC/AHA/HRS guidelines are used to guide pacemaker therapy and divide indications into three classes: class I—definite benefit, class II—possible benefit, and class III—no benefit or evidence of harm.
3. The degree to which the patient is symptomatic, in addition to the specific medical condition requiring a pacer, ultimately determines whether permanent cardiac pacing is indicated.

DISCUSSION

The indications for pacemaker placement have changed since the advent of implantable cardiac pacemakers more than 60 years ago. Early research into and the development of cardiac pacemakers examined their use in complete heart block and bradycardia. Over the years, with the development of new technology, the role of cardiac pacemakers has expanded dramatically to include multiple arrhythmias as well as heart failure.

The two most important factors in determining whether a pacemaker is necessary are (1) whether the patient is symptomatic (as assessed by poor exercise tolerance, fatigue, dizziness, or syncope) and (2) the specific underlying arrhythmia. Permanent cardiac pacers are indicated for the following: atrioventricular (AV) block, bifascicular/trifascicular block, AV block after myocardial infarction, sinus node dysfunction, tachy-brady syndrome, hypersensitive carotid sinus syndrome, anticipated use of beta blockers in pediatric patients with congenital long QT syndromes, obstructive hypertrophic cardiomyopathy, dilated cardiomyopathy, reentrant tachycardias, and refractory class III/IV heart failure.

AV block, categorized as first-, second-, and third-degree AV block on the basis of ECG patterns, is an indication for pacing with the exception of first-degree AV block. Permanent pacing is recommended for second- or third-degree AV block that is either congenital or associated with MI. Syncope as a symptom of AV block or bifascicular/trifascicular block is also an indication for permanent pacing, given the associated high incidence of injury or sudden death. Sinus node dysfunction includes sick sinus or tachy-brady syndrome, sinus arrest, sinus pauses, and any symptomatic bradycardia or sinus node–related syncope. Any bradycardia that consistently causes a heart rate (HR) less than 40 beats per minute (bpm) and results in symptoms should be treated with permanent cardiac pacing. Symptomatic medication–induced dysfunction in which the medication cannot be changed or discontinued also demands placement of a permanent pacer.

Given the many conditions for which permanent pacemakers play an important role in medical management, the American College of Cardiology, the American Heart Association, and the Heart Rhythm Society (ACC/AHA/HRS) published a set of guidelines to guide pacemaker therapy. Indications are divided into three classes: class I—definite benefit, class II—possible benefit, and class III—no benefit or evidence of harm. Class I includes conditions that clearly benefit from pacemaker therapy. Class II indications are conditions where permanent pacing may be beneficial but the evidence is not clear in favor of or against pacing. Class II is divided further into class IIA conditions where the majority of evidence is in favor of pacing and class IIB conditions where the evidence for the efficacy of pacing is not well established. Class III conditions are those where pacing is not indicated and/or may be harmful.

115

C

The following table is an outline of the common conditions in which permanent cardiac pacing may be indicated along with the ACC/AHA/HRS class designation supporting permanent cardiac pacing in those conditions:

Class I indications	• Symptomatic sinus bradycardia • Complete heart block (symptomatic HR <40 bpm, or abnormal left ventricular function) • Advanced second-degree AV block • Symptomatic Mobitz I or Mobitz II • Mobitz II block with intraventricular conduction delay or bifascicular block • Exercise-induced 2nd or 3rd degree AV block • Cardiac resynchronization in atrial fibrillation, class III/IV heart failure
Class IIA indications	• Sinus node dysfunction w/HR <40 bpm w/possible link to symptoms or syncope • Unexplained syncope w/possible sinus node pathology • Congenital long-QT syndrome
Class IIB indications	• HOCM • Refractory AV reentrant SVT
Class III indications	• Transient conduction abnormalities due to infection, drugs, etc. • Asymptomatic 1st degree AV block • Asymptomatic Mobitz type I AV block • Asymptomatic sinus bradycardia

Adapted from Libby P. *Braunwald's Heart Disease: A Textbook of Cardiovascular Medicine.* 8th ed. Philadelphia, PA: Elsevier; 2007:34, 831–841.

SUGGESTED READINGS

Epstein AE, Di Marco JP, Ellenbogen KA, et al. ACC/AHA/HRS 2008 guidelines for device-based therapy of cardiac rhythm abnormalities: a report of the American College of Cardiology/American Heart Association task force on practice guidelines. *Circulation.* 2008;117:350–408.
Kaplan JA. *Essentials of Cardiac Anesthesia.* Philadelphia, PA: Elsevier; 2008:19, 445–447.
Libby P. *Braunwald's Heart Disease: A Textbook of Cardiovascular Medicine.* 8th ed. Philadelphia, PA: Elsevier; 2007:34, 831–841.

Cardiac Tamponade: Pulsus Paradoxus

Organ-based Clinical: Cardiovascular

Brooke Albright

Edited by Benjamin Sherman

KEY POINTS

1. Pulsus paradoxus is a clinical finding associated with pericardial tamponade and is defined as a decrease in systolic blood pressure greater than 10 mm Hg on inspiration.
2. The pericardial space can normally hold 15 to 50 mL of pericardial fluid. Acute fluid accumulation may cause signs and symptoms of cardiac tamponade with as little as 100 mL of fluid, whereas chronic slow accumulation may not be symptomatic until as much as 2 L of fluid accumulate.
3. ECG findings of pericardial effusions may show signs of pericarditis, but classically, a pattern of electrical alternation of the P and QRS waves due to swinging of the heart in the pericardial fluid can be seen.
4. Pericardial effusions can be visualized on echocardiography. Signs of pericardial tamponade on echocardiography include early diastolic collapse of the right ventricle and late diastolic collapse of the right atrium. Pulse Doppler measurements of transmitral blood flow will be decreased during inspiration, whereas transtricuspid flow will be increased during inspiration.
5. Right heart catheterization shows an equalization of right atrial pressures and right ventricular end diastolic pressures. Without this pressure gradient, flow through the heart will be seriously impeded and cardiovascular collapse will ensue.

DISCUSSION

Pulsus paradoxus is a clinical finding associated with pericardial tamponade and is defined as a systolic pressure decrease of greater than 10 mm Hg on inspiration. Depending on the speed of fluid accumulation, pericardial effusions may or may not develop into tamponade. If pericardial fluid rapidly increases and exceeds the ability of the pericardium to stretch and accommodate the fluid, a steep increase in intrapericardial pressure will occur. However, if the fluid accumulates chronically over time, compensatory mechanisms are activated, and the pericardium is allowed to slowly stretch to accommodate the fluid over time; therefore, more volume is accepted before pericardial pressure is exceeded. The steep rise of the pressure–volume curve in acute tamponade explains the "last drop phenomenon," which is when the final "drop" of fluid collected leads to critical cardiac compression, and how the first "drop" of fluid drained produces the largest relative decompression.

Pericardial effusions can be visualized on echocardiography. Signs of pericardial tamponade on echocardiography include early diastolic collapse of the right ventricle and late diastolic collapse of the right atrium. Pulse Doppler measurements of transmitral blood flow will be decreased during inspiration, leading to decreased left ventricular filling and pulsus paradoxus (Figs. 1–3).

Right heart catheterization shows an equalization of right atrial pressures and right ventricular end diastolic pressures. Without this pressure gradient, flow through the heart will be seriously impeded, and cardiovascular collapse will ensue. Some other catheterization findings associated with tamponade are shown below.

- Respiratory reversal of cardiac pressures
- Elevated RA pressure with an X descent, but blunting of the Y descent (panel A, solid arrow)

- LVEDP and PAWP tracings (panel B) show pulsus paradoxus as a result of LV under-filling during inspiration
- **Pulsus paradoxus** greater than 10 mm Hg decrease in systolic pressure on inspiration (refer to Fig. 1, panel A open arrows)

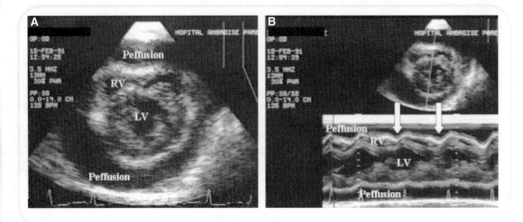

Figure 1. Diastolic collapse of the right ventricle on a parasternal short axis view **(A)**. The use of the time motion study **(B)** allowed detection of the diastolic collapse of the right ventricle *(arrows)* because of the elevation of the pericardial pressure. LV, left ventricle; $P_{effusion}$, pericardial effusion; RV, right ventricle (reused with permission from Bodson L, Bouferrache K, Vieillard-Baron A. Cardiac tamponade. *Curr Opin Crit Care*. 2011;17(5):416–424.)

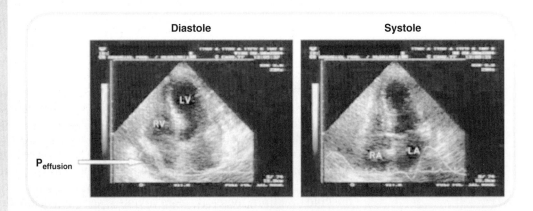

Figure 2. Apical four-chamber view demonstrating a diastolic collapse of the right atrium in a patient with a pericardial effusion. In systole, because of the decrease in pericardial pressure, the right atrium is filling once again. LA, left atrium; LV, left ventricle; $P_{effusion}$, pericardial effusion; RA, right atrium; RV, right ventricle (Reused with permission from Bodson L, Bouferrache K, Vieillard-Baron A. Cardiac tamponade. *Curr Opin Crit Care*. 2011;17(5):416–424.)

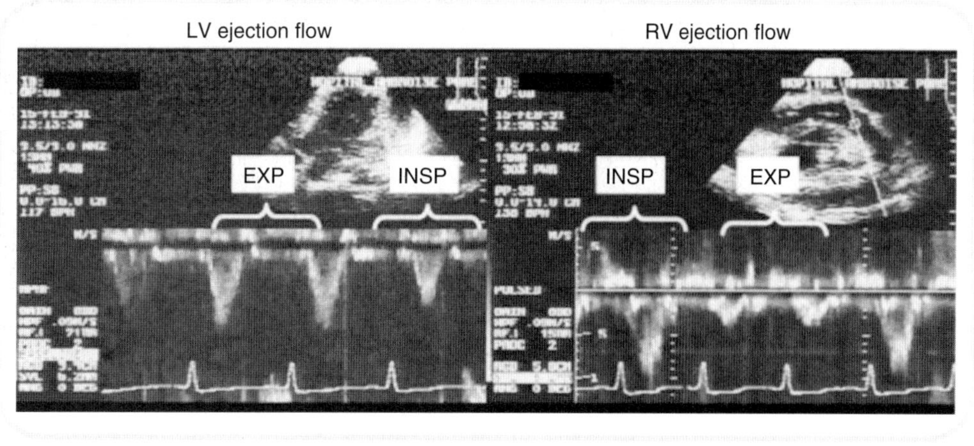

Figure 3. Pulsed Doppler in the left and in the right ventricular outflow track. During expiration, the left ventricular ejection flow was maximal and the right ventricular ejection flow was minimal. It was the opposite during inspiration. EXP, expiration; INSP, inspiration. (Reused with permission from Bodson L, Bouferrache K, Vieillard-Baron A. Cardiac tamponade. *Curr Opin Crit Care*. 2011;17(5):416–424.)

SUGGESTED
READINGS

Bodson L, Bouferrache K, Vieillard-Baron A. Cardiac tamponade. *Curr Opin Crit Care*. 2011;17(5):416–424.
Hines R, Marschall K. *Stoelting's Anesthesia and Co-existing Disease*. 5th ed. Saunders Elsevier; 2002:127–128.
Spodick DH. Acute cardiac tamponade. *N Engl J Med*. 2003;349:684–690.

Cardiopulmonary Bypass Management
Organ-based Clinical: Cardiovascular

Veronica Matei

Edited by Qingbing Zhu

1. Cardiopulmonary bypass (CPB) replaces heart and lung function during the period of cardiorespiratory arrest.
2. CPB management involves multiple steps, the most critical ones being initiation of CPB and termination of bypass.
3. The first step before initiation of CPB is administration of heparin through a central line.
4. CPB initiation requires insertion of two cannulas: a venous cannula and an arterial cannula.
5. During arterial cannula insertion (occurring mostly in the ascending aorta), controlled hypotension is used to avoid aortic dissection.
6. Preparation for weaning from bypass begins during CPB, and checklists before separation of bypass are very helpful (see below).

Initiation of CPB involves the following steps:

- The first step before initiation of CPB is administration of heparin through a central line. Systemic anticoagulation is accomplished and thrombosis of the CPB is avoided. The dose of heparin varies between 300 and 400 U per kg. Anticoagulant activity of heparin is checked by measurements of activated clotting time (ACT). Most ACTs greater than 450 are acceptable for initiation of CPB. Serial measurements of ACTs are required not only for initiation of CPB, but also for the entire period of CPB, and redosing of heparin may be required to maintain ACT.
- CPB initiation requires insertion of the two basic cannulas, creating the CPB circuit: venous cannula and arterial cannula. Additional cannulas can be inserted to optimize the CPB circuit.
- During arterial cannula insertion, controlled hypotension is used to avoid aortic dissection. During venous cannulation, arrhythmias should be anticipated and promptly treated if hemodynamically significant.

After initiation of CPB, the following aspects are monitored:

- Oxygenation/ventilation by serial Arterial Blood Gases (ABGs)
- Perfusion by maintenance of Mean Arterial Pressure (MAP), serial ABGs, and mixed venous saturation monitoring
- Electrolyte/acid–base status by serial ABGs
- Systemic anticoagulation by serial ACTs
- Maintenance of mild to moderate hypothermia
- Maintenance of moderate hemodilution by serial hematocrit levels
- Maintenance of anesthetic depth.

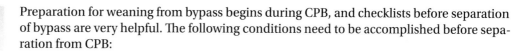

Preparation for weaning from bypass begins during CPB, and checklists before separation of bypass are very helpful. The following conditions need to be accomplished before separation from CPB:

- Airway is confirmed.
- Breathing is resumed with mechanical ventilation.
- Circulation parameters are in normal range, including heart rate, rhythm, contractility, preload, and afterload.
- Hematocrit (Hct), electrolyte, and acid–base status are acceptable.
- Temperature is normal.
- Deaired heart.
- No major bleeding in the field.

SUGGESTED READINGS

Barash PG, Cullen BF, Stoelting RK, et al, eds. *Clinical Anesthesia*. 6th ed. Philadelphia, PA: Lippincott Williams & Wilkins; 2009.

Yao FS. *Yao & Artusio's Anesthesiology*. 7th ed. Philadelphia, PA. Lippincott Williams & Wilkins; 2011.

Carotid Body: Hypoxic Drive
Physiology

Bijal Patel

Edited by Veronica Matei

KEY POINTS

1. Carotid bodies are peripheral chemoreceptors located at the bifurcation of the common carotid arteries.
2. These receptors are primarily stimulated by decreased PaO_2 and only to a small degree by decreased pH or changes in $PaCO_2$. Carotid bodies stimulation results in increased ventilation through increased respiratory rate and tidal volume.
3. One begins to see increased neural activity from the carotid bodies as the PaO_2 falls below 100; however, significant changes in ventilation are not actually seen until the PaO_2 falls below 65.
4. The response of the carotid bodies to hypoxia is blunted by the use of potent inhaled anesthetics.

DISCUSSION

Carotid bodies are peripheral chemoreceptors located at the bifurcation of the common carotid arteries. When stimulated, they send neural signals via the afferent glossopharyngeal nerves to the central respiratory centers to mediate ventilation. These receptors are primarily stimulated by decreased arterial blood oxygen *tension* (PaO_2). Reduced arterial blood oxygen *content* is not a primary stimulant, and thus there is little stimulation in anemia, methemoglobinemia, or carboxyhemoglobinemia. Decreased pH, changes in $PaCO_2$, hypoperfusion of the carotid bodies, and increase in temperature and certain chemicals, such as nicotine and acetylcholine, have also been known to stimulate the carotid bodies but to a lesser degree.

One begins to see increased neural activity from the carotid bodies as the PaO_2 falls below 100; however, significant changes in ventilation are not actually seen until the PaO_2 falls below 65. This point becomes extremely important when dealing with patients who rely on hypoxic ventilatory drive. For example, after terminating mechanical ventilation on these patients, they do not begin spontaneously breathing until the PaO_2 reaches below 65, which will in turn stimulate the carotid bodies.

Stimulation of the carotid bodies results in increased ventilation through increasing both the respiratory rate and the tidal volume. This response is blunted by the use of potent inhaled anesthetics. Also of note, after bilateral carotid endarterectomy, the patient has almost no hypoxic ventilatory drive because the carotid bodies are usually ablated during the procedure.

SUGGESTED READINGS

Barash PG, Cullen BF, Stoelting RK, et al, eds. *Clinical Anesthesia.* 6th ed. New York, NY: Lippincott Williams & Wilkins; 2009:221, 240.

Miller RD, Stoelting RK. *Basics of Anesthesia.* 5th ed. Philadelphia, PA: Churchill Livingstone; 2007:319.

Carotid Endarterectomy: CNS Monitoring
Organ-based Clinical: Neurologic and Neuromuscular

Terrence Coffey

Edited by Ramachandran Ramani

c

KEY POINTS

1. During carotid endarterectomies, the anesthesiologist must assess cerebral perfusion to determine whether a shunt is necessary while the diseased artery is clamped.
2. Under regional anesthesia, cerebral perfusion is best assessed through checking contralateral handgrip strength and continual verbal communication with patient.
3. The gold standard for assessing cerebral perfusion under general anesthesia is the electroencephalogram (EEG).
4. Several other methods, including somatosensory evoked potential (SSEP), transcranial Doppler (TCD), infrared spectroscopy, and jugular venous oxygen saturation, may be useful, but currently appear to be less reliable intraoperatively compared with EEG.

DISCUSSION

Assessment of adequate cerebral circulation is critical during carotid endarterectomy (CEA). A monitoring technique is needed to evaluate perfusion to the ipsilateral brain while the diseased artery is clamped. If CEA is performed under regional anesthesia, frequent examination of strength using contralateral handgrip and verbal communication with the patient are used to assess the motor function, level of consciousness, and ultimately cerebral perfusion. Assessment is completed every 2 to 5 minutes.

If CEA is performed under general anesthesia, there are several methods to assess cerebral perfusion. The current gold standard is 12-lead EEG. Although it is the gold standard, EEG cannot monitor perfusion to deep brain structures. SSEP may evaluate deep brain structures, but it is unclear whether the technique is sensitive or specific enough for clinical use at this time.

TCD ultrasound provides another noninvasive approach to determining the amount of blood flow in the middle cerebral artery by insonating it through the temporal bone. However, this method's reliability is also controversial, and it may be more effective for postoperative monitoring of stroke. It is more effective in evaluating the presence of emboli in the artery.

Another noninvasive technique to measure blood flow during CEA is near infrared spectroscopy. It allows continuous monitoring of regional cerebral oxygen saturation via the scalp and skull. However, it should not be used solely for determining placement of a shunt because it has a low sensitivity and specificity. Jugular venous oxygen saturation can be measured, but is not reliable because it does not measure regional/focal cerebral ischemia; rather, it serves as a global measure of ischemia.

SUGGESTED READINGS

Barash PG, Cullen BF, Stoelting RK. *Clinical Anesthesia*. 5th ed. Philadelphia, PA: Lippincott Williams & Wilkins; 2006:946–954.

Morgan GE, Mikhail MS, Murray MJ. *Clinical Anesthesiology*. 4th ed. New York, NY: McGraw-Hill; 2005:627–628.

Carotid Sinus Stim: Post-Heart Transplant Physiology

Nicholas Dalesio

Edited by Qingbing Zhu

KEY POINTS

1. The carotid sinus contains arterial baroreceptors at the bifurcation of the common carotids.
2. The afferent signal is via the glossopharyngeal nerve.
3. The efferent signal is via the vagus nerve.
4. Carotid massage in a normal heart causes baroreceptor stimulation that leads to an increased efferent signal via the vagus nerve to the heart. This acts indirectly on pacemaker cells and conducting pathways to slow down the heart.
5. After heart transplant surgery, these innervations are interrupted and the response from carotid manipulation is absent.

DISCUSSION

The carotid sinus contains arterial baroreceptors at the bifurcation of the common carotids. These receptors have tonic activity at baseline. With a sudden rise in arterial blood pressure, baroreceptors stretch and activate sodium channels. Activation of sodium channels sends an afferent signal via the glossopharyngeal nerve to the central nuclei, including the nucleus tractus solitarius. From the central nuclei, an efferent signal propagates to the heart from the vagus nerve. The vagus sends long preganglionic fibers to the heart to synapse on postganglionic neurons in the myocardial tissue. These postganglionic neurons act directly on pacemaker cells and conducting pathways to slow down the heart.

When a heart is transplanted, the postganglionic parasympathetic fibers traveling within the vagus nerve are cut and the heart becomes denervated (Fig. 1). The transplanted heart

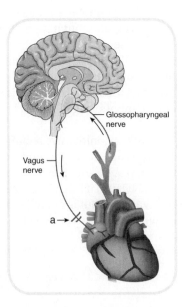

Figure 1. Carotid baroreceptor reflex. The afferent pathway is via the glossopharyngeal nerve. The efferent pathway is via the vagus nerve. Heart transplantation *(a)* disrupts the efferent pathway via the vagus nerve. (Modified from http://www.mightysworld.com/unity-companies/neural-pathways.html.)

no longer responds to indirect-acting medications. Furthermore, carotid massage to simulate stretch at the carotid baroreceptors is no longer effective. The preganglionic neurons to the heart are severed and will not signal to their postganglionic counterpart in the heart. Similarly, Valsalva maneuvers are also ineffective.

SUGGESTED READING

Barash PG, Cullen BF, Stoelting RK, et al, eds. *Clinical Anesthesia*. 6th ed. Philadelphia, PA: Lippincott Williams & Wilkins; 2009:220–221, 1414.

Carotid Stent: Bradycardia Cause
Physiology

Trevor Banack

Edited by Shamsuddin Akhtar

1. The baroreceptors located in the carotid sinus are innervated by a branch of the glossopharyngeal nerve called the carotid sinus nerve or nerve of Hering.
2. Increased baroreceptor firing leads to a temporary inhibition of sympathetic output and increase in parasympathetic activity, which results in bradycardia and hypotension.
3. Stretching of the carotid sinus baroreceptor during carotid artery stenting (CAS) by the angioplasty balloon and stent mimics an increase in systemic arterial blood pressure and increased carotid sinus barorecptor firing.
4. Additional factors leading to hypotension and bradycardia during CAS include coronary disease, increased age, and low ejection fraction.

The human body regulates blood pressure within a narrow range to ensure blood flow to organs. The blood pressure is regulated by arterial pressure receptors, called barorecptors. One of these receptors, the carotid sinus, is located at the bifurcation of the external and internal carotid arteries. If the carotid sinus senses a drop in blood pressure by a decrease in arterial wall stretch, the receptor will decrease firing. The baroreceptors located in the carotid sinus are innervated by a branch of the glossopharyngeal nerve called the carotid sinus nerve or nerve of Hering. The carotid sinus nerve synapses via the glossopharyngeal nerve in the nucleus tractus solitaries located in the medulla of the brainstem. This synaptic area in the medulla is responsible for the regulation of the sympathetic and parasympathetic output of the medulla. Increased baroreceptor firing leads to a temporary inhibition of sympathetic output and increase in parasympathetic activity. This increase parasympathetic activity results in bradycardia and a decrease in blood pressure.

Stretching of the carotid sinus baroreceptor during CAS by the angioplasty balloon and stent mimics an increase in systemic arterial blood pressure. This stretching results in an increased firing of the baroreceptor via the carotid sinus nerve and the resultant inhibition of sympathetic activity and increase of parasympathetic activity. A 33% incidence of significant bradycardia and hypotension has been reported in patients during CAS.

There have been numerous studies that have discovered other factors that put patients at risk of bradycardia and hypotension during CAS. Taha et al. and Gupta et al. reported carotid bulb lesions to be predictive of CAS-induced instability when compared with lesions outside this region. Stretching of the carotid bulb, which is located near carotid sinus baroreceptors, is more likely to cause hemodynamic instability because of barorecptor activation. Additional factors leading to hypotension and bradycardia during CAS include coronary disease, increased age, and low ejection fraction.

Cayne NS, Faries PL, Trocciola SM, et al. Carotid angioplasty and stent-induced bradycardia and hypotension: impact of prophylactic atropine administration and prior carotid endarterectomy. *J Vasc Surg.* 2005;41:956–961.

Cayne NS, Rockman CB, Maldonado TS, et al. Hemodynamic changes associated with carotid artery interventions. *Perspect Vasc Surg Endovasc Ther.* 2008;20(3):293–296.

Gupta R, Abou-Chebl A, Bajzer CT, et al. Rate, predictors, and consequences of hemodynamic depression after carotid artery stenting. *J Am Coll Cardiol.* 2006;47:1538–1543.

Lin PH, Zhou W, Kougias P, et al. Factors associated with hypotension and bradycardia after carotid angioplasty and stenting. *J Vasc Surg.* 2007;46:846–853.

Taha MM, Toma N, Sakaida H, et al. Periprocedural hemodynamic instability with carotid angioplasty and stenting. *Surg Neurol.* 2008;70(3):279–285.

Categorical Data: Chi-square

Mathematics, Statistics, Computers

Holly Barth

Edited by Raj K. Modak

KEY POINTS

1. The chi-square test is a nonparametric statistical test.
2. Chi-square test is used to compare ratios or proportions, commonly used in Mendelian genetic analysis.
3. Chi-square test determines whether observed frequencies are significantly different from expected frequencies.

DISCUSSION

The chi-square test is a nonparametric statistical test. It is used in the comparison of data that is ordinal or nominal, when the distribution of the data is unknown and when transformations applied to the data fail to normalize the data. Chi-square test can be used on one-sample, two-sample or multiple-sample tests. It is used to determine whether observed frequencies are significantly different from expected frequencies. The chi-square test is testing the null hypothesis, which states that there is no significant difference between the expected and observed result.

To calculate chi-square value, the following formula is used:

$$\chi^2 = \sum \frac{(\text{observed} - \text{expected})^2}{\text{expected}},$$

where the chi-square value is the sum of the squares of the observed values minus expected values divided by the expected values.

The ability to accept or reject the null hypothesis is based on a chi-square table, where the calculated chi-square value is compared with critical chi-square values based on probability and the number of degrees of freedom in the system. If the calculated value is **less than** the critical value, then the null hypothesis is accepted and **no significance** is stated between the values. If the calculated chi-square value is **greater than** the critical tabled value, then the null hypothesis is rejected and a **significant** difference is noted between the values. By convention, a probability value of 0.05 is used as a level of significance. It is important to note that the chi-square test is dependent upon the expected values being not too small and that the degree of freedom can be properly evaluated. The test requires a large amount of data, but when a significant result is found, it is most likely correct.

Miller RD, ed. *Miller's Anesthesia*. 6th ed. Philadelphia, PA: Elsevier Churchill Livingstone; 2005:70.

SUGGESTED READING

Caudal Anesthesia

Subspecialties: Regional Anesthesia

Glenn Dizon

Edited by Thomas Halaszynski

1. The caudal space, where caudal anesthesia is performed, is the sacral portion of the epidural space.
2. Caudal anesthesia is one of the most commonly employed regional techniques, especially in pediatric patients, and is also commonly used for postoperative analgesia for urogenital, rectal, inguinal, and lower extremity surgery.
3. Choosing local anesthetics for caudal anesthesia should be the same set of considerations as those used for epidural anesthesia, and it must be recognized that volumes in the 25 to 30 mL range are typically necessary to provide predictable sensory levels to thoracic 10 to 12 levels with a caudal injection.
4. Complications include total spinal seizure or cardiac arrest from intravascular injection of local anesthetic.

The caudal space is defined as the sacral level of the epidural space. To achieve access to the caudal space, a needle and/or catheter penetrates into the sacrococcygeal ligament covering the sacral hiatus, with subsequent injection of medication.

Performance of caudal anesthesia:

a. Lateral decubitus or prone positioning of the patient.
b. The caudal space can be entered through the sacral hiatus, which can be palpated as a midline groove above the coccyx and between the palpable sacral cornua on either side of the midline.
c. After sterile skin preparation, a needle is directed at a 45° angle to the skin, piercing the sacrococcygeal ligament.
d. Needle angle is then flattened and advanced an additional 2 cm in adults or 1 cm in children.
e. Injection of local anesthetic (0.5 to 1.0 mL per kg of 0.125% to 0.25% bupivacaine or ropivacaine) can proceed after negative aspiration for cerebrospinal fluid (CSF) and blood.

Caudal block is used commonly for regional anesthesia, especially in pediatric cases. It is commonly used for postoperative analgesia in children and most commonly performed after the induction of general anesthesia. Common procedures where caudal anesthesia is indicated include urogenital, rectal, inguinal, and lower extremity surgery. In adults, caudal anesthesia may also be used for anorectal surgery and can be used in the second stage of labor when the epidural does not adequately block sacral nerves. In addition, caudal anesthesia can be used when epidural placement has failed or is ineffective in obstetric patients.

For performance of this block (caudal anesthesia), adults are placed in the lateral decubitus or prone position. Children are typically placed in the lateral decubitus position after induction of general anesthesia. From these positions, the caudal space can be entered through the sacral hiatus at the unfused sacral-4 (S4) and sacral-5 (S5) laminae. The hiatus can be palpated as a midline groove above the coccyx and between the palpable sacral cornua on either side of the midline. It may also be located at the apex of an equilateral triangle created by the two posterior superior iliac spines and the sacral hiatus. After sterile preparation, the needle is directed cephalad at a 45° angle. With needle advancement,

a pop can often be felt as the needle penetrates the sacrococcygeal ligament. The needle angle is then flattened and advanced an additional 2 cm in adults or 1 cm in children. Injection of local anesthetics can proceed after negative aspiration for CSF and blood. Test dosing with local anesthetic medications will also help rule out subarachnoid or intravenous injection.

Typical dosing of local anesthetics is 0.5 to 1.0 mL per kg of 0.125% to 0.25% bupivacaine or ropivacaine with or without epinephrine. Opioids such as 50 to 70 μg per kg of morphine may also be added. Analgesia can extend for hours postoperatively on a single dose, or a catheter can be placed for more prolonged analgesia.

Complications associated with caudal anesthesia are similar to those associated with epidural analgesia and include total spinal and seizures or cardiac arrest from an intravascular injection of local anesthetic.

SUGGESTED READINGS

Morgan GE, Mikhail MS, Murray MJ. *Clinical Anesthesiology*. 4th ed. New York, NY: McGraw-Hill; 2005:314–316.
Rathmell JP, Neal JM, Viscomi CM. *Regional Anesthesia: The Requisites in Anesthesiology*. Philadelphia, PA: Elsevier Mosby; 2004:111–112.

Celiac Plexus Block: Side Effects and Complications

Subspecialities: Pain

Meredith Brown and Dan Froicu

Edited by Jodi Sherman

C

KEY POINTS

1. Celiac plexus blocks are utilized to aid in relief of cancer pain originating from the upper abdomen.
2. Side effects and complications to the celiac plexus block include orthostatic hypotension, retroperitoneal hematoma, abdominal aortic dissection, interscapular back pain, hiccups, reactive pleurisy, hematuria, transient diarrhea, pneumothorax, transient motor paralysis, paraplegia.

DISCUSSION

Celiac plexus blocks are performed to relieve cancer pain in the upper abdomen. The celiac plexus is located anterior to the crura of the diaphragm, at approximately T12-L1, and surrounds the abdominal aorta, superior mesenteric artery, and celiac artery. It provides the innervation to the abdominal viscera with the exception of the descending colon and pelvic structures. The celiac plexus includes sympathetic innervation, originating from the splanchnic nerves, and parasympathetic innervation, originating from the vagus nerve. A celiac block can be performed under direct visualization at the end of a laparotomy or laparoscopy, or more commonly by fluoroscopy-guided percutaneous techniques. Initially, the block is performed with local anesthetic; if pain relief is achieved, then the block is repeated with a neurolytic agent for prolonged effects.

There are three approaches to blocking the celiac plexus block: classic retrocrural approach, anterocrural approach, and neurolysis of the splanchnic nerves. On the basis of the location of the celiac plexus, many of the side effects and complications can be predicted. These side effects include orthostatic hypotension, retroperitoneal hematoma, abdominal aortic dissection, interscapular back pain, hiccups, reactive pleurisy, hematuria, transient diarrhea, pneumothorax transient motor paralysis, and paraplegia. Most common side effects include hypotension and diarrhea. Hypotension occurs in 35% to 60% of cases without preprocedure fluid load or pressor agents and is due to acute vasodilatation from sympathetic blockade. Some episodes of hypotension can manifest up to 48 hours after block placement. Diarrhea is due to parasympathetic action lacking sympathetic counterbalance. It occurs acutely in 20% to 40% of cases and may last days, but rarely longer. Somatostatin can be used together with fluid replacement as treatment for prolonged diarrhea.

The complications of celiac plexus block vary with the technique and the agent used. Neurologic complications include inadvertent intrathecal injection of agents. This can cause permanent paraplegia when neurolytic agents are employed. Compression or chemical injury of the artery of Adamkiewicz may cause an anterior spinal artery syndrome, which includes transient and possibly permanent motor paralysis. Seizures can be caused by the intravascular injection of agents as well. Finally, infection is a known complication of celiac plexus blockade. Retroperitoneal abscesses have been reported after celiac plexus blockade.

131

C

SUGGESTED
READINGS

Barash PG, Cullen BF, Stoelting RK, et al, eds. *Clinical Anesthesia*. 6th ed. Lippincott Williams & Wilkins; 2009:1518–1519.

Morgan GE, Mikhail MS, Murray MJ. *Clinical Anesthesiology*. 4th ed. New York, NY: McGraw-Hill Companies, Inc; 1996:385.

Central Line Infections: Prevention

Subspecialties: Critical Care

Xing Fu

Edited by Ala Haddadin

KEY POINTS

1. It has been estimated that there are approximately 250,000 instances of central line–associated bacteremia in the United States each year.
2. In 2000, an infection-control advisory committee convened, and soon after established a multifaceted intervention aimed at eliminating central venous catheter associated infections, which included the use of maximum sterile barrier precautions during insertion, avoiding the femoral vein site, use of chlorhexidine for cleaning the skin before catheter insertion, and removing the catheter when not needed and appropriately dressing the catheter site.
3. Antimicrobial-coated catheters have also shown benefit in preventing central line–associated infections, with the combination of minocycline and rifampin displaying up to 4 weeks of antimicrobial activity.

DISCUSSION

It has been estimated that there are approximately 250,000 instances of central line–associated bacteremia in the United States each year. The mortality for these infections is estimated to be 12% to 15% for each infection. In light of these numbers, much attention has been given to preventing central line–associated infections. In 2000, an infection-control advisory committee convened, and soon after established a multifaceted intervention aimed at eliminating central venous catheter associated infections. These interventions included evidence-based catheter insertion practices, such as maximum sterile barrier precautions during insertion, avoiding the femoral vein site, use of chlorhexidine for cleaning the skin before catheter insertion, and removing the catheter when not needed and appropriately dressing the catheter site.

Additional interventions mentioned by the committee were a module providing information about central line–associated infections and how to prevent them, a way of standardized recording of adherence to these infection control practices, a standardized list of supplies necessary to follow evidence-based practices, and measurement of central line infection rates and distribution of this data. According to one study, these interventions resulted in the reduction of the pooled mean rate of central line–associated bacteremia by 68%.

An additional method used to prevent central line–associated infections is through the use of antimicrobial-coated catheters. Two types of coated catheters are the one with the combination of chlorhexidine and silver sulfadiazine and the other coated with minocycline and rifampin. The former has been reported to display antimicrobial activity for 1 week, whereas the latter has been reported to show this activity for up to 4 weeks.

SUGGESTED READINGS

Marino PL. *The ICU Book.* 3rd ed. Philadelphia, PA: Lippincott Williams & Wilkins; 2007:114.

Muto C, Herbert C, Harrison E, et al. Reduction in central line–associated bloodstream infections among patients in intensive care units—Pennsylvania, April 2001–March 2005. *JAMA.* 2006;295:269–270.

Cerebral Aneurysm Clipping: Anesthetic Management

Organ-based Clinical: Neurologic and Neuromuscular

Jorge Galvez

Edited by Ramachandran Ramani

1. Patients with ruptured aneurysms are at a high risk for rebleeding, approximately 25% during the first 14 days.
2. Anesthetic goals for intracranial aneurysm surgery are as follows
   a. Avoid aneurysm rupture.
   b. Maintain cerebral perfusion pressure while avoiding a high transmural aneurysm pressure.
   c. Provide a "slack" brain for optimal surgical access.
3. Transmural pressure is related to the difference between the mean arterial pressure and the intracranial pressure.
4. Ensure adequate depth of anesthesia for laryngoscopy and intubation, placement of head pins, skin incision, turning bone flap, and opening the dura.

The rupture of intracranial aneurysms affects approximately 27,000 Americans (women > men), with peak incidence in the fifth and sixth decades of life, and has a mortality rate of 25%, with significant morbidity affecting 50% of patients. Most aneurysms involve the structures in the circle of Willis, but may involve the ophthalmic artery. Risk factors include tobacco use, hypertension, alcohol use, cocaine, oral contraceptive use, hyperlipidemia, genetic conditions, and affected first-degree relatives.

The size and location of the aneurysm, along with the severity of subarachnoid hemorrhage and clinical status of the patient, impact the decision among the available therapeutic interventions.

Patients presenting with subarachnoid hemorrhage suffer from abrupt increases in intracranial pressure that may result in neurologic impairment, severe systemic hypertension, and dysrhythmias. Patients classically complain of sudden onset of severe headache, nuchal rigidity, photophobia, nausea/vomiting, and possibly loss of consciousness. After initial aneurysm rupture, disorganized clot can tamponade the bleeding temporarily. However, the risk of rebleeding is significant, approximately 4% in the first 24 hours, then about 1.5% per day, with a cumulative risk of 25% in 2 weeks. Rebleeding after the initial rupture of an aneurysm is often catastrophic, as it is more likely to result in brain parenchymal damage because blood cannot dissect through the cerebrospinal fluid (CSF) space that is filled with clot.

Patients suffering from subarachnoid hemorrhage after aneurysm rupture may develop hyponatremia. This occurs either from the syndrome of inappropriate antidiuretic hormone secretion (SIADH) or from cerebral salt wasting syndrome due to the release of a natriuretic peptide from the damaged brain. These patients typically have contracted intravascular volume despite hyponatremia. Electrolyte abnormalities should be optimized before proceeding with operative management.

Vasospasm can occur within the first 12 days after aneurysm rupture (peak incidence from day 4 to 9). Patients suffering from vasospasm may become lethargic or have focal neurologic deficits corresponding to the arterial territory involved. Diagnosis is confirmed by angiography, and transcranial Doppler may be used to assess the severity and evaluate the effectiveness of therapy. Treatment for cerebral vasospasm is targeted at improving cerebral blood flow to affected areas until neurologic symptoms are improved with medical management or interventional procedures (angioplasty, intraarterial papaverine, or calcium channel blockers). This is achieved with triple-H therapy:

- Hypervolemia—central venous pressure (CVP) 10 to 12 mm Hg or pulmonary artery wedge pressure (PACWP) 12 to 18 mm Hg.
- Hypertension—achieved with vasopressors (typically phenylephrine or dopamine); end point of systemic hypertension is improvement of neurologic symptoms.
- Hemodilution—goal of reducing viscosity to improve cerebral blood flow and oxygen delivery (goal hematocrit is variable among centers).

The goals of intraoperative management include the following:

1. Avoid aneurysm rupture.
2. Maintain cerebral perfusion pressure and avoid high transmural aneurysm pressure.
3. Provide a "slack" brain for optimal surgical access.
4. Systemic hypertension is gradually lowered with care to prevent development of neurologic deficits (preoperative evaluation should elicit this information if available).

ECG abnormalities (ST elevation/depression, T-wave inversion, U waves, QT prolongation, arrhythmias) are common in patients suffering from subarachnoid hemorrhage and may not be indicative of myocardial ischemia. If warranted, evaluation for myocardial ischemia and appropriate therapy may be indicated.

The transmural pressure of the aneurysm, which is the difference between mean arterial pressure and intracranial pressure, should not be high. Wall tension of the aneurysm increases linearly with increase in transmural pressure, thus increasing the likelihood of aneurysm rupture.

Precise control of mean arterial pressure is of paramount importance, and it may be achieved with a variety of agents. Typically, beta antagonists, calcium channel blockers, intravenous and inhaled anesthetics, and arterial vasodilators may be used. Intracranial pressure may be monitored with a ventriculostomy if available. CSF may be drained to reduce intracranial pressure if needed (usually under surgical guidance). Adequate depth of anesthesia is mandatory for all stimulating parts of the surgery including laryngoscopy and intubation, placement of head pins, skin incision, turning bone flap, and opening the dura.

Patients with Hunt–Hess grades 1 to 2 who are awake before surgery may be candidates for extubation at the conclusion of the surgery, in contrast with patients with grades 3 to 4 who may remain intubated in the ICU until neurologic symptoms begin to improve (Table 1). If extubation is planned, anesthetic agents should be titrated to ensure an expeditious emergence. Thiopental is beneficial for cerebral protection when temporary arterial clips are used, but it may be associated with prolonged emergence and systemic hypotension.

Table 1. Hunt–Hess Classification for Patients with SAH

Grade	Criteria
0	Unruptured aneurysm
1	Asymptomatic, minimal headache, and slight nuchal rigidity
2	Moderate to severe headache, nuchal rigidity, no neurologic deficit other than cranial nerve palsy
3	Drowsiness, confusion, or mild focal deficit
4	Stupor, moderate to severe hemiparesis, early decerebration, vegetative disturbance
5	Deep coma, decerebrate rigidity, moribund

Controlled hypotension may be used during dissection of the aneurysm to facilitate manipulation of arteries and aneurysm clip placement, although this technique has been replaced largely by the use of temporary clips. If temporary clips are used, normotension should be maintained to optimize collateral circulation. Thiopental may be administered before the placement of temporary clips to reduce cerebral metabolic rate in the regions distal to the temporary clips. Ischemic damage has been reported with the use of temporary clips longer than 15 minutes. Emergence must be smooth, minimizing hypercarbia, hypertension, coughing, and straining.

SUGGESTED READINGS

Barash PG, Cullen BF, Stoelting RK, eds. *Clinical Anesthesiology.* 5th ed. Philadelphia, PA: Lippincott Williams & Wilkins; 2005:chap 27.
Miller RD. *Miller's Anesthesia.* 6th ed. Philadelphia, PA: Elsevier; 2005:chap 53:2147.

Cerebral Blood Flow: Temp Effect
Organ-based Clinical: Neurologic and Neuromuscular

Anna Clebone

Edited by Ramachandran Ramani

1. "Flow-metabolism coupling" refers to the fact that cerebral blood flow (CBF) and cerebral metabolic rate ($CMRO_2$) change in parallel.
2. CBF and $CMRO_2$ decrease when brain temperature decreases.

"Flow-metabolism coupling" refers to the fact that CBF and $CMRO_2$ change in parallel. The $CMRO_2$ at 37° C is approximately 3.5 mL/100 g/min. $CMRO_2$ decreases when brain temperature decreases. There is a 7% decrease in the metabolism for every 1° C drop in temperature. The brain has decreased oxygen requirements during cooling, reflecting a decreased cerebral metabolic rate. CBF is normally 50 mL/100 g/min, whereas it can be 20 to 25 mL/100 g/min during moderate hypothermia (28° to 30° C).

Greeley WJ, Ungerleider RM, Kern FH, et al. Effects of cardiopulmonary bypass on cerebral blood flow in neonates, infants, and children. *Circulation.* 1989;80(suppl I):1209–1215.

Schell RM, Kern FH, Greeley WJ, et al. Cerebral blood flow and metabolism during cardiopulmonary bypass. *Anesth Analg.* 1993;76:849–865.

Cerebral Ischemia: Deep Hypothermia
Organ-based Clinical: Neurologic and Neuromuscular

Amit Mirchandani

Edited by Ramachandran Ramani

KEY POINTS

1. Hypothermia could potentially be protective to the brain, particularly in patients undergoing operations that place the patient at high risk for global or focal cerebral ischemia.
2. Hypothermia optimizes the oxygen supply and demand relationship by decreasing cerebral metabolic rate ($CMRO_2$).
3. Recent evidence demonstrates potential cerebral protective benefit from even milder reductions in temperature.

DISCUSSION

Although the value of intraoperative hypothermia remains unproven, many practitioners institute hypothermia for cerebral protection during certain operations. The goal of clinical cerebral protection against ischemia is to maximize cerebral oxygen delivery and preserve cerebral blood flow while decreasing oxygen demand.

Candidates for deep hypothermia are those who are scheduled for intracranial vascular procedures, including cerebral aneurysm coiling/clipping. Patients undergoing cardiac bypass who may be at risk for global or focal ischemia secondary to low flow states or small emboli may also be candidates for deep hypothermia.

Hypothermia is beneficial because it diminishes both metabolic and functional activities of the brain. Hypothermia decreases $CMRO_2$ by approximately 7% for each degree Celsius decrease in temperature, but this correlation is not definitively linear. Reductions in temperature that correlate with an isoelectric electroencephalogram, between 18° and 21° C, parallel loss of neuronal function and the ability for the brain to tolerate a more prolonged ischemia.

Although deep hypothermic circulatory arrest (DHCA) at temperatures between 15° and 18° C has been shown to demonstrate the protective cerebral effects against ischemia, recent evidence points to the fact that even milder decreases in temperature (25° to 32° C) offer brain protection during both focal and global ischemia.

In addition to reducing both the functional and the cellular framework of cerebral metabolism, the mechanism of action of cerebral protection in the setting of hypothermia potentially involves decreasing free radicals and increasing blood–brain barrier stability. On the basis of outcome studies, the only two clinical indications for hypothermia are found in post–cardiac arrest survivors and in neonatal cerebral hypoxia.

SUGGESTED READINGS

Barash PG, Cullen BF, Stoelting RK, eds. *Clinical Anesthesia*. 5th ed. Philadelphia, PA: Lippincott Williams & Wilkins; 2006:780.

Newfield P. *Handbook of Neuroanesthesia*. 4th ed. Philadelphia, PA: Lippincott Williams & Wilkins; 2007:60–62.

Cerebral Vasospasm: Rx

Organ-based Clinical: Neurologic and Neuromuscular

Frederick Conlin and Thomas Gallen

Edited by Ramachandran Ramani

KEY POINTS

1. Cerebral vasospasm is the most common complication of subarachnoid hemorrhage (SAH), which can lead to significant morbidity and mortality.
2. Cerebral vasospasm typically has an onset of 3 to 5 days after SAH.
3. Nimodipine (60 mg PO every 4 hours for 21 days) is recognized as effective prophylaxis for cerebral vasospasm and improves neurologic outcome and mortality.
4. Current treatment strategies include the use of nimodipine (a calcium channel blocker), "triple-H therapy" (hypertension, hypervolemia, and hemodilution), and angioplasty.
5. No other pharmacologic therapies aside from statins have been shown to reduce the incidence or morbidity of cerebral vasospasm in clinical trials.

DISCUSSION

Patients who survive subarachnoid hemorrhages frequently have their courses complicated by cerebral vasospasm. It is caused by the presence of blood in the subarachnoid space surrounding the cerebral arteries, and occurs anywhere from 3 to 5 days after the hemorrhage. The artery constricts, resulting in decreased blood flow, which may lead to cerebral ischemia in the distribution of the affected vessel. Patients may present with altered mental status, followed by focal deficits, and finally cerebral infarction. The diagnosis is made on the basis of the patient's symptoms and/or cerebral angiography or transcranial Doppler.

Nimodipine, a calcium channel blocker, is the drug of choice for the treatment of cerebral vasospasm, and it improves neurologic outcome and mortality as well. The mechanism of action could be through its vasodilatory and/or cytoprotective properties. Should clinically significant vasospasm occur despite nimodipine therapy, clinicians will often next employ "triple-H therapy" (hypertension, hypervolemia, and hemodilution). As autoregulation does not apply to the vasospastic vessel, triple-H therapy attempts to drive flow through the compromised vessel by increasing the pressure gradient (hypertension) and decreasing the resistance (hemodilution/hypervolemia). Common goals are to keep systolic blood pressure >160 mm Hg and central venous pressure 12 to 16 mm Hg. This approach has limited evidence supporting its use and can come at the cost of severe complications such as pulmonary and cerebral edema, increased myocardial burden, electrolyte abnormalities, and problems related to the placement of central venous or pulmonary arterial catheters. For these reasons, triple-H therapy is not employed prophylactically.

Statins are the only other pharmacologic agents with significant evidence to be effective at treating cerebral vasospasm, although further trials are needed before a final conclusion is made. In addition, balloon angioplasty may be performed to dilate the affected vessel. There is also increasing evidence that statins may have a role in the treatment of cerebral vasospasm.

SUGGESTED READINGS

Drummond JC, Patel PM. Neurosurgical anesthesia. In: Miller RD, ed. *Miller's Anesthesia*. 6th ed. Philadelphia, PA: Elsevier; 2005:2147–2148.

Lee KH, Lukovits T, Friedman JA. "Triple-H" therapy for cerebral vasospasm following subarachnoid hemorrhage. *Neurocrit Care*. 2006;4:68–76.

Morgan GE, Mikhail MS, Murray MJ. *Clinical Anesthesiology*. 4th ed. New York, NY: McGraw Hill; 2005:624, 642.

Sulek CA. Increased intracranial pressure. In: Lobato EB, ed. *Complications in Anesthesiology*. Philadelphia, PA: Lippincott Williams & Wilkins; 2008:319.

Treggiari MM, Deem S. Critical care medicine. In: Barash PG, Cullen BF, Stoelting RK, et al, eds. *Clinical Anesthesia*. 6th ed. Lippincott Williams & Wilkins; 2009:1449–1450.

C

Cervical Cerclage: Anes Mgmt
Subspecialties: Obstetric Anesthesia

Nehal Gatha

Edited by Lars Helgeson

KEY POINTS

1. Cervical cerclage is a treatment for cervical incompetence. The cervix is sutured closed (purse string) during pregnancy to prevent preterm delivery.
2. This is most commonly done between 12 and 24 weeks' gestational age.
3. General or spinal anesthesia are common anesthesia solutions although low dose epidural and pudendal nerve blocks can be utilized.
4. Cervical cerclage is usually a very quick (<30 minutes), outpatient procedure, done in the lithotomy position, all of which must be taken into account for choice of the anesthetic.

DISCUSSION

Cervical cerclage is a common treatment for cervical incompetence in pregnancy. If a woman has a history of early miscarriages, previous gynecologic surgery (i.e., LEEP procedure) or D&E, her cervix can become incompetent and shorten or open too early, resulting in preterm labor. A cerclage can prevent this by suturing the cervix os closed to lessen these changes. A cerclage is placed ideally from 12 to 15 weeks of pregnancy. Occasionally, there is a need for urgent cerclage later in pregnancy if there is concern for preterm opening or shortening of the cervix. The cerclage is usually removed around 37 weeks of pregnancy in an office procedure not usually requiring anesthesia.

Cervical cerclage placement is quite a painful procedure. General anesthesia can be utilized; however, as with all pregnant patients, there are multiple concerns. There is risk to the mother, particularly because of aspiration. There is an increased risk of preterm labor, and several potential pharmacologic risks to the fetus. The fetal concerns are less pronounced after the first trimester, but maternal ones become more so. Because of many of these concerns, a spinal anesthetic is the technique of choice. One of the short-acting local anesthetics such as bupivacaine, lidocaine, mepivacaine, or prilocaine can be used. Lidocaine is less commonly used secondary to concerns of transient neurologic symptoms (TNS). A level of T10 is required for surgical anesthesia. Small amounts of opioid can be used to decrease the amount of local anesthetic needed. There is usually a very little visceral stimulation, so systemic opioids are usually unnecessary.

It is possible to use an epidural block or even a pudendal block with adequate anesthesia. These are less common techniques that may not be as fast-acting or reliable as a spinal anesthetic. However, in a patient where a general or spinal anesthetic is not desirable or possible, these options can be considered.

SUGGESTED READINGS

Beilin Y, Zahn J, Abramovitz S, et al. Subarachnoid small-dose bupivacaine versus lidocaine for cervical cerclage. *Anesth Analg.* 2003;97(1):56–61.

McCulloch B, Bergen S, Pielet B, et al. McDonald cerclage under pudendal nerve block. *Am J Obstet Gynecol.* 1993;168(2):499–502.

Morgan GE, Mikhail MS, Murray MJ. *Clinical Anesthesiology.* 4th ed. New York, NY: Lange Medical Books/McGraw-Hill; 2005:chap 17:890–910.

Schumann R. Low-dose epidural anesthesia for cervical cerclage. *Can J Anaesth.* 2003;50(4):424–425.

Cervical Fracture: Intubation Techniques
Anatomy

Jinlei Li

Edited by Ramachandran Ramani

C

KEY POINTS

1. With a documented or potential cervical fracture, the neck is to be maintained in neutral position to avoid excessive axial traction, extension, flexion, or rotation. Neck hyperflexion is proven to be more detrimental to the spinal cord than is neck hyperextension.
2. Commonly used techniques of neck stabilization include manual in-line stabilization (MILS), axial traction, sandbags, forehead tape, soft collar, and hard collar.
3. Neck positioning will make intubation more difficult. Among techniques used to maintain neutral neck position, MILS is the most effective; however, it is also the one that makes intubation the most difficult.
4. A variety of intubation techniques have been used: oral or nasal, direct laryngoscopy or blind, awake or asleep, videolaryngoscopy or fiberoptic bronchoscopy, depending on the clinical situation. Nasal intubation should be avoided in patients with midface or basilar skull fractures. In severe facial or neck injury that precludes endotracheal intubation, tracheostomy will be indicated.

DISCUSSION

In head trauma patients, cervical spine instability rate is anywhere between 2% and 10% on the basis of the severity of trauma overall. Head injuries with low Glasgow Coma Scores and/or focal neurologic deficits are more likely to be associated with C-spine injuries. On the other hand, cervical fracture or injury is less likely in an awake, alert patient without midline neck pain or tenderness. Cervical injury rate is significantly higher in patients with brain injuries, and vice versa. Confirmed or potential cervical fractures and injuries demonstrated by history, physical examination, X-ray, CT scan, or MRI should be treated with cervical spine precaution such as C-collar. Additional factors that may complicate the clinical evaluation of cervical fracture includes (1) neck pain, midline rather than paramedian; (2) severe distracting pain other than the neck; (3) any new onset neurologic signs and symptoms; (4) intoxicated patients; and (5) history of or current loss of consciousness. Any one of these factors will necessitate C-collar until C-spine fracture or injury is ruled out conclusively by imaging techniques. Cervical precautions are also exercised in nontrauma patients such as patients with rheumatoid arthritis or trisomy 21.

Almost all airway maneuvers during ventilation and intubation such as chin lift, jaw thrust, oral airway, and head tilt theoretically may result in cervical spine movement, although clinical evidence is lacking. The standard practice is to maintain the neck in neutral position in any acutely injured patients in whom neck injury has not been ruled out yet.

Among the various ways to maintain neutral neck position, MILS is performed by holding down the occiput (to prevent head and neck rotation, hyperflexion, or hyperextension) by two to three operators. The neck positioning will evidently make oral intubation more difficult. Nasal intubation either blind or fiberoptic can be used under circumstances when midface or basilar skull fractures are not involved or suspected. Video-guided techniques such as videolaryngoscopy and fiberoptic bronchoscopy may minimize the requirement of mouth opening or head/neck movement. In trauma patients, rapid sequence induction is frequently indicated. When difficult intubation in anticipated

C

and/or multiple neck injuries are involved, awake intubation, retrograde intubation, or elective tracheotomy may be warranted. It is important to document existing neurologic injuries in preoperative evaluation before any maneuvers of the head and neck.

Capan LM, Miller SM. Anesthesia for trauma and burn patients. In: Barash PG, Cullen BF, Stoelting RK, et al, eds. *Clinical Anesthesia*. 6th ed. Philadelphia, PA: Lippincott Williams & Wilkins; 2009:890–903.
Morgan GE, Mikhail MS, Murray M. *Clinical Anesthesiology*. 4th ed. New York, NY: McGraw-Hill; 2005:860–863.

SUGGESTED READINGS

Chloroprocaine: Onset and Metabolism

Pharmacology

Tori Myslajek and Archer Martin

Edited by Jodi Sherman

KEY POINTS

1. Local anesthetic pKa greatly influences the rate of onset. Those with a pKa closer to physiologic pH have a more rapid onset.
2. Local anesthetic onset is most rapid when the drugs are in their lipid-soluble form, thus facilitating diffusion across lipid cellular walls.
3. Chloroprocaine is a local anesthetic with a relatively high pKa of 9.0, and so the fast onset is likely due to the high concentration of chloroprocaine used clinically.
4. Chloroprocaine is an ester-type local anesthetic and is metabolized by pseudocholinesterase.
5. Systemic toxicity of ester-type local anesthetics is inversely proportional to the rate of hydrolysis. Within this class, chloroprocaine is hydrolyzed the quickest.
6. Pseudocholinesterase enzymes are not present in cerebrospinal fluid, so metabolism of intrathecal administration of chloroprocaine and other ester-type local anesthetics depends on systemic absorption.
7. Metabolism of ester-type local anesthetics is slowed in patients with liver disease, neonates, parturients, or patients with a genetically abnormal pseudocholinesterase.

DISCUSSION

Local anesthetics are composed of three structural groups: a lipophilic group (an aromatic ring), a hydrophilic group (usually a tertiary amine), and a connecting hydrocarbon chain (either an ester or amide). The ester or amide linkage determines the local anesthetic group classification. The two major differences in the ester and amide groups are their metabolism and allergic potential, with esters being a greater allergen than amides (Table 1).

Local anesthetic pKa greatly influences the rate of onset. Those with a pKa closer to physiologic pH have a more rapid onset. The onset of local anesthetics is most rapid when the drugs are in their lipid-soluble form, thus facilitating diffusion across lipid cellular walls. Chloroprocaine has a pKa of 9.0, well above physiologic pH, and in fact higher than nearly every other local anesthetic. However, the rapid onset of chloroprocaine in vivo is likely due to the high concentration (3%) used clinically. As a result of the rapid metabolism of chloroprocaine by plasma cholinesterase, there is less toxicity when compared with amides despite the large concentration of drug used clinically.

Table 1. List of Local Anesthetics

Esters	Amides
Benzocaine	Lidocaine
Cocaine	Mepivacaine
Procaine	Bupivacaine
Chloroprocaine	Etidocaine
Tetracaine	Prilocaine
	Ropivacaine

After injection, local anesthetics are systemically absorbed and the majority of metabolism is either in the liver (amides) or by pseudocholinesterase (esters). Ester-type local anesthetics undergo hydrolysis by pseudocholinesterase, either plasma cholinesterase or butyrylcholinesterase, which mostly occurs in the plasma and to a lesser extent in the liver itself. The exception is cocaine, which undergoes significant metabolism in the liver.

Chloroprocaine is an ester-type local anesthetic that, like others in its class, is metabolized by pseudocholinesterase. Pseudocholinesterase enzymes are not present in cerebrospinal fluid, so metabolism of intrathecal administration of chloroprocaine and other ester-type local anesthetics depends of systemic absorption. It is rarely used intrathecally because of the potential for prolonged deficit, although this may be related more to the preparation of the drug in a low pH solution containing sodium bisulfite rather than from chloroprocaine itself.

Systemic toxicity of ester-type local anesthetics is inversely proportional to the rate of hydrolysis. Within this class, chloroprocaine is hydrolyzed the quickest. Metabolism of these drugs is slowed in patients with liver disease, neonates, parturients, or patients with a genetically abnormal pseudocholinesterase. This implies that toxicity may be enhanced and duration of blockade may be prolonged secondary to decreased metabolism in these patient populations.

Hydrolysis at the ester linkage results in water-soluble derivatives, 2-chloroaminobenzoic acid and 2-diethylaminoethanol, and are excreted in the urine. Benzocaine and procaine also result in para-aminobenzoic acid (a PABA derivative). The metabolites are inactive, but para-aminobenzoic acid may be antigenic and responsible for allergic reactions.

For comparison, amide-type local anesthetics are metabolized in the liver by microsomal enzymes via aromatic hydroxylation, N-dealkylation, and amide hydrolysis. Compared with ester anesthetics, this is a more complicated and slower process. The slower metabolism implies that systemic toxicity and cumulative drug effects are more likely in this drug class when compared with the ester class.

SUGGESTED READINGS

Cousins MJ, Bridenbaugh PO, Carr DB, et al, eds. *Cousins & Bridenbaugh's Neural Blockade in Clinical Anesthesia and Pain Medicine*. 4th ed. Philadelphia, PA: Lippincott Williams & Wilkins; 2008.

Miller RD. *Miller's Anesthesia*. 6th ed. Philadelphia, PA: Churchill Livingstone; 2005:573–576, 592.

Morgan GE, Mikhail MS, Murray MJ. *Clinical Anesthesiology*. 4th ed. Philadelphia, PA: McGraw-Hill Professional; 2005:265–269.

Stoelting RK, Hillier SC. *Pharmacology & Physiology in Anesthetic Practice*. 4th ed. Philadelphia, PA: Lippincott Williams & Wilkins; 2006:179–188.

Chloroprocaine Placental Transfer

Subspecialties: Obstetric

Donald Neirink

Edited by Lars Helgeson

C

KEY POINTS

1. Factors that influence the placental transfer of local anesthetics include the concentration of free drug in the maternal blood, placenta permeability, and the chemical characteristics of the local anesthetic itself.
2. The duration of action of chloroprocaine is short lived, and its rapid metabolism by plasma pseudocholinesterase results in almost no drug crossing the placenta.

DISCUSSION

Many drugs, including local anesthetics, readily cross the placenta. Factors that influence the placental transfer of local anesthetics include the concentration of free drug in the maternal blood, placenta permeability, and the chemical characteristics of the local anesthetic itself. Local anesthetics cross the placenta by passive diffusion. The rate of actual transfer is determined in part by the degree of ionization, molecular size, and lipid solubility. Of note, 95% of chloroprocaine is ionized at physiologic pH, one of the highest compared with other local anesthetics.

Chloroprocaine is an ester local anesthetic, with a rapid onset and short-time duration of action. The intravascular half-life is approximately 45 seconds. The rapid metabolism by plasma pseudocholinesterase allows for no accumulation, and therefore almost no drug crosses the placenta. This rapid metabolism, along with its quick onset, makes chloroprocaine an excellent choice for safely establishing epidural anesthesia quickly in the event of an emergency caesarean section.

SUGGESTED READINGS

Barash PG, Cullen BF, Stoelting RK, et al. *Clinical Anesthesia*. 6th ed. New York, NY: Lippincott Williams & Wilkins; 2009:536.

Chestnut DH. *Obstetric Anesthesia: Principles and Practice*. 3rd ed. Philadelphia, PA: Elsevier and Mosby; 2004:199–200.

Miller RD. *Miller's Anesthesia*. 6th ed. Philadelphia, PA: Elsevier, Churchill, and Livingstone; 2006:2323.

Chronic Opioids: Side Effects
Subspecialties: Pain

Adrianna Oprea

Edited by Thomas Halaszynski

KEY POINTS

1. Opioids are the most commonly used analgesic in the postoperative period, including patients with chronic opioid use.
2. Side effects from high doses and chronic use may limit successful use of these medications in the treatment of pain.
3. Adverse effects associated with chronic opioid use can predominate over the therapeutic pain-relieving properties of such drugs and cause sedation, respiratory depression, impaired cognition, nausea and vomiting, loss of appetite, pruritus, urinary retention, impaired orthostatic tolerance, and ileus and constipation.
4. Patients may develop tolerance to some of the adverse effects of opioids, but not to others, such as constipation.

DISCUSSION

Opioid analgesics can generate numerous side effects that complicate their use in postoperative care, in the treatment of pain associated with advanced cancer, for chronic pain patients, and in numerous other uses and illnesses. Side effects from these medications are among the most common reasons cited for the failure of opioids to relieve pain in patients taking opioids chronically. Physician concerns regarding the risk of certain side effects, such as respiratory depression, might dissuade prescribing opioids or may lead to suboptimal opioid dosing. The incidence and severity of side effects from the administration of opioids can be an important factor in the success or failure of pain management in patients taking opioids chronically. These side effects include sedation, respiratory depression, impaired cognition, nausea and vomiting, loss of appetite, pruritus, urinary retention, impaired orthostatic tolerance, and ileus and constipation.

Constipation is a common adverse effect associated with opioid administration. Although patients may develop tolerance to some of the associated opioid side effects, this does not usually hold true in the case of chronic opioid use. Nausea and vomiting sometimes seen with opioid administration may also be associated with constipation. Constipation is best treated prophylactically at the initiation of opioid therapy.

Nausea may occur with or without vomiting. Tolerance to nausea usually develops after several days of opioid therapy. Vomiting accompanies nausea more often when constipation is not well controlled. Any complaint of nausea or vomiting warrants a thorough bowel assessment. It may be necessary to use antiemetic therapy on a scheduled basis for the first week of opioid therapy, after which it can be discontinued if nausea disappears or opioids are used on an as-needed basis.

Sedation may occur at the onset of opioid therapy but usually disappears after a few days. The patient may complain of feeling drowsy. Patients and their families should be cautioned to expect this and be reassured that should the problem persist, it can usually be managed without sacrificing pain control through the reduction of the dose gradually or by changing the opioid. Occasionally, sedation continues to be a problem; however, it can be effectively managed with the judicious use of central nervous system stimulants, such as methylphenidate (Ritalin) or dexamphetamine (Dexedrine).

Respiratory depression is perhaps the most serious side effect from opioid administration. Chronic opioid users are usually tolerant to this effect. Pain is a natural antagonist to the respiratory depressant effects of opioids; therefore, as long as the patient is experiencing pain, it is less likely that respiratory depression will occur.

Close monitoring is warranted in patients taking chronic opioids or when another pain intervention, such as an anesthetic block, effectively takes away the pain stimulus. Care must be taken in these situations to titrate the opioid dose downward without precipitating an opioid withdrawal reaction. Withdrawal can be avoided by administering approximately 33% of the previous opioid dose.

Myoclonus is a fairly common side effect seen most often with chronic opioid use or administration of higher opioid doses. The patient may experience mild to moderate muscle jerks, most commonly during sleep, but occasionally throughout the day. If persistent, low doses of a benzodiazepine or muscle relaxant may help.

Other side effects from chronic opioid use include confusion, hallucinations, and dizziness. Like sedation, these are most often temporary and tolerance frequently develops. However, progressive worsening of these symptoms on stable opioid dosing usually indicates an alternate cause and should be evaluated.

SUGGESTED READINGS

Barash PG, Cullen BF, Stoelting RK. *Clinical Anesthesia*. 5th ed. Philadelphia, PA: Lippincott Williams & Wilkins; 2006:353–379.

Morgan GE, Mikhail MS, Murray MJ. *Clinical Anesthesiology*. 4th ed. New York, NY: McGraw-Hill; 2005:195–196.

Circ Arrest: pH-Stat Implications
Subspecialties: Critical Care

Roberto Rappa

Edited by Benjamin Sherman

KEY POINTS

1. During hypothermic conditions, the solubility of CO_2 in plasma increases, resulting in a lower $PaCO_2$ and a higher plasma pH.
2. Hypothermic hypocarbia causes cerebral vasoconstriction and decreased blood flow to the brain.
3. pH-stat management promotes the maintenance of a constant blood pH and CO_2 during hypothermia with temperature-*corrected* blood gas values.
4. Alpha-stat management promotes the maintenance of electrochemical neutrality by maintaining a constant OH^-/H^+ ratio and uses temperature-*uncorrected* blood gas values.
5. In adults, alpha-stat management during moderate hypothermia produces better neurologic outcomes.
6. In infants, pH-stat management may be more beneficial than alpha-stat management because of more homogeneous brain cooling, less oxygen consumption, and better cerebral metabolic recovery.

DISCUSSION

Alpha-stat and pH-stat are blood gas management modalities used when patients undergo hypothermic cardiopulmonary bypass or deep hypothermic circulatory arrest. There exists some controversy regarding which management strategy is best under deep hypothermic conditions. The following discussion will illustrate the differences in alpha and pH stat management strategies and present advantages and disadvantages of each.

Temperature has a profound impact on the solubility of gasses in solution. In general, as temperature decreases, the solubility of gasses in solution (i.e., plasma) increases. The most notable effect of this phenomenon is seen with carbon dioxide gas tensions under hypothermic or deep hypothermic cardiopulmonary bypass and/or circulatory arrest. There exists considerable debate whether temperature-corrected or temperature-uncorrected blood gas values should be used to manage the patient during cardiac surgery.

Under hypothermic conditions, the solubility of CO_2 in plasma increases, resulting in a lower partial pressure of CO_2 ($PaCO_2$). Plasma bicarbonate concentrations, however, remain unchanged. Therefore, as the $PaCO_2$ decreases, the pH tends to increase. For example, blood with a CO_2 tension of 40 mm Hg and pH of 7.40 at 37° C will have a CO_2 tension of 23 mm Hg and pH of 7.60 when cooled to 25° C.

It is useful to review briefly the definition of temperature *corrected* when discussing blood gas analysis. All blood gas analysis machines warm the blood sample to 37° C, regardless of what the patient's actual temperature is. As a result, the measured pCO_2 level does not reflect the true pCO_2 levels in the hypothermic patient. Yet these machines can *correct* for this over measurement if the technician enters the patient's true temperature (i.e., 25°) into the machine. The blood gas machine will then *correct* the temperature by subtracting the amount of pCO_2 that is due to the warming of the sample and then give a reading that corresponds to the patient's true temperature and hypothermic pCO_2.

The pH-stat management strategy promotes the maintenance of a constant blood pH and CO_2 tension, despite changes in body temperature. It involves managing blood gas parameters with temperature-*corrected* values. As a result, pH-stat management requires the perfusionist to add CO_2 to the oxygenator gas inflow as body temperature and $PaCO_2$ decreases. Total CO_2 content in the patient's blood subsequently increases.

Theoretic advantages include more homogeneous brain cooling and decreased brain O_2 consumption. This is achieved because the increase in CO_2 content during pH-stat management uncouples cerebral autoregulation. CO_2 is a potent cerebral vasodilator, and therefore cerebral blood flow increases despite decreased O_2 consumption during general anesthesia and hypothermia. The increased cerebral blood flow is thought to confer neuroprotection for infants maintained on cardiopulmonary bypass (CPB) and to promote deep homogeneous cooling of the brain before circulatory arrest. The disadvantage of this technique, however, is that the higher cerebral blood flow during rewarming may increase the embolic load sent to the brain.

The alpha-stat management strategy attempts to achieve electrochemical neutrality by maintaining a constant OH^-/H^+ ratio. It involves managing blood gas parameters with temperature-*uncorrected* values. It does not call for the addition of CO_2 to the oxygenator and, consequently, does not alter total CO_2 content in the blood. Theoretical advantages include the preservation of enzymatic function and the maintenance of cerebral autoregulation.

Despite the purported benefits of pH-stat management, several prospective randomized trials have demonstrated that alpha-stat management during moderate hypothermia produces better neurologic outcomes. Current recommendations, therefore, promote the use of alpha-stat management in adults undergoing moderate hypothermic CPB. It is unclear which strategy is best when deep hypothermia is used with or without circulatory arrest.

In the pediatric literature, a single prospective randomized trial showed no significant neurologic outcome benefit of the pH-stat management strategy. Other studies, however, suggest that pH-stat management may be more beneficial than alpha-stat management for infants because of more homogeneous cooling, less oxygen consumption, and better cerebral metabolic recovery. The current trend in pediatric CPB is to use pH-stat alone or in combination with alpha-stat when deep hypothermia is used.

SUGGESTED READINGS

Morgan GE, Mikhail MS, Murray MJ. *Clinical Anesthesiology*. 4th ed. New York, NY: Lange Medical Books/McGraw-Hill; 2005:chap 21:514–515.

Nussmeier NA, Hauser MC, Sarwar MF, et al. *Miller's Anesthesia*. 7th ed. Philadelphia, PA: Churchill Livingstone; 2009:chap 60.

Cirrhosis: NMB Pharmacokinetics

Pharmacology and Generic Clinical Sciences: Anesthesia Procedures, Methods, Techniques

Gabriel Pitta and Marianne Saleeb

Edited by Thomas Halaszynski

KEY POINTS

1. Cirrhosis of the liver can result in decreased hepatic blood flow along with a hyperdynamic circulation and an increased volume of distribution.
2. Cirrhosis of the liver can affect what the body does to medications (metabolism) that may alter the kinetics of nondepolarizing muscle relaxants.
3. Succinylcholine and mivacurium are usually acceptable alternatives for use in cirrhotic patients who may otherwise be unable to properly tolerate nondepolarizing muscle relaxants.
4. Dosage and administration of nondepolarizing neuromuscular blockers (NMB) need to take into consideration both the increased volume of distribution that accompanies cirrhosis as well as the decreased hepatic clearance and metabolism of such drugs inherent in these patients.

DISCUSSION

The physiology of the cirrhotic patient presents with several challenges for anesthesiologist. The extent of liver scarring and parenchymal damage coupled with portal hypertension will affect hepatic perfusion and clearance of metabolites. In addition, it is expected that cirrhosis of the liver will influence the volume of distribution of medications that will typically be increased in such patients. The hypoproteinemic state of the cirrhotic patient will also play a part in pharmacokinetics, with an example being the smaller degree of midazolam protein binding in these patients that results in an increase in the free fraction of drug and an enhancement of its pharmacologic effect.

Succinylcholine and mivacurium are generally well accepted and safe to use on the cirrhotic patient unlike other nondepolarizing muscle relaxants. Severe liver dysfunction can decrease plasma cholinesterase activity and theoretically prolong the action of these drugs, although this has rarely caused a clinical problem or concern.

Several factors affect the pharmacologic effects of nondepolarizing muscle relaxants like age, temperature, acid–base balance, intravascular protein concentration, and electrolyte status. Hypothermia decreases the metabolism of some drugs and also prolongs the excretion of some medications, and this may also prove evident in patients with cirrhosis (prolongs the block from NMB agents). Hypocalcemia, hypermagnesemia, and hypokalemia can all potentiate neuromuscular blockade. Acidosis can augment the neuromuscular blocking effect of several muscle relaxants and also plays an antagonistic role in the reversal of these medications.

The increased volume of distribution of medications administered that accompanies cirrhosis, particularly in those patients with ascites, results in the need for a larger initial dose of nondepolarizing neuromuscular agents. Besides the increased volume of distribution required in these patients, an increase in the concentration of gamma-globulin may also contribute to the increased initial dose required to achieve an appropriate plasma concentration of these particular NMB. Rocuronium, atracurium, and pancuronium are more likely to require an increased initial dose than vecuronium. Subsequent doses of NMB may in turn need to be smaller than usual due to decreased hepatic clearance and metabolism of nondepolarizing muscle relaxants. There is some variability among NMBs, with the half-time of atracurium and cisatracurium remaining unaffected and vecuronium's half-time increasing in excess of 0.1 mg/kg/dose in patients with cirrhosis.

SUGGESTED READINGS

Barash PG, Cullen BF, Stoelting RK, eds. *Clinical Anesthesia*. 5th ed. Philadelphia, PA: Lippincott Williams & Wilkins; 2006:1104.

Hines RL, Marschall KE, eds. *Stoelting's Anesthesia and Co-existing Disease*. 5th ed. Philadelphia, PA: Elsevier; 2008:271.

Mikhail GE, Morgan M, Murray M. *Clinical Anesthesiology*. 4th ed. New York, NY: McGraw-Hill Companies; 2006:155, 205–219.

C

Closed Claims: Brain Damage

Generic Clinical Sciences: Anesthesia Procedures, Methods, Techniques

Neil Sinha

Edited by Ramachandran Ramani

1. American Society of Anesthesiologists (ASA) Closed Claim Project is a study of 8,594 closed insurance claims resulting from a primary anesthetic complication.
2. Permanent brain damage or death was the resulting outcome in 2,613 of 6,750 claims between 1975 through 2000.
3. The major mechanisms of injury resulting in brain damage or death were respiratory and cardiovascular.

The ASA Closed Claim Project is an in-depth study of 8,594 closed insurance claims resulting from a primary anesthetic complication. Case summaries are generated from each claim, which include patient demographic information, ASA physical status, surgical procedure, anesthetic technique, events leading to claim, type and severity of injury, outcome of litigation, and potential to prevent the adverse outcomes. Dental injury and claims in which the basic sequence of events cannot be constructed are excluded from the database. The ASA Closed Claims Project collects data on a continual basis.

Permanent brain damage or death was the resulting outcome in 2,613 of 6,750 claims between 1975 through 2000. Claims for brain damage or death were 56% in 1976; this dropped approximately 1% per year until 2000, at which time 27% of total claims were from death or brain damage.

The major mechanisms of injury resulting in brain damage or death were respiratory and cardiovascular (68% of damaging events from 1975 to 2000). The respiratory causes were further subdivided into difficult intubation (23% of respiratory events), inadequate ventilation and/or oxygenation (22%), esophageal intubation (13%), and premature extubation (12%). The cardiovascular causes included multifactorial (35%), pulmonary embolism (16%), inadequate fluid (14%), stroke (13%), hemorrhage (11%), and myocardial infarction (11%) (see Table 1).

The proportion of claims for death or permanent brain damage has been declining from 1975 through 2000. Increased uses of SpO_2 and $ETCO_2$, and increased claims for "lesser" issues have been hypothesized as the causes of the steady decline, although no causality has been established at this point.

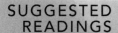

Table 1. Damaging Events Associated with Death and Permanent Brain Damage, 1986 to 2000 ($n = 1,411$)

Respiratory Damaging Events	n	Total Respiratory Events (%)	Less Than Appropriate Care, n (%)
Difficult intubation	115	23	58 (50)
Inadequate ventilation/ oxygenation	111	22	82 (74)
Esophageal intubation	66	13	60 (91)
Premature extubation	58	12	47 (81)
Aspiration	50	10	21 (42)
Airway obstruction	47	9	25 (53)
Other respiratory	56	11	29 (52)
Total	503	100	322 (64)*

Cardiovascular Damaging Events	n	Total Cardiovascular Events (%)	Less Than Appropriate Care, n (%)
Multifactorial/miscellaneous	154	35	28 (18)
Pulmonary embolism	70	16	10 (14)
Inadequate fluid therapy	63	14	48 (76)
Stroke	58	13	14 (24)
Hemorrhage	49	11	9 (18)
Myocardial infarction	48	11	23 (27)
Total	442	100	122 (28)*

Medication-Related Damaging Events	n	Total Medication-Related Events (%)	Less Than Appropriate Care, n (%)
Wrong drug/dose	68	55	52 (76)
Allergic or adverse drug reaction	51	41	12 (24)
Malignant hyperthermia	5	4	4 (80)
Total	124	100	68 (55)

Equipment-Related Damaging Events	n	Total Equipment-Related Events (%)	Less Than Appropriate Care, n (%)
Central lines	54	60	22 (41)
Gas delivery	16	18	13 (81)
Miscellaneous/other	20	22	10 (50)
Total	90	100	45 (50)

Block-Related Damaging Events	n	Total Block-Related Events (%)	Less Than Appropriate Care, n (%)
Neuraxial cardiac arrest	47	53	23 (49)
High spinal/epidural	19	22	12 (63)
Intravenous injection/local absorption	9	10	5 (56)
Other	13	15	10 (77)
Total	88	100	50 (57)

* $P < 0.01$ difference between % less than appropriate care in respiratory *versus* cardiovascular events (chi-square).
Miscellaneous categories of damaging events are not shown ($n = 164$).

ASA Closed Claims Project. www.asaclosedclaims.org. Accessed November 14, 2010.
Cheney FW, Posner KL, Lee LA, et al. Trends in anesthesia-related death and brain damage: a closed claims analysis. *Anesthesiology*. 2006;105(6):1081–1086.

SUGGESTED READINGS

Clostridium tetani Infection
Subspecialties: Critical Care

Margaret Rose

Edited by Hossam Tantawy

KEY POINTS

1. *Clostridium tetani* is an anaerobic bacillus producing tetanospasmin, which prevents the release of inhibitory neurotransmitters GABA and glycine, leading to widespread muscle spasm and a hypersympathetic state. Its binding in synaptic terminals is irreversible, and recovery requires generation of new synapses.
2. Tetanus is characterized by descending muscle rigidity, "lock-jaw," muscle spasms, and excessive circulating catecholamines (causing blood pressure instability and cardiac arrhythmias).
3. Complications include respiratory compromise due to laryngospasm or tetanic diaphragm contraction, dislocated joints, broken long bones or vertebrae, rhabdomyolysis, seizure, cardiac arrhythmias, and nosocomial infections.
4. Recommended treatment includes airway stabilization, mechanical ventilation, intrathecal immunoglobulin, benzodiazepines, nondepolarizing neuromuscular blockade, antibiotics (metronidazole or clindamycin), Labetolol, and prevention of metabolic complication and nosocomial infections.

DISCUSSION

Clostridium tetani is an obligate anaerobic gram-positive spore-forming bacillus, commonly found in the soil. The disease-state tetanus remains widespread in developing nations due to lack of or inadequate vaccinations, with more than 50% of deaths occurring in neonates. In developed nations, infections have become rare due to widespread immunization since 1924. However, infections in the United States have been reported, generally following acute trauma (more than 80% in puncture wounds or lacerations), in patients who are most commonly diabetic, elderly, or Hispanic.

Clostridium tetani bacteria produce tetanospasmin, one of the most potent toxins known, with the lethal dose for a 70 kg human estimated to be 175 ng. The primary effect of tetanospasmin is to block the release of inhibitory neurotransmitters glycine and GABA by preventing the fusion of the neurotransmitter vesicle with the presynaptic neuron membrane, leading to widespread neuronal excitation. In addition to well-known effects on skeletal muscle, also of critical importance is the hypersympathetic state resulting from excessive (uninhibited) catecholamine release.

The incubation period is between 3 and 21 days, with the duration of incubation being related to the distance of the site from the central nervous system, and also correlates inversely with disease severity. The shorter efferent nerves are affected first accounting for the early characteristic "lock-jaw" and neck rigidity. In a descending progression, it causes difficulty swallowing and abdominal rigidity. Commonly, spasms result in arm flexion and leg extension and may include laryngospasm and tetanic diaphragm contraction, causing respiratory compromise. The spasms may be so severe as to cause joint dislocations, rhabdomyolysis, and even long bone and vertebral fractures. These spasms are excruciatingly painful, particularly as the patient remains conscious. Excessive catecholamine release causes extremes of blood pressure as well as cardiac arrhythmias, including arrest.

Since no laboratory test is currently available, tetanus remains a diagnosis of exclusion. The simple bedside "spatula test" has been reported to have greater than 90% specificity and sensitivity for tetanus: the insertion of a spatula into the mouth of a patient with tetanus will result in masseter spasm (rather than gag reflex), causing the patient to bite the spatula. The differential diagnoses are limited, but include strychnine poisoning, hypocalcemia, neuroleptic drug toxicity, and dystonic reactions from central dopamine antagonist.

TREATMENT

Patients suspected of having tetanus must be monitored in an intensive care setting with minimal stimulation. Treatment is directed toward the treatment of muscle spasms, respiratory support, and prevention of complications arising from autonomic dysfunction, respiratory compromise, metabolic derangements, and nosocomial infections.

Early airway stabilization is crucial, and tracheotomy may well be necessary (due to laryngospasm). With the disease course being predictably over 2 weeks, mechanical ventilation and nutritional support should be instituted. As GABA agonists, benzodiazepines are an important intervention, helping to reduce muscle rigidity and prevent spasm as well as seizure. If the appropriate dose is not effectively controlling muscle spasm, a nondepolarizing neuromuscular blocker can be added. Autonomic instability arising from excessive circulating catecholamines should be treated with both alpha and beta blockade (i.e., Labetolol). The infection of *C. tetani* itself should be treated with metronidazole or clindamycin, antibiotics with activity against anaerobic organisms. Any wound suspected to be the portal of entry should be debrided.

Since the toxin appears to irreversibly affect nerve terminals, and recovery is dependent on the formation of new synapses, a crucial component of therapy is the protection of unaffected neurons. Therefore antitoxin therapy should be instituted early, with intrathecal administration being the preferred route, owing to a relative reduction in the rate of respiratory complications and decreased duration of spasm, when compared with intravenous administration.

Preventing and treating metabolic complications and nosocomial infections is an important facet of these patients' care. In particular, they have an increased risk of hospital-acquired pneumonia and rhabdomyolysis.

SUGGESTED READING

Irwin RS, Rippe JM, eds. *Irwin and Rippe's Intensive Care Medicine*. Philadelphia, PA: Lippincott Williams & Wilkins; 2008:chap 89:1139–1141.

CO$_2$ Absorbers: Volatile Anesthetics Toxicity

Physics, Monitoring, and Anesthesia Delivery Devices

Robert Schonberger

Edited by Raj K. Modak

KEY POINTS

1. Several volatile anesthetics react with CO$_2$ absorbents.
2. Both Baralyme and soda lime degrade sevoflurane into Compound A, a substance that has been shown to exhibit nephrotoxicity in laboratory studies.
3. Most anesthesia practitioners avoid low fresh-gas flows when using sevoflurane, and the Food and Drug Administration (FDA)-approved package insert follows this recommendation.
4. Volatile anesthetics react with strong bases to form carbon monoxide. This is of clinical relevance only in the case of desiccated absorbers.
5. Degradation of volatile anesthetics in a desiccated absorber is an exothermic reaction. Particularly in the case of sevoflurane, this reaction can in extreme circumstances lead to operating room fires.

DISCUSSION

Both Baralyme and soda lime degrade sevoflurane into fluoromethyl-2-2-difluoro-1-(trifluoromethyl) vinyl ether, which is better known, for obvious reasons, as Compound A. While Compound A has been demonstrated to exhibit nephrotoxicity in laboratory rats, no study has ever shown clinically significant changes in human kidney function after exposure to sevoflurane. Nevertheless, many practitioners avoid low fresh-gas flows when using sevoflurane, and the FDA-approved package insert follows this recommendation. Amsorb, in contrast to soda lime and Baralyme, is not known to cause the formation of Compound A.

The strong bases sodium and potassium hydroxide found in many absorbers can react with volatile anesthetics to form carbon monoxide. Desiccated absorbents are much more efficient at carbon monoxide production than hydrated absorbents. Although all volatile anesthetics will form some carbon monoxide, desflurane will produce the highest concentration, followed by enflurane and isoflurane. Both sevoflurane and halothane will produce only very small amounts of carbon monoxide. Amsorb is not known to catalyze the formation of carbon monoxide. Desiccated absorbers are commonly encountered in so-called "Monday morning syndrome" after machines have been flushed with high fresh-gas flows for 2 days. Clinically relevant carbon monoxide toxicity can be prevented by the use of hydrated absorbents.

Degradation of volatile anesthetics in a desiccated absorber is an exothermic reaction. Particularly in the case of sevoflurane, this reaction can in extreme circumstances lead to operating room fires. The best way to avoid such an outcome is to use hydrated absorbents by changing them regularly.

SUGGESTED READING

Miller RD. *Miller's Anesthesia.* 6th ed. Philadelphia, PA: Elsevier Churchill Livingstone; 2005:251–256.

Compensated Respiratory Acidosis: ABG
Subspecialties: Critical Care

Chi Wong

Edited by Ala Haddadin

KEY POINTS

1. The most common cause of respiratory acidosis is alveolar hypoventilation.
2. Compensation is by renal elimination of H^+, increased HCO_3^- reabsorption and HCO_3^- production.
3. In acute respiratory acidosis, plasma HCO_3^- will increase 1 mEq per L for each 10 mm Hg increase in $PaCO_2$ above 40.
4. In chronic respiratory acidosis, plasma HCO_3^- will increase 4 mEq per L for each 10 mm Hg increase in $PaCO_2$ above 40.

DISCUSSION

Respiratory acidosis is an arterial blood pH < 7.35 (normal 7.35 to 7.45) with an increase in $PaCO_2 > 40$ and $HCO_3^- \geq 24$. This occurs when there is a rise in $PaCO_2$ due to ventilatory elimination (e.g., hypoventilation) and/or overproduction (e.g., hypermetabolic state such as malignant hyperthermia, large caloric loads, thyroid storm, intense shivering, prolonged seizure activity).

Acute respiratory acidosis is present before renal compensation is complete. The pH will decrease 0.08 for every acute 10 mm Hg increase in $PaCO_2$. The compensation is limited to the buffering capacity of primarily hemoglobin, as well as plasma proteins and phosphates. Transcellular shifts of extracellular H^+ for intracellular K^+ also occur. In the acute setting, there is limited renal effect by retaining HCO_3^-. Hence, plasma HCO_3^- will increase 1 mEq per L for each acute 10-mm Hg increase in $PaCO_2$ above 40.

Chronic respiratory acidosis occurs after complete renal compensation via elimination of H^+, increased renal HCO_3^- reabsorption, and HCO_3^- production. These effects are not immediate and take hours (12 to 24 hours) to days (maximum response at 3 to 5 days) to return the pH toward normal. Hence, plasma HCO_3^- will increase 4 mEq per L for each chronic 10-mm Hg increase in $PaCO_2$ above 40.

For severe respiratory acidosis (pH < 7.2) treatment requires mechanical ventilation to increase alveolar ventilation. Respiratory parameters such as respiratory rate and tidal volume are guided by the arterial blood gas analysis. Definitive treatment is aimed at correcting the underlying cause. During compensation, the pH will return toward normal, but never back to normal in respiratory acidosis. Correction of pH back to normal occurs only after the initial insult that caused the acid–base disorder is resolved.

SUGGESTED READINGS

Miller RD. *Miller's Anesthesia.* 7th ed. Philadelphia, PA: Elsevier, Churchill Livingstone; 2009:1560, 1562.

Morgan GE, Mikhail MS, Murray MJ. Obstetric anesthesia. In: *Clinical Anesthesiology.* 4th ed. New York, NY: McGraw Hill; 2006:715–716.

Stoelting RK, Miller RD. *Basics of Anesthesia.* 5th ed. Philadelphia, PA: Churchill Livingstone; 2005:320–321.

Congenital Heart Disease: Prostaglandin Rx

Subspecialties: Pediatric Anesthesia

Margo Vallee

Edited by Mamatha Punjala

C

1. Prostaglandin (PGE_1) is primarily used for therapy in infants with congenital cardiac anomalies that require a patent ductus arteriosus for survival, including pulmonary stenosis and atresia, aortic coarctation, tetralogy of Fallot, and transposition of the great arteries.
2. The mechanism of PGE_1 is through relaxation of the smooth muscle of the ductus arteriosus.
3. Side effects of PGE_1 therapy include apnea, flushing, and fever.

DISCUSSION

PGE_1 is primarily used for therapy in infants with congenital cardiac anomalies that require a patent ductus arteriosus for survival. There are several kinds of ductal-dependent lesions, including pulmonary stenosis or pulmonary atresia, severe coarctation of the aorta, transposition of the great arteries, tetralogy of Fallot, and interrupted aortic arch. This drug is utilized in patients who have ductus-dependent cardiac lesions such as aortic stenosis and hypoplastic left heart syndrome, where systemic flow is obtained through the ductus. It is also indispensable in patients with cyanotic lesions such as pulmonary atresia as well as transposition of the great arteries, where pulmonary blood flow is supplied by the ductus. The goal of treatment is to achieve an increased PO_2, an increased systemic blood pressure, and an improved pH.

The mechanism of PGE_1 is through relaxation of the smooth muscle of the ductus arteriosus. It is a potent vasodilator of both the pulmonary and the systemic vascular beds, although it may produce less systemic vasodilation than other nonspecific vasodilators. However, PGE_1 was shown to reduce pulmonary vascular resistance and systemic vascular resistance by a similar amount when given to children after cardiopulmonary bypass. PGE_1 also has a positive inotropic effect and therefore increases cardiac output. This explains why a slight increase in blood pressure is seen in awake humans. Additional effects include inhibition of platelet aggregation (although this is not appreciated at clinical doses) and stimulation of intestinal and uterine smooth muscle. It also increases renal blood flow, urine flow, and sodium excretion. The starting dose of PGE_1 is 0.05 to 0.1 μg/kg/minute. Maintenance infusion rate is between 0.05 and 0.4 μg/kg/minute. At low doses (0.1 μg/kg/minute), it serves to maintain the patency of the ductus arteriosus. It can also reopen a closed ductus in some cases. Approximately 80% of PGE_1 is bound to albumin. Approximately 80% is metabolized in one pass through the lung vasculature. PGE_1 metabolites are excreted through the kidneys; about 90% of an intravenous dose is excreted in the urine within 24 hours. The neonate generally responds with an increase in PaO_2 10 to 15 minutes after initiation of the drug. Some patients may not respond until after several hours of drug infusion. The half-life of the drug is one circulation time, so continuous uninterrupted infusion must be maintained. Once the patient responds, the dose can be reduced to one-half or less of the initial effective dose.

About 20% of infants who receive PGE_1 have one or more adverse reactions. Three of the most common side effects are apnea, fever, and flushing. Apnea is more common in neonates weighing less than 2 kg at birth and is usually appreciated during the first hour of the treatment. It is important to continuously monitor respiratory status throughout the treatment. Apnea is an indication for assisted or mechanical ventilation. Non–central nervous system twitching, fever, and peripheral flushing will usually stop with reduction of the dose by half. Less common side effects include tachycardia or bradycardia, hypotension, and cardiac arrest. A decrease in systolic arterial pressure of greater than 20% is an indication for volume expansion. Hypoglycemia may also develop after several hours of the treatment. In addition to monitoring respiratory rate, temperature, and blood pressure, glucose should also be monitored throughout the treatment. Assessment of response to the treatment by measuring PaO_2 and pH should be evaluated with serial arterial blood gases.

SUGGESTED READINGS

Lake CL, Booker PD. *Pediatric Cardiac Anesthesia*. 4th ed. Philadelphia, PA: Lippincott Williams & Wilkins; 2005:110, 545–546.

Lerman J, Cote C, Steward D. *Manual of Pediatric Anesthesia*. 6th ed. Philadelphia, PA: Churchill Livingstone; 2010:407–408, 639.

Miller R. *Miller's Anesthesia*. 6th ed. Philadelphia, PA: Churchill Livingstone; 2005:2838–2839.

Motoyama EK, Davis PJ. *Peter Smith's Anesthesia for Infants and Children*. 7th ed. Philadelphia, PA: Mosby Inc; 2006:409, 1202.

Congenital Long QT: Management

Organ-based Clinical: Cardiovascular and Subspecialties: Pediatrics

Michael Tom

Edited by Mamatha Punjala

KEY POINTS

1. Syncope is the most common symptom, which can be triggered during times of sympathetic stimulation.
2. The most common rhythm seen during syncopal episodes is polymorphic ventricular tachycardia (torsades de point).
3. Treatment includes normalizing electrolytes, beta-blockers, pacemaker/defibrillators, and avoiding drugs that prolong the QT interval.

DISCUSSION

Long QT syndrome is a group of disorders characterized by syncope and sudden death due to episodic cardiac arrhythmias, particularly torsades de point. Most individuals with long QT syndrome show no manifestations of the disease, and arrhythmias are relatively rare except in severe cases. Long QT syndromes can be either congenital or acquired. Jarvell and Lange-Nielsen described the familial syndrome in association with congenital deafness and Romano-Ward syndrome without associated deafness.

Syncopal events usually occur during times of sympathetic stimulation, such as stress, intense emotion, or exercise. On ECG, prolonged QT is defined as a QTc greater than 460 to 480 milliseconds. The most common finding on ECG during a syncopal episode is polymorphic ventricular tachycardia. The manifestation of the polymorphic ventricular tachycardia results from an abnormality in repolarization in patients with long QT syndrome. This abnormality enables after depolarizations to trigger a premature ventricular complex (PVC), which can initiate a ventricular reentry rhythm creating the polymorphic ventricular tachycardia.

The treatment of long QT syndrome starts with correction of electrolyte abnormalities, especially derangements in magnesium and potassium. Drugs that can prolong the QT interval should also be avoided. Pharmacologic treatment includes beta-blockers, which have been shown to decrease the incidence of ventricular dysrhythmias associated with long QT syndrome. Another treatment option is cardiac pacing, as polymorphic ventricular tachycardia often occurs after an episode of bradycardia, which the pacemaker can prevent.

Anesthetic management of patients with prolonged QT syndrome includes avoiding medications that can prolong the QT interval. Droperidol and other antiemetic drugs can increase the QT interval. Events known to increase the QT interval, such as abrupt increases in sympathetic stimulation and hypokalemia associated with hyperventilation, should be avoided. A defibrillator should be available in the event the patient goes into unstable ventricular rhythm during surgery.

SUGGESTED READING

Hines RL, Marschall KE, eds. *Stoelting's Anesthesia and Co-existing Disease*. 5th ed. Philadelphia, PA: Churchill Livingstone; 2008:73.

Constrictive Pericarditis: Venous Waveform

Organ-based Clinical: Cardiovascular

C

Francis vanWisse

Edited by Benjamin Sherman

KEY POINTS

1. Constrictive pericarditis is present when a fibrotic pericardium restricts diastolic filling of the heart.
2. The characteristic central venous pressure (CVP) waveform in pericardial constriction (M or W configuration) contains prominent *a* and *v* waves, steep *x* and *y* descents, and a mid-diastolic plateau wave or *h* wave.
3. The symmetrical constricting effect of the pericardium results in elevation and equilibrium of diastolic pressure in all the four cardiac chambers.

DISCUSSION

Constrictive pericarditis is present when a fibrotic pericardium restricts diastolic filling of the heart. It usually begins with an initial episode of acute pericarditis, slowly progresses to a subacute stage of organization and resorption of effusion, followed by a chronic stage consisting of fibrous scarring and thickening of the pericardium with obliteration of the pericardial space, producing uniform restriction to filling of all heart chambers.

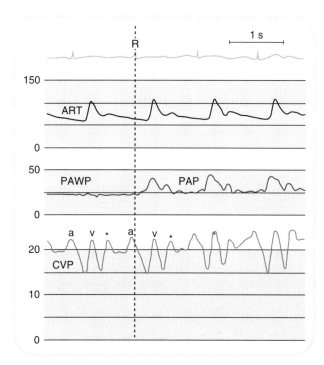

Figure 1. Pericardial constriction. This condition causes elevation and equalization of diastolic filling pressure in the PAP, PAWP, and CVP traces. The CVP waveform reveals tall *a* and *v* waves with steep *x* and *y* descents and a mid-diastolic plateau wave *(star)* or *h* wave. ART, arterial blood pressure; PAP, pulmonary artery pressure; PAWP, pulmonary artery wedge pressure. (From Mark JB. *Atlas of Cardiovascular Monitoring*. New York, NY: Churchill Livingstone; 1998:Fig. 18-1.)

The symmetrical constricting effect of the pericardium results in elevation and equilibrium of diastolic pressure in all the four cardiac chambers, as well as of the pulmonary capillary wedge pressure. In early diastole, when intracardiac volume is less than that defined by the stiff pericardium, diastolic filling is unimpeded, and early diastolic filling is more rapid than normal because venous pressure is elevated. Rapid early diastolic filling is abruptly halted when the intracardiac volume reaches the limit set by the noncompliant pericardium.

The characteristic CVP waveform in pericardial constriction (M or W configuration) contains prominent a and v waves, steep x and y descents, and a mid-diastolic plateau wave or h wave. Impaired venous return decreases end-diastolic volume, stroke volume, and cardiac output (Fig. 1).

The early diastolic dip corresponds to the period of excessively rapid filling, whereas the plateau corresponds to the period of mid and late diastole, when there is little additional ventricular volume expansion. Because the atria are equilibrated with the ventricles in early diastole, the jugular venous waveform and right and left atrial waveforms show a prominent and deep y descent.

Miller R. *Miller's Anesthesia*. 7th ed. Orlando, FL: Churchill Livingston; 2009:1307–1308, 1951.

SUGGESTED READING

CO Poisoning/Toxicity: Clinical Features, Dx, Rx, and Burn Mgmt

Subspecialties: Critical Care and Generic, Clinical Sciences: Anesthesia Procedures, Methods, Techniques

Gregory Albert, Garth Skoropowski, Christian Scheps, Anjali Vira, and Chi Wong

Edited by Hossam Tantawy

C

KEY POINTS

1. Suspect carbon monoxide (CO) poisoning in any patient exposed to smoke in an enclosed space.
2. CO causes tissue hypoxia by binding to hemoglobin and displacing oxygen as well as interfering with oxygen release from hemoglobin.
3. CO impairs oxidative metabolism and can cause metabolic acidosis.
4. Pulse oximetry does not differentiate between oxyhemoglobin (HbO_2) and carboxyhemoglobin (COHb). Conventional pulse oximetry interprets the COHb as HbO_2, giving a falsely elevated SpO_2.
5. Diagnose with CO-oximeter spectrophotometer using either venous or arterial samples.
6. The half-life of CO is inversely related to the inspired oxygen concentration (FiO_2).
7. Treatment of CO toxicity is 100% oxygen and possibly hyperbaric oxygen therapy (HBO).

DISCUSSION

Combustion of carbon-containing compounds produces CO. CO poisoning may accompany smoke exposure and occurs when the COHb level in the blood is greater than 15%.

CO causes tissue hypoxia by avidly binding to hemoglobin and displacing oxygen, causing a decrease in oxygen-carrying capacity as well as functional anemia. The affinity of CO for hemoglobin is more than 230 times greater than the affinity of oxygen. CO also increases the affinity of oxygen already bound to hemoglobin, preventing oxygen dissociation and shifting the oxygen dissociation curve to the left. Furthermore, CO uncouples oxidative phosphorylation by binding to mitochondrial cytochrome oxidase and interferes with ATP production, causing metabolic acidosis.

Side effects of CO are proportional to the amount bound to hemoglobin (Table 1). When COHb levels approach 10% to 20% saturation, headache, visual changes, and light-headedness occur. When COHb levels approach 50% to 60%, seizure, coma, and death can occur.

CO poisoning can be difficult to diagnose initially because of its nonspecific symptoms. The classic picture of the patient with cherry-red lips is actually rarely seen. Again, neurologic and cardiac effects are most prominent. Most often, the first signs and symptoms include headache, nausea, dizziness, confusion, weakness, and difficulty concentrating. These symptoms can lead to angina, cardiac dysrhythmias, and pulmonary edema. Cardiac manifestations result from an increase in cardiac output as a compensatory mechanism for tissue hypoxia. Further neurologic consequences include syncope and seizures, and one can see delayed and persistent neurologic impairment. Severe impairments can include memory loss, cognitive dysfunction, mutism, blindness, psychosis, and frank coma. The severity and extent of presenting signs and symptoms seems to directly correlate with length of CO exposure.

CO poisoning is most reliably detected by direct measurement of COHb levels via CO-oximetry of arterial or venous blood. A CO-oximeter spectrophotometer measures HbO_2 and COHb on two light paths. A regular pulse oximeter will not differentiate between HbO_2 and COHb and will likely yield a normal reading. Conventional pulse oximetry measures COHb and HbO_2 with the same wavelength of 660 nm and will overestimate the SpO_2 when COHb levels are elevated. Hence, pulse oximetry is inaccurate in the presence of COHb because the measurement is interpreted as saturated hemoglobin, yielding a normal oxygen saturation. Arterial blood gas samples will also likely not help to diagnose CO poisoning, as the PaO_2 does not measure the oxygen bound to hemoglobin but instead measures the oxygen in the plasma that will be normal.

The half-life of CO is inversely related to the inspired oxygen concentration (Table 2). It is 300 to 360 minutes when breathing room air ($FiO_2 = 0.21$), 60 to 90 minutes with $FiO_2 = 1$, and 20 to 30 minutes at 3 atmospheres in a hyperbaric chamber.

Patients with exposure to smoke in an enclosed space should be placed on a 100% non-rebreather mask until CO poisoning is ruled out by measuring CO levels in an arterial or venous blood gas. COHb levels of <20% may be treated with 100% mask ventilation, with the expectation that concentrations will fall to nontoxic levels (<10%) within 60 minutes. A COHb level of >20% implies an oxygen saturation of <80% and endotracheal intubation with delivery of 100% oxygen while maintaining adequate ventilation should be considered.

Specialized care facilities such as those with burn units may have hyperbaric oxygen chambers. These chambers deliver 100% oxygen at a pressure of up to 3 atmospheres. This pressure further reduces the half-life of CO and according to some studies the severity of injury. HBO is recommended in nonpregnant women when COHb levels are >30% and in pregnant women when COHb levels are >15% as long as the treatment of life-threatening problems is not compromised. Early HBO may prevent delayed neuropsychiatric disorders secondary to elevated levels of COHb. HBO is also recommended when there are neurologic impairments such as dizziness, loss of consciousness, and coma, and when there are cardiac abnormalities such as ischemia, dysrhythmias, and ventricular failure.

Table 1. Symptoms of CO Toxicity as a Function of Blood COHb Level

Blood COHbc Level (%)	Symptoms
<15–20	Headache, dizziness, confusion
20–40	Nausea, vomiting, disorientation, visual impairment
40–60	Agitation, combativeness, hallucinations, coma, shock
>60	Death

Referenced from Barash PG, Cullen BF, Stoelting RK, et al, eds. *Clinical Anesthesia*. 6th ed. Philadelphia, PA: Lippincott Williams & Wilkins; 2009:909–910.

Table 2. Half-life of CO as a Function of FiO_2

Fraction of Inspired Oxygen	Half-life of COHb
Room air	4 hours
100% inspired oxygen	60–90 minutes
100% inspired oxygen at 3 atmospheres hyperbaric	20–30 minutes

SUGGESTED READINGS

Barash PG, Cullen BF, Stoelting RK, et al, eds. *Clinical Anesthesia*. 6th ed. Philadelphia, PA: Lippincott Williams & Wilkins; 2009:909–910.

Hines RL, Marschall KE. *Stoelting's Anesthesia and Coexisting Disease*. Philadelphia, PA: Saunders Elsevier; 2008:550–551.

McPhee S, Papadakis M. *Current Medical Diagnosis and Treatment*. New York, NY: The McGraw-Hill Company; 2007:1653.

Miller RD. *Miller's Anesthesia*. 7th ed. Philadelphia, PA: Elsevier, Churchill Livingstone; 2009:2490–2501.

Morgan GE, Mikhail MS, Murray MJ. *Clinical Anesthesiology*. 4th ed. New York, NY: McGraw-Hill; 2006:1044–1045.

Coronary Artery: Anatomy

Anatomy

Jeffrey Widelitz

Edited by Qingbing Zhu

1. The heart is supplied with blood via the right coronary artery (RCA) and the left main coronary artery (LMCA).
2. The main branches of the LMCA are the left anterior descending artery (LAD) and the circumflex artery (CX).
3. In approximately 85% of people, the RCA gives rise to the posterior descending artery (PDA), which is called *right dominant circulation*.

The aorta supplies the heart with blood through two major arteries, the LMCA and RCA. The LMCA is the major supplier of blood to the left atrium, and a large proportion to the interventricular septum and left ventricle. After a very short distance, the LMCA branches into the LAD and CX. The LAD is a continuation of the LMCA and can be found in the interventricular septum, giving rise to diagonal and septal branches supplying the anterior wall and septum. The CX travels in the left atrioventricular (AV) groove, bifurcating into one to three obtuse marginal branches (Fig. 1).

Atherosclerotic disease in the LMCA affects blood supply to the LAD and CX. Proximal atherosclerotic disease in the LAD and CX simultaneously causes effects similar to disease in the LMCA. This type of proximal disease in both the LAD and the CX is called *left main equivalent*.

The RCA can be found in the right AV groove, giving rise to acute marginal branches. The RCA supplies the sinoatrial (SA) node in 60% of people and the AV node in 85% to 90% of people. The LAD supplies the SA node in the remaining 40%, and the CX supplies the AV node in 10% to 15% of people. In approximately 85% of people, the RCA gives rise to the PDA. This is called *right dominant circulation*. But in the remaining 15%, the PDA comes from the CX (left dominant) or the RCA and CX combined (codominant).

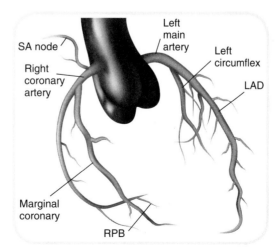

Figure 1. Anatomical distribution of the coronary arteries. (Adapted from Valentine RJ, Wind GG. *Anatomic Exposures in Vascular Surgery.* 1st ed. Philadelphia, PA: Lippincott Williams & Wilkins; 1991.)

SUGGESTED READINGS

Hensley FA, Martin DE, Gravlee GP. *Cardiac Anesthesia*. 4th ed. Philadelphia, PA: Lippincott Williams & Wilkins; 2008:291–292.

Morgan GE, Mikhail MS, Murray MJ. *Clinical Anesthesiology*. 4th ed. New York, NY: McGraw-Hill; 2006:430–431.

Valentine RJ, Wind GG. *Anatomic Exposures in Vascular Surgery*. 1st ed. Philadelphia, PA: Lippincott Williams & Wilkins; 1991.

C

Coronary Perfusion Pressure: Definition and L vs. R
Physiology

Caroline Al Haddadin and Martha Zegarra

Edited by Benjamin Sherman

KEY POINTS

1. Coronary perfusion pressure (CPP) is defined by the difference between diastolic blood pressure (DBP) and left ventricular end-diastolic pressure (LVEDP).
2. Coronary blood flow (CBF) is autoregulated when CPP is between 50 and 150 mm Hg.
3. Coronary perfusion of the left ventricle occurs almost exclusively in diastole.
4. Coronary perfusion of the right ventricle (RV) occurs in both systole and diastole.

DISCUSSION

The critical factors that modify CBF are the coronary perfusion pressure, perfusion time, vascular tone of the coronary circulation, and the presence or absence of collateral circulation or intraluminal obstruction.

CPP is determined by the difference between the aortic pressure and the intraventricular pressure. Coronary perfusion in the left ventricle occurs almost exclusively during diastole and can be calculated by the following formula: CPP = DBP – LVEDP. There is no CBF to the left ventricle during systole because the CPP = 0 (systolic blood pressure [SBP] = left ventricular systolic intracavitary pressure [LVSP], therefore SBP – LVSP = 0). If there is no pressure gradient, there will be no flow.

The RV, however, receives coronary perfusion during both systole and diastole. This occurs because there is a pressure gradient in the coronary arteries during both systole and diastole. For example, in a patient with normal BP (120/70 mm Hg) and normal RV pressures (25/5 mm Hg), RV CPP during systole and diastole equals SBP – RV systolic pressure (RVSP) (120 – 25 mm Hg = 95 mm Hg) and DBP – RV end-diastolic pressure (RVEDP) (70 – 5 mm Hg = 65 mm Hg), respectively.

When CPP is between 50 and 150 mm Hg, CBF is autoregulated by factors affecting coronary vascular resistance (CVR). This can be represented by the equation CBF = CPP/CVR. Factors affecting CVR include autonomic, hormonal, anatomic, and metabolic variables. Metabolic factors include concentrations of hydrogen, CO_2, lactate, and adenosine, whose levels may fluctuate with increased cardiac workload. Hormones that affect CVR include vasopressin, prostaglandin I_2, thromboxane, and angiotensin. An anatomic variable that may affect CVR is the presence of collateral coronary circulation.

Because of high intramural pressures during systole, the endocardium is more susceptible to ischemia, especially at lower perfusion pressures. Furthermore, with tachycardia, there is a proportionally lesser amount of time spent in diastole and thus less time available for coronary flow; this is particularly significant in patients with coronary artery disease, where coronary flow reserve (maximal flow capacity) is reduced. Conditions that cause an increase in the LVEDP or a decrease in the DBP may also result in a drop in coronary perfusion pressure, potentially resulting in perioperative ischemia.

SUGGESTED READINGS

Barash PG, Cullen BF, Stoelting RK, et al, eds. *Clinical Anesthesia*. 6th ed. Philadelphia, PA: Lippincott Williams & Wilkins; 2009:1074–1075.

Marino PL. *The ICU Book*. 3rd ed. Philadelphia, PA: Lippincott Williams & Wilkins; 2007:287.

Miller RD, Eriksson LI, Fleisher LA, et al. *Miller's Anesthesia*. 7th ed. Philadelphia, PA: Churchill Livingstone/Elsevier; 2010:1924.

Morgan G, Mikhail M, Murray M. Cardiovascular physiology and anesthesia. In: *Clinical Anesthesiology*. 4th ed. New York, NY: McGraw-Hill Medical; 2005:chap 19:376.

CRPS: Dx Nerve blk

Subspecialities: Pain

Jonathan Tidwell

Edited by Jodi Sherman

KEY POINTS

1. Pain is classified into malignant and nonmalignant pain, with complex regional pain syndrome (CRPS) being a neuropathic pain in the nonmalignant pain group.
2. CRPS has three types: type I (reflex sympathetic dystrophy [RSD], generic), type II (causalgia with obvious nerve injury), and type III.
3. Injuries usually preclude the development of CRPS.
4. Treatment for CRPS is often difficult and includes techniques such as nerve blocks and/or medications such as antidepressants, anticonvulsants, alpha antagonists, and nonsteroidal anti-inflammatory drugs (NSAIDs).

DISCUSSION

CRPS is used to describe a constellation of symptoms of neuropathic pain. It is a definition that was coined in 1994 to replace the former descriptor of RSD. Current taxonomy divides CRPS into type I (RSD, generic), type II (causalgia with obvious nerve injury that typically manifests regionally and that is out of proportion to the injury), and type III (not otherwise specified). The exact mechanism of CRPS is unknown, but appears to involve the central and peripheral nervous systems. CRPS usually presents as pain, but a host of other symptoms typically accompany CRPS and include weakness, hyperpathia, allodynia, hyperalgesia, sweating, color change, and dystonia (Table 1).

No diagnostic tests define CRPS; however, several laboratory tests and measurements may support the clinical diagnosis. These tests include temperature measurement, laser Doppler peripheral blood flowmetry, sweat and sensory testing, bone scans, and muscle/joint testing. Often, blood tests can help rule out other conditions such as infection or rheumatic disorders.

Treatment of CRPS involves physical rehabilitation, pharmacotherapy, and psychological treatment. These comprehensive treatment modalities can require significant amounts of time and patient rapport. Medications that have been utilized in the treatment of CRPS are targeted at modulation of clinical manifestations of the disease, including pain, insomnia, mood disturbances and others. NSAIDs, opioids, anticonvulsants, antiarrhythmics, tricyclic antidepressants, adrenergic agonists, and corticosteroids have been employed. Patients who respond poorly to the above treatments are often treated with regional

---

Table 1. International Association for the Study of Pain Diagnostic Criteria for CRPS

1. Presence of an initiating noxious event or cause of immobilization.
2. Continuing pain, allodynia, or hyperalgesia, with pain disproportionate to any inciting event.
3. Evidence at some time of edema, changes in skin blood flow, or abnormal sudomotor activity in the region of pain.
4. Diagnosis is excluded by the existence of conditions that would otherwise account for the degree of pain and dysfunction.

Type I: Without evidence of major nerve damage.
Type II: With evidence of major nerve damage.

From Wilson PR, Stanton-Hicks M, Harden RN, eds. CRPS: Current Diagnosis and Therapy. Seattle, WA: IASP Press, 2005: 47.

anesthesia such as regional nerve blockade techniques and spinal cord stimulation. All treatment courses must be individualized and modified if insufficient improvement is demonstrated.

SUGGESTED READINGS

Hamid B. Common pain syndromes. In: Longnecker DE, Brown DL, Newman MF, et al, eds. *Anesthesiology.* New York, NY: McGraw-Hill; 2008:2020–2041.

Warfield CA, Bajwa ZH. *Principles and Practice of Pain Medicine.* 2nd ed. New York, NY: McGraw-Hill; 2004:405–420.

Wilson PR, Stanton-Hicks M, Harden RN, eds. *CRPS: Current Diagnosis and Therapy.* Seattle, WA: IASP Press; 2005:47.

C

CRPS I: Early Sx and Diagnosis
Subspecialties: Pain

Lisbeysi Calo and Tiffany Denepitiya-Balicki

Edited by Thomas Halaszynski

1. Complex regional pain syndrome type I (CRPS I) is a state of sympathetically driven pain that can have multiple triggers, where specific criteria to arrive at the diagnosis have been developed.
2. There are two types of CRPS. Type I was originally called *reflex sympathetic dystrophy*, whereas type II was originally termed *causalgia*. Although the clinical presentation of these two types may seem the same, in CRPS type II, there was a previous nerve injury, whereas in CRPS I, there is no evidence of a preceding nerve injury.
3. The risk factors for CRPS include previous trauma, previous surgery, work-related injuries, and female sex, with evaluation to include a history and physical along with diagnostic imaging.
4. The International Association for the Study of Pain (IASP) standardized criteria for the diagnosis of CRPS suggest that there should be at least one sign and one symptom from the following categories: sensory, vasomotor, sudomotor, or motor dystrophy.
5. Treatment of CRPS I early symptoms include sympathetic blockade, physical therapy, alpha adrenergic antagonists, antidepressants, anticonvulsants, and spinal cord stimulation.

DISCUSSION

The following are the IASP diagnostic criteria for CRPS:

- The presence of an initiating noxious event, or a cause of immobilization.
- Continuing pain, allodynia, or hyperalgesia in which the pain is disproportionate to any known inciting event.
- Evidence at some time of edema, changes in skin blood flow, or abnormal sudomotor activity in the region of pain (can be a sign or symptom).
- This diagnosis is excluded by the existence of other conditions that would otherwise account for the degree of pain and dysfunction.

The most common symptom in CRPS is spontaneous burning or stinging pain (81%); however, burning pain is often nonspecific. Patients may also report hyperesthesia (65%) in response to mechanical stimuli such as the touch of a cloth to the affected site, or increased sensitivity to temperature changes, or bathing. In addition, color and temperature changes to the affected area may also occur. In CRPS, sweating asymmetry is present in 53% of patients, whereas trophic changes such as altered skin, hair, or nail growth are present in 24% of patients. A significant number of patients with CRPS (80%) may also report decreased range of motion as well as muscle weakness. In some instances, a tremor will accompany the clinical presentation (20%), and other common symptoms are myofascial pain.

On physical examination, the examiner can elicit evidence of allodynia (innocuous stimuli that is perceived as painful). Using a light brush for tactile examination, or cold and warm tubes of water for temperature examination, the examiner can determine which type of allodynia the patient is exhibiting. Although CRPS clearly affects both the peripheral and the central nervous systems, the exact mechanism by which these changes occur is still in debate.

Table 1. Phases of Reflex Sympathetic Dystrophy

	Phase		
Characteristic	**Acute**	**Dystrophic**	**Atrophic**
Pain	Localized, severe, and burning	More diffuse, throbbing	Less severe; often involves other extremities
Extremity	Warm	Cold, cyanotic, and edematous; muscle wasting	Severe muscle atrophy; contractures
Skin	Dry and red	Sweaty	Glossy and atrophic
X-ray	Normal	Reveals osteoporosis	Reveals severe osteoporosis, and ankylosis of joints
Duration	1–3 mo	3–6 mo	

Reused with permission from Morgan G, Mikhail M, Murray M. Clinical Anesthesiology. 4th ed. New York, NY: McGraw-Hill Medical; 2005: 406-407

Autonomic dysfunction may also be present in the affected area of CRPS patients. In CRPS, skin changes are more common than nail or hair changes. The examiner should determine any sudomotor involvement, and findings should be thoroughly described as hypofunction (red, hot, dry) or hyperfunction (cold, blue, pale, sweaty). The presence of tremor, myoclonus, weakness, or decreased range of motion should also be assessed.

There are three phases associated with this syndrome and are termed *acute*, *dystrophic*, and *atrophic*. Early symptoms of the acute phase last for 1 to 3 months, with pain described as severe burning with an identifiable location. The extremity involved may be warm to touch, with a dry and erythematous appearance. Radiographic imaging at this point, however, usually appears normal (Table 1).

SUGGESTED READINGS

Barash PG, Cullen BF, Stoelting RK, et al, eds. *Clinical Anesthesia*. 6th ed. Philadelphia, PA: Lippincott Williams & Wilkins; 2009:1517–1518.

Harden RN, Bruehl SP. Diagnosis of complex regional pain syndrome. Signs, symptoms, and empirically derived diagnostic criteria. *Clin J Pain*. 2006;22(5):415–419.

Morgan G, Mikhail M, Murray M. *Clinical Anesthesiology*. 4th ed. New York, NY: McGraw-Hill Medical; 2005:406–407.

Stanton-Hicks M. Complex regional pain syndrome. *Anesthesiol Clin North America*. 2003;21(4):733–744.

Cryoprecipitate: Fibrinogen Content
Organ-based Clinical: Hematologic

Jennifer Dominguez

Edited by Benjamin Sherman

KEY POINTS

1. Cryoprecipitate contains concentrates of high molecular weight glycoproteins including factor VIII, fibrinogen, fibronectin, factor XIII, and von Willebrand factor (vWF).
2. It is primarily used to treat fibrinogen-deficient states or conditions.
3. Cryoprecipitate is no longer the treatment of choice for hemophilia A or von Willebrand deficiency (vWD), as it can transmit viruses.

DISCUSSION

Cryoprecipitate is a blood product produced by the slow thawing of fresh frozen plasma at 4° C. It contains concentrates of high molecular weight glycoproteins, including factor VIII (antihemophilic factor), fibrinogen, fibronectin, and factor XIII, as well as clinically effective amounts of vWF.

Cryoprecipitate is indicated for microvascular bleeding associated with low fibrinogen levels such as disseminated intravascular coagulation (DIC), or after massive transfusion with fibrinogen levels less than 80 to 100 mg per dL. It can be given to patients with hemophilia A (factor VIII deficiency) and vWD in urgent situations for the treatment or prevention of bleeding if virus-inactivated or recombinant factor VIII concentrate is not available or effective. However, because cryoprecipitate may carry live viruses, factor VIII concentrate is the preferred blood product for these patients. Cryoprecipitate is also used for prophylaxis or treatment of bleeding in patients with congenital dysfibrinogenemias, as well as those with factor XIII deficiency. It can also be used to treat bleeding in the setting of uremia where DDAVP has not been helpful. Lastly, it can be given as a fibrin sealant if virus-inactivated concentrate is not available.

One unit contains concentrated factor VIII (>80 IU), vWF, fibrinogen (>150 mg), fibronectin, and factor XIII (about 30% of content of original plasma) and can increase fibrinogen levels by 5 to 10 mg per dL. It is usually available in bags that contain 10 to 20 units each. The typical therapeutic adult dose of cryoprecipitate is usually 80 to 150 mL, or about 8 to 10 pooled units. ABO compatibility is not necessary because the associated plasma vehicle contains little antibody (10 to 20 mL of plasma). It is stored at –20° C, and thawed just before use. Cryoprecipitate can be kept at room temperature for up to 6 hours. Once pooled, it must be transfused within 4 hours.

Calculating the cryoprecipitate dose:

$$\frac{\text{(Desired – Initial fibrinogen level [mg per dL])} \times \text{Patient's plasma volume}}{250 \text{ mg (Amount of fibrinogen per bag)}}$$

Average adult plasma volume:

$$(1 - [\text{Hct\%}/100] \times \text{Patient's weight [kg]} \times 70 \text{ mL per kg})$$

Plasma Volume (PV) of infants and children below 40 kg:

$$([\{1 - \text{Hct\%}\}/100] \times \text{Patient's weight in kg}) \times (80–85 \text{ mL per kg})$$

SUGGESTED READINGS

Barash PG, Cullen BF, Stoelting RK, et al, eds. *Clinical Anesthesia*. 6th ed. Philadelphia, PA: Lippincott Williams & Wilkins; 2009:381.

Young NS, Gerson SL, High KA. *Clinical Hematology*. Philadelphia, PA: Mosby; 2006:1261.

Denervated Heart: Exercise Physiology
Organ-based Clinical: Cardiovascular

Juan Egas
Edited by Qingbing Zhu

KEY POINTS

1. Heart innervation consists of sympathetic and parasympathetic systems that maintain an adequate hemodynamic status.
2. Parasympathetic innervation of the heart is governed by the vagus nerve. The main effect of cardiac vagal stimulation is a negative chronotropic effect with little or no effect on inotropism.
3. Sympathetic stimulation will have a positive chronotropic effect, enhance atrioventricular (AV) node conduction, and cause a positive inotropism effect.
4. Heart transplantation involves denervation of the heart. The transplanted heart will have intact alpha and beta receptor activity without evidence of denervation hypersensitivity.
5. The normal heart during exercise increases the cardiac output (CO) (to meet the rise in metabolic demands) by increasing the heart rate with little change in the stroke volume. After heart transplantation, the increase in the CO associated with exertion occurs mainly by increasing the stroke volume and not the heart rate.
6. In the absence of vagal tone, the denervated heart has a greater resting rate of approximately 90 to 100 beats per minute. The denervated heart is free of baroreceptor reflex stimulation; therefore, there are no associated changes in the heart rate secondary to hypovolemia or direct laryngoscopic stimulation, but it responds to the effect of circulating catecholamines.

DISCUSSION

Heart innervation consists of sympathetic and parasympathetic systems that regulate its main functions (i.e., inotropism, chronotropism) for maintaining an adequate hemodynamic status by complex integration of impulses secondary to hemodynamic changes. Heart's sympathetic fibers originate from intermediolateral column preganglionic neurons in the first four to five thoracic segments. These first-order neurons send their white myelinated communicating rami into the cervicothoracic ganglia (stellate ganglia) synapsing with a second-order postganglionic neurons. Parasympathetic innervation of the heart is governed by the vagus nerve. Parasympathetic fibers of the vagus will join the sympathetic fibers at the level of stellate ganglion. Therefore, past this level, the vagus nerve is a mixed nerve containing both preganglionic parasympathetic and sympathetic postganglionic fibers (unmyelinated) that travel together and innervate the heart and lungs.

Parasympathetic fibers are distributed mainly to the sinoatrial, atrioventricular nodes, and to a lesser extent to the atria, with little or no distribution to the ventricles. The main effect of cardiac vagal stimulation is a negative chronotropic effect with little or no effect on inotropism. The negative chronotropic effect is due to a slowing of the rate of spontaneous sinoatrial discharge, and will also slow down impulse conduction at the level of the AV node. Intense vagal stimulation could potentially arrest the sinoatrial (SA) node and block impulse conduction through the AV node with little compromise of the inotropism.

Sympathetic fibers share the same supraventricular distribution of the parasympathetic fibers, but they differ in that they provide an extensive innervation to the ventricles. Sympathetic stimulation, besides having a positive chronotropic effect and enhancing AV node conduction, will have a major effect in inotropism.

D

The first heart transplant was done in 1967 at Cape Town, South Africa, by Christiaan Barnard. The second heart transplant was done at Stanford University 1 month later. Since the 1960s, the surgical technique has not changed dramatically except for the introduction of the bicaval anastomosis, which better preserves the integrity of the sinus node and architecture of the right atrium.

Heart transplantation inevitably involves denervation of the heart remaining free of autonomic reinnervation. The transplanted heart will have intact alpha and beta receptor activity without evidence of denervation hypersensitivity. The denervated heart retains its intrinsic control mechanisms such as Normal Frank-Starling response to changes in preload, normal impulse formation, and conductivity, and will respond to the effect of circulating catecholamines.

In the absence of vagal tone, the denervated heart has a greater resting rate of approximately 90 to 100 beats per minute. The denervated heart is free of baroreceptor reflex stimulation; therefore, there are no associated changes in the heart rate secondary to hypovolemia or direct laryngoscopic stimulation. Maneuvers or drugs that produce changes in heart rate mediated by the autonomic nervous system (ANS) (i.e., valsalva, carotid massage, atropine, neostigmine) will have no effect in the denervated heart, but will respond to direct acting drugs such as beta adrenergic agonists (i.e., isoprenaline).

The normal heart during exercise increases the CO (to meet the rise in metabolic demands) by increasing the heart rate with little change in the stroke volume. This happens in association with an unchanged to diminished left ventricular end diastolic (LVED) volume/pressure. Cardiac catheterization studies in posttransplanted heart patients reported the hemodynamic changes during exertion in this patient subgroup. In the denervated heart, during resting conditions, the LVED pressure is normal and CO tends to be in the lower end of normal range. During exercise, there is an increase of venous return to the heart with a prompt elevation of LVEDP to an average of 10 mm Hg. There is a subsequent increase of the stroke volume ranging from 36% after 5 minutes and 49% after 10 minutes of exertion. The heart rate increases gradually and almost linearly after the start of exercise, reaching steady levels after 5 to 6 minutes ranging from 3 to 36 bpm. This latter effect is associated to a parallel increase in contractility (dp/dt) and systolic pressure. It was concluded that in these patients, the increase in the CO associated with exertion occurs mainly by increasing the stroke volume and not the heart rate.

SUGGESTED READINGS

Barash PG, Cullen BC, Stoelting RK, et al, eds. *Clinical Anesthesia*. 6th ed. Philadelphia, PA: Lippincott Williams & Wilkins; 2009.

Demas K. Anaesthesia for heart transplantation. A retrospective study and review. *Br J Anaesth*. 1986;58(12):1357–1364.

Hunt SA. Taking heart-cardiac transplantation past, present, and future. *N Engl J Med*. 2006;355(3):231–235.

Samuels SI. Anaesthesia for major surgery in a patient with a transplanted heart. *Br J Anaesth*. 1977;49(3):265–267.

Shaw IH. Anaesthesia for patients with transplanted hearts and lungs undergoing non-cardiac surgery. *Br J Anaesth*. 1991;67(6):772–778.

Stinson EB. Hemodynamic observations one and two years after cardiac transplantation in man. *Circulation*. 1972;45(6):1183–1194.

Desmopressin for Von Willebrand

Organ-based Clinical: Hematologic

Jammie Ferrara

Edited by Qingbing Zhu

D

KEY POINTS

1. Von Willebrand Disease (vWD) is a bleeding disorder characterized by abnormal or insufficient amounts of von Willebrand factor (vWF), a protein important in primary hemostasis and coagulation.
2. Desmopressin is the first-line treatment in most patients with vWD.
3. Desmopressin increases factor VIII and vWF levels.
4. Desmopressin is contraindicated in patients with type IIb vWD, as it is known to cause marked thrombocytopenia.
5. A significant limitation of desmopressin is the subsequent tachyphylaxis that can be seen after several days of administration secondary to depletion of factor VIII and vWF.

DISCUSSION

vWD is the most common hereditary bleeding disorder occurring in approximately 1% of the general population. vWF is a protein synthesized by platelets, megakaryocytes, and endothelial cells, and is important in primary hemostasis and coagulation. vWD is characterized by abnormal vWF or normal vWF in a reduced quantity (Table 1).

Table 1. Summary of vWD

Type	Defect	Incidence	Presentation	Effect of Desmopressin
I	Quantitative	70%–80%	Bleeding abnormalities of primary hemostasis	Treatment
IIa	Qualitative	20%–30%	IIb—abnormal aggregation of platelets and thrombocytopenia	IIa—ineffective
IIb			IIn—normal platelet activity however decreased factor VIII coagulant activity (often misdiagnosed as hemophilia A)	IIb—thrombocytopenia
IIm				IIn—treatment
IIn				
III	Complete absence	Very rare	Severe abnormality of primary hemostasis and coagulation	Ineffective

Desmopressin is an exogenous analog of the endogenous antidiuretic hormone (ADH). It acts on V_2 receptors, which cause conservation of water and release of blood coagulation factors such as factor VIII and vWF levels. By elevating vWF, desmopressin shortens bleeding time. Desmopressin is the first-line therapy for most patients with type I vWD and in some with type IIn vWD. However, desmopressin is generally ineffective in patients with types IIa, IIb, and III vWD. Desmopressin causes thrombocytopenia in individuals with type IIb vWD and is therefore contraindicated in those patients.

A test dose of nasal spray desmopressin should be given to patients with type I vWD 1 to 2 weeks before elective surgery to evaluate the increase in factor VIII or vWF. Given intravenously, desmopressin will increase factor VIII and vWF for more than 6 hours, and should be given in 12- to 24-hour intervals depending on the clinical response and the severity of bleeding. A significant limitation of desmopressin is the tachyphylaxis secondary to depletion of factor VIII and vWF that can be seen after several days of administration. The usefulness of desmopressin for preoperative preparation, postoperative bleeding, excessive menstrual bleeding, and emergency situations is therefore limited. A major adverse effect mediated by the V_2 receptor is water intoxication.

SUGGESTED READINGS

Barash PG, Cullen BF, Stoelting RK, et al, eds. *Clinical Anesthesia*. 6th ed. Philadelphia, PA: Lippincott Williams & Wilkins; 2009:397–398.

Brunton LL, Lazo JS, Parker KL, eds. *Goodman and Gilman's The Pharmacological Basis of Therapeutics*. 11th ed. New York, NY: McGraw-Hill; 2005:785–878.

Diabetes Insipidus Intracranial Surg

Organ-based Clinical: Neurologic and Neuromuscular

Gabriel Jacobs

Edited by Ramachandran Ramani

KEY POINTS

1. Trauma and neurosurgery are the most common causes of central diabetes insipidus (DI).
2. Edema and inflammation of the hypothalamus or posterior pituitary is the primary mechanism by which perioperative DI develops.
3. Patients suspicious for perioperative DI should be closely monitored for electrolyte disturbances (hypernatremia) and hypovolemia (hypotension, tachycardia).
4. Appropriate fluid management and hormone replacement are the mainstays of treatment of DI.

DISCUSSION

Trauma and neurosurgery are the most common causes of central DI. Twelve percent of neurosurgery patients may experience transient post-op DI, and up to 3% of cases become permanent. Brain death and lesions at the level of the hypothalamus and pituitary stalk can also be causes of DI.

Pathophysiology

DI is caused by damage to the neurohypophysis. The hypothalamus is the sight of antidiuretic hormone (ADH) production and storage, and the hormone is released by the posterior pituitary. Postsurgical DI is caused by inflammation and edema at the hypothalamus or posterior pituitary.

Sometimes postsurgical DI can be observed in three different phases:

1. *Polyuric phase*—can start within the first 24 hours and last for several days. This is due to acute hypothalamic dysfunction and loss of ADH production.
2. *Antidiuretic phase*—can start 6 to 11 days post-op. This phase involves the release of stored ADH from dying cells in the posterior pituitary. Patient can have excessive water retention and may clinically resemble SIADH (syndrome of inappropriate secretion of antidiuretic hormone).
3. *Permanent DI*—this phase is dependent on the extent of damage done to the hypothalamus.

Clinical Signs of DI

In patients prone to DI, it is very important to watch them closely early in the postoperative period. Patients can develop severe electrolyte disturbances. Owing to the nature of neurosurgical disease, some patients may have impaired cognition, and thus, they may not be able to compensate for the free water loss they experience from DI. As a result of free water loss, the patients may develop postoperative hypotension, tachycardia, hypernatremia, and high output of dilute urine without glycosuria. Polydipsia is seen in patients with adequate cognition.

Treatment
Fluid Replacement

Some patients may be able to make up for the free water losses through oral fluid replacement, although many neurosurgical patients must be managed with careful intravenous (IV) fluid replacement. Two aspects must be considered with regard to fluid replacement in DI—urine output and hypernatremia.

Replacement of fluid volume deficit should be adjusted to three-fourth the previous hour's urine loss. Half-normal saline is usually used. Fluids containing dextrose must be used cautiously, as high volume of glucose containing fluid can lead to hyperglycemia and osmotic diuresis. To correct hypernatremia to a normal level of 140, one must replace the free water deficit, which can be calculated from the following equation:

$$\text{Free water deficit} = 0.5 \times \text{Body weight (kg)} \times [(\text{Serum sodium} - 140)/140]$$

When correcting hypernatremia, sodium levels must be closely monitored. Rapid corrections can be deleterious (central pontine myelinolysis).

Hormone Replacement

Intranasal desmopressin can be used in cases where urine output becomes greater than 300 mL per hour. Desmopressin is dosed and titrated in 5 to 10 μg increments to the desired effect. ADH replacement can be given intramuscularly. Once hormone replacement is initiated, urine osmolarity will increase. Patients who have known DI can be treated intraoperatively with IV ADH given at a rate of 100 to 200 mU per hour with concurrent infusion of isotonic solution.

SUGGESTED READINGS

Barash PG, Cullen BF, Stoelting RK, eds. *Clinical Anesthesia*. 6th ed. Philadelphia, PA: Wolters Kluwer Lippincott Williams & Wilkins; 2009: 1301–1302.

Morgan GE Jr, Mikhail MS, Murray MJ. *Lange Clinical Anesthesiology*. 4th ed. New York, NY: Lange Medical Books/McGraw-Hill; 670.

Williams MV, Flanders SA, Whitcomb WF, eds. *Comprehensive Hospital Medicine*. 1st ed. Philadelphia, PA: Saunders, 2007: Chapter 65.

Doxorubicin: Complications

Pharmacology

Tomalika Ahsan-Paik

Edited by Zhu

KEY POINTS

1. Doxorubicin and daunorubicin are antineoplastic agents, which are anthracycline or cytotoxic antibiotics.
2. These drugs are most commonly used for acute myleloid leukemia (AML), Hodgkin lymphoma, breast cancer, and other solid tumors.
3. These compounds bind to DNA at the guanine–cytosine base pair and block topoisomerase I from binding to the double-stranded DNA.
4. The use of doxorubicin and daunorubicin is significantly limited because of their well-known cardiotoxicity involved with a cumulative dose higher than 550 mg per m^2.
5. There are two subtypes of cardiotoxicity: acute and chronic.

DISCUSSION

Doxorubicin and daunorubicin are antineoplastic agents, which are anthracycline or cytotoxic antibiotics. These are chromopeptides derived from *Streptomyces*, a kind of fungal species. Anthracyclines are four-member anthracene rings (responsible for its red color) with attached sugars. These drugs are most commonly used for AML, Hodgkin lymphoma, breast cancer, and other solid tumors.

These compounds bind to DNA at the guanine–cytosine base pair and block topoisomerase I from binding to the double-stranded DNA. This creates breaks in the DNA chains. They also form free radicals by undergoing reduction.

The use of doxorubicin and daunorubicin is significantly limited because of their well-known cardiotoxicity involved with high dose usage. These drugs show a dose-response relationship in terms of efficacy. Cardiotoxicity is more likely to occur with a cumulative dose higher than 550 mg per m^2. Some of the other side effects of anthracyclines include myelosuppression, nausea, vomiting, alopecia, mucosal ulceration, and extravasation at the site of injection.

The exact mechanism by which doxorubicin causes cardiotoxicity is not clearly understood, but it is most likely multifactorial. It is believed that doxorubicin undergoes redox cycling and produces free radicals that lead to myocardial damage. Cytochrome P450 reductase is the enzyme responsible for reducing the quinone form of doxorubicin to the free radical form of semiquinone within myocardial cells. Anthracyclines have also been shown to cause changes in myocellular protein transcription.

There are two subtypes of cardiotoxicity: acute and chronic.

The acute type can manifest within a week or after one dose of initiating therapy. The overall incidence of acute cardiotoxicity is 0.7%. ECG changes such as ST-T wave changes can be the first sign. Other signs include flattening of T waves, decrease in QRS voltage, or QT prolongation. Arrhythmias can also be present, but are not as common. Arrhythmias include ventricular, supraventricular, or junctional tachycardia. Patients can also experience subacute toxicity such as left ventricular failure and pericarditis.

The chronic subtype is more recognized and clinically more significant. The chronic form can be subdivided into early and late onset cardiomyopathy. Patients developed congestive heart failure symptoms anywhere between 1 and 231 days after completion of therapy. In many cases, symptoms were subclinical during the initial follow-up and progressed to become "clinical" over time. Another study observed that the incidence and severity of left systolic dysfunction increased over time.

Risk factors for anthracycline-related chronic progressive cardiotoxicity include the following:

1. Total cumulative dose is the most important factor. The incidence of congestive heart failure secondary to doxorubicin use is only 0.14% with a dosage of 440 mg per m^2, compared with 7% with a dosage of 550 mg per m^2.
2. Rate of administration. Less incidence of cardiotoxicity was reported when doxorubicin was delivered as an infusion over 48 to 96 hours.
3. Age at which anthracycline was administered. Patients younger than 4 years at the time of exposure seem to be at greater risk for developing cardiac dysfunction. The association is linked with the effect of doxorubicin on decreased left ventricular wall thickness, leading to increased afterload.
4. Female gender.
5. Any preexisting heart condition or hypertension.
6. Mediastinal irradiation. Radiation is often used in conjunction with chemotherapy for treating solid neoplasm.
7. Interval dosing schedule since receiving chemotherapy, particularly if received during childhood.
8. Concurrent cyclophosphamide use, which by itself, can also induce cardiotoxicity.

SUGGESTED READINGS

Brenner G, Stevens C. DNA intercalating drugs. In: *Pharmacology.* 3rd ed. Philadelphia, PA: Saunders; 2009:502–503.

Burnett AK, Gharib MI. Cardiac complication. In: Chang A, Ganz PA, Hayes DF, et al, eds. *Oncology: An evidence Based Approach.* New York, NY: Springer; 2006:1411–1416.

Burton L, Lazo J, Parker K, eds. Antineoplastic agents. *Goodman and Gilman's Pharmacology.* 11th ed. New York, NY: McGraw-Hill; 2006:1357–1359.

Raya J, Mikhail M. Anesthesia for orthopedic surgery. In: Morgan G, Mikhail M, eds. *Clinical Anesthesiology.* 4th ed. New York, NY: McGraw-Hill; 2006:860.

Dural Sac: Caudal Extent

Anatomy

Tomalika Ahsan-Paik

Edited by Thomas Halaszynski

KEY POINTS

1. The spinal cord is covered with a protective membrane called the meninges; there are three meningeal layers: the pia mater, the arachnoid mater, and the dura mater.
2. The dural sac (composed of the dura mater) extends rostrally from the foramen magnum to the termination of the periosteal dura.
3. The filum terminale is a strand of fibrous tissue that extends down from the conus medullaris to the closed end or caudal end of the dural sac.
4. The filum terminale helps hold the spinal cord to the sacrum and terminates at the level of sacral 2 vertebrae in adults and sacral 3 vertebrae in children.

DISCUSSION

The spinal cord is covered with a protective membrane called the meninges. There are three meningeal layers: the pia mater, the arachnoid mater, and the dura mater. The pia mater (the innermost layer) adheres to the spinal cord, whereas the arachnoid mater adheres to the dura mater. Space between the pia mater and the arachnoid mater is called the subarachnoid space, containing cerebrospinal fluid. Space between the dura mater and the arachnoid mater is the subdural space and is a poorly defined area. Epidural space is defined as the space between the ligamentum flavum and the dura mater composed of venous channels, lymphatics, and fat.

The dural sac is the outermost and thickest meningeal membrane consisting of collagen and elastin fibers along with elongated fibroblasts. The dura mater consists of only one layer of cells between itself and the arachnoid mater, but is highly vascular, which makes it an important route for drug clearance. The distal spinal cord is attached to the dura by two ligaments: the denticulate ligament and the filum terminale internum (Fig. 1). The dural blood supply comes from the branches of major arteries such as the vertebral, the intercostal, and the lumbar arteries. The dural nerves are the recurrent branches of the spinal nerves at that level, which enter through the intervertebral foramina. There are no venous sinuses in the spinal dura.

The dural sac is composed of the dura mater and extends from the foramen magnum to where the periosteal dura terminates. Caudally, it narrows down significantly and forms an investing sheath for the filum terminale, which is an extension of the pia mater. There are two parts to the filum terminale: the filum terminale externum and the filum terminale internum. The conus medullaris is the most distal cone shaped end portion of the spinal cord located at lumbar vertebral levels 1 and 2 of the vertebrae column. The filum terminale is a strand of fibrous tissue that extends down from the conus medullaris to the closed end or caudal end of the dural sac, where it terminates at the sacral 2 vertebrae level in adults and sacral 3 vertebrae level in children. The filum terminale externum anchors the caudal closed end of the dural sac to the inner attachment to the coccyx. Laterally, the dura mater extends along nerve roots leaving the spinal cord and becomes the epineurium, which is the outermost connective tissue layer of the peripheral nerves.

The spinal cord ends at the level of lumbar 1 or 2 vertebrae. Lumbar, sacral, and coccygeal anterior and posterior nerve roots that exit the vertebrae at a lower level than lumbar 1 or 2 are connected to the spinal cord at a higher level. These spinal nerve roots form the cauda equina.

182

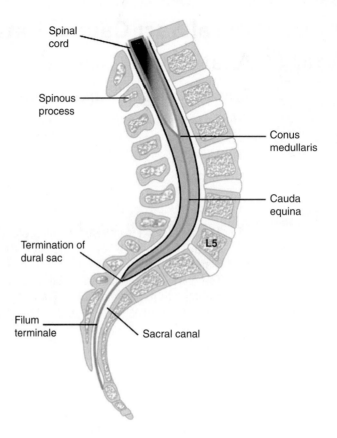

Spinal cord

Spinous process

Conus medullaris

Cauda equina

Termination of dural sac

L5

Filum terminale

Sacral canal

Figure 1. Contents of dural sac. (Courtesy of http://www.nysora.com/regional_anesthesia/neuraxial_techniques/3119-spinal_anesthesia.html.)

The lumbar cistern is an enlarged part of the subarachnoid space, extending from the conus medullaris to the caudal end of the dural sac that forms the lower border of the outer meninges (dura/subarachnoid). The cistern consists of sweeping nerve roots of the cauda equina, filum terminale, and a large volume of cerebrospinal fluid (the cistern is a location for lumbar puncture or spinal tap, and local anesthetic can be injected through this caudal potion of the dura with low risk of nerve injury).

SUGGESTED READINGS

Bernards C. Epidural and spinal anesthesia. In: Barash P, Cullen B, Stoelting R, et al, eds. *Clinical Anesthesia.* 6th ed. Philadelphia, PA: Lippincott Williams & Wilkins 2009: chap 37: 929–930.

Drake RB. Arrangement of structures in vertebral canal. In: *Gray's Anatomy.* 2nd ed. Philadelphia, PA: Elsevier, 2010:104–109.

Haines DE. The meninges. In: *Fundamental Neuroscience for Basic and Clinical Application.* 3rd ed. Philadelphia, PA: Churchill Livingstone, 2006: 108–112.

Haines DE, Mihailoff GA, Yezierski RP. The spinal cord. In: *Fundamental Neuroscience for Basic and Clinical Application.* 3rd ed. Philadelphia, PA: Elsevier, 2006: 143–145.

Kleiman W, Mikhail M. Spinal, epidural and caudal blocks. In: Morgan G, Mikhail M, Murray M, eds. *Clinical Anesthesiology.* 4th ed. New York, NY: Large Medical Books McGraw Hill, 2006:293–294.

ECG: Loose Lead Effect

Physics, Monitoring, and Anesthesia Delivery Devices

Rongjie Jiang

Edited by Qingbing Zhu

KEY POINTS

1. The main source of artifact from ECG leads is loss of the integrity of the lead insulation.
2. Patient movement is a common source of ECG artifact.
3. Loose lead artifact can mimic wide complex tachycardia, atrial flutter, Q waves, or inverted T waves.
4. To identify loose lead effect, it is useful to see regular QRS complexes "marching through" the artifact.

DISCUSSION

The main source of artifact from ECG leads is loss of the integrity of the lead insulation. To identify loose lead effect, it is useful to see regular QRS complexes "marching through" the artifact. The patient is asymptomatic, and satisfactory recording from other leads may be seen.

Figure 1 shows an example of the strip from a patient who had an episode of "asymptomatic ventricular fibrillation" that was captured through telemetry monitoring. Regular QRS complexes appearing in the strip suggest that the background "ventricular fibrillation" waves are artifacts. The waveforms of arterial line, central line, and/or pulse oximeter may help differential the artificial effects.

There are several common practices that may help reduce artifacts secondary to the loose ECG lead effect. Always use fresh electrodes to provide the best signal from the skin to the monitor. It is also important to always replace loose, cracked, and damaged cables. Patient movement is a common source of ECG artifact that can be easily controlled. It is also critical to avoid electromagnetic interference if possible. Surgical electrocautery is the main source of electromagnetic interference in the operating room.

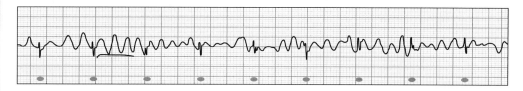

Figure 1. "Ventricular fibrillation"—black dots mark QRS complexes "marching through" the artifact in the background.

SUGGESTED READINGS

Estefanous FG, Barash PG, Reeves JG. *Cardiac Anesthesia: Principles and Clinical Practice.* Philadelphia, PA: Lippincott Williams & Wilkins; 1994:181.

Jafary FH. The "incidental" episode of ventricular fibrillation: a case report. *J Med Case Rep.* 2007;1:72.

Kusumoto F. *ECG Interpretation: From Pathophysiology to Clinical Application.* New York, NY: Springer; 2009:270.

ECG Leads: P-Wave Detection

Physiology

Sharif Al-Ruzzeh

Edited by Benjamin Sherman

E

KEY POINTS

1. P waves are the ECG tracings that arise from the right and left atrial contractions.
2. Changes in P-wave morphology may indicate the presence of various pathologies, such as right atrial enlargement, left atrial enlargement, atrial flutter/fibrillation, etc.
3. The idea of analyzing P waves to diagnose diseases is not new. Although the standard approach deals mainly with the analysis of the duration or amplitude of the P wave, there is an increasing interest in the study of the P-wave morphology.
4. Detailed analysis of the low-voltage P wave will require a hardware setup that enables high-quality signal acquisition with low noise interference in combination with an ECG subtraction technique.
5. The feasibility of the surface ECG to detect the presence of an abnormal electrophysiologic substrate in the atrial myocardium, as well as to localize ectopic atrial rhythms, will be enhanced by use of P-wave morphologic analysis.

DISCUSSION

P waves are the ECG tracings that arise from the contraction of the atria and are composed of the right and left atrial contractions. The first portion of the P wave represents the depolarization of the right atrium, whereas the latter portion represents the depolarization of the left atrium. P-wave morphology can indicate various pathologies within the heart, including right atrial enlargement, left atrial enlargement, which can be signs of various cardiac pathologies.

Right atrial enlargement, indicated by a peaked P wave of greater than 0.2 mV, can be a sign of underlying cardiac pathologies including tricuspid insufficiency, atrial septal defect, or pulmonary hypertension. Left atrial enlargement, indicated by widening of the P wave greater than 0.1 seconds, can be a sign of underlying cardiac pathologies including mitral stenosis, mitral regurgitation, and aortic insufficiency.

The problem of automatic P-wave detection and classification is not a new one in computer-assisted ECG processing and interpretation. The difficulties in automatic P-wave detection are due to low amplitudes, widely varying shapes, low signal-to-noise ratio and adjacent QRS complexes or T waves. Many sophisticated methods have been proposed and investigated for P-wave detection and classification; however, none have yet achieved satisfactory accuracy. The emphasis of the solution is directed to detection, localization, and classification of the P waves, and probably additional filtration and quantification to give a true representation of the wave energy and disease-specific characteristics like being monophasic, M-shaped or biphasic.

The success of any automatic detection system of characteristic ECG waves is based on locating the waveform boundaries, that is, the onsets and offsets of P, QRS, and T waves in generalized single-lead ECG signals. This is where many algorithms are being developed and tested for accuracy and performance with successes approaching 98% in many of them. The recent technologic advances in computer-assisted ECG processing are aimed to combine useful facilities from different signal processing fields, thus creating new tools for improving diagnostic precision and decreasing computation time.

SUGGESTED READINGS

Haberl R. *ECG Pocket.* Hermosa Beach, CA: Borm Bruckmeier Publishing LLC, 2007:31–33.

Stoelting R, Miller R. *Basics of Anesthesia.* 5th ed. Philadelphia, PA: Churchill Livingstone; 2007:305–306.

Sun Y, Chan K, Krishnan S. Characteristic wave detection in ECG signal using morphological transform. *BMC Cardiovasc Disord.* 2005;5:28. http://www.biomedcentral.com/content/pdf/1471-2261-5-28.pdf.

Thakor N, Zhu Y. Application of adaptive filtering to ECG analysis: noise cancellation and arrhythmia detection. *IEEE Trans Biomed Eng.* 1991;38(8):785–793.

E

ECT: Side Effects

Generic, Clinical Sciences: Anesthesia Procedures, Methods, Techniques

Ashley Kelley

Edited by Ramachandran Ramani

1. Electroconvulsive therapy (ECT) is the induction of seizure activity as therapy for psychiatric illnesses such as depression.
2. The most commonly observed side effects of ECT result from parasympathetic and sympathetic discharges that accompany the seizure activity and include initial bradycardia and increased secretions followed by hypertension and tachycardia.

ECT is the induction of seizure activity as therapy for psychiatric illnesses such as depression. Anesthesiologists play a key role in ECT by administering medications to produce hypnosis, amnesia, and muscle relaxation. Muscle relaxation is necessary because patients are at high risk for musculoskeletal injury during the induced seizure activity.

The most commonly observed side effects of ECT result from parasympathetic and sympathetic discharges that accompany the seizure activity. The parasympathetic discharge accompanies the tonic phase of the seizure, whereas the sympathetic discharge is associated with the clonic seizure activity. The parasympathetic nervous system is activated first and followed by a longer period of sympathetic nervous system discharge. The parasympathetic discharge can cause bradycardia and even asystole as well as increased secretions. These effects can be attenuated by administering glycopyrrolate before the onset of seizure activity. If parasympathetic effects are still seen, treatment with atropine can be initiated. The longer sympathetic discharge that occurs after the initial parasympathetic discharge can lead to hypertension and tachycardia, which can precipitate cardiac arrhythmias and myocardial ischemia. Hypertension and tachycardia are commonly limited and abate with the termination of seizure activity. For this reason, agents to attenuate the effects of the sympathetic discharge can also be administered before the onset of seizure activity. Commonly used drugs include esmolol, labetalol, calcium channel blockers, clonidine, and dexmedetomidine.

Less commonly observed side effects of ECT include muscle aches, musculoskeletal injury, agitation, headache, status epilepticus, and sudden death. Because of direct muscle stimulation, masseter spasm is also seen, and therefore a bite block is usually necessary to prevent tongue injury. Airway protection equipment is also necessary, although most patients do not require endotracheal intubation.

Barash PG, Cullen BF, Stoelting RK, et al, eds. *Clinical Anesthesia*. 6th ed. Philadelphia, PA: Lippincott Williams & Wilkins; 2009:871–872.

Morgan GE, Mikhail MS, Murray MJ. *Clinical Anesthesiology*. 4th ed. New York, NY: McGraw-Hill; 2006:659–660.

Stoelting RK, Miller RD, eds. *Basics of Anesthesia*. 5th ed. Philadelphia, PA: Churchill Livingstone; 2007:556–558.

Electrolyte Homeostasis: Hormones

Physiology

Dallen Mill

Edited by Ala Haddadin

E

1. Sodium, potassium, and calcium constitute the key hormonally regulated electrolytes.
2. Sodium homeostasis is regulated primarily by aldosterone and vasopressin.
3. Potassium homeostasis is regulated primarily by aldosterone.
4. Calcium homeostasis is regulated primarily by parathyroid hormone (PTH) and possibly calcitonin.

Several hormones are instrumental in the maintenance of electrolyte homeostasis. Sodium, potassium, and calcium constitute the key hormonally regulated electrolytes.

Sodium Homeostasis

Aldosterone

In response to a decrease in intravascular volume or an increase in sympathetic tone, renin is released from the juxtaglomerular apparatus of the kidney. Renin converts angiotensinogen to angiotensin I. In the lung and other tissues, angiotensin-converting enzyme converts angiotensin I to angiotensin II, resulting in the synthesis and release of aldosterone from the zona glomerulosa of the adrenal cortex. Aldosterone modifies sodium channels in the distal convoluted tubule and collecting duct of the kidney. As a result, sodium transport across cell membranes is enhanced, leading to sodium retention.

Vasopressin

Osmoreceptors in the hypothalamus and elsewhere in the brain direct the release of vasopressin from the posterior pituitary gland. Increases in osmolality of as little as 1% will result in the release of vasopressin. This hormone, also known as antidiuretic hormone, acts at the collecting duct of the kidney to promote solute-free water resorption. As the kidney absorbs solute-free water, plasma sodium concentration, and ultimately plasma osmolality, declines.

Potassium Homeostasis

Aldosterone

As described above, aldosterone favors resorption of sodium from the distal convoluted tubule and collecting duct. The departure of positively charged sodium ions from the lumen of these renal structures results in a negatively charged environment, favoring the secretion of positively charged potassium. Aldosterone thus participates in the lowering of plasma potassium concentration.

Calcium Homeostasis

Parathyroid Hormone

Hypocalcemia triggers the release of PTH from the chief cells of the parathyroid glands. PTH increases absorption of calcium from the gastrointestinal tract and reabsorption from the renal tubules. The conversion of 25-hydroxyvitamin D to 1,25-dihydroxyvitamin D is also stimulated by PTH. Both osteoblast and osteoclast activity are stimulated by the release of PTH; however, under normal physiologic conditions, PTH release favors osteoblast activity and thus bone formation. In contrast, the pathologic levels of PTH seen in hyperparathyroidism typically result in decreased bone mineral density.

Calcitonin

Calcitonin is released from the C cells of the thyroid gland in response to elevated plasma calcium concentrations. Calcitonin has been shown to decrease renal tubular calcium resorption, and decreases bone resorption through direct osteoclast inhibition. The importance of calcitonin in the regulation of calcium homeostasis in humans, however, remains unclear.

SUGGESTED READINGS

Barash PG, Cullen BF, Stoelting RK, et al, eds. *Clinical Anesthesia.* 6th ed. Philadelphia, PA: Lippincott Williams & Wilkins; 2009:1301.

Behrman R, Jenson H, Kliegman R, et al. Physiology of the adrenal glands. *Nelson Textbook of Pediatrics.* 18th ed. Philadelphia, PA: Saunders Elsevier; 2007:575.

Chambers TJ, McSheehy PM, Thomason BM, et al. The effect of calcium-regulating hormones and prostaglandins on bone resorption by osteoclasts disaggregated from neonatal rabbit bones. *Endocrinology.* 1985;116(1):234–239.

Hamann KL, Lane NE. Parathyroid hormone update. *Rheum Dis Clin North Am.* 2006;32:703–719.

Kronenberg H, Larsen P, Melmed S, et al. Posterior pituitary and in hormones and disorders of mineral metabolism. *Williams Textbook of Endocrinology.* 11th ed. Philadelphia, PA: Saunders Elsevier; 2008:263–286, 1203–1224.

Elevated INR: Factor Rx
Organ-based Clinical: Hematologic

Stephanie Cheng

Edited by Benjamin Sherman

KEY POINTS

1. The international normalized ratio (INR) is a standardized prothrombin time (PT) among the different laboratories. INR is a calculated ratio, calculated by taking the patient's PT and dividing it by a control PT.
2. PT is the actual time of fibrin formation with factors of the classic extrinsic coagulation cascade.
3. PT, and therefore, INR, will be prolonged with low levels of VII, X and V, prothrombin, and fibrinogen.
4. An elevated INR is treated with fresh frozen plasma, which is a type of blood-product that contains all clotting factors and plasma proteins except platelets.
5. Perioperative clinical situations necessitating correction of elevated INR with FFP include coumadin use, deficiency of factors X and V and prothrombin, or hypocoagulation due to disseminated intravascular coagulopathy.

DISCUSSION

In the recent past, hemostasis was thought to be a result of a cascade where two pathways activated a series of enzymes, resulting in the formation of fibrin from fibrinogen. It is now understood that coagulation occurs on the surface of cells as a series of events, rather than within the plasma as two distinct pathways and mechanisms. When there is an injury at a vascular site, factor VII causes a conformational change and binds to the extracellular portion of tissue factor of the cell. This complex, factor VIIa will then activate factor IX and X. Factor Xa then activates and joins factor V, forming the prothrombinase complex. This factor Xa–Va complex will catalyze prothrombin into thrombin. The thrombin will cleave factor VIII from von Willebrand factor. Thrombin also activates factor XIII that will stabilize the cross-linked fibrin (Fig. 1).

Blood tests for coagulation include PT and partial thromboplastin time (PTT). PT will be prolonged with low levels of VII, X and V, prothrombin, and fibrinogen. PT is the actual time of fibrin formation with factor of the classic extrinsic coagulation cascade (TF, factor VII, X, V, II, and I). PT, although useful, is only a laboratory value and thus does have limitations. Factor deficiency must be fairly significant (down 30%) before PT will be prolonged. It is most sensitive in detecting a deficiency of factor VII (due to its short half-life) and least sensitive to a factor II deficiency. PTT will be prolonged with decreased factor VIII, IX, XI, and XII along with X, V, prothrombin and fibrinogen. Like PT, the sensitivity of PTT is limited, also requiring decreases by 30% of normal factor levels before PTT will be prolonged. If PT is elevated but PTT is normal, the factor deficiency lies with factor VII as the other factors affected by PT are also shared with PTT.

PT and PTT are unfortunately, not standardized between laboratories. Thus, hospitals that use different laboratories cannot compare values. INR is a standardized PT among the different laboratories. INR is a calculated ratio, calculated by taking the patient's PT and dividing it by a control PT. There is no standard for PTT. INR is elevated in the setting of coumadin use, deficiencies of factors X, V, and prothrombin, or in coagulopathies associated with disseminated intravascular coagulopathy, which can be a result of infection, trauma, shock, or burns. At least four to six units of FFP are required to attain 20% to 30% levels of any missing factor, and the duration of efficacy of replacement is dependent on the individual factor's half-lives.

190

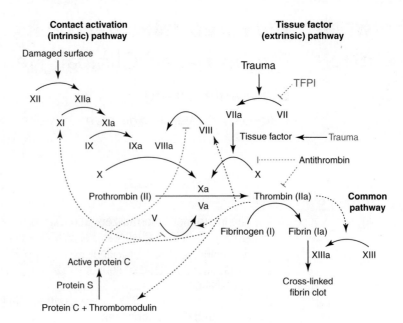

Figure 1. Coagulation cascade. (Courtesy of http://en.wikipedia.org/wiki/File:Coagulation_full.svg.)

SUGGESTED
READINGS

Barash PG, Cullen BF, Stoelting RK. *Clinical Anesthesia.* 6th ed. Philadelphia, PA: Lippincott Williams & Wilkins; 2009:386–396.

Hines R, Marschall K. *Anesthesia and Co-existing Disease.* 5th ed. Philadelphia, PA: Churchill Livingstone; 2008:418–422.

Miller RD, Robert KS. *Basics of Anesthesia.* 5th ed. Philadelphia, PA: Churchill Livingstone; 2007:331–337.

Epidural Anesthetics: Respiratory Effects
Regional Anesthesia

Kellie Park

Edited by Jodi Sherman

E

KEY POINTS

1. Ideally placed epidural anesthetics can improve respiratory function by decreasing the incidence of shallow breathing, low-tidal volumes, and resultant atelectasis secondary to pain splinting, along with a decreased need for opioids.
2. However, an epidural where the injectate results in a high block can lead to impaired ventilation, thus necessitating airway equipment to be readily available at all times.

DISCUSSION

Epidural anesthesia provides a segmental sensory blockade. Height of epidural anesthesia, unlike spinal, depends greatly on the site of initial injection, volume of injectate, drug dosage, and less on baricity and patient position. When blocks are placed at the level of the mid-thorax, pulmonary function is rarely affected in people with normal healthy lungs. In fact, epidural anesthesia can improve respiratory function as it decreases the incidence of low-tidal volumes secondary to pain splinting, and also decreases the need for opioids.

After high-level epidural blocks, patients may perceive the numbness of their chest wall as difficulty breathing or shortness of breath. Assessment of the patient should be performed to determine if the patient has appropriate tidal volumes, has good SpO_2 measurements, shows no changes in mental status, and is able to speak in a strong voice. If these quantitative and qualitative measurements are present, the patient and anesthesiologist should be reassured that respiratory function is not compromised; however, standard airway equipment should always be readily available.

Intercostal muscles can be anesthetized with a high block, with a very large volume, or with a dense concentration of local anesthetic. Patients who depend on accessory muscles may require ventilatory support if the intercostal muscles are anesthetized. High blocks affecting C_3–C_5 impair the diaphragm and will necessitate endotracheal intubation in any patient.

SUGGESTED READINGS

Barash PG, Cullen BF, Stoelting RK, et al, eds. *Clinical Anesthesia*. 6th ed. Philadelphia, PA: Lippincott Williams & Wilkins; 2009:947.
Stoelting RK, Miller RD, eds. *Basics of Anesthesia*. 5th ed. Philadelphia, PA: Churchill Livingstone; 2007:268.

Epidural Test Dose: Symptom
Pharmacology

Bijal Patel

Edited by Jodi Sherman

1. Negative aspiration does not exclude intravascular or intrathecal placement of epidural needle or catheter.
2. Since spinal anesthesia has a much faster onset than epidural anesthesia, failure to produce motor and sensory anesthesia within 3 minutes may rule out intrathecal placement, although not with absolute certainty.
3. Administration of epinephrine in the test dose will allow assessment for possible intravascular placement—one may see a rapid increase in heart rate of approximately 20 to 30 beats per minute (bpm) within 30 seconds.
4. Patients taking beta-blockers may not experience an increase in heart rate with test dose administration intravascularly. In these patients, a systolic blood pressure rise of greater than 20 may indicate intravascular placement.
5. Intravascular placement may also lead to systemic symptoms such as ringing in the ears and numbness of the lips, from intravascular dosing of local anesthetic.
6. When administering therapeutic doses of local anesthetic solution, one must do so in incremental doses with close monitoring for any adverse effects, as no test dose is 100% conclusive.

Before anesthetic use, one must confirm proper placement of the needle or catheter into the epidural space. The first step in this process is to aspirate to assess for blood (indicating possible intravascular placement) or cerebrospinal fluid (indicating possible intrathecal placement). However, proper placement cannot solely rely on negative aspiration. One must administer a test dose of local anesthetic solution, for example, 3 mL of 1.5% lidocaine with 1:200,000 epinephrine. Since spinal anesthesia has a much faster onset than epidural anesthesia, failure to produce motor and sensory anesthesia within 3 minutes may rule out intrathecal placement, although not with absolute certainty.

Administration of epinephrine (isoproterenol has also been used) in the test dose will allow assessment for possible intravascular placement. One may see a rapid increase in heart rate of approximately 20 to 30 bpm within 30 seconds if administered intravascularly, with the patient occasionally complaining of palpitations. However, it is possible that this increase may not be seen in patients taking beta-blockers, and in fact, it may result in a reflexive bradycardia. In these patients, a systolic blood pressure rise of greater than 20 may indicate intravascular placement. ECG monitoring should also be present during this time and can demonstrate characteristic increases in T-wave amplitude (up to 25%) with intravascular placement. Systemic symptoms of intravascular placement should also be assessed. These include tinnitus, perioral paresthesias, a metallic taste, blurry vision, and seizures.

It is again important to note that the test dose will not assure 100% certainty that the catheter/needle is in the appropriate position. As such, when administering therapeutic doses of local anesthetic solution, one must do so in incremental doses with close monitoring for any adverse effects.

Barash PG, Cullen BF, Stoelting RK, et al, eds. *Clinical Anesthesia*. 6th ed. New York, NY: Lippincott Williams & Wilkins; 2009:700.

Hughes SC, Levinson G, Rosen MA, eds. *Shnider and Levinson's Anesthesia for Obstetrics*. 4th ed. Philadelphia, PA: Lippincott Williams & Wilkins; 2001:209–210.

Stoelting RK, Miller RD, eds. *Basics of Anesthesia*. 5th ed. Philadelphia, PA: Churchill Livingstone Elsevier; 2007:241, 265.

Epiglottitis: Anes Mgt and Inhal Induction
Subspecialties: Pediatric Anesthesia

Christina Biello and Michael Archambault
Edited by Mamatha Punjala

E

KEY POINTS

1. The classic finding on X-ray of a patient with epiglottitis is the "thumb print sign" seen with epiglottic enlargement.
2. Patients with epiglottitis present with a recent onset high fever, sore throat, and drooling due to difficulty swallowing.
3. Patients may require intubation secondary to airway obstruction; surgical staff should be prepared to perform a surgical airway if necessary.

DISCUSSION

Acute epiglottitis presents rapidly, can cause airway obstruction, and if not treated appropriately can be fatal. It is usually infectious in nature with *Haemophilus influenzae* type B being the most frequent pathogen, although *Streptococcus pneumoniae* and group A β-hemolytic streptococci are also known pathogens. Epiglottitis most commonly occurs in children ages 3 to 5 years, but can occur at any age. Owing to the routine immunization with *H. influenzae* B vaccine, the incidence of epiglottitis decreased from 3.47 per 100,000 in 1980 to 0.63 per 100,000 in 1990.

Patients with epiglottitis present with a recent onset high fever, sore throat, and drooling due to difficulty swallowing. These patients appear toxic, sitting upright in the sniffing position to optimize their airways, and may be very anxious. As the infection progresses, patients may become dyspneic and develop inspiratory stridor. Patients can appear flushed, sweaty, and tachycardic (Table 1).

The rapid progression of the illness makes swift intervention mandatory. Depending on the appearance of the child, a workup may include a lateral X-ray, MRI, or laboratory data. The classic finding on lateral X-ray demonstrates a "thumb print sign" seen with epiglottic enlargement. This differs from the steeple sign seen on X-ray in patients with croup due to subglottic airway inflammation.

Once the diagnosis is confirmed or clinical suspicion is high enough, the child should be brought to the operating room. Before proceeding to the operating room, the airway should not be instrumented because this can cause acute obstruction. Every effort should be made to keep the child calm, including delaying an intravenous line until after induction. The parent may accompany the child to the operating room to help alleviate anxiety.

A surgeon should be available and ready to perform a surgical airway if acute obstruction occurs at any point during the induction. Standard ASA monitors should be applied, including a pulse oximeter, ECG, and blood pressure cuff. The patient should be pre-oxygenated with 100% oxygen. Inhalation induction with sevoflurane and spontaneous ventilation is chosen over a rapid sequence induction. Keeping the patient spontaneously ventilating helps to stent open the airway, which could be lost during a rapid sequence induction. Sevoflurane is chosen as the inhalation agent because it is less pungent than other inhalational agents and is not associated with laryngospasm, coughing, or airway irritation. Halothane formerly was the inhalation induction agent of choice, but is no longer routinely used because of hepatic injury and the possibility of ventricular arrhythmias when used with catecholamines. The inhalation agent should be slowly increased as the patient maintains spontaneous ventilation. Once the patient is deeply anesthetized, intravenous access is obtained. Intubation is performed with direct laryngoscopy along with either an oral or a nasal endotracheal tube to secure the airway. An air leak at 20 to 25 cm H_2O demonstrates an appropriately sized endotracheal tube.

Patients remain intubated and sedated if needed for several days in the intensive care unit with intravenous antibiotics, frequent suctioning, and acetaminophen for high fever. After 24 to 48 hours when children no longer appear toxic, they can usually be extubated. Some controversy exists concerning whether patients should undergo direct laryngoscopy before extubation to visualize the larynx.

Epiglottitis should be distinguished from laryngotracheobronchitis. See the following table for comparison of the two diseases:

Table 1. Features of Epiglottitis

	Epiglottitis	Laryngotracheobronchitis
Incidence	Less common	More common
Obstruction	Supraglottic	Subglottic
Etiology	Bacterial	Viral
Onset	Sudden (hours)	Gradual (days)
Fever	High	Low grade
Dysphagia/drooling	Present	None
Posture	Sitting	Recumbent
Toxemia	Present	None
Cough	None	Barking
Voice	Clear or muffled	Hoarse
Respiratory rate	Slow	Rapid
Larynx palpation	Tender	Not tender
Radiographs	Lateral: thumb print	Anterior posterior: steeple
Clinical course	Shorter	Longer
Primary treatment	Secure airway first	Medical management
Oxygen and humidity	Harmful	Essential
Racemic Epi	Not helpful	Helpful
Antibiotics	Effective	Not indicated
Intubation	Always indicated (100%)	Occasionally indicated (3%)

SUGGESTED READINGS

Cote CJ, Lerman J, Todres ID, eds. *A Practice of Anesthesia for Infants and Children.* 4th ed. Philadelphia, PA: Saunders-Elsevier; 2009:675–677, 772.

Jenkins IA, Saunders M. Infections of the airway. *Paediatr Anaesth.* 2009;19(suppl 1):118–130.

Verghese ST, Hannallah RS. Pediatric otolaryngologic emergencies. *Anesthesiol Clin North Am.* 2001;19:237–256.

Yao FS. *Yao and Artusio's Anesthesiology: Problem Oriented Patient Management.* 6th ed. Philadelphia, PA: Lippincott Williams & Wilkins; 2008:1038–1048.

Ethics: Speaker Disclosure

Generic Clinical Sciences: Anesthesia Procedures, Methods, Techniques

Mary DiMiceli

Edited by Raj K. Modak

E

KEY POINTS

1. Conflicts of interest (COI) are defined as "circumstances that create a risk that professional judgments or actions regarding a primary interest will be unduly influenced by a secondary interest."
2. Many recommendations have been proposed to limit the influence and presence of COI; however, to date there is no universal system.
3. COI policies are governed by four universal principles: proportionality, transparency, accountability, and fairness.
4. Recommends include that a universal disclosure statement format must be enforced not only by research institutions, but also by academic institutions and medical professional organizations, to ensure that disclosure is not only indicated, but also to what extent the COI are involved in the research, in order to accurately assess whether bias plays a potential role.

DISCUSSION

The Committee on Conflict of Interest in Medical Research, Education, and Practice was appointed by the Institute of Medicine (IOM) in 2007 to examine COI in medicine and to recommend steps that would be able to identify, limit, and manage COI without negatively impacting beneficial associations and the progress of science and medicine. In the committee's report, COI is defined as "circumstances that create a risk that professional judgments or actions regarding a primary interest will be unduly influenced by a secondary interest." In the case of medical research, the primary interest is advancing medical knowledge and protecting its integrity and the safety of patients under clinical research, and the secondary interest is anything that one may receive in return, whether financial or other personal gain. Therefore, the presence of COI cannot be underappreciated because it is not just whether or not they are present that is significant, but also to what degree. Depending on the degree of influence a COI has on a particular researcher, the institution or foundation will determine how much the reader can trust the results. However, not all COI's result in bias. Often in order to undertake certain medical research initiatives, one must be equipped with the funding. Thus, the relationship between scientists and clinicians with industry is born. A lot of good may come from financial support of research from industry, but the many negatives ultimately foster unethical practices and biased conclusions.

In their report, the IOM recommends that a universal policy or strategy be used to assess COI in medical research, using certain criteria to ensure that the said policy/policies are governed by universal principles. These include (1) proportionality—addresses whether the policy is "effective, efficient, and directed at the most important and common conflicts"; (2) transparency—the policy must be "comprehensible and accessible to all individuals and institutions" affected by it; (3) accountability—the COI policy must indicate who is responsible for monitoring, enforcing, and revising it; and, finally, (4) fairness—the policy must apply equally to all applicable groups within and between institutions. Furthermore, the IOM also recommended that a universal disclosure statement format must be enforced not only by research institutions but also by academic institutions and medical professional organizations, not only to ensure that disclosure is indicated, but also to find out to what extent the COI are involved in the research, in order to accurately assess whether bias plays a potential role.

Recently, recommendations have been proposed to oversee some of the legal and moral aspects of COI, including the development of ethical review committees. These proposed committees would comprise experts, including scientists; "lay" members with expertise in law, ethics, or theology; and subject representatives, that is, representatives of the group of individuals who may benefit from research of interest (e.g., HIV patients who may benefit from a stage 4 clinical trial in an experimental drug). Every member involved is a stakeholder in research and represents his/her own interests, and it is the discussion of the committee that determines whether a particular research endeavor should be allowed to proceed. Furthermore, this report also delineates that a separate committee should be created to determine funding versus ethical review of the research.

In attempting to manage and limit COI, disclosure of financial relationships is essential; however, an evaluation of the risk of bias or influencing research results must also be completed to determine the ethics of the said research. Subsequently, research committees should determine whether or not it can then proceed or whether additional measures should be undertaken to improve or limit COI influence on research and the results, and thus improve the quality and integrity of research results and the judgments of researchers and institutions.

SUGGESTED READINGS

Kofke WA. Disclosure of industry relationships by anesthesiologist: is the conflict of interest resolved? *Curr Opin Anaesthesiol.* 2010;23:177–183.

Little M. Research, ethics and conflict of interest. *J Med Ethics.* 1999;25:259–262.

Lo B, Field MJ, eds. *Conflict of Interest in Medical Research, Education and Practice.* Washington, DC: National Academies Press, Institute of Medicine (US) Committee on Conflict of Interest in Medical Research, Education and Practice; 2009.

Evoked Potentials and SSEP Latency: Anesthetic Effects

Physics, Monitoring, and Anesthesia Delivery

Alexey Dyachkov and Tiffany Denepitiya-Balicki

Edited by Ramachandran Ramani

KEY POINTS

1. Evoked potentials (EPs) are techniques allowing monitoring of functional integrity of neural pathways in the spinal cord and is often used during surgeries on the spinal cord or vertebral column. It EP monitoring is also indicated during vascular surgeries where blood supply to neural structures can be compromised.
2. The EPs may be either sensory or motor.
3. Sensory evoked responses are further subdivided to somatosensory evoked potentials (SSEPs), brainstem auditory evoked potentials (BAEPs), and visual evoked potentials (VEPs).
4. The two key characteristics of all EP are latency and amplitude. Usually, "clinically significant" change means a decrease in amplitude of 50% and/or an increase in latency of more than 10%.

DISCUSSION

EPs are techniques allowing monitoring of functional integrity of neural pathways, and is often used during neurosurgical interventions as well as during vascular surgeries, when blood supply to neural structures can be compromised. The technique is based on an electrical stimulation of a peripheral nerve, or rarely cranial nerve (sensory EP) or cerebral cortex (MEP), and recording response up or down the nerve (the spinal cord, cortex) stimulated, or muscle response.

The EPs may be either sensory or motor. Sensory evoked responses (SER) are further subdivided to SSEPs, BAEPs, and VEPs depending on the sensory modality being stimulated. VEP has several limitations: It is the most affected by anesthetic agents and is not frequently used intraoperatively.

The two key characteristics of an EP tracing are latency and amplitude. Latency is the time from the application of the stimulus to the onset of the response. The amplitude is the voltage of the recorded response. According to convention, deflections below the baseline are labeled "positive (P)" and deflections above the baseline "negative (N)." Because amplitude and latency change with recording circumstances, normal values must be established for each neurologic monitoring laboratory, and may differ from values recorded in other laboratories. The third characteristic of EPs sometimes mentioned is the central conduction time, which is the time needed for the signal to travel from the cervico-medullary junction to the contralateral cerebral cortex.

Usually, "clinically significant" change means decrease in amplitude of 50% and/or more than 10% prolongation in latency. Such changes are associated in clinical series and in case reports with onset of new postoperative neurologic deficits. Baseline tracings must always be obtained for comparison.

Anesthetic Effects

The capability of anesthetics effects to elicit changes in SSEP and motor evoked potential (MEP) that may confound the surgically induced changes is summarized in the following table:

Ability of an individual anesthetic drug to produce a change in SSEP and MEP that could be mistaken for a surgically induced change.

Drugs	SSEPs		BAEPs		VEPs		Transcranial MEPs	
	LAT	AMP	LAT	AMP	LAT	AMP	LAT	AMP
Isoflurane, enflurane, halothane, nitrous oxide[a]	Yes	Yes	No	No	Yes	Yes	Yes	Yes
Barbiturates, benzodiazepines, propofol	Yes	Yes	No	No	Yes	Yes	Yes	Yes
Etomidate, ketamine	No	No	No	No	Yes	Yes	No	No
Droperidol	No	No	No	No	—	—	Yes	Yes
Opiates	No	No	No	No	No	No	No	No
Dexmedetomidine	No	No	No	No	No	ND	ND	No

[a]Increases the effect of the agent(s) with which it is used.

Note: This table is not quantitative in any way. "Yes" or "no" designations indicate whether an individual drug is capable of producing an effect on any portion of the evoked response that could be mistaken for a surgically induced change.

AMP, amplitude; LAT, latency; ND, no data available from the literature.

(Modified from Miller RM, ed, et al. Miller's Anesthesia. 7th Edition. Philadelphia: Elsevier, 2009.)

Volatile anesthetics. The volatile anesthetics isoflurane, sevoflurane, desflurane, enflurane, and halothane have similar effects on all types of SERs (an increase in latency, a decrease in amplitude). VEPs are the most sensitive to the effects of volatile anesthetics, and BAEPs are the most resistant to anesthetic-induced changes. Spinal and subcortical SSEP responses are significantly less affected than cortical potentials.

In neurologically normal patients, up to 0.5 minimum alveolar concentration (MAC) of any of the potent inhaled agents in the presence of nitrous oxide, or up to 1 MAC without nitrous oxide, is compatible with monitoring of cortical SSEPs. The key point is to keep anesthetic concentration constant to avoid alteration in the SSEPs that potentially may be caused by the anesthetic, the surgical procedure, or both.

Neurologically impaired patients may show a significantly greater sensitivity to inhaled agents, even to the point of not tolerating any recordable level of inhaled agent.

Nitrous oxide. N_2O decreases SSEPs amplitude without significant changes in latency when used alone or when added to a narcotic-based or volatile anesthetic. For example, adding 50% (0.5 MAC) nitrous oxide to a fentanyl-based anesthetic resulted in a greater decrease in amplitude than adding 1% (0.8 MAC) isoflurane, especially in patients with abnormal preoperative SSEP.

During opioid-based anesthetics, nitrous oxide depressed cortical SSEP amplitude more than propofol when substituted for nitrous oxide.

BAEPs—no change, unless gas accumulates in the middle ear.
VEPs—increase in latency and a decrease in amplitude.

Intravenous agents. Intravenous (IV) anesthetics generally affect SSEPs less than inhaled anesthetics. Low doses of IV agents have minimal effects on SSEPs, whereas high doses of most agents cause mild-to-moderate decreases in amplitude and increases in latency. With very few exceptions, subcortical potentials are unaffected.

Barbiturates. Cause dose-dependent increases in latency, decreases in amplitude of SSEPs, and progressive increases in latency of BAEPs, but allow for intraoperative monitoring of early cortical and subcortical SSEPs and BAEPs even at doses greater than needed for isoelectric electroencephalogram.

Etomidate. Cortical SSEP amplitude: Increased up to 400% above preinduction baseline in some patients, possibly due to an altered balance between inhibitory and excitatory influences at the level of the cerebral cortex, resulting in increased signal synchronization at the thalamic level.

Subcortical SSEP amplitude: Decreased up to 50%.
SSEP latency: Increased.
BAEPs: Dose-dependent increases in latency and decreases in amplitude that are not clinically significant.

Ketamine. Cortical SSEP amplitude: increased; cortical latency: no effect; subcortical amplitude and latency: no effect.

Propofol. Propofol is a convenient drug because it can be infused in anesthetic concentrations during prolonged neurosurgical operations and can allow for rapid emergence for timely postoperative neurologic assessment. As a hypnotic, in the equivalent concentrations, propofol reduces SSEP amplitude less than nitrous oxide or midazolam.

Amplitude: 2.5 mg per kg of propofol produced no changes in the amplitude of the cortical and subcortical SSEPs.

Cortical latency and central conduction time: increased by 8% and 20%, respectively.

TIVA: propofol and sufentanil. SSEP amplitude: 50% decrease; cortical latency: increased up to 10% to 15%.

However, SSEP waveforms stabilized within 30 minutes after anesthetic administration and were compatible with intraoperative monitoring.

Benzodiazepines. They have only mild-to-moderate depressant effects on SSEPs.

Diazepam—0.1 to 0.25 mg per kg.
Cortical amplitude: mild-to-moderate decreases in amplitude.
Latency: very long latency peaks (200 to 400 milliseconds) were abolished.
Midazolam—0.2 to 0.3 mg per kg.
Amplitude: modest or no reduction in amplitude.
Latency: slight prolongation of median nerve SSEP latency.

Midazolam and propofol appear to be better agents (in terms of SSEP suppression) to combine with opioids or nitrous oxide as compared with thiopental, etomidate, or ketamine.

Opioids. Minimal and no significant effects on amplitude (decrease) and latency (increase).

Droperidol. Used for premedication causes a decrease in amplitude and prolongation of conduction time. Effects are not clinically significant.

Clonidine and dexmedetomidine seem to be compatible with all types of EP monitoring, including MEPs.

Adenosine. No effects

Neuromuscular blocking drugs. No direct influence on SSEP, VEP, or BAEP; in fact, they can improve waveform, decreasing noise.

Anesthesia and MEPs. Except in the case of neurogenic MEPs, effects of anesthetics are prominent, particularly on MEP recordings from muscle produced by either single-pulse transcranial electric, or especially magnetic, stimulation. IV agents produce significantly less depression, and techniques using any of a combination of ketamine, opiates, etomidate, and propofol have been described.

The excellent experience was described with a combination of propofol and remifentanil. Anesthetic effects on MEP responses recorded at spinal levels seem to be less affected by propofol–remifentanil combination. When response is recorded from muscle, quantitative monitoring of neuromuscular blocking agents must be instituted to keep T1 twitch height at around 30% of control values. It is preferable to totally avoid using neuromuscular blocking agents during MEP monitoring.

SUGGESTED READINGS

Barash PG, Cullen BF, Stoelting RK, et al, eds. *Clinical Anesthesia.* 6th ed. New York, NY: Lippincott Williams & Wilkins; 2009:1010–1012.

Mark B, John ET, Armin S. Pharmacologic and physiologic influences affecting sensory evoked potentials. *Anesthesiology.* 2003;99:716–737.

Ronald DM, Lars IE, Lee AF, et al. Neurologic monitoring. In: *Miller's Anesthesia.* 7th ed. Philadelphia, PA Churchill Livingstone; 2009: 1481–1487.

EXIT Procedure: Uterine Atony
Subspecialties: Obstetric Anesthesia

Johnny Garriga

Edited by Lars Helgeson

E

1. The ex utero intrapartum treatment (EXIT) is an extension of the standard classical C-section, requiring careful coordination between the obstetricians and the specialists operating on the newborn baby.
2. The difficulty lies in preserving enough blood flow through the umbilical cord by protecting the placenta and by avoiding uterine contractions, so that there is sufficient time to establish the neonatal airway.
3. Uterine atony is an uncommon, but serious, complication in the EXIT procedure.

The EXIT is a specialized surgical delivery procedure used to temporize establishment of a definitive airway in babies with airway compromise at the time of cesarean delivery. The EXIT procedure was originally developed to reverse temporary tracheal occlusion in infants. Causes of airway compression in neonates include bronchopulmonary sequestration, congenital cystic adenomatoid malformation, mouth or neck teratomas, and pleuropulmonary blastoma. Airway compression is often discovered during prenatal ultrasound examinations, allowing sufficient time to plan for a safe delivery via the EXIT procedure.

The EXIT procedure often begins with a standard rapid-sequence induction. Epidural anesthesia is also an option, maintaining good placental perfusion. A midline incision is generally the best approach. The neonate is then partially delivered through the opening, but the umbilical cord remains attached to the neonate. During this time, the neonate's blood supply is still being provided by the placenta, the mother acting as a maternal "heart–lung machine" for the fetus. At this point, it is critical to maintain fetal anesthesia and to ensure adequate fetal oxygenation and fetal monitoring.

To maintain good uteroplacental blood flow, the uterus must be kept relaxed. Placental gas exchange can be maximized by optimizing uterine blood flow, which is affected by uterine tone, maternal blood pressure, and myometrial vasoconstriction. Maintenance of anesthesia with high concentrations of volatile anesthetic agents provides for uterine relaxation. However, high inspired inhalational anesthesia often results in maternal hypotension. Therefore, volume loading and/or the use of ephedrine may be required to ensure adequate uteroplacental blood flow. Often, use of a phenylephrine infusion is required. Use of volatile anesthetic concentrations less than 2 minimum alveolar concentration (MAC) is recommended to minimize untoward effects on uterine blood flow. Tocolytics (indomethacin, terbutaline) may be given to augment the uterine relaxation. Intravenous (IV) nitroglycerine is also highly effective. Uterine relaxation is confirmed by direct palpation before any uterine manipulation.

During the period of fetal manipulation, fetal heart rate and oxygenation can be monitored by sterile ultrasound and pulse oximetry. During this critical period, the pediatric ENT or neonatal general surgeon can then establish an airway. The second phase begins immediately before clamping of the cord, at which point the uterine relaxation must be reversed to avoid uterine atony after delivery. Uterine relaxation must be reversed rapidly by decreasing the inspired concentration of inhalation agent, discontinuing IV nitroglycerine, and administering uterotonic agents, such as oxytocin, so as to minimize maternal blood loss.

Uterine atony results from the loss of tone in the uterine musculature. This invariably leads to maternal hemorrhage because uterine tone compresses the blood vessels and reduces blood flow. Uterine atony often results from an overdistended uterus, a fatigued uterus, an obstructed uterus, or in this case, overrelaxation by pharmacologic agents such as volatile anesthetics and tocolytics. Before clamping the umbilical cord, the volatile anesthetic is decreased to 0.5 MAC or turned off entirely to allow uterine tone to return to normal. This is followed by administration of oxytocin 20 U in 500 mL of normal saline IV as a bolus and then 10 U in 1,000 mL drip titrated to enhance uterine contraction. Additional measures to decrease uterine atony include uterine massage and administration of methergine, ergotamine, or carboprost (F2-alpha prostaglandin). Carboprost tromethamine is effective in treating about 90% of uterine atony patients. If medical means fail to correct the atony, then surgical intervention is undertaken (uterine compression sutures, arterial embolization, and hysterectomy)

An FIO_2 of 1.0 helps maximize oxygen delivery to the placenta. Inhalational anesthetics rapidly cross the placenta and contribute to fetal anesthesia; IV opioids may be used to provide additional fetal anesthesia. Intramuscular anesthetic agents, neuromuscular blocking agents, and atropine are administered to the fetus as needed after partial delivery. Once the EXIT procedure is completed and the baby is off the surgical field, the remainder of the C-section is completed.

SUGGESTED READINGS

Adzick NS. Management of fetal lung lesions. *Clin Perinatol.* 2003;30(3):481–492.

Gaiser RR, Cheek TG, Kurth CD. Anesthetic management of cesarean delivery complicated by ex utero intrapartum treatment of the fetus. *Anesth Analg.* 1997;84:1150–1153.

Hirose S, Farmer DL, Lee H, et al. The ex utero intrapartum treatment procedure: looking back at the EXIT. *J Pediatr Surg.* 2004;39(3):375–380; discussion 375–380.

Oleen MA, Mariano JP. Controlling refractory atonic postpartum hemorrhage with Hemabate sterile solution. *Am J Obstet Gynecol.* 1990;162:205–208.

Factor VIII Concentrate: Indications
Organ-based Clinical: Hematologic

Kristin Richards

Edited by Qingbing Zhu

Kristin Richards

Edited by Qingbing Zhu

KEY POINTS

1. Factor VIII deficiency results in hemophilia A.
2. Hemophilia A can be classified as mild, moderate, or severe.
3. Factor VIII is transfused according to its level in the patient, with minimal hemostatic level of 0.3 U per mL for mild bleeding episodes and 0.5 U per mL for serious bleeding episodes.
4. Factor VIII may be necessary after massive transfusion.

DISCUSSION

Deficiency of, or defective, factor VIII (antihemophilic factor) results in hemophilia A. It is typically thought of as an X-linked recessive genetic condition, but can also result secondary to genetic mutations.

Hemophilia A can be classified as mild, moderate, or severe depending on the detectability of factor VIII levels. Laboratory tests provide confirmation of the diagnosis, and these abnormal laboratory tests include a normal platelet count, normal PT, and prolonged PTT. Specific assays are needed to determine the specific deficiency.

Treatment of hemophilia A is with factor VIII concentrates, and the amount that is required is dependent on the factor level needed to treat the specific bleeding episode. To determine the amount of indicated factor VIII, it is important to know that infusion of factor VIII 1 U per kg increases its level by 0.02 U per mL. Minimal hemostatic levels of 0.3 U per mL are usually necessary to treat mild bleeding episodes; however, levels of 0.5 U per mL are considered minimum for treating serious bleeding into joints or muscles. The halftime is about 8 hours, so that repeated doses are needed, unless it is administered by continuous infusion.

After massive transfusion, factor VIII level may be decreased, as this factor decreases significantly in stored blood. However, only 30% of factor VIII is necessary for hemostasis, so deficiencies are usually only after massive blood loss.

Factor VIII is a protein complex of two factors, von Willebrand factor and factor VIII antigen. In von Willebrand disease, there is a decrease in both factor VIII and von Willebrand factor. Therefore, factor VIII is indicated in von Willebrand disease; however, it is often not the first line of treatment.

Stoelting RK, Dierdorf SF. *Anesthesia and Co-existing Disease*. 4th ed. Philadelphia, PA: Churchill Livingstone; 2002:490–492.

SUGGESTED READING

Factors Affecting Turbulent Flow
Physics, Monitoring, and Anesthesia Delivery Devices

Kimberly Slininger
Edited by Raj K. Modak

F

KEY POINTS

1. Turbulent flow can be predicted by calculating the Reynolds number.
2. Turbulent flow tends to occur at high flow rates, flow through branch points, abrupt changes in airway diameter, or flow through irregular tubing—that is, corrugated tubing of an anesthesia circuit.

DISCUSSION

Gas flow is either defined as laminar or turbulent. Random movement of gas molecules, in this case throughout the airway, characterizes turbulent flow. Predicting laminar versus turbulent flow is usually done by calculating the Reynolds number of the gas.

$$\text{Reynolds number} = \frac{velocity \times diameter \times density}{viscosity}$$

Reynolds number less than 1,000 generally means that flow will be laminar, and a Reynolds number greater than 1,500 indicates that flow will be turbulent. Values between 1,000 and 1,500 mean it is uncertain whether flow will be laminar or turbulent.

Velocity is the rate of gas flow through the anesthesia circuit. High gas flow results in a transition from laminar to turbulent gas flow. Likewise, anything that changes the diameter of the tubing (including airways) that the gas is flowing through can cause flow to transition from laminar to turbulent. Examples of changes in diameter are valves, circuit tubing to endotracheal tube diameter, tubing irregularities, and changes in patients' airway diameters. Turbulent flow is therefore more common in the larger airways, whereas laminar flow is more common in distal to small bronchioles. Gas density is relatively similar between the various gas mixtures that are commonly used by anesthesiologists. The only exception to this is helium–oxygen combinations, which is significantly less dense than 100% oxygen or oxygen-and-nitrogen mixtures. For this reason, helium–oxygen (heliox) mixtures are used in cases of severe upper airway obstruction. Gas viscosities do not vary enough to be clinically significant.

SUGGESTED READINGS

Dorsch JA, Dorsch SE. *Understanding Anesthesia Equipment.* 5th ed. Philadelphia, PA: Lippincott Williams & Wilkins; 2008:192–193.
Morgan GE, Mikhail MS, Murray MJ. *Clinical Anesthesiology.* 4th ed. New York, NY: McGraw-Hill; 2006:546–547.

Fat Embolism: Dx
Subspecialties: Critical Care

Kevan Stanton

Edited by Hossam Tantawy

1. Fat embolism syndrome (FES) is a physiologic response and is not equivalent to fat embolization.
2. Presentation of signs/symptoms can be gradual or acute.
3. Petechial rash, diffuse alveolar infiltrates, and hypoxemia are the most common presenting signs.
4. FES affects multiple organ systems, including respiratory, cardiovascular, and central nervous systems.
5. The two diagnostic tools for diagnosing FES are Gurd's diagnostic criteria of FES and the Schonfeld FES index.

FES is a physiologic reaction to fat in the systemic circulation. FES is not the same as fat embolization. Fat embolization can be detected in almost all patients with pelvic or femoral fractures, but only a small portion of these patients manifest the signs/symptoms associated with FES. The incidence of FES is somewhere between less than 1% and 4%, depending on the source. Risk factors for developing FES include male sex, age 20 to 30 years, hypovolemic shock, intramedullary instrumentation, rheumatoid arthritis, long-bone fractures, total hip replacement using bone cement, and bilateral total knee replacement.

Signs and symptoms of FES involve multiple organ systems, including respiratory, cardiovascular, and central nervous system. Symptoms may include change in mental status such as confusion, respiratory distress, hypotension, or cardiovascular compromise. Disseminated intravascular coagulation (DIC) can also occur in conjunction with FES. Presentation can be gradual, appearing 12 to 72 hours after embolization, or can be acute, leading to adult respiratory distress syndrome (ARDS) and cardiac arrest. Diagnosis can be aided by the use of Gurd's diagnostic criteria of FES or the Schonfeld FES index.

Gurd's Criteria

Major criteria

- Respiratory insufficiency
- Cerebral involvement (can range from drowsiness and confusion to obtundation and coma)
- Petechial rash (pathognomonic—usually on the conjunctiva, oral mucosa, and skin folds of the neck and axilla)

Minor criteria

- Pyrexia
- Tachycardia
- Retinal changes
- Jaundice
- Renal changes

Laboratory features

- Fat microglobulinemia—required (this feature is often criticized given that it can be found in healthy volunteers and trauma patients without FES)
- Anemia

- Thrombocytopenia
- High erythrocyte sedimentation rate

To make the diagnosis of FES using Gurd's criteria, the patient must have at least one major criterion and at least four minor criteria as well as fat microglobulinemia. However, the quantity of fat in the blood does not correlate with the severity of signs or symptoms.

The Schonfeld FES index is based on a scoring system in which a score of greater than 5 is required for the diagnosis of FES. The scoring system is as follows:

Sign	Score
Petechial rash	5
Diffuse alveolar infiltrates	4
Hypoxemia—PaO_2, 70 mm Hg on 100% FiO_2	3
Confusion	1
Fever >38° C	1
Heart rate >120 bpm	1
Respiratory rate >30	1

Although 75% of patients with FES present with diffuse alveolar infiltrates and hypoxemia, less than 10% of them progress to ARDS.

SUGGESTED READINGS

Barash PG, Cullen BF, Stoelting RK, et al, eds. *Clinical Anesthesia.* 6th ed. Philadelphia, PA: Lippincott Williams & Wilkins; 2009:1388.

Miller RD, Eriksson LI, Fleisher LA, et al, eds. *Miller's Anesthesia.* 7th ed. Philadelphia, PA: Churchill Livingstone; 2010:2243.

FB Aspiration: Physical Exam
Organ-based Clinical: Respiratory

Alexander Timchenko

Edited by Shamsuddin Akhtar

F

1. Aspiration of foreign body (FB) may occur in any age group, but is most common in children 1 to 2 years of age. Nevertheless, adults account for 20% of reported cases.
2. Risk factors for aspiration in children are children in early age and immature dentition.
3. Risk factors for aspiration in adults include altered mental status, trauma, impaired airway reflexes secondary to neurologic disease, and dental procedures.
4. In cases of complete obstruction, attempts should be made to remove FB by Heimlich maneuver in adults, whereas younger children should be administered five back blows followed by five chest blows until the object is expelled or patient becomes unresponsive.
5. If the above fails, an attempt at mask ventilation should be made, followed by endotracheal intubation or other invasive ventilation techniques. Definitive management requires rigid bronchoscopy and removal of FB.

FB aspiration most commonly occurs in young children and is associated with a high rate of airway distress, morbidity, and mortality. The peak age for FB aspiration is 1 to 2 years. Adults account for 20% of reported FB aspiration cases. Risk factors for aspiration in children include early age and immature dentition. In adults, risk factors are altered mental status from alcohol or sedative use, trauma with decreased level of consciousness, impaired airway reflexes associated with neurologic disease, and dental procedures. The prevalence of FB aspiration in adults increases with age, beginning in the sixth decade.

Symptoms of FB aspiration vary depending on its location, size, and chronicity. Symptoms are nonspecific, range from none to severe airway obstruction. Coughing, choking (known as penetration syndrome) along with wheezing, shortness of breath, fever, and recurrent pneumonia may each be representing symptom.

Clinical findings of acute FB aspiration are nonspecific, may include diminished breath sounds, wheezing, or even a clear chest. Fourteen percent to 45% of patients with abnormal bronchoscopic findings present with normal physical exam. Chest X-ray provides definitive diagnosis if the object is radiopaque. Most commonly aspirated objects, however, are organic and unlikely to be visualized on chest X-ray.

Pathogenesis of acute aspiration describes four types of airway obstruction:

- *Bypass valve*—Partial obstruction on both phases of respiration. Chest X-ray is normal because obstruction allows for aeration distal to FB.
- *Check valve*—Air is trapped during exhalation. On chest X-ray, hyperinflation of ipsilateral lung segment is found with possible mediastinal shift to normal side.
- *Ball valve*—FB intermittently prolapses and obstructs the affected bronchus, thereby blocking aeration of lung segment. Early atelectasis/lung collapse may develop. On chest X-ray, mediastinal shift to affected side.
- *Stop valve*—FB obstructs bronchus, blocking air passage on both inspiration and expiration. This leads to consolidation and subsequent collapse of bronchopulmonary segment.

Management of FB aspiration depends on the severity, location, and chronicity of symptoms. If obstruction is *mild* (when the patient can cough and phonate), no active management is indicated. Patient should be allowed to clear the obstruction by coughing, and should be observed for worsening of airway obstruction.

In *severe* cases (when the patient is not able to make a sound), subdiaphragmatic abdominal thrusts (Heimlich maneuver) are performed until the object is expelled or the patient becomes unresponsive. Infants should receive five back blows followed by five chest thrusts repeatedly until the object is expelled or the infant becomes unresponsive. Abdominal thrusts in infants are not recommended because of the possibility of damage to the relatively large liver. In case of complete obstruction of trachea, if airway potency is not restored within 3 to 5 minutes, death or anoxic brain injury may occur. In cases of life-threatening asphyxiation, usually central airway obstruction, attempts to ventilate with a bag valve mask or mouth-to-mouth should be performed initially. This should be followed by immediate endotracheal intubation. If symptoms of asphyxiation persist, a cricothyrotomy can be performed by inserting an 18G needle or catheter to allow for oxygen and positive pressure ventilation en route to the operating room for definitive intervention.

The definitive management of FB aspiration includes bronchoscopy. Success rates are higher with rigid bronchoscopy than with flexible fiberoptic bronchoscopy. Flexible bronchoscopy can be performed in awake individuals, whereas rigid bronchoscopy necessitates general anesthesia. Following induction of general anesthesia, the ventilating bronchoscope is introduced. When the bronchoscope is under the subglottis, the anesthesia circuit is connected to allow oxygen delivery and positive pressure ventilation. If FB is localized in the subglottis or trachea, it must be pushed distally into a bronchus to allow ventilation through the healthy lung. If FB cannot be retrieved, preparations for thoracotomy should be made. After FB is safely retrieved, the follow-up bronchoscopy is immediately performed to rule out the presence of additional FB and airway injury. Postoperative chest X-ray is performed to document resolution of trapped air or atelectasis.

Anesthetic considerations

Prior to induction

1. nebulized bronchodilator may be used to improve lower airway ventilation, especially when edema and bronchospasm are present.
2. intravenous atropine or glycopyrrolate may be given to dry airway secretions and to prevent vagal-induced bradycardia from insertion of the bronchoscope.
3. sedative medications should be used with caution, as they may exacerbate existing upper airway obstruction and lead to life-threatening hypoxemia.

Induction and maintenance

1. Induction can be performed using inhaled anesthetic or IV hypnotics, with or without maintenance of spontaneous ventilation, depending on the anesthetic or surgical plan.

   - *Spontaneous ventilation* may provide better ventilation and oxygenation for some obstructions. However, more superficial anesthesia is used that may be insufficient to obliterate airway reflexes and to prevent patient movement. Topical anesthesia is important.

   - *Controlled ventilation* necessitates utilization of deeper anesthesia along with neuromuscular blocker administration. Airway reflexes and patient movement are controlled. Positive pressure ventilation may cause unintentional movement of the object distally and further pulmonary compromise.

2. Rapid sequence induction and intubation is used when there is suspicion for full stomach; otherwise, if respiratory status is stable, routine fasting guidelines apply.
3. Total Intravenous Anaesthesia (TIVA) may be preferrable in these situations as it can provide greater control of depth of anesthesia during bronchoscopy.

SUGGESTED READINGS

Boyd M, Chatterjee A, Chiles C, et al. Tracheobronchial foreign body aspiration in adults. *South Med J.* 2009;102(2):171–174.

Cataneo AJ, Cataneo DC, Ruiz RL Jr. Management of tracheobronchial foreign body in children. *Pediatr Surg Int.* 2008;24:151–156.

Paintal HS, Kuschner WG. Aspiration syndromes: 10 clinical pearls every physician should know. *Int J Clin Pract.* 2007;61(5):846–852.

Sersar SI, Rizk WH, Bilal M, et al. Inhaled foreign bodies: presentation, management and value of history and plain chest radiography in delayed presentation. *Otolaryngol Head Neck Surg.* 2006;134:92–99.

Zur KB, Litman RS. Pediatric airway foreign body retrieval: surgical and anesthetic perspectives. *Pediatr Anesth.* 2009;19:109–117.

Femoral Nerve Block Anatomy

Anatomy

Ira Whitten and Emilio Andrade

Edited by Thomas Halaszynski

F

1. Understanding of femoral nerve block anatomy is necessary for a host of surgical procedures involving the anterior, medial, or lateral aspect of the thigh above the knee, the knee itself, and also the medial aspect of the leg below the knee.
2. Knowing the anatomy and distribution of the femoral nerve is crucial to avoid femoral artery puncture/trauma during femoral nerve blockade and to achieve a successful nerve block.
3. The femoral nerve block can be combined with a sciatic nerve block to often provide adequate anesthesia for any surgical procedure of the lower extremity.
4. A mnemonic for the typical anatomical organization of the femoral nerve block in the inguinal groove is Nerve → Artery → Vein → Lymphatics → Symphysis (NAVLS), beginning laterally and progressing medially.

The femoral nerve arises from the lumbar plexus and is composed of nerve roots from lumbar levels 2 to 4 (L2 to L4). The femoral nerve travels between the psoas major muscle and the iliacus muscle, exiting behind/deep to the inguinal ligament, lateral to the femoral artery and vein within the "femoral triangle."

The first step in performing a femoral nerve block involves understanding the anatomy and identifying the boundaries and contents of the "femoral triangle"—specifically, the anterior superior iliac spine, inguinal ligament, and the femoral artery (Fig. 1). The inguinal ligament runs from the anterior superior iliac spine to the pubic tubercle and lies 1 to 2 cm above the femoral skin crease. The inguinal ligament makes up the superior border of the femoral triangle. The remaining sides of the femoral triangle are made up of the adductor longus muscle medially and the sartorius muscle laterally. The femoral triangle contents from the lateral aspect to the medial aspect include the femoral nerve, femoral artery, femoral vein, lymphatics, and lastly pubic symphysis (commonly remembered by the acronym "NAVLS," pronounced navels). The femoral artery should be palpated at the level of the femoral skin crease and clearly marked, to avoid possible puncture from needle insertion during femoral nerve blockade.

The procedure needle should be inserted perpendicular to the skin, immediately inferior to the inguinal ligament, and approximately 1 to 2 cm (thumb with) lateral to the pulsation of the femoral artery. The direction of the procedure needle should take a slight medial-to-lateral fashion of passage as it is inserted. Once the nerve has been identified and the needle is positioned properly, either by ultrasound guidance or by a nerve stimulator technique, the needle should be held stable and local anesthetic injected (applied in a medial-to-lateral fashion to achieve proper anesthetic spread) around the nerve sheath to avoid femoral artery puncture. Twitch monitor (nerve stimulation technique) may elicit contraction of the quadriceps femoris, resulting in patellar twitch that can be easily seen or palpated (even often under a cast/knee immobilizer).

210

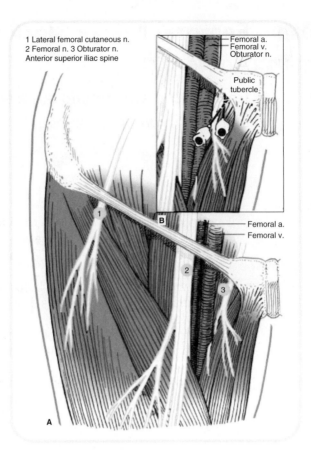

Figure 1. A: Anatomic landmarks for the lateral femoral cutaneous, femoral, and obturator nerve blocks. Before an obturator nerve block, the needle is walked off the inferior pubic ramus in a medial and cephalad direction until it passes into the obturator canal. (From Miller RD. Nerve blocks. *Miller's Anesthesia.* 7th ed. Philadelphia, PA: Churchill Livingstone, 2009:1695.)

SUGGESTED READINGS

Barash PG, Cullen BF, Stoelting RK, et al, eds. *Clinical Anesthesia.* 6th ed. Philadelphia, PA: Lippincott Williams & Wilkins; 2009:988–992.
Brown DL. *Atlas of Regional Anesthesia.* 2nd ed. Philadelphia, PA: W.B. Saunders Company; 1999:104–110.
Hadzic A. *Hadzic's Regional Anesthesia.* New York: McGraw-Hill Professional; 2006:85.
Miller RD, Eriksson LI, Fleisher LA, et al, eds. *Miller's Anesthesia.* 7th ed. Philadelphia, PA: Churchill Livingstone; 2009:1695.

KEYWORD

Fenoldopam: Renal Effects

SECTION

Organ-based Clinical: Renal Urinary/Electrolytes

Zhaodi Gong

Edited by Qingbing Zhu

F

KEY POINTS

1. Fenoldopam is a drug specific to dopamine-1 receptors in the kidneys.
2. Fenoldopam exhibits many desirable renal effects that support its use for the prophylaxis and attenuation of contrast-induced nephropathy.
3. At high doses, systemic vasodilation, decreases in systemic vascular resistance, and a reduction in systemic blood pressure can occur in a dose-dependent fashion.
4. A meta-analysis of randomized clinical trials showed a beneficial effect of fenoldopam in critically ill patients with or at risk for acute renal failure.
5. More studies are needed to evaluate fenoldopam's renoprotective effect.

DISCUSSION

Fenoldopam is a selective dopamine-1 agonist, produces renal vasodilation, and increases renal blood flow, while maintaining normal hemodynamics throughout the body in lower doses. Higher doses may effect hemodynamics systemically, but maintain renal perfusion pressures. In contrast to dopamine, fenoldopam does not display effects on alpha- or beta-adrenergic receptors. Selective agonism of the dopamine-1 receptor at high doses causes systemic vasodilation, decrease in systemic vascular resistance, and a reduction in systemic blood pressure in a dose-dependent fashion.

Fenoldopam exhibits many desirable renal effects that support its use for the prophylaxis of contrast-induced nephropathy, including decreases in renal vascular resistance, increases in renal blood flow, increase in glomerular filtration, and increase in sodium and water excretion. Several reports have also documented a beneficial effect of fenoldopam administration in attenuating contrast-induced nephropathy.

In contrast, a recent multicenter, randomized study did not demonstrate a renoprotective effect of fenoldopam against contrast-induced nephropathy. The presence of multiple confounders, however, precludes a definitive conclusion regarding the ability of fenoldopam to protect against contrast-induced nephropathy. Additional studies are needed to properly evaluate the role of fenoldopam in contrast-induced nephropathy prophylaxis.

Fenoldopam has also been studied in critically ill patients with or at risk for acute renal failure. In a study on hemodynamically stable patients undergoing cardiac surgery with preserved renal function, fenoldopam showed a beneficial effect of a dose-dependent increase in renal flow, and a reduction in the resistances of the renal circulation.

SUGGESTED READINGS

Landoni G, Biondi-Zoccai GG, Tumlin JA, et al. Beneficial impact of fenoldopam in critically ill patients with or at risk for acute renal failure: a meta-analysis of randomized clinical trials. *Am J Kidney Dis.* 2007;49(1):56–68.
Meco M, Cirri S. The effect of various fenoldopam doses on renal perfusion in patients undergoing cardiac surgery. *Ann Thorac Surg.* 2010;89:497–503.
Stoelting RK, Hillier SC. *Pharmacology & Physiology in Anesthetic Practice.* 4th ed. Philadelphia, PA: Lippincott Williams & Wilkins; 2006:495.

Fetal Blood Gas Values
Subspecialties: Obstetric

Trevor Banack

Edited by Lars Helgeson

KEY POINTS

1. The P_{50} of hemoglobin of term infants ranges between 19 and 24 mm Hg as opposed to 26 mm Hg in adult hemoglobin.
2. The normal pH of the umbilical vein is 7.3 to 7.35.
3. The normal pH of the umbilical artery is 7.24 to 7.29.
4. A pH cutoff of less than 7.00 is associated with a significantly increased frequency of low Apgar scores, early neonatal seizures, and neonatal deaths.

DISCUSSION

The placenta is the location of gas exchange between the fetus and the mother. The umbilical vein carries the highest oxygen saturation, which delivers 50% of its circulation to the inferior vena cava and 50% to the hepatoportal system. From the inferior vena cava, the blood flow is divided into two distinct streams: oxygenated blood enters the left atrium via the foramen ovale, and deoxygenated blood enters the right atrium. The left heart blood supplies oxygenated blood to the brain, and the right atrium deoxygenated blood returns to the placenta through the umbilical artery. Table 1 displays the fetal blood gas and acid–base values between the umbilical artery and the umbilical vein.

Table 1. Fetal Blood Gas and Acid–Base Values

	PO_2	PCO_2	Saturation (%)	pH
Umbilical vein	30	40	70	7.3–7.35
Umbilical artery	20	50	28	7.24–7.29

Adapted from Andres RL, Saade G, Gilstrap LC, et al. Association between umbilical blood gas parameter and neonatal morbidity and death in neonates with pathologic fetal acidemia. *Am J Obstet Gynecol.* 1999;181:867–871.

Because of the lower affinity of 2,3-diphosphoglycerate to fetal hemoglobin, there is a higher hemoglobin oxygen saturation in the fetal blood compared with the adult blood at the same oxygen tension. The P_{50} of hemoglobin of term infants ranges between 19 and 24 mm Hg as opposed to 26 mm Hg in adult hemoglobin.

During labor, events such as repeated uterine contractions, cord compression, aortocaval compression, and maternal hypotension may decrease uteroplacental blood flow sufficiently to produce fetal hypoxia and acidosis. Respiratory acidosis with a buildup of carbon dioxide occurs with placental hypoperfusion. If asphyxia is prolonged, a metabolic acidosis can result from anaerobic metabolism. Traditionally, newborn academia is defined as an umbilical artery pH less than 7.20.

Recent studies have shown the traditional pH cutoff of 7.20 may be too high. A pH cutoff of less than 7.00 was associated with a significantly increased frequency of low Apgar scores, early neonatal seizures, and neonatal deaths. Other studies have shown that a metabolic component to the acidemia increased the incidence of death or significant morbidity. Andres et al. found the median base deficit in neonates who either died or had any morbidity was 19 mmol per L.

SUGGESTED READINGS

Andres RL, Saade G, Gilstrap LC, et al. Association between umbilical blood gas parameter and neonatal morbidity and death in neonates with pathologic fetal acidemia. *Am J Obstet Gynecol.* 1999;181:867–871.

Barash PG, Cullen BF, Stoelting RK, et al, eds. *Clinical Anesthesia.* 6th ed. Philadelphia, PA: Lippincott Williams & Wilkins; 2009:1160.

Goldaber KG, Gilstrap LC III, Leveno KJ, et al. Pathologic fetal acidemia. *Obstet Gynecol.* 1991;78:1103–1107.

Sanjay D. *Obstetric Anesthesia Handbook.* 4th ed. New York, NY: Springer; 2006:87.

Fetal HR: Maternal Hypotension

Subspecialties: Obstetric Anesthesia

Christina Mack

Edited by Lars Helgeson

F

KEY POINTS

1. Electronic fetal heart rate (FHR) monitoring is standard for obstetric practice.
2. Late decelerations are indicative of maternal hypotension.
3. Causes of maternal hypotension include compression of the inferior vena cava (IVC) and regional anesthesia.

DISCUSSION

Continuous electronic FHR monitoring became a part of routine obstetric care in the 1970s to aid in recognizing fetal hypoxia during labor. Electronic FHR monitoring can be accomplished by either internal (scalp electrode) or external (ultrasound Doppler) monitoring.

The normal baseline FHR ranges from 110 to 160 beats per minute. For a change in baseline to be established, the change in FHR must occur for at least 10 minutes. Periodic FHR changes are interpreted in relation to maternal contractions and fall into the following general categories: accelerations, early decelerations, variable decelerations, and late decelerations.

Accelerations are abrupt increases in FHR. They are usually due to fetal movement or stimulation, and indicate fetal well-being. Early decelerations are gradual decreases in FHR that mirror uterine contractions. They are usually benign and indicate fetal head compression. Variable decelerations are an abrupt decrease in FHR that last between 15 seconds and 2 minutes. They vary in timing, shape, and depth relative to uterine contractions, and usually indicate cord compression. Atypical variable decelerations may be indicative of fetal hypoxia. Late decelerations are gradual decreases in FHR that occur at or after the peak of uterine contractions. Late decelerations are indicative of fetal hypoxia from any cause, including maternal hypotension or any other cause of poor placental perfusion (Figs. 1 and 2).

The causes of maternal hypotension are important to identify because it is often a preventable cause of fetal distress. Supine hypotension syndrome results from compression of the IVC from a gravid uterus, which decreases venous return to the heart. This syndrome is seen in up to 20% of women at term. In addition to hypotension, patients may show symptoms of light headedness, pallor, diaphoresis, nausea, and vomiting. Compression of the IVC is exacerbated by the Trendelenburg position, and is relieved by positioning for left uterine displacement.

The aorta can also be compressed by the gravid uterus, which will reduce blood flow to the uterus and lower extremities. Contraction of the uterus relieves IVC compression; however, it worsens aortic compression. Women who are at 28 weeks of gestation or later should have left uterine displacement when being placed in the supine position. This can be accomplished by placing a wedge, with at least 15° of elevation, under the right hip.

Physiologic changes that occur with regional anesthesia are another cause of hypotension in parturient patients. Hypotension is the most common side effect of epidural and spinal anesthesia. For this reason, patients are often given a fluid bolus before regional anesthesia is initiated, and the BP is monitored every 2 to 3 minutes after these techniques are employed. Boluses of ephedrine (5 to 15 mg) or phenylephrine (25 to 50 μg) can be used to treat maternal hypotension.

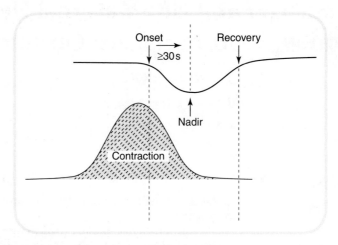

Figure 1. Schematic of late deceleration. (Source: Cunningham FG, Leveno KJ, Bloom SL, et al. *Williams Obstetrics*. 23rd ed. New York, NY: McGraw-Hill. http://www.accessmedicine.com.)

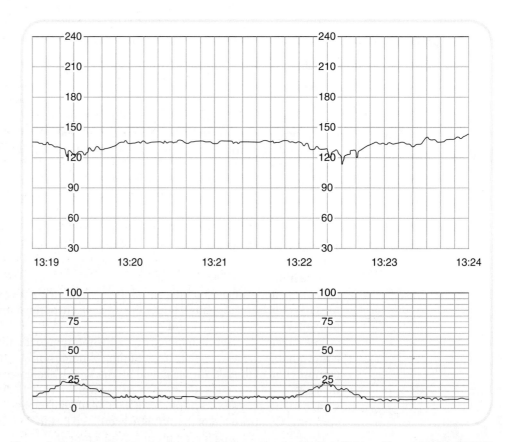

Figure 2. Example of late deceleration occurring from uteroplacental insufficiency. The top graph is the FHR tracing, and the bottom graph is the tracing of uterine contractions. (Source: Cunningham FG, Leveno KJ, Bloom SL, et al. *Williams Obstetrics*. 23rd ed. New York, NY: McGraw-Hill. http://www.accessmedicine.com.)

SUGGESTED READINGS

Bailey RE. Intrapartum fetal monitoring. *Am Fam Physician*. 2009;80(12):1388–1396.

Cunningham FG, Leveno KJ, Bloom SL, et al. Intrapartum assessment. In: *Williams Obstetrics*. 23rd ed. New York, NY: McGraw-Hill; 2010: chap 18. http://www.accessmedicine.com/content.aspx?aID=6024243. Accessed on 31st September 2012.

Morgan GE, Mikhail MS, Murray MJ. Maternal & fetal physiology & anesthesia. *Clinical Anesthesiology*. 4th ed. New York, NY: McGraw-Hill; 2006: chap 42: 876–883.

Fetal HR Pattern: Normal Labor

Subspecialties: Obstetric Anesthesia

Shaun Gruenbaum

Edited by Lars Helgeson

F

1. The approach to fetal heart rate (FHR) patterns must be systematic to avoid misinterpretation. Baseline heart rate, the presence of variability, and periodic patterns must always be assessed.
2. Changes in the baseline FHR range are determined by the autonomic nervous system and may reflect internal or external sources.
3. Loss of beat-to-beat variability reflect central nervous system (CNS) depression by asphyxia, and may therefore be an ominous sign.
4. Early decelerations and variable decelerations, two FHR patterns with a favorable outcome, reflect fetal head compression during maternal contractions and umbilical cord compression, respectively.
5. Late decelerations and a sinusoidal pattern, two ominous FHR patterns, reflect myocardial ischemia caused by uteroplacental insufficiency and severe anemia, or hypoxia, respectively.

FHR monitoring is commonly used to assess fetal well-being during labor. A reassuring FHR tracing correlates with a good fetal outcome and includes good beat-to-beat variability without decelerations. A nonreassuring FHR tracing correlates with a poor fetal outcome and includes lack of variability and persistent, severe, or prolonged decelerations. Other FHR patterns may be difficult to interpret. Thus, the approach to FHR patterns must be systematic to avoid misinterpretation. Baseline heart rate, the presence of variability, and periodic patterns must always be assessed.

The normal FHR range is from 120 to 160 beats per minute, which is determined by the autonomic nervous system. The baseline FHR is considered changed if an alteration in rate persists for more than 15 minutes. Changes in FHR reflect internal or external sources. Fetal tachycardia is associated with prematurity, maternal anxiety, maternal fever, and the administration of drugs such as atropine or ephedrine. Fetal bradycardia may be associated with congenital heart block, fetal hypoxia, or acidosis.

Beat-to-beat variability in FHR reflects a healthy nervous system, which is mediated by the CNS, peripheral nervous system (PNS), and cardiac conduction system. Loss of variability may reflect CNS depression by asphyxia, and may therefore be an ominous sign. Other causes of decreased variability include a calm or sleeping behavioral state (usually transient, with variability increasing within 30 to 40 minutes) and administration of CNS depressants (i.e., barbiturates and opioids), parasympatholytic agents (i.e., atropine), or centrally acting adrenergic agents (i.e., methyldopa). Administration of ephedrine may increase variability.

Important periodic FHR patterns include early, late, and variable decelerations and sinusoidal pattern. Early decelerations reflect fetal head compression during maternal contractions. Early decelerations are U-shaped, starting at the beginning of a contraction and returning to baseline at the end of the contraction. Thus, they are characteristically a "mirror image" of the contraction tracing (Fig. 1). This FHR pattern is usually transient, is not indicative of fetal distress, and is tolerated well by the fetus.

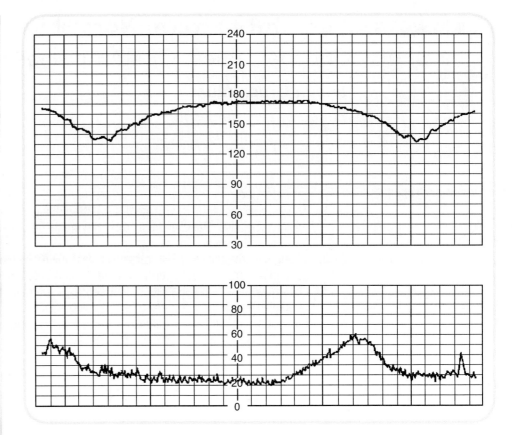

Figure 1. Early deceleration FHR pattern, which usually reflects fetal head compression during maternal contractions. (Adapted from Sweha A, Hacker TW, Nuovo J. Interpretation of the electronic fetal heart rate during labor. *Am Fam Physician*. 1999;59:2487–2500.)

Late decelerations reflect myocardial ischemia caused by uteroplacental insufficiency, and are provoked by maternal contractions. Late decelerations can be the result of placental dysfunction or decreased uterine blood flow. Late decelerations are U-shaped, and they begin at or after the peak of uterine contraction and return to baseline after the contraction has ended (Fig. 2). Late decelerations are nonreassuring and are an ominous sign, especially if they are persistent and show decreased beat-to-beat variability.

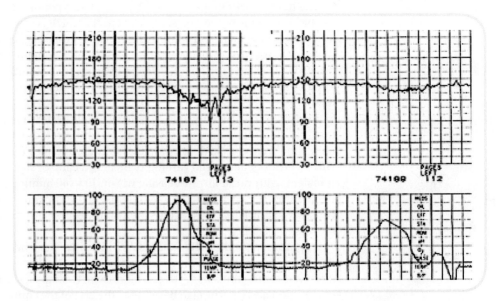

Figure 2. Late deceleration FHR pattern, which usually reflects uteroplacental insufficiency. (Adapted from Sweha A, Hacker TW, Nuovo J. Interpretation of the electronic fetal heart rate during labor. *Am Fam Physician*. 1999;59:2487–2500.)

Variable decelerations are the most common periodic FHR pattern observed. They typically vary in duration, intensity, and timing, and may be U-, V-, or W-shaped (Fig. 3). Variable decelerations reflect umbilical cord compression, and may or may not be associated with maternal contractions. They are associated with a favorable outcome.

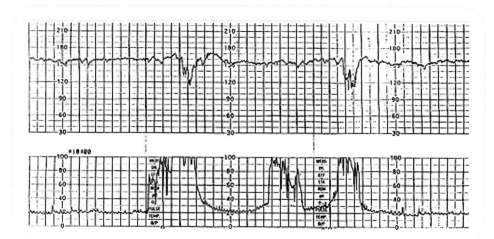

Figure 3. Variable deceleration FHR pattern, which usually reflects umbilical cord compression during maternal contractions. (Adapted from Sweha A, Hacker TW, Nuovo J. Interpretation of the electronic fetal heart rate during labor. *Am Fam Physician.* 1999;59:2487–2500.)

A sinusoidal FHR pattern is a rare but ominous sign. The pattern is a regular, smooth sine wave with a frequency of two to five cycles per minute, amplitude range of 15 beats per minute, and absent beat-to-beat variability (Fig. 4). This pattern reflects severe anemia or hypoxia, neither of which is associated with maternal contractions.

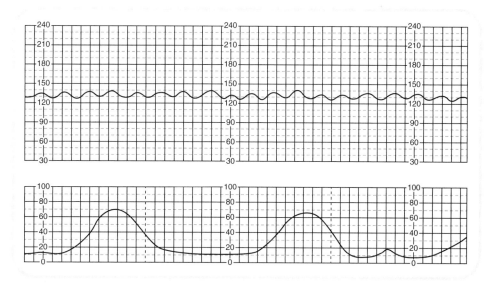

Figure 4. Sinusoidal FHR pattern, which usually reflects severe fetal anemia or severe hypoxia. (Adapted from Sweha A, Hacker TW, Nuovo J. Interpretation of the electronic fetal heart rate during labor. *Am Fam Physician.* 1999;59:2487–2500.)

SUGGESTED READINGS

Barash PG, Cullen BF, Stoelting RK. *Clinical Anesthesia.* 5th ed. Philadelphia, PA: Lippincott Williams & Wilkins; 2009:1160–1161.

Sweha A, Hacker TW, Nuovo J. Interpretation of the electronic fetal heart rate during labor. *Am Fam Physician.* 1999;59:2487–2500.

Flowmeter: Gas Properties
Physics, Monitoring, and Anesthesia Delivery

Adnan Malik
Edited by Raj K. Modak

KEYWORD SECTION

KEY POINTS

1. Flowmeters are gas specific and calibrated based on various characteristics of a given gas.
2. Viscosity and density influence flow through a flowmeter.
3. The higher the Reynolds number (>1,500), the more turbulent the flow, and the lower the Reynolds number (<1,000), the more laminar the flow.

DISCUSSION

Flowmeters are a key component to the anesthesia machine, allowing for monitoring of the amount of flow through the circuit for a specific gas. Flow through the tapered flowmeter (Thorpe Tube) and the constriction, caused by the float device (bobbin), can be either laminar or turbulent in nature (depending on the flow rate). Each flowmeter is thus calibrated for each gas due to differing gas properties.

The flow rate across the flowmeter is directly dependent upon the specific gas's viscosity at low laminar flows. Alternatively, during high turbulent flows, flow through the flowmeter is determined by the gas's density.

The degree of laminar flow versus turbulent flow can be predicted by analyzing the Reynolds number:

$$\mathrm{Re} = \frac{\rho V L}{\mu}$$

ρ represents density, μ is viscosity, V is linear velocity, and L is length. The greater the density, the higher the Reynolds number and thus, the greater the turbulent flow. Conversely, the greater the viscosity, the lower the Reynolds number and the more laminar the flow.

The densities (mass/volume) of the three most common flowmeter gases are as follows: 1.2 g per L for air, 1.429 g per L for oxygen, and 1.977 g per L for nitrous oxide.

Clinically, helium has a very low density-to-viscosity ratio (0.31), making it very useful during states of severe turbulent flow (i.e., upper airway obstruction).

SUGGESTED READINGS

Barash PG, Cullen BF, Stoelting RK, et al. *Clinical Anesthesia*. 6th ed. Philadelphia, PA: Lippincott Williams & Wilkins; 2009:656.
Morgan GE, Mikhail MS, Murray MJ. *Clinical Anesthesiology*. 4th ed. New York, NY: Lange/McGraw-Hill; 2006:58.

Fluid Replacement in Pediatrics

Subspecialties: Pediatrics

Meredith Brown

Edited by Mamatha Punjala

F

1. Clinical signs of adequate perfusion must be monitored to effectively manage fluid replacement in pediatric patients.
2. Maintenance fluids should be calculated using the "4-2-1 Rule" (Table 1).

Table 1. "4-2-1" Rule for Calculating Maintenance Fluids Requirements

Weight (kg)	Hourly Fluid
<10	4 mL/kg
11–20	40 mL + 2 mL/kg
>20	60 mL + 1 mL/kg

3. Volume deficits can be accomplished with an initial 10 mL per kg bolus of isotonic fluid, with the remaining deficit replaced over the subsequent 1 to 2 hours.
4. Third space losses should be calculated and replaced hourly (Table 2).

Table 2. Estimation of Intraoperative Third Space Volume Losses

Surgical Site	Third Space Losses (mL/kg/h)
Intraabdominal	6–15
Intrathoracic	4–7
Cutaneous/intracranial	6–15

5. When significant blood loss is expected, the patient's estimated blood volume (EBV) and maximal allowable blood loss (MABL) should be calculated to help determine the need for blood transfusions.

The goal of fluid therapy is to maintain adequate perfusion and tissue oxygenation. Clinical signs of perfusion and oxygenation include blood pressure, urine output (goal 0.5 to 1 mL per kg), capillary refill, blood gases, etc. The discussion below provides a guideline for volume replacement in pediatric patients.

In replacing fluids in pediatric patients, it is necessary to account for fluid deficits, maintenance fluid requirements, and translocation of fluids and blood loss during surgery. Metabolic demand dictates the calculation for maintenance fluids: one calorie of energy expended requires 1 mL of H_2O for metabolism. Maintenance fluid requirements can be calculated on the basis of the patient's weight, as illustrated in Table 1.

Volume deficit from NPO status can be calculated by multiplying maintenance fluid rate by hours of NPO (volume replacement therapy prior to the operating room must be considered).

Replacement of volume deficit can be accomplished with an initial 10 mL per kg bolus of isotonic fluid, with the balance of the deficit replaced over the subsequent 1 to 2 hours. Neonates, former preterm infants, and other high-risk pediatric patients may require a dextrose solution to prevent dangerous hypoglycemia. The recommended 2.5% dextrose in isotonic crystalloid is not always available. Alternatively, 5% dextrose with 0.45% normal saline can be given, although care must be taken to avoid hyperglycemia.

During surgery, stimulation and manipulation may result in extravasation of isotonic fluids from the extracellular fluid compartment to the interstitial compartment, that is, third-spacing. Third-spacing losses should be replaced hourly with isotonic salt solution. See Table 2 for a guide to estimating third space losses by surgical site.

Estimated blood losses (EBL) should be carefully calculated and replaced to maintain adequate perfusion (3 mL crystalloid per 1 mL EBL). Significant blood loss in pediatric patients may necessitate transfusion of blood or blood products, although the risks and benefits of blood transfusion are carefully considered.

Calculation of the maximum allowable blood loss (MABL) aids in the determination of when to transfuse a pediatric patient.

$$MABL = \frac{[EBV \times (\text{starting Hct} - \text{lowest acceptable Hct})]}{\text{starting Hct}},$$

where EBV is estimated blood volume, an age dependent factor (see Table 3).

Table 3. EBV by Age

Age	EBV (mL/kg)
Preterm infant	100
Term infant	90
3–12 mo of age	80
>1 y of age	70

Transfusion of 1 mL per kg of packed red blood cells can be expected to increase the hematocrit approximately by 1.5%.

Barash PG, Cullen BF, Stoelting RK, et al, eds. *Clinical Anesthesia*. 6th ed. Philadelphia, PA: Lippincott Williams & Wilkins; 2009:1214–1215.

SUGGESTED READING

F

FRC: Definition

Physiology

Jordan Martin

Edited by Veronica Matei

KEY POINTS

1. Functional residual capacity (FRC) is the lung volume at the end of a normal passive expiration.
2. FRC serves as a reservoir of oxygen during apnea.
3. FRC is increased by height and chronic obstructive pulmonary disease (COPD).
4. FRC is reduced in atelectasis, obesity, pregnancy, pulmonary edema, pleural effusions, pulmonary fibrosis, positioning (upright vs. supine vs. Trendelenburg).

DISCUSSION

The physiologic definition of FRC is the volume remaining in the lungs after a passive expiration. This occurs at the point where the force of the collapsing lung (elastic recoil) equals the force of the chest wall muscles to remain open. As there are no external forces acting on the lung, the pressure in the alveoli will equal the ambient pressure, and hence there will be no airflow.

As exemplified in the depiction of a spirometry tracing (Fig. 1), FRC can also be defined as the sum of the expiratory reserve volume or ERV (volume that can be forcefully exhaled after passive expiration) and the residual volume or RV (volume remaining in the lungs after forceful expiration). Because RV cannot be measured using simple spirometry, the same is true for FRC. Thus, both require other techniques such as the multiple breath nitrogen washout test to determine their values.

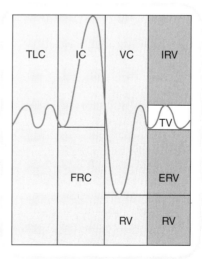

Figure 1. Spirometry tracing. (Obtained from Barash PG, Cullen BF, Stoelting RK, et al, eds. *Clinical Anesthesia*. 6th ed. Philadelphia, PA: Lippincott Williams & Wilkins; 2009:248.)

It is important for anesthesiologists to understand FRC because when a patient is apneic, such as during induction of anesthesia, this lung volume serves as a reserve of oxygen. The duration of a patient remaining properly oxygenated while apneic is determined by how large or small each individual's FRC is. Many conditions can affect a patient's FRC, and a properly prepared anesthesiologist should be able to anticipate potential changes in

the FRC given a patient's past medical history. Patients, who are tall or have COPD, exemplify situations where FRC can be increased. Some instances where FRC is reduced are atelectasis (including high inspired oxygen leading to absorption atelectasis), pulmonary edema, pleural effusions, obesity, pregnancy, pulmonary fibrosis, and respiratory muscle weakness. Positioning can also play a role; Trendelenburg position decreases FRC, and simply lying prone, in a healthy individual, can cause a 10% decrease in FRC. Induction of anesthesia can cause a 15% to 20% reduction in FRC, partially due to the rising diaphragm, loss of muscle tone, and increased blood volume in the lungs. This reduction in FRC from anesthesia can be further exacerbated by the addition of some of the above-mentioned conditions (obesity and anesthesia induction can result in 50% decline in FRC).

SUGGESTED READINGS

Barash PG, Cullen BF, Stoelting RK, et al, eds. *Clinical Anesthesia*. 6th ed. Philadelphia, PA: Lippincott Williams & Wilkins; 2009:234, 247–248, 1232.

Miller RD, ed. *Miller's Anesthesia*. 6th ed. Philadelphia, PA: Elsevier; 2005:693–694, 708–712.

Morgan GE, Mikhail MS, Murray MJ. *Clinical Anesthesiology*. 4th ed. New York, NY: McGraw-Hill; 2006:537–584.

FRC: Vent Settings Effects

Physiology

Harika Nagavelli

Edited by Shamsuddin Akhtar

1. Functional residual capacity (FRC) is the volume of air that remains after a normal exhalation.
2. Respiratory physiology and systemic oxygenation are affected by FRC.
3. Respiratory care for a patient on mechanical ventilation is often adjusted in order to increase a patient's FRC.
4. Positive end-expiratory pressure (PEEP) and end-expiration time are key factors in determining a patient's FRC during mechanical ventilation.

FRC is the volume of air that remains in the lungs after a normal exhalation. In an average person, this volume may range from 2 to 4 L; however, gender, age, height, and weight affect FRC. FRC, also termed functional reserve capacity, is the summation of residual volume (RV) and expiratory reserve volume (ERV), and is approximately 2,300 mL in an average adult. At the end of normal exhalation, the inward pull of the lung is equally counterbalanced by the outward pull of the chest. This point defines elastic recoil, and takes into account the airway smooth muscle fibers, elastic fibers of the lung, and the tension of the alveoli. The lung volume at the balance of all the elastic recoil is FRC. Resistance increases during exhalation as airways narrow, and at the level of FRC, may be approximately 1 cm $H_2O/L/s$. With additional exhalation of air toward RV, the resistance exponentially increases.

During anesthesia, muscle tone is decreased, and resistance is reduced to the point where FRC is closer to the RV of an awake patient. When supine, the abdominal organs displace the diaphragm cephalad. This creates additional loss of FRC, besides that lost secondary to decreased muscle tone from anesthetics. In the supine position, the FRC lung volumes are lower and may even be lower then the closing capacity.

Alveoli and small airways in the dependent areas of the lung are prone to atelectasis. Furthermore, preoxygenation with 100% oxygen also contributes to atelectasis (absorption atelectatsis). Intraoperatively, the high oxygen concentration used during assisted ventilation, lower functional residual capacities from anesthetics, and being in supine position also contributes to airway closure and atelectasis. Well-perfused but atelectatic lung areas lead to increased intrapulmonary shunt, which then produces hypoxemia. Compensatory hypoxic pulmonary vasoconstriction is diminshed by higher doses of volatile anesthetics.

Mechanical ventilation can also be adjusted to counteract hypoxemia and decreased lung volumes. Two manuevers that can improve lung volumes in mechanically ventilated patients are PEEP and inspiration-to-expiration (I:E) ratios. Five to 8 cm H_2O of PEEP helps maintain FRC, thereby decreasing shunting and hypoxemia. PEEP is maintained usually by the expiratory valve during mechanically ventilation. The airway pressures during exhalation must equal or exceed the preset PEEP amount, thus allowing the basal or dependent airway structures that lack cartilaginous support, to remain patent for gas exchange.

The second tool that can be used to improve FRC during mechanical ventilation is the I:E ratio. In a normal breathing individual, alveolar pressure is zero at end expiration. By controlling the expiration time, one can artificially increase FRC, by increasing air trapping and increasing time for gas exchange. By shortening the expiration period of time-cycled ventilation, one artificially allows for air trapping, thus increasing the volume remaining in the lungs after exhalation. This is also termed intrinsic PEEP (PEEPi) or auto-PEEP. This tool is especially useful in patients with lung pathology.

F

SUGGESTED
READINGS

Barash PG, Cullen BF, Stoelting RK, et al, eds. *Clinical Anesthesia*. 6th ed. New York, NY: Lippincott Williams & Wilkins; 2009:234–238, 247–253.

Miller RD, Eriksson LI, Fleisher LA, et al, eds. *Miller's Anesthesia*. 7th ed. Philadelphia, PA: Elsevier, Churchill Livingstone; 2009: chap 15: 363–367.

Fresh Frozen Plasma: Indications and Warfarin Reversal

Organ-based Clinical: Hematologic

Holly Barth and Soumya Nyshadham

Edited by Qingbing Zhu

KEY POINTS

1. Fresh frozen plasma (FFP) is a type of blood product that is the fluid component of a unit of whole blood, and is frozen in the first 6 hours after separation. It consists of plasma proteins and all clotting factors except platelets.
2. Indications for FFP include treatment of specific clotting factor deficiencies; warfarin therapy reversal; liver failure–related coagulopathies; patients receiving large blood transfusions in which platelet transfusions are not successful in slowing bleeding; thrombotic thrombocytopenic purpura; and heparin resistance, the final two resulting from antithrombin III deficiency.
3. A unit of FFP essentially raises each clotting factor level by roughly 2% to 3% in adults, with the therapeutic dose being 10 to 15 mL per kg.
4. The goal of therapy is to reach 30% of normal coagulation factor levels so as to accomplish effective hemostasis.
5. Warfarin acts by depleting vitamin K–dependent coagulation factors II, VII, IX, and X, and proteins C and S.
6. FFP contains all the coagulation factors depleted by warfarin, and can reverse warfarin quicker than vitamin K in an emergency situation; however, its effect is not permanent, and thus FFP may have to be redosed.

DISCUSSION

FFP is a type of blood product that is the fluid component of a unit of whole blood, and is frozen in the first 6 hours after separation. It consists of plasma proteins and all clotting factors except platelets. A unit of FFP essentially raises each clotting factor level by roughly 2% to 3% in adults, with the therapeutic dose being 10 to 15 mL per kg. The goal of therapy is to reach 30% of normal coagulation factor levels so as to accomplish effective hemostasis. Although most research indicates that use of FFP and platelets should be only in the context of clinical coagulopathies, clinically both are often used even without such evidence.

Indications for FFP include treatment of specific clotting factor deficiencies; warfarin therapy reversal; liver failure–related coagulopathies; patients receiving large blood transfusions in which platelet transfusions are not successful in achieving hemostasis; thrombotic thrombocytopenic purpura; and heparin resistance. Deficiencies of coagulation factors are indicated by prothrombin time and/or partial thromboplastin time, that is, greater than 1.5 times upper limit of normal. This deficiency can occur secondary to many physiologic events, for instance, disseminated intravascular coagulation (DIC). This is a pathologic systemic overactivity of the body's coagulation pathways. Fibrinolysis, platelet activation, and consumption of coagulation factors occur, often resulting in profound hemorrhage. DIC can be the result of infection, trauma, shock, burn, or embolism. Replacement blood products including platelets, FFP, and cryoprecipitate are indicated.

The liver is responsible for the synthesis and clearance of most coagulation factors. Those with liver dysfunction or failure may have decreased synthesis of new coagulation factors and decreased clearance of activated factors. As a result, there is a deficiency of coagulation factors as well as an ongoing consumptive coagulopathy that is similar to that seen in DIC. Hence, FFP is often necessary to replenish the low levels of these coagulation factors. Coagulopathy can also occur secondary to massive transfusion, generally only after 1 to 1.5 times blood volume replacement. Transfusion in such high volume can lead to coagulopathy, most often resulting from decreased levels of factors V, VIII, or IX and fibrinogen. Platelet therapy is often the initial therapy, as thrombocytopenia is more often the cause of hemorrhage after massive transfusion. If coagulopathy is refractory to this treatment, FFP is initiated. Finally, FFP is also often used for the treatment of thrombotic thrombocytopenic purpura as well as heparin resistance, which results from antithrombin III deficiency.

Warfarin is an anticoagulant that is routinely used for the treatment of existing thrombi or the prevention of formation of new thrombi. Common indications include treatment or prophylaxis for deep venous thrombosis (DVT) and pulmonary embolism (PE), as well as therapy for patients with atrial fibrillation, and prosthetic heart valves to reduce the incidence of embolic cerebrovascular accidents. Ultimately, the risk of reversing the anticoagulation effect of warfarin needs to be weighed with the consequences of development of thrombi and their consequences, before administering reversal. Typically, life-threatening bleeding requires urgent reversal, whereas super-therapeutic international normalized ratio (INR) without evidence of bleeding or requirement for reversal such as invasive procedures/surgery may be managed more conservatively.

Warfarin functions by inhibiting vitamin K epoxide reductase, resulting in a deficiency of vitamin K, which in turn prevents factors II, VII, IX, and X, and proteins C and S from achieving their active forms. Vitamin K can be used to reverse the effects of warfarin, but this requires at least 6 hours. Urgent reversal of warfarin therapy can be achieved with FFP doses as small as 8 to 10 mL per kg, or often can be more effectively achieved with the use of prothrombin complex concentrate, which contains factors II, VII, IX, and X.

If the need for reversal of the anticoagulant effect of warfarin is anticipated, simply stopping administration of warfarin for approximately 5 to 7 days is adequate to achieve normalization of the INR. Patients with therapeutic INR on warfarin therapy returned to INR of 1.6 by approximately 2.7 days after cessation of warfarin, and to INR of 1.2 after 4.7 days.

Reversal of anticoagulation with warfarin may be achieved by administration of either vitamin K or FFP. Patients taking warfarin are deficient in the vitamin K coagulation factors. Therefore, this deficiency can be reversed by the administration of vitamin K. If the patient is actively bleeding or needs emergency surgery, FFP can be used for hemostasis.

FFP is the separated plasma from whole red blood cells that contains all the coagulation factors, specifically those depleted by therapy with warfarin. Administration of FFP results in temporary normalization of the INR, typically in the range of 4 to 6 hours. Therefore, this therapy should be reserved for severe bleeding episodes in the setting of warfarin anticoagulation or before surgical interventions that may become complicated with hemorrhage secondary to warfarin-induced coagulopathy. Note that patients requiring anticoagulation with warfarin may have existing comorbidities, and may not tolerate plasma volume expansion with repeated doses of FFP.

SUGGESTED READINGS

Barash PG, Cullen BF, Stoelting RK, et al, eds. *Clinical Anesthesia*. 6th ed. New York, NY: Lippincott Williams & Wilkins; 2009:380–381.

Crowther MA, Julian J, McCarty D, et al. Treatment of warfarin-associated coagulopathy with oral vitamin K: a randomized controlled trial. *Lancet*. 2000;356(9241):1551–1553.

Dezee KJ, Shimeall WT, Douglas KM, et al. Treatment of excessive anticoagulation with phytonadione (vitamin K): a meta-analysis. *Arch Intern Med*. 2006;166(4):391–397.

Dunn PF. *Clinical Anesthesia Procedures of the Massachusetts General Hospital*. 7th ed. Philadelphia, PA: Lippincott Williams & Wilkins; 2007:615–617.

Kasper DL, Braunwald E, Fauci AS, et al. *Harrison's Principles of Internal Medicine*. 16th ed. New York, NY: McGraw-Hill; 2005:409.

Miller RD, Stoelting RK, eds. *Basics of Anesthesia*. 5th ed. Philadelphia, PA: Churchill Livingstone; 2007:358.

Morgan GE, Mikhail MS, Murray MJ. *Clinical Anesthesiology*. 4th ed. Philadelphia, PA: McGraw-Hill Professional; 2006:699.

Glasgow Coma Scale: Definition and Components

Organ-based Clinical: Neurologic and Neuromuscular

Frederick Conlin and Tara Paulose

Edited by Ramachandran Ramani

KEY POINTS

1. The Glasgow Coma Scale (GCS) is intended to be used as a standardized measure to assess a patient's neurologic status.
2. The scale is broken down into three categories: eye-opening ability, verbal response, and motor response.
3. Scores range from 3 to 15, with a score less than or equal to 8 representing severe head injury and associated with poor prognosis.

DISCUSSION

The GCS was developed to assess the level of consciousness of patients after traumatic brain injuries. It is used to evaluate patients during initial assessment and follow-up. The popularity of the scale can be attributed to its high correlation with outcome, its simplicity, and strong interobserver reliability.

Patients are scored on the basis of their best responses in three categories: eye opening, verbal response, and motor response. The lowest score for each category is 1, and thus the lowest possible total score is 3 with the highest achievable score being 15. Of patients with GCS scores of 3 to 4, 85% will die within 24 hours, although comorbid conditions and age also influence outcome (see Table 1).

Table 1. Glasgow Coma Scale

Sign	Evaluation	Score
Eye opening	Spontaneous	4
	To speech	3
	To pain	2
	None	1
Best verbal response	Oriented	5
	Confused	4
	Inappropriate	3
	Incomprehensible	2
	None	1
Best motor response	Obeys commands	6
	Localizes pain	5
	Withdrawal to pain	4
	Flexion to pain	3
	Extension to pain	2
	None	1

Despite the attempt to make an objective assessment, the efficacy of the GCS scale is affected by subjectivity of clinicians, as well as factors that diminish a patient's ability to demonstrate eye, motor, and verbal responses, that is, sedating medications and intubation. Although these factors are limiting, the GCS still represents an organized and standardized measure of neurologic status.

SUGGESTED READINGS

Barash PG, Cullen BF, Stoelting RK, et al, eds. *Clinical Anesthesia*. 6th ed. Philadelphia, PA: Lippincott Williams & Wilkins; 2009:898–901.

Evans C, Tippans E. *Foundations of Emergency Care*. Berkshire, England: Open University Press; 2006:189–196.

Kasper DL, Braunwald E, Fauci AS, et al. *Harrison's Principles of Internal Medicine*. 16th ed. New York, NY: McGraw-Hill; 2005:2450–2451.

Miller RD, ed. *Miller's Anesthesia*. 7th ed. Philadelphia, PA: Churchill Livingstone; 2009:2068.

Morgan GE, Mikhail MS, Murray MJ. *Clinical Anesthesiology*. 4th ed. New York, NY: McGraw-Hill Medical; 2006:639–641.

Gas Laws: Temp/pressure Changes

Physics, Monitoring, and Anesthesia Delivery Devices

Anna Clebone

Edited by Raj K. Modak

G

KEY POINTS

1. The ideal gas equation ($PV = nRT$) defines the relationship between pressure, volume, and temperature of gases.
2. Boyle's Law demonstrates an inverse relationship between the pressure and volume of a gas.
3. Gay-Lussac's Law demonstrates a direct relationship between the pressure and temperature of a gas.
4. Charles' Law describes a direct relationship between the volume and temperature of a gas.
5. These gas laws apply to ideal gases, and humidity or extreme pressures will affect accuracy.

DISCUSSION

The *Ideal Gas Equation* defines the relationship between the pressure, volume, and temperature of ideal gases.

$$PV = nRT,$$

where P = pressure, R = constant, V = volume, T = temperature, and n = moles.

To clarify the relationships, simplify the equation by omitting the constant and assuming a constant number of moles:

$$PV = T.$$

The Ideal Gas Equation was developed by combining the relationships described by the following three laws:

Boyle's Law: A gas at a constant temperature will exhibit an inverse relationship between pressure and volume. More pressure = less volume.

Gay-Lussac's Law: A gas with a constant volume will exhibit a direct relationship between pressure and temperature. Higher pressure = higher temperature.

Charles' Law: A gas held at a constant pressure will exhibit a direct relationship between volume and temperature. Increased temperature = increased volume.

Gas density is calculated by dividing its mass by its volume. The density of a gas varies directly with pressure and inversely with temperature. More pressure = more density. Higher temperature = less density.

SUGGESTED READINGS

Kotz JC, Treichel PM, Townsend JM. *Chemistry and Chemical Reactivity*. Belmont, CA: ThompsonBrooks/Cole; 2009:517–531.

Walker J. *Introduction to Physical Chemistry*. London, UK: MacMillan; 1907:26–28.

H$_2$ Blockers: Onset Time

Pharmacology

Hyacinth Ruiter

Edited by Lars Helgeson

KEY POINTS

1. H$_2$ blockers reduce the perioperative risk of aspiration pneumonitis.
2. H$_2$ blockers competitively inhibit histamine binding to H$_2$ receptors, hence decreasing gastric acid production and thereby increasing gastric pH.
3. Patients should be pretreated with H$_2$ blockers at bedtime and again at least 2 hours before surgery.
4. Typical onset of action of H$_2$ blockers occurs within 1 to 2 hours, but duration time can vary between the different H$_2$ blockers.

DISCUSSION

Histamine is involved in the secretion of hydrochloric acid by parietal cells in the stomach. H$_1$ and H$_2$ receptors mediate the effects of histamine. The H$_1$ receptor activates phospholipase C, and the H$_2$ receptor raises intracellular cyclic adenosine monophosphate (cAMP). H$_2$ blockers competitively inhibit histamine binding to H$_2$ receptors, hence decreasing gastric acid production, and thereby increasing gastric pH. H$_2$ blockers effectively treat gastroesophageal reflux disease (GERD), Zollinger–Ellison syndrome, and peptic duodenal and gastric ulcers.

H$_2$ blockers include cimetidine, famotidine, nizatidine, and ranitidine. They all effectively reduce gastric fluid volume and hydrogen ion content and prevent the perioperative risk of aspiration pneumonia. Importantly, H$_2$ blockers only change the pH of gastric secretions, but do not affect the lower esophageal sphincter tone or alter gastric emptying.

Patients should be pretreated with H$_2$ blockers at bedtime and again at least 2 hours before surgery. Their onset of action occurs within 1 to 2 hours when taken orally, but duration of action can vary between the different H$_2$ blockers. Cimetidine lasts 3 to 4 hours, whereas the duration of action of ranitidine, famotidine, and nizatidine ranges from 10 to 12 hours. Therefore, cimetidine is suitable only for those operations of that duration. Famotidine in a dose of 40 mg orally 1.5 to 3 hours preoperatively has been shown to effectively increase gastric pH. Nizatidine 150 to 300 mg orally 2 hours before surgery has also demonstrated decreased gastric acidity. Most H$_2$ blockers, when administered parenterally, will be effective within 1 hour of administration.

H$_2$ blockers are eliminated primarily by the kidneys; therefore, patients with renal dysfunction should have reduced dosages of all four drugs. Rare adverse side effects of rapid intravenous injection of cimetidine and ranitidine are bradycardia, hypotension, arrhythmias, and cardiac arrest.

SUGGESTED READINGS

Barash PG, Cullen BF, Stoelting RK, et al, eds. *Clinical Anesthesia*. 6th ed. Philadelphia, PA: Lippincott Williams & Wilkins; 2009:590–591.

Miller RD, ed. *Miller's Anesthesia*. 6th ed. Philadelphia, PA: Churchill Livingstone; 2005:2598–2600.

Morgan GE, Mikhail MS, Murray MJ. *Clinical Anesthesiology*. 4th ed. New York, NY: McGraw-Hill; 2006:279–280.

Haldane Effect

Physiology

Thomas Gallen

Edited by Hossam Tantawy

H

KEY POINTS

1. The Haldane effect describes the increased affinity of deoxyhemoglobin for carbon dioxide (3.5 times greater than oxyhemoglobin).
2. Deoxyhemoglobin buffers hydrogen ions formed by dissociation of carbonic acid, thereby allowing increased transport of carbon dioxide as bicarbonate ions.
3. The Bohr effect explains that during periods of increased hydrogen ion concentration (acidosis), hemoglobin releases oxygen and will bind hydrogen ions, shifting the CO_2-bicarbonate equilibrium in favor of greater bicarbonate formation.

DISCUSSION

Carbon dioxide is carried in the blood in four forms: physical solution, carbonic acid, bicarbonate (the majority approximately 60%), and carbamino compounds. Although the primary function of hemoglobin is to carry oxygen, it also binds carbon dioxide. The Haldane effect describes the increased affinity of deoxyhemoglobin for carbon dioxide. In fact, deoxygenated hemoglobin has a 3.5 times greater affinity for carbon dioxide than does oxygenated hemoglobin.

The Bohr effect explains the effect of $PaCO_2$ and pH on the oxyhemoglobin dissociation curve. During periods of increased hydrogen ion concentration (acidosis), hemoglobin releases oxygen and will bind hydrogen ions, shifting the CO_2–bicarbonate equilibrium in favor of greater bicarbonate formation:

$$CO_2 + H_2O + HbO_2 \rightarrow HbH^+ + HCO_3^- + O_2$$

A rightward shift of the oxyhemoglobin dissociation curve denotes a decreased affinity of hemoglobin for oxygen, permitting unloading of oxygen to tissues. This occurs during increased $PaCO_2$, acidosis, hyperthermia, and increased 2,3-diphosphoglycerate.

A leftward shift of the oxyhemoglobin dissociation curve indicates an increased affinity of hemoglobin for oxygen, allowing the hemoglobin to bind more oxygen at the lungs, but decreased unloading at the tissue level. This occurs with alkalosis, hypothermia, and variant hemoglobin (methemoglobin, carboxyhemoglobin, etc.).

SUGGESTED READINGS

Levitzky MG. *Pulmonary Physiology.* 6th ed. New York, NY: McGraw-Hill; 2003:158–161.
Morgan GE, Mikhail MS, Murray MJ. *Clinical Anesthesiology.* 4th ed. New York, NY: McGraw-Hill; 2005:564–567.

Head Down Position: Hypoxemia
Organ-based Clinical: Respiratory

Nehal Gatha

Edited by Veronica Matei

H

KEY POINTS

1. Head down (Trendelenburg) positioning, although beneficial for surgical exposure, has detrimental effects on respiratory physiology at times, resulting in hypoxemia.
2. Trendelenburg positioning promotes a cephalad shifting of the abdominal viscera, severely limiting diaphragmatic excursion, and thereby reducing functional residual capacity (FRC), total lung volume, and pulmonary compliance.

DISCUSSION

Trendelenburg positioning is used in many surgeries, particularly abdominal and gynecologic procedures to facilitate surgical exposure; however, it has multiple effects on respiratory physiology and may cause hypoxemia.

Trendelenburg positioning promotes a cephalad shifting of the abdominal viscera, severely limiting diaphragmatic excursion, and thereby reducing FRC, total lung volume, and pulmonary compliance. This decrease in pulmonary compliance also leads to atelectasis while patients are in this position. The Trendelenburg position can also cause V/Q mismatch, contributing to hypoxemia.

The Trendelenburg position theoretically may increase pulmonary capillary hydrostatic pressure, causing an increase in interstitial fluid and oxygen diffusion impairment. Furthermore, while in the Trendelenburg position, the lungs and carina may shift cephalad, potentially causing the endotracheal tube to slide into the right mainstem bronchus.

SUGGESTED READINGS

Barash PG, Cullen BF, Stoelting RK, et al, eds. *Clinical Anesthesia.* 5th ed. Philadelphia, PA: Lippincott Williams & Wilkins; 2006:800–802.

Morgan GE, Mikhail MS, Murray MJ. *Clinical Anesthesiology.* 4th ed. New York, NY: McGraw-Hill; 2006:580–585.

Perilli V, Sollazzi L, Bozza P, et al. The effects of the reverse Trendelenburg position on respiratory mechanics and blood gases in morbidly obese patients during bariatric surgery. *Anesth Analg.* 2000;91(6):1520–1525.

Heart Block: Coronary Occlusion
Anatomy

Jonathan Tidwell

Edited by Benjamin Sherman

H

KEY POINTS

1. The myocardial blood supply is derived almost entirely from the right and left coronary arteries. The endocardium receives some of its blood supply directly from blood within the cardiac chambers.
2. *Coronary dominance* is a term to describe which coronary artery supplies blood to the posterior descending artery (PDA). The PDA supplies blood to the atrioventricular (AV) node.
3. Coronary dominance is as follows:
   a. Right coronary artery (RCA) dominance is 70%.
   b. Left coronary artery dominance is 10%.
   c. Codominance is found in 20% of patients.
4. RCA occlusion is the most common coronary artery occlusion that produces AV nodal block.
5. Treatment of AV nodal block in the setting of acute myocardial infarction (MI) is dependent on the location of occlusion.
   a. Symptomatic heart block at the level of the AV node to include third and second degree blocks can be treated with atropine.
   b. Block below the AV node requires pacemaker utilization and can be worsened by administration of atropine.

DISCUSSION

The myocardial blood supply is derived almost entirely from the right and left coronary arteries. Some perfusion of the endocardium is through direct supply from blood in the cardiac chamber itself. The AV node is supplied by the RCA (right dominant circulation) in 70% of people and by the left circumflex artery (left dominant circulation) in 10% of people, and codominance is present in 20% of people. RCA occlusion with right heart dominance produces an inferior wall MI and ischemia of the node and occasionally increased vagal tone. Although RCA occlusion is the most common one resulting in AV node block, the left anterior descending artery can also become occluded and lead to AV node block. Left anterior descending artery occlusion resulting in AV node block from anterior wall MI has a poor prognosis and often requires pacemaker insertion.

It is critical to determine the location of AV nodal block in the setting of an acute MI because the treatment varies drastically. Third degree block at the level of the AV node and symptomatic second degree block are treated with atropine; however, atropine can worsen AV infranodal block. Acute anterior wall MIs resulting in heart block are treated with a pacemaker.

SUGGESTED READINGS

Fuster V, Walsh R, Harrington R. *Hurst's the Heart.* 13th ed. New York, NY: McGraw-Hill; 2010:53.

Goldberger AL. *Clinical Electrocardiography: A Simplified Approach.* 7th ed. Philadelphia, PA: Mosby; 2006:34.

Goldman L, Ausiello DA, Arend W, et al, eds. *Cecil's Textbook of Medicine.* 23rd ed. Philadelphia, PA: Saunders; 2007:412–415, 513.

Marx JA, Hockberger RS, Walls RM, et al, eds. *Rosen's Emergency Medicine.* 7th ed. Philadelphia, PA: Mosby; 2009:947–957.

Heart Transplant: Autonomic Effects and Pharmacology

Organ-based Clinical: Cardiovascular

Jinlei Li and K. Karisa Walker

Edited by Benjamin Sherman

H

KEY POINTS

1. Heart transplantation results in a totally denervated donor heart, resulting in a high fixed heart rate and loss of parasympathetically mediated reflexes.
2. Indirect drug effects requiring intact autonomic innervation to the heart are ineffective in transplanted hearts; drugs acting directly on cardiac tissue remain effective (see Tables 1 and 2).
3. Cardiac denervation increases adrenergic sensitivity through an increase in beta-receptor density (as opposed to affinity).
4. Atropine is ineffective as a treatment for bradycardia.
5. Isoproterenol is the inotrope and chronotrope of choice; norepinephrine and epinephrine should be reserved for refractory hypotension.
6. Beta-blockers have an increased antagonist effect.
7. Transplanted hearts also do not respond to carotid massage and Valsalva maneuvers.

Table 1. Effect of Denervation on Cardiac Pharmacology

Substance	Effect on Recipient	Mechanism
Digitalis	Normal increase of contractility, minimal effect on AV node	Direct myocardial effect, denervation
Atropine	None	Denervation
Adrenaline	Increased contractility Increased chronotropy	Denervation hypersensitivity
Noradrenaline	Increased contractility Increased chronotropy	Denervation No neuronal uptake
Isoproterenol	Normal increase in contractility, normal increase in chronotropy	
Quinidine	No vagolytic effect	Denervation
Verapamil	AV block	Direct effect
Nifedipine	No reflex tachycardia	Denervation
Hydralazine	No reflex tachycardia	Denervation
Beta-blocker	Increased antagonist effect	Denervation

From Deng MC. Cardiac transplantation. *Heart.* 2002;287:177.

DISCUSSION

Heart transplantation includes more than 98% orthotopic transplantation (recipient heart removed and replaced with donor heart) and 1% to 2% heterotopic transplantation (recipient heart left intact and donor heart transplanted and anastomosed to the failing recipient heart, "double heart"). Orthotopic biatrial or bicaval implantation has been performed with very good success. Heterotopic cardiac transplantation is rarely performed because of high operative mortality and the requisite ongoing medical care of the still present native heart.

Autonomic innervation of the heart, much like most organ systems, comprises both parasympathetic and sympathetic innervation. Cholinergic parasympathetic fibers (vagus nerve) primarily innervate the atria and electrical conducting system. Adrenergic sympathetic fibers originating at the T1–T4 spinal levels, via the stellate ganglia, innervate the

Table 2. Drug Effects on Denervated Hearts

Drug	Action	Heart Rate	Blood Pressure
Atropine	Indirect	−	−
Digoxin	Direct	−/↓	−
Dopamine	Indirect and direct	↑	↑
Ephedrine	Indirect and direct	−/↑	−/↑
Fentanyl	Indirect	−	−
Isoproterenol	Direct	↑	−/↑
Neostigmine	Indirect	−/↓	−
Norepinephrine	Direct	↑	↑
Pancuronium	Indirect	−	−
Phenylephrine	Direct	−	↑
Verapamil	Direct	↓	↓

From Hensley FA Jr, Martin DE, Gravlee GP. *A Practical Approach to Cardiac Anesthesia.* 4th ed. Philadelphia, PA: Lippincott Williams & Wilkins; 2008:439–463.

heart in a generalized fashion. After cardiac transplantation, there is a total denervation of the recipient's heart. There is a loss of parasympathetic-mediated slowing of the sinoatrial (SA) node pacemaker cells, resulting in a relatively fixed heart rate of 90 to 110 beats per minute. Reflexes mediated by the vagal nerves (i.e., reflex bradycardia from carotid sinus massage or Valsalva) are absent in a transplanted heart. Sympathetic-mediated cardiac responses, however, are often normal or enhanced. This is due to an increased adrenergic receptor density in the heart. It is important to understand these changes because they result in different physiologic responses to various common medications.

Atropine is an anticholinergic drug that normally exerts its effect on the heart by blocking parasympathetic input to the SA and atrioventricular (AV) node, leaving sympathetic stimulation unopposed, thus causing an increase in heart rate. Atropine and other anticholinergic medications (glycopyrrolate) are ineffective in the transplanted heart because of the lack of vagal innervation. Therefore, the treatment of bradycardia in cardiac transplant patients should include pacing and/or beta-adrenergic medications such as isoproterenol or epinephrine. It is important to note that in patients who have recovered from the acute phase of heart transplantation, reinnervation of the vagus nerve is possible. This phenomenon is infrequent, but is important to consider while administering medications or performing maneuvers that augment vagal tone, with potential unexpected bradycardia.

Direct beta-adrenergic medications (isoproterenol, norepinephrine, epinephrine, dobutamine) may exhibit enhanced beta effects on the heart in transplant patients because of denervation hypersensitivity (resulting from increased adrenergic receptor expression). Isoproterenol is frequently used in heart transplantation because of its direct and reliable effect on cardiac beta-receptors. If there is concurrent hypotension, epinephrine and norepinephrine should be considered because they include alpha-receptor stimulation with subsequent vasoconstriction. Dopamine and ephedrine work through both direct and indirect mechanisms, and therefore, reduced efficacy may occur.

Beta blocking drugs exhibit an increased effect and should be used with care. They can be the mainstay of therapy for sinus tachycardia in transplant patients (who do not have vagal tone), but have a heightened response compared with normal controls.

Tables 1 and 2 outline some other medications with the expected responses in cardiac transplantation patients.

SUGGESTED READINGS

Barash PG, Cullen BF, Stoelting RK, et al. *Clinical Anesthesia.* 6th ed. Philadelphia, PA: Lippincott Williams & Wilkins; 2009:1412.

Deng MC. Cardiac transplantation. *Heart.* 2002;287:177.

Hensley FA Jr, Martin DE, Gravlee GP. *A Practical Approach to Cardiac Anesthesia.* 4th ed. Philadelphia, PA: Lippincott Williams & Wilkins; 2008:439–463.

Morgan GE, Mikhail MS, Murray MJ. *Clinical Anesthesiology.* 4th ed. New York, NY: McGraw-Hill; 2006:420.

H

Helium Advantage: Small-Bore Tube

Generic Clinical Sciences: Anesthesia Procedures, Methods, Techniques

Suzana Zorca

Edited by Mamatha Punjala

H

KEY POINTS

1. Helium is a nontoxic, inert, colorless, nonflammable gas with unique physicochemical properties, which include very low density, low solubility, and high thermal conductivity.
2. Helium–oxygen mixes (as high as 78% to 22%) can be used to reduce airway resistance in patients with obstructive pathology, for example, laryngeal obstruction, postintubation stridor, tracheobronchitis, or airway narrowing due to compressive laryngeal and mediastinal tumors.
3. Although heliox mixtures reduce Reynolds number and favor laminar flow, thereby reducing work of breathing and decreasing respiratory muscle fatigue, they are not curative.

DISCUSSION

Helium is the first of the noble gas series in the periodic table, and is the lightest and least dense gas after hydrogen. It is also the second most abundant element in the universe, although present in only minute amounts in the earth's atmosphere (0.00052% in air). Commercially available helium, therefore, must be distilled from other sources (e.g., from natural gas by fractional distillation after being formed by radioactive decay of alpha particles). Discovered over 100 years ago by William Ramsey, it has been described as an inert, odorless, colorless, tasteless, nonflammable agent. Unlike most other gases, it exists in a monoatomic state. It is extremely unreactive because it has a maximum number of valence electrons in its outer shell. Under all but the most extreme conditions, helium behaves like an ideal gas (obeying $PV = nRT$, the ideal gas equation). The main physical characteristics of He, N_2, O_2,

Table 1. Main physical Characteristics of Helium, Nitrogen, Oxygen, and Air at 20° C

Gas	Density (ϑ), g/L	Viscosity (η), miscropoises	Thermal conductivity ($\varkappa$), lcal/cm/sec/°K
Helium	0.1785	188.7	352.0
Nitrogen	1.251	167.4	58.0
Oxygen	1.429	192.6	58.5
Air	1.293	170.8	58.0

Adapted from Jolliet P, Tassaux D. Usefulness of helium-oxygen mixtures in the treatment of mechanically ventilated patients. *Curr Opin Crit Care.* 2003;9:46.

and air are compared in Table 1.

As an inert gas, helium is nontoxic and nonirritant to the respiratory tract. It can change the phonation/resonance of speech by increasing the speed of sound (voice sounds thin and squeaky) (Harris and Barnes, p. 285). In the airways, helium again changes the rate of gas flow and affects the patterns of gas flow, known as laminar, turbulent, or transitional regimens. Flow pattern is influenced by many factors, including airway shape/angulation/branching, rate of gas flow, and the density and viscosity of the inspired gas. Reynolds number describes and can predict flow type—laminar, turbulent, or transitional.

$$\text{Reynolds number} = \frac{2 \times \text{Flow rate (mL/s)} \times \text{Gas density (g/mL)}}{\pi \times \text{Radius (cm)} \times \text{Gas viscosity (g/cm/s)}},$$

with Reynolds no. less than or equal to 2,000 predicting laminar flow, Reynolds no. greater than or equal to 4,000 predicting turbulent flow, and transitional flow occurring in between (Reynolds nos. of 2,000 to 4,000).

Factors that decrease Reynolds number, and therefore favor laminar flow, are low gas density (e.g., use of helium, which is eight times less dense than oxygen, or clinically available heliox mixtures, which are at least three times less dense than air), or increasing breathing tube radius (i.e., using an endotracheal tube (ETT) with as large of an internal diameter as possible). Of note, the viscosity of helium and helium mixtures is only slightly higher than that of air, so viscosity does not play a significant role here.

Gas flow pattern (turbulent vs. laminar) is important because it affects the inspiratory effort required to achieve a desired inspiratory flow rate and therefore affects alveolar ventilation and oxygen delivery. Alveolar ventilation depends on the pressure gradient between atmospheric gas and gas pressure in the lower-bronchial tree. This pressure gradient/driving pressure depends on flow conditions: higher driving pressures are required during turbulent flow conditions to achieve the same gas flow rate than during laminar flow conditions. Higher driving pressures translate into higher work of breathing and increased respiratory muscle fatigue.

During calm, quiet breathing, laminar flow predominates in the human airways after the second generation of bronchi, with turbulent flow occurring in the larynx and trachea (primarily due to high gas flows in the large upper airways). The transition between laminar and turbulent flow depends critically on gas flow rate; that is, low flow rates (0.5 L per second) allow laminar flow to exist as far up as the proximal conducting airways, whereas increased flow rate of 2 L per second keeps flow turbulent down to the fifth generation of bronchi (Jolliet and Tassaux, p. 46). Use of heliox favors laminar flow and allows higher flow rates to be generated with the same driving pressure/inspiratory muscle effort. Alternatively, during turbulent airway conditions (e.g., obstruction and stridor), helium allows smaller driving pressures/inspiratory efforts to generate a necessary gas flow rate. Overall, heliox mixtures reduce airway resistance and thereby reduce the work of breathing and the risk of dynamic hyperinflation.

This becomes important in patients struggling to breathe against narrowed or obstructed airways, for example, in chronic obstructive pulmonary disease (COPD) or asthma exacerbations, laryngeal obstruction, postintubation croup, or airway narrowing due to an impinging mediastinal or laryngeal tumor. This also applies to healthy patients who must undergo mechanical ventilation with small ETT, for example, in pediatric populations, or during ENT surgery that necessitates the use of ETT with the smallest internal diameter possible because of surgical work on the vocal cords or internal airways (Fig. 1).

Use of helium–oxygen mixtures has been studied in spontaneously ventilating pediatric and adult populations, as well as in mechanically ventilated patients. Several relatively small studies of patients in status asthmaticus have conclusively shown benefit in terms of improved feeling of dyspnea, decreased respiratory rate, increased expiration times, and reduction in peak airway pressures with heliox. However, these beneficial effects are reversed almost immediately upon cessation of heliox use. This highlights the obvious drawback that heliox is an adjunctive but not curative therapy in airway obstruction and bronchospasm. It has no intrinsic reversal benefit on the root cause of increased airway resistance, and can provide only symptomatic relief until bronchodilators, corticosteroids, surgery, laser therapy, or other curative interventions can be used to definitively address the obstructive pathology.

Similarly, in COPD patients, heliox can decrease inspiratory and expiratory resistance, allowing better alveolar ventilation and improved CO_2 elimination. Improved expiratory flow can improve lung emptying, prevent air trapping, and decrease the risk of dynamic hyperinflation. This can decrease hyperinflation and the buildup of intrinsic positive end-expiratory pressure (PEEP). Potentially, this can improve nebulized bronchodilator delivery to the distal airways. Again, the reduced work of breathing, respiratory muscle fatigue, and dynamic hyperinflation all disappear once heliox use is stopped. Although not yet proven in sufficiently large randomized studies, heliox use combined with noninvasive ventilation methods in awake, spontaneously ventilating COPD patients has the potential to reduce rates of intubation and length of hospital stay.

It is worth remembering, however, that the same properties (low density, increased thermal conductivity) that make helium attractive for improving gas flow in spontaneously ventilating patients can interfere with monitoring and function of mechanical ventilators.

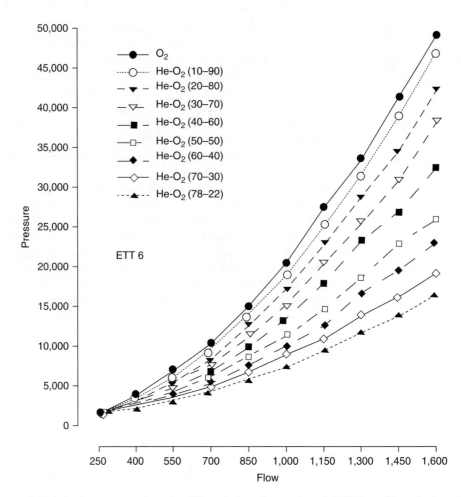

Figure 1. Resistive flow-pressure curves for different heliox mixtures through ETT 6.0 cm. (From Gerbeaux P, Gainnier M, Arnal JM, et al. Effects of helium-oxygen mixtures on endotracheal tubes: an in vitro study. *J Biomech.* 2005;38:33–37.)

Heliox delivery can create confusion in terms of delivered tidal volume (underestimating actually delivered V_t), fraction of inspired O_2, and malfunction of hot-wire pneumotachometers (Jolliet and Tassaux, p. 48). Correction factors must be carefully applied. Cost is also a factor, with 78:22 heliox pressurized to 200 bar costing US \$200 to \$300 per 50 L tank (provides 10,000 L heliox at atmospheric pressure). Therefore, heliox is typically considered only for patients with severe airway obstruction and persistent respiratory compromise, despite adequate corticosteroid/bronchodilator treatment and optimal ventilator settings.

Barash P, Cullen BF, Stoelting RK, et al, eds. *Clinical Anesthesia.* 6th ed. Philadelphia, PA: Wolters Kluwer/ Lippincott Williams & Wilkins; 2009:237.

Gerbeaux P, Gainnier M, Arnal JM, et al. Effects of helium-oxygen mixtures on endotracheal tubes: an in vitro study. *J Biomech.* 2005;38:33–37.

Harris PD, Barnes R. The use of helium and xenon in current clinical practice. *Anaesthesia.* 2008;63:284–293.

Jolliet P, Tassaux D. Usefulness of helium-oxygen mixtures in the treatment of mechanically ventilated patients. *Curr Opin Crit Care.* 2003;9:45–50.

SUGGESTED READINGS

Hemolysis: Bilirubin Levels
Organ-based Clinical: Hematologic

Archer Martin

Edited by Hossam Tantawy

H

1. Normal bilirubin levels in the body range from 0.5 to 1.0 mg per dL.
2. Hemolysis results in the destruction of red blood cells, within the extravascular or intravascular compartments, and has many causes (e.g., sickle cell, autoimmunity, disseminated intravascular coagulation, thrombotic thrombocytopenic purpura, valvular hemolysis, infection, drugs).
3. Other tests for hemolysis include haptoglobin, peripheral blood smear, reticulocyte count, lactate dehydrogenase.

Bilirubin is a product of heme metabolism, with 80% of the daily production being derived from heme breakdown. The rest of the bilirubin comes from catabolism of heme proteins and ineffective erythropoiesis. Causes of unconjugated hyperbilirubinemia include overproduction, impaired hepatic uptake, and impaired conjugation. Overproduction results from hemolysis. The production reaction of bilirubin involves cleavage of heme ring to biliverdin by heme oxygenase, followed by production of bilirubin from biliverdin by the enzyme biliverdin reductase. The unconjugated bilirubin is highly protein bound (albumin) and is lipid soluble, so it can cross the blood–brain barrier.

Bilirubin is taken up by hepatocytes (phase 1 uptake), conjugated intrahepatically (phase 2 conjugation), and then excreted (phase 3 excretion). The final step of bilirubin excretion involves bacterial conversion in the intestine. Therefore, the levels of bilirubin in the setting of hemolysis are greatly dependent on hepatic function. The serum bilirubin will rarely exceed 5 mg per dL in those with normal liver function; however, even in the setting of mild hepatic dysfunction, severe hyperbilirubinemia can be seen.

Andreoli TE, Carpenter CCJ, Griggs RC, et al, eds. *Andreoli and Carpenter's Cecil Essentials of Medicine.* 7th ed. Philadelphia, PA: Saunders; 2007:chap 41:437–439.

Hepatic Dysfunction: Dx

Generic, Clinical Sciences: Anesthesia Procedures, Methods, Techniques

Roberto Rappa

Edited by Ala Haddadin

H

KEY POINTS

1. Liver disease is commonly grouped into two categories: parenchymal liver disorders and cholestatic (obstructive) liver disorders.
2. Liver function tests (LFTs) can help delineate parenchymal liver disease versus obstructive pathology.
3. The ratio of the aspartate aminotransferase (AST) to alanine aminotransferase (ALT) elevation can also be used diagnostically to help differentiate among specific hepatocellular processes.
4. Obstructive liver disorders often present with jaundice, a conjugated (direct) hyperbilirubinemia, and marked elevations in alkaline phosphatase.
5. The most sensitive indicator of cholestatic liver disease is gamma-glutamyl transferase (GGT).
6. The most specific indicator of cholestatic liver disease is 5'-nucleotidase (5'-NT).
7. Measurement of liver synthetic capacity often involves the serum assay of albumin, prothrombin time/international normalized ratio (PT/INR), cholesterol, and pseudocholinesterase.

DISCUSSION

The liver is responsible for a number of vital physiologic processes in the human body. Some of its most important activities include nutrient metabolism and glucose homeostasis, the production of plasma proteins and clotting factors, drug metabolism and biotransformation, bilirubin formation and bile excretion. It is not surprising that it is one of the largest organs in the human body. Fortunately, it has a high degree of functional reserve. Therefore, clinically significant hepatic dysfunction becomes only apparent when a large degree of hepatic physiologic capacity is affected.

Hepatic dysfunction is a broad topic that encompasses a number of disease states and pathologies. It can present as an acute process (i.e., acute viral hepatitis) or as a more insidious chronic process (i.e., alcoholic cirrhosis). Liver disease is commonly grouped into two categories: parenchymal (hepatocellular) liver disorders and cholestatic (obstructive) liver disorders. Cholestatic liver pathology can be further classified as intrahepatic disease or extrahepatic disease (often distinguished by the type of hyperbilirubinemia). The diagnostic workup should include studies that suggest the etiology of the specific hepatic pathologic processes. The following discussion will provide a brief overview on how to diagnose liver dysfunction.

The ability to identify and successfully diagnose liver disease always starts with a good history and physical examination. General signs and symptoms of liver disease include fatigue, anorexia, pruritus, steatorrhea, abdominal distention, dyspnea, upper gastrointestinal bleeding, mental confusion, irritability, oliguria, easy bruising, peripheral edema, osteoporosis, and muscle wasting. Physical examination findings of liver disease include hepatomegaly, splenomegaly, ascites, jaundice, caput medusae (visibly dilated abdominal veins), asterixis, fetor hepaticus, spider angiomas, hypogonadism (male), gynecomastia, palmar erythema, and Dupuytren contractures.

A laboratory workup for the presence of hepatic dysfunction often consists of the evaluation of LFTs. LFTs often include analysis of the aminotransferases (AST and ALT), alkaline phosphatase, total bilirubin, direct (conjugated) bilirubin, serum albumin/serum proteins, and prothrombin time. Trends in LFTs can help group liver disorders in terms of hepatocellular disease, obstruction liver disease, and disorders of hepatic synthetic function (see Table 1).

Table 1. Blood Tests and the Differential Diagnosis of Hepatic Dysfunction

	Bilirubin Overload	Parenchymal Dysfunction	Cholestasis
Aminotransferases	Normal	Increased (may be normal or decreased in advanced stages)	Normal (may be increased in advanced stages)
Alkaline phosphatase	Normal	Normal	Increased
Bilirubin	Unconjugated	Conjugated	Conjugated
Serum proteins	Normal	Decreased	Normal (may be decreased in advanced stages)
Prothrombin time	Normal	Decreased (may be normal in early stages)	Normal (may be prolonged in advanced stages)
Blood urea nitrogen	Normal	Normal (may be decreased in advanced stages)	Normal

From Gelman S. Anesthesia and the liver. In: Barash P, Cullen B, Stoelting R, eds. *Clinical Anesthesia*. 3rd ed. Philadelphia, PA: Lippincott-Raven; 1997:1011.

Elevation of the aminotransferases is often seen in the setting of hepatocellular injury and necrosis. It is important to note that ALT is localized primarily to the liver, and AST is present in a variety of nonhepatic tissues. An isolated elevation in AST is generally not an indication of a hepatic process. The ratio of the AST to ALT elevation can also be used diagnostically to help differentiate among specific hepatocellular processes. For example, an AST/ALT ratio of greater than 2 may indicate the presence of alcoholic liver disease, whereas a ratio of less than 1 may alert the clinician to the presence of viral hepatitis. The degree of aminotransferase elevation may also indicate the severity and/or acuity of the underlying hepatic process (i.e., mild elevations in the setting of fatty liver disease and greater elevations in the setting of acute hepatitis).

Obstructive liver disorders often present with jaundice, a conjugated (direct) hyper-bilirubinemia, and marked elevations in alkaline phosphatase. Alkaline phosphatase is normally concentrated in the microvilli of the bile canaliculi and the sinusoidal surface of the hepatocytes. Like AST, it is found in a variety of nonhepatic tissues. In the presence of cholestatic disease, it is often elevated in disproportionate concentrations to the aminotransferases.

A more precise measure of cholestatic liver disease could be made by the analysis of 5'-NT and GGT. 5'-NT is the most specific marker for liver disease and is markedly increased in the presence of intrahepatic or extrahepatic cholestasis. It is often used to confirm that elevations in alkaline phosphatase are secondary to liver disease. The most sensitive indicator of biliary tract pathology includes the serum analysis of GGT. It is found in high concentrations in the epithelial cells lining the biliary ductules. Its poor specificity, however, still makes 5'-NT the confirmatory test of choice.

With progressive liver disease, hepatic functional capacity may be compromised and may result in decreased hepatic synthetic function. This phenomenon is mostly manifested in markers for hepatic synthetic function. Because the liver synthesizes a variety of plasma proteins, analysis of serum albumin and assays of coagulation function provide useful measures in assessing hepatic synthetic function. The simple analysis of serum albumin and the PT/INR can be a useful starting point in the assessment of hepatic synthetic function.

SUGGESTED READINGS

Barash PG, Cullen BF, Stoelting RK, et al, eds. *Clinical Anesthesia*. 6th ed. Philadelphia, PA: Lippincott Williams & Wilkins; 2009:1247–1255.

Morgan GE, Mikhail MS, Murray MJ. *Clinical Anesthesiology*. 4th ed. New York, NY: Lange Medical Books/ McGraw-Hill; 2005:chap 34:773–788.

Hepatitis B: Needlestick Rx

Generic Clinical Sciences: Anesthesia Procedures, Methods, Techniques

Lisbeysi Calo

Edited by Hossam Tantawy

1. Risk of hepatitis B virus (HBV) transmission increases with the type of exposure, for example, needlestick with a hollow bore needle versus needle puncture with solid needle, and type of infected fluid one comes in contact with, for example, blood versus cerebrospinal fluid versus synovial fluid.
2. Risk of HBV transmission increases with exposure to hepatitis B surface antigen (HBsAg) and hepatitis B "e" antigen (HBeAg) positive blood when compared with HBsAg-positive and HBeAg-negative blood.
3. Hepatitis B immune globulin (HBIG) initiated within 1 week after percutaneous exposure to HBeAg-positive blood provides approximately 75% protection from HBV infection.
4. Because health-care providers are at increased risk for exposure to HBV, all should receive HBV vaccination.

HBV is a well-recognized occupational risk for health-care providers. Fortunately, in the United States, most of the general population and medical community are prophylactically vaccinated against this disease. The risk of infection is primarily related to the degree of contact with infected body fluid, to the HBeAg status of the source person, and, of course, to the vaccination status of the exposed person.

Exposures that place health-care personnel (HCP) at risk for HBV include (1) percutaneous injury (e.g., needlestick injury or cut with a sharp object), and (2) contamination/contact of mucous membranes with infected fluids. Cerebrospinal, pleural, amniotic, pericardial, synovial, and peritoneal fluids are potentially infectious, but the risk of transmission from these fluids is unknown and has not been evaluated in epidemiologic studies. The risk of transmission from contact with feces, nasal secretions, saliva, and sputum is low. HBV has been demonstrated to survive in dried blood at room temperature on environmental surfaces for at least 1 week.

Recommendations for HBV postexposure management include initiation of the hepatitis B vaccine series to any unvaccinated person who sustains an occupational blood or body fluid exposure. Postexposure prophylaxis (PEP) with HBIG and/or hepatitis B vaccine series should be considered for occupational exposures after evaluation of the HBeAg status of the source person and the vaccination status of the exposed person.

In studies of unvaccinated HCP who sustained needlestick injuries contaminated with blood containing HBV, the risk of developing clinical hepatitis if the blood was both HBsAg- and HBeAg-positive was 22% to 31%. The risk of developing serologic evidence of HBV infection, with or without clinical evidence of hepatitis, was higher ranging from 37% to 62%. The risk of developing clinical hepatitis from a needle contaminated with HBsAg-positive and HBeAg-negative blood was lower at 1% to 6%, but the risk of developing serologic evidence of HBV infection was still 23% to 37%.

In the occupational setting, multiple doses of HBIG initiated within 1 week after percutaneous exposure to HBeAg-positive blood provide an estimated 75% protection against HBV infection. Although the postexposure efficacy of combined HBIG and the hepatitis B vaccine series has not been evaluated in the occupational setting, the increased efficacy of this regimen in the perinatal setting compared with HBIG alone likely applies to the occupational setting as well. Because HCP are at increased risk for exposure to HBV, they should all receive HBV vaccination prophylactically.

The most common side effects of HBV vaccination are pain at the site of injection and fever. Angioedema and anaphylaxis are rare. The common side effects are not higher in patients receiving vaccine versus placebo. The vaccine is contraindicated in patients with a history of anaphylaxis to the HBV vaccine.

HBIG is prepared from human plasma known to contain a high titer of antibody to HBsAg. No evidence exists that HBV, HCV, or HIV has ever been transmitted through the administration of HBIG in the United States. Serious effects from HBIG when administered as recommended are rare.

SUGGESTED READINGS

Barash P, Cullen BF, Stoelting RK, et al. *Clinical Anesthesia*. 6th ed. Philadelphia, PA: Lippincott Williams & Wilkins; 2009:70–71.

Bartlett J. Updated U.S. Public Health Service Guidelines for the management of occupational exposures to HVB, HVC, and HIV and recommendations for post-exposure prophylaxis. *Infect Dis Clin Pract*. 2001;10(6):338–340.

Hepatic Synthetic Capacity and Impairment: Dx

Generic, Clinical Sciences: Anesthesia Procedures, Methods, Techniques, and Organ-based Clinical: Hematologic

Caroline Al Haddadin and Marianne Saleeb
Edited by Hossam Tantawy

KEY POINTS

1. The liver plays a role in the metabolism of glucose, fats, proteins, and several drugs, which may be affected by liver dysfunction.
2. Given large functional reserve, patients may have significant hepatocellular damage/dysfunction, including cirrhosis without change in laboratory values.
3. The biosynthetic functions of the liver include serum albumin, serum globulins, and coagulation factors and may be tested by obtaining serum values.
4. Albumin and coagulation factors are the most widely used methods of assessing hepatic synthetic function.
5. Only 20% to 30% of normal coagulation factor activity is required for normal coagulation, and therefore changes in coagulation function tests indicate severe liver disease. As such, measured prothrombin time (PT) serves as an excellent indicator of liver dysfunction.

DISCUSSION

The liver serves a variety of metabolic functions, most importantly of which include the metabolism of carbohydrates, fats, proteins, and several drugs. Given the liver's large functional reserve, the effect of anesthesia rarely impacts the liver's synthetic and metabolic capacity; however, preexisting liver disease/dysfunction may alter the pharmacokinetics of some anesthetics and impact anesthetic management of these patients. In preoperative evaluation for such a patient, knowing the degree of dysfunction, or rather functional reserve of the liver, may help in guiding anesthetic management.

Given the liver's role in synthesizing a variety of proteins, including those involved in the coagulation cascade and albumin, performing certain liver tests to ascertain the plasma level of such proteins is warranted to determine the degree of liver dysfunction. Furthermore, additional values and liver tests may be obtained to determine whether it is acute or chronic. Serum albumin (normal 3.5 to 5.0 g per dL) is exclusively synthesized by liver cells, called hepatocytes. It has a half-life of 15 to 20 days, with approximately 4% being degraded daily, and therefore a value below 2.5 g per dL is indicative of chronic liver disease, acute stress or severe malnutrition. Owing to the many differential diagnoses for hypoalbuminemia, and the fact that serum albumin has a long half-life, albumin is not a reliable indicator for hepatic synthetic function, and interpretation of its level should take into consideration the patient's overall status. Acute liver dysfunction will affect the albumin levels only mildly. One must also keep in mind, however, that hypoalbuminemia can also occur with protein-losing enteropathies, nephrotic syndrome, and chronic infections that are associated with increased tumor necrosis factor or interleukin 1, which suppresses the production of albumin, and therefore is not specific to liver dysfunction.

Hepatocytes also form bile acids that aid in the intestinal absorption of lipids and in emulsifying fats. With hepatocellular dysfunction and decreased bile acid formation, the intestinal absorption of lipids and therefore lipid-soluble fats, including vitamins A, D, E, and K, is interrupted. Finally, with vitamin K deficiency, one may become coagulopathic since it is involved in the formation of coagulation factors VII, IX, and X, which will be manifested by an increased PT level.

Coagulation factors are commonly tested and are the single best measure of liver synthetic function. The blood clotting factors have a short half-life compared with albumin (e.g., factor VII has half-life of ~4 to 6 hours) and therefore can be used in acute or chronic liver disease. Only 20% to 30% of normal coagulation factor activity is required for normal coagulation and therefore changes in coagulation function tests indicate severe liver disease. As such, measured PT serves as an excellent indicator of liver dysfunction. However, elevated PT levels may also occur with vitamin K deficiency, Disseminated Intravascular Coagulation (DIC), congenital clotting factor deficiencies, and certain drugs.

SUGGESTED READINGS

1. Barash P, Cullen B, Stoelting RK, et al, eds. *Clinical Anesthesia.* 6th ed. Philadelphia, PA: Lippincott Wilkins & Williams; 2009:1253–1254.
2. Morgan GE Jr, Mikhail MS, Murray MJ. *Clinical Anesthesiology.* 4th ed. New York, NY: Lange Medical Books/McGraw Hill; 2006:780.
3. Longo D, Fauci A, Kasper D, et al, eds. *Harrison's Principles of Internal Medicine.* 18th ed. Philadelphia, PA: Elsevier; 2011:1713–1714.
4. Stoelting RK, Miller RD. *Basics of Anesthesia.* 5th ed. Philadelphia, PA: Churchill Livingstone/Elsevier; 2007:334.

Herbals: Garlic

Pharmacology

Svetlana Sapozhnikova

Edited by Thomas Halaszynski

H

KEY POINTS

1. Common side effects of garlic ingestion include gastrointestinal upset, allergic reactions, and dermatitis.
2. Garlic may inhibit platelet aggregation in a dose-dependent manner and therefore increases the risk of perioperative bleeding.
3. Garlic may potentiate the effects of warfarin, heparin, nonsteroidal anti-inflammatory drugs (NSAIDs), and aspirin.
4. Garlic may have dose-dependent blood pressure and heart rate lowering properties; however, studies do not support its use for treatment of hypertension.

DISCUSSION

Garlic, whose scientific name is *Allium sativum*, is sometimes used (alone or in combination with other medications) for treatment of hypertension, dyslipidemia, and cardiovascular disease. Garlic has also been used to reduce oxidative stress and incidence of sepsis, to prevent thrombus formation, and to decrease platelet aggregation.

Some of garlic's known side effects include gastrointestinal upset, allergic reactions, and dermatitis. Smell from garlic ingestion is related to sulfur content of allicin, which is the main active ingredient of garlic.

Garlic may inhibit platelet aggregation in a dose-dependent and potentially irreversible manner. This platelet inhibitory effect may increase the risk of perioperative bleeding. It has been suggested that garlic supplements should be stopped at least 7 days before elective surgery. Garlic may also potentiate the effects of warfarin, heparin, NSAIDs, and aspirin that may be reflected in abnormal coagulation tests and increased bleeding time.

There is a lack of strong evidence to support the use of garlic for the sole treatment of hypertension. Human studies on the hypotensive effects of garlic are small and are not very well designed. The dosages of garlic needed to decrease blood pressure in some study subjects were large and were not well tolerated. Meta-analysis of these studies has shown a reduction in both systolic and diastolic blood pressures from the administration of garlic herbal drugs. However, currently, it is not recommended to treat hypertension with garlic alone. Clinicians need to be aware of garlic's dose-dependent blood pressure and heart rate lowering properties.

As evidenced from rat studies, garlic may prevent development of acute cardiotoxicity associated with doxorubicin use. Other animal studies suggest that garlic may be a vasodilator to pulmonary vessels. Garlic may decrease efficacy of HIV protease inhibitor drugs such as saquinavir, possibly via induction of the cytochrome P450 system. Mice studies suggest that garlic may confer protection against methicillin-resistant *Staphylococcus aureus* infection.

SUGGESTED READINGS

American Society of Anesthesiologists. *What You Should Know about Your Patients' Use of Herbal Medicines and Other Dietary Supplements.* 2003.

Barash PG, Cullen BF, Stoelting RK, et al, eds. *Clinical Anesthesia.* 6th ed. Philadelphia, PA: Lippincott Williams & Wilkins, a Wolters Kluwer Business; 2009:399, 562.

Fleisher LA. *Anesthesia and Uncommon Diseases.* 5th ed. Philadelphia, PA: Saunders, an Imprint of Elsevier; 2005:495, 497–498.

Jaffe RA, Samuels SI, eds. *Anesthesiologist's Manual of Surgical Procedures.* 4th ed. Philadelphia, PA: Lippincott Williams & Wilkins, a Wolters Kluwer Business; 2009:Appendix F-11.

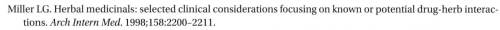

Miller LG. Herbal medicinals: selected clinical considerations focusing on known or potential drug-herb interactions. *Arch Intern Med*. 1998;158:2200–2211.

Miller RD, Eriksson LI, Fleisher LA, et al. *Miller's Anesthesia*. 7th ed. Philadelphia, PA: Churchill Livingstone, an Imprint of Elsevier; 2010:959–961.

Stoelting RK, Hillier SC. *Pharmacology and Physiology in Anesthetic Practice*. Philadelphia, PA: Lippincott Williams & Wilkins, a Wolters Kluwer Business; 2006:608.

Hetastarch: Platelet Function

Generic, Clinical Sciences: Anesthesia
Procedures, Methods, Techniques

Neil Sinha

Edited by Benjamin Sherman

KEY POINTS

1. Hetastarch consists of 6% hydroxyethyl starch in a physiologic medium of electrolytes, glucose, and lactate.
2. Hetastarch has been shown to decrease the availability of the glycoprotein (GP) IIb-IIIa complex on activated platelets in both in vivo and in vitro studies, possibly leading to platelet dysfunction.
3. The degree of platelet dysfunction caused by hetastarch in clinically relevant situations still remains unclear.

DISCUSSION

Hetastarch is an artificial colloid created by the addition of hydroxyethyl ether groups into amylopectin containing solutions. Hetastarch (Hespan and Hextend) consists of 6% hydroxyethyl starch in a physiologic medium of electrolytes, glucose, and lactate. In general, hetastarch is a physiologically balanced plasma expander that is reserved for large volume resuscitation and major surgery. Administration of 500 mL of 6% hetastarch will expand intravascular volume by 800 mL and is sustained for up to 8 hours. Comparatively, 1,500 mL of crystalloid would need to be administered for a similar effect.

Hetastarch has been shown to decrease the availability of the GP IIb-IIIa complex on activated platelets in both in vivo and in vitro studies. This decreased availability of the GP IIb-IIIa complex results in the inability of the platelet to achieve a conformational state that is competent for the binding of fibrinogen and ultimately platelet aggregation. The suspected mechanism for this phenomenon is through a direct platelet inhibiting effect of the hetastarch or through a direct modification of the platelet cytoplasmic membrane structure. DDAVP has been shown to reverse this phenomenon.

The degree of platelet dysfunction caused by hetastarch in clinically relevant situations still remains unclear. Factors such as hemodilution and systemic changes such as shock are confounding factors that may distort the full picture. Nevertheless, platelet dysfunction should be considered when hetastarch is used.

SUGGESTED READINGS

Stogermuller B, Stark J, Willschke H, et al. The effect of hydroxyethyl starch 200 kD on platelet function. *Anesth Analg.* 2000;91:823–882.

Strauss RG, Stansfield C, Henriksen RA, et al. Pentastarch may cause fewer effects on coagulation than hetastarch. *Transfusion.* 1988;28(3):257–260.

HOCM/IHSS: Hypotension and Rx Treatment

Organ-based Clinical: Cardiovascular

Glenn Dizon and Garth Skoropowski

Edited by Benjamin Sherman

KEY POINTS

1. Hypertrophic cardiomyopathy (HCM) is a genetically linked condition causing severe hypertrophy of the myocardium with a disruption of the normal myocyte arrangement (myocardial disarray) and a disruption to the conduction system.
2. HCM is a well-known cause of sudden cardiac death in young athletes.
3. HCM can further be categorized as obstructive or nonobstructive.
4. Hypertrophic obstructive cardiomyopathy (HOCM) is characterized by a dynamic left ventricular outflow tract (LVOT) obstruction produced by asymmetric hypertrophy of the intraventricular septum and systolic anterior motion (SAM) of the anterior mitral leaflet.
5. Certain factors tend to worsen the obstruction of HOCM:
   a. Enhanced contractility
   b. Decreased ventricular volume
   c. Decreased left ventricular (LV) afterload
6. Treatment focuses on improving diastolic filling, reducing LV outflow obstruction, and decreasing myocardial ischemia:
   a. Beta-blockers
   b. Calcium channel blockers
   c. Amiodarone for arrhythmias
   d. Surgical myomectomy

DISCUSSION

HCM is a genetically linked condition causing severe hypertrophy of the myocardium, with a disruption of the normal myocyte arrangement (myocardial disarray) and a disruption of the conduction system. It is most well known as a leading cause of sudden cardiac death in young athletes. HCM can further be categorized as obstructive or nonobstructive. HOCM is characterized by LV outflow obstruction produced by asymmetric hypertrophy of the intraventricular septum. Other names for HOCM are asymmetric septal hypertrophy (ASH), idiopathic hypertrophic subaortic stenosis (IHSS), and muscular subaortic stenosis.

Most patients with HCM are asymptomatic at rest. With activity, patients who are symptomatic generally complain of shortness of breath, fatigue, syncope, near-syncope, or angina. This occurs as a result of a dynamic outflow obstruction across the LVOT. As the hypertrophied septum moves closer to the mitral valve during systole, narrowing of the LVOT causes a Venturi effect to bend the mitral valve into the LVOT. This motion of the mitral valve is called *systolic anterior motion* or *SAM*. As SAM worsens, the LVOT becomes severely obstructed and mitral regurgitation develops with a posteriorly directed jet.

Certain factors tend to worsen the obstruction of HCM. These include enhanced contractility, decreased ventricular volume, and decreased LV afterload. As a result, medical treatment of this pathology will focus on avoiding these hemodynamic changes, overall improvement of diastolic filling, reducing LV outflow obstruction, and decreasing myocardial ischemia. Pharmacologically, beta-blockers and calcium channel blockers are a mainstay of treatment. Both medications can decrease heart rate and contractility, which lengthens the time of diastole and prolongs passive ventricular filling. Beta-blockers also decrease myocardial oxygen requirements. Calcium channel blockers increase ventricular filling while lessening myocardial ischemia. Atrial fibrillation may develop in these patients. Normal sinus rhythm is important in these patients because adequate ventricular filling is dependent on left atrial contraction, making amiodarone the treatment choice for arrhythmias. Patients at high risk for sudden death may require placement of an internal cardioverter/defibrillator. Patients with severe outflow tract gradients and symptoms of congestive heart failure, even on medications, may benefit from surgical treatment. Surgery involves removal of the excess hypertrophied muscle from the ventricular septum (myomectomy).

During the induction of anesthesia, care must be made to ensure adequate preload, maintain afterload, keep heart rate low to promote increased ventricular filling time, and avoid increases in sympathetic stimulation with increased myocardial contraction. Historically, halothane has been the inhalational agent of choice because of its myocardial depressant effects.

SUGGESTED READINGS

Barash PG, Cullen BF, Stoelting RK, et al. *Clinical Anesthesia*. 6th ed. Philadelphia, PA: Lippincott Williams & Wilkins; 2009:1080–1081.

Fifer MA, Vlahakes GJ. Management of symptoms in hypertrophic cardiomyopathy. *Circulation*. 2008;117:429–439.

Hines RL, Marschall KE. *Stoelting's Anesthesia and Co-existing Disease*. 5th ed. Philadelphia, PA: Churchill Livingstone; 2008:117–118.

Morgan GE, Mikhail MS, Murray MJ. *Clinical Anesthesiology*. 4th ed. New York, NY: McGraw-Hill; 2005:475.

Stoelting RK, Miller RD. *Basics of Anesthesia*. Philadelphia, PA: Elsevier Churchill Livingstone; 2007:382.

H

Hormonal Stress Response
Physiology

Anjali Vira

Edited by Ala Haddadin

1. Surgery and anesthesia produce a state of metabolic stress characterized by the release of various hormones and measurable changes in the patient's physiologic state.
2. The effects of neurohumoral stress may be detrimental to the patient if not recognized and treated.
3. Patients with adrenal insufficiency are unable to mount a hormonal response to physical stress.

Any type of physical stress including surgery, trauma, and the induction of general anesthesia leads to the release of catecholamines and various hormones including cortisol, antidiuretic hormone, renin, and endorphins from the adrenal gland and the hypothalamic–pituitary axis. This response is mediated in part by neuronal factors such as pain and anxiety, but also by changes in the patient's physical state such as acidosis and hypoxia. The release of these substances leads to a cascade of changes. For example, chronically elevated levels of catecholamines inhibit insulin release, and can therefore lead to hyperglycemia. In general, the overall state of physiologic stress is indirectly measured by monitoring of vital signs such as blood pressure and heart rate, and also by invasive monitors and intraoperative laboratory tests such as serum glucose levels.

The many effects of the humoral stress response can be detrimental to the patient, and therefore, anesthesiologists attempt to block this response using various techniques. Regional anesthesia is used in part to blunt the stress response accompanied by surgery. This can be accomplished by interruption of the neural communication from the surgical site to the central nervous system. General anesthesia may blunt the stress response in a dose-related fashion. Endorphins have been shown to be secreted in large amounts by the anterior pituitary during times of pain and during surgery, and to help transmit the sensation of pain by binding to opiate receptors in the brain and spinal cord. Various pain management techniques are aimed at the disruption of this communication.

Patients with primary or secondary adrenal insufficiency are unable to mount a stress response to physical stress, including surgical stimulation, and may require hormone and steroid replacement pre-, post-, and intraoperatively.

Barash PG, Cullen BF, Stoelting RK, et al. *Clinical Anesthesia*. 6th ed. Philadelphia, PA: Lippincott Williams & Wilkins; 2009:283, 1302.
Marino PL. *The ICU Book*. 3rd ed. Philadelphia, PA: Lippincott Williams & Wilkins; 2007:871–880.

Hydrochlorothiazide: Blood Chem Effect

Pharmacology

Tiffany Denepitiya-Balicki

Edited by Benjamin Sherman

KEY POINTS

1. Hydrochlorothiazide (HCTZ) is an agent whose mechanism of action is largely focused on the distal tubule of the nephron.
2. Because thiazide diuretics inhibit sodium reabsorption, an increased sodium load reaches the collecting tubule, thus causing it to increase reabsorption of sodium, with subsequent increase in potassium excretion. As a result, patients taking thiazide diuretics may develop *hypokalemia*.
3. Other transport mechanisms within the collecting duct may also increase H⁺ secretion (compensatory when sodium is being reabsorbed), and patients may also develop *metabolic alkalosis*.

DISCUSSION

HCTZ is a commonly used diuretic agent used to treat hypertension. The physiologic action of HCTZ largely occurs within the distal tubule of the nephron (Fig. 1). HCTZ inhibits the sodium-chloride carrier protein on the luminal membrane, and therefore inhibits sodium reabsorption with the net effect of increasing the concentration of sodium in the filtrate at the distal tubule. Since this part of the nephron is impermeable to water, reabsorption of urine becomes more dilute. When used as a single agent, HCTZ increases sodium excretion by approximately 3% to 5%. In addition, with the increased concentration of sodium reaching the distal tubule, more potassium is exchanged for sodium, resulting in increased potassium wasting and *hypokalemia*.

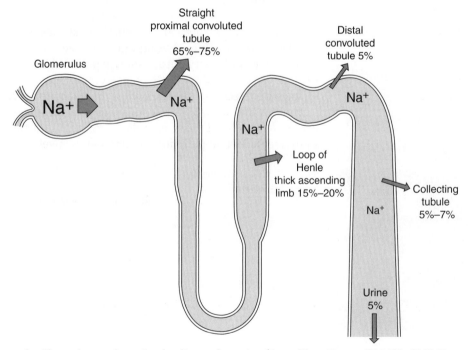

Figure 1. The nephron and associated sodium reabsorption. (Reused from Morgan GE, Mikhail MS, Murray MJ. *Clinical Anesthesiology.* 4th ed. http://www.accessmedicine.com)

In addition, since sodium reabsorption is inhibited, an increased sodium load is delivered to the collecting duct, which results in a compensatory reabsorption of sodium. As a result, other transport mechanisms within the collecting duct increase H^+ secretion in response to this compensatory reabsorption, and patients may also develop a *metabolic alkalosis*.

Recall that the distal tubule is an important site of action for vitamin D and parathyroid hormone induced calcium reabsorption. Thiazide diuretics, including HCTZ, also cause calcium reabsorption at the distal tubule, thus resulting in decreased urinary calcium with the possibility of causing *hypercalcemia*, and accordingly, should not be used, or used, with caution, in patients with hyperparathyroidism. (Loop diuretics cause increased urine calcium concentration and therefore are useful for emergent treatment of hypercalcemia.) Hypomagnesemia may also occur.

In addition to electrolyte abnormalities, jaundice, diarrhea, pancreatitis, and aplastic anemia have been reported with HCTZ administration.

SUGGESTED READINGS

Barash P, Cullen B, Stoelting R, et al, eds. *Clinical Anesthesia*. 6th ed. Philadelphia, PA: Lippincott Williams & Wilkins; 2009:1359–1360.

Harvey RA, Champe PC, Howland RD, et al. *Pharmacology*. 3rd ed. Philadelphia, PA: Lippincott Williams & Wilkins; 2006:217–218.

Morgan GE, Mikhail MS, Murray MJ. *Clinical Anesthesiology*. 4th ed. New York, NY: McGraw-Hill; 2006:726–728, 738.

Hyperbaric Chamber: MAC Effect
Generic Clinical Sciences: Anesthesia Procedures, Methods, Techniques

Jennifer Dominguez
Edited by Raj K. Modak

KEY POINTS

1. The potency of volatile anesthetics and their anesthetic effects on patients are proportional to the partial pressure of the anesthetic in the body.
2. Because partial pressure changes with ambient pressure, at ambient pressures above 1 atmosphere (atm), a similar effects on minimum alveolar concentration (MAC) can be obtained at a lower concentration of anesthetic.
3. The MAC of an inhalational anesthetic is the concentration of that vapor at 1 atm that prevents movement in response to a surgical stimulus (usually a skin incision) in 50% of patients.
4. Under hyperbaric conditions, nitrous oxide can be used at partial pressures at or above its MAC (104%) without hypoxia.

DISCUSSION

The potency of volatile anesthetics and their anesthetic effects on patients are proportional to the partial pressure of the anesthetic in the body. Within approximately 15 minutes of constant exposure to a given concentration of volatile anesthetic, a steady state is reached in which the partial pressure of brain, blood, and alveoli are in equilibrium.

$$P_{CNS} = P_{blood} = P_{alveoli}$$

Thus, the alveolar concentration of an inhalational anesthetic as measured by end-tidal partial pressure becomes an indicator of its partial pressure in the brain. Partial pressure is dependent on ambient pressure (usually 1 atm or 760 mm Hg). Because of this property, the potency of volatile anesthetics is affected by ambient pressure.

The MAC of an inhalational anesthetic is the concentration of that vapor at 1 atm that prevents movement in response to a surgical stimulus (usually a skin incision) in 50% of patients. However, because it depends on atmospheric pressure, MAC is affected by ambient pressures above and below 1 atm (such as at high altitude or in a hyperbaric chamber). For example, the effect of 2% sevoflurane (1 MAC) with a partial pressure of 15.2 mm Hg at 1 atm will be equivalent to 1.0% sevoflurane concentration at 2 atm because the partial pressure will not change. In fact, under hyperbaric conditions, nitrous oxide can be used at partial pressures at or above its MAC (104%) without hypoxia.

SUGGESTED READINGS

Barash PG, Cullen BF, Stoelting RK, et al, eds. *Clinical Anesthesia*. 6th ed. Philadelphia, PA: Lippincott Williams & Wilkins; 2009:413–425.
Longnecker DE, Brown DL, Newman MF, et al, eds. *Anesthesiology*. New York, NY: McGraw-Hill; 2008:1136–1138.
Miller RD, Eriksson LI, Fleisher LA, et al, eds. *Miller's Anesthesia*. 7th ed. Philadelphia, PA: Churchill Livingstone; 2009: chap 39:1235–1236: chap 80: 1242–1244:2499–2504.

Hyperbaric Oxygen: Indications

Generic, Clinical Sciences: Anesthesia Procedures, Methods, Techniques

Chi Wong

Edited by Ala Haddadin

KEY POINTS

1. Hyperbaric oxygen (HBO) therapy increases the amount of oxygen dissolved in the plasma by increasing the ambient pressure of oxygen to 2 to 3 atmospheres absolute (ATA).
2. HBO therapy is indicated in severe carbon monoxide (CO) poisoning (carboxyhemoglobin [COHb] > 30%) and in pregnant patients with COHb greater than 15%.
3. The half-life of CO is inversely related to the inspired oxygen concentration.
4. HBO therapy is the standard of care for decompression sickness, and it is the treatment of choice for air or gas embolism.
5. HBO therapy is recommended as adjuvant therapy for soft-tissue necrotizing infections such as clostridial myonecrosis and osteoradionecrosis prevention.
6. HBO therapy provides temporary support in treating exceptional blood loss anemia.

DISCUSSION

HBO therapy increases the amount of oxygen (O_2) dissolved in the plasma by increasing the ambient pressure of oxygen to 2 to 3 ATA. The physiologic effects of O_2 under pressure will increase blood O_2 content, which is useful for the treatment of ischemic conditions. Another physiologic effect is vasoconstriction that directly increases systemic vascular resistance (SVR) and causes hypertension, bradycardia, and decreased cardiac output. Despite decreased blood flow to the periphery, total oxygen delivery is increased because oxygen diffusion away from the vascular bed is greatly enhanced. HBO therapy also causes inhibition of endothelial neutrophil adhesion in injured tissue, allowing for greater WBC mobilization.

HBO therapy is indicated in severe CO poisoning when COHb is greater than 30% and in pregnant patients with COHb greater than 15%. It improves tissue oxygenation by decreasing COHb half-life, by increasing the amount of O_2 dissolved in plasma, and by increasing the rate of release of CO from cytochrome oxidase. The half-life of CO is inversely related to the inspired oxygen concentration. Treatment is guided by the severity of symptoms and response to the therapy. Clinical indications include a patient presenting with a history of neurologic impairment (dizziness, obtundation, unconsciousness) and evidence of cardiac abnormality (ST-segment depression on ECG and ventricular failure).

Gas bubble diseases such as gas embolism and decompression sickness respond well to HBO therapy. Such illnesses may occur in airplane pilots, scuba divers, patients on cardio-pulmonary bypass, and patients undergoing neurosurgical procedures in sitting position who develop venous gas embolism. HBO therapy increases tissue perfusion and tissue O_2 tension, and it is the treatment of choice for air or gas embolism. The rapid increase in ambient pressure decreases bubble volume and improves blood flow immediately. The standard of care for decompression sickness is HBO therapy.

HBO therapy is recommended as an adjuvant therapy during antibiotic treatment before emergency surgical debridement for the management of soft-tissue necrotizing infections, such as clostridial myonecrosis. *Clostridium perfringens* is the most common cause of gas gangrene that is mediated by alpha-toxin, a lecithinase that injures cell membranes, causing RBC lysis and damage to muscle and renal tubules. Anaerobic bacteria are sensitive to increased tissue PO_2 because they lack antioxidant enzymes, such as superoxide dismutase and catalase. High O_2 tensions also inhibit clostridial alpha-toxin production. Other mechanisms include reversal of hypoxia-induced neutrophil dysfunction, enhancement of macrophage interleukin-10 expression, and anti-inflammatory effects. HBO therapy induces hyperoxic vasoconstriction that decreases edema and improves perfusion to swollen ischemic tissue. It also increases tissue oxygen tension and improves survival of marginally viable tissues.

Intracranial abscesses are generally caused by anaerobic bacteria. The mode of action of HBO therapy is through enhancement of WBC killing.

Chronic ischemia and radiation necrosis occurs after 6 to 18 months, when blood vessels in the radiated area begin to progressively sclerose, with resultant decrease in blood flow. Treatment with HBO therapy will stimulate neovascularization of radiated tissue, allowing for subsequent bone or tissue grafting. HBO therapy is indicated for soft-tissue radiation necrosis, radiation cystitis, and osteoradionecrosis prevention.

HBO therapy provides temporary support in treating exceptional blood loss anemia when blood transfusion is unavailable, or when a Jehovah's Witness refuses blood. Life can be supported solely by increasing the O_2 content through dissolved oxygen in plasma at FIO_2 of 100% and 3 atm, even with a hemoglobin of 1 g per dL. Concurrently, patients should receive epoetin alpha, iron, and folate to maximize marrow production. HBO therapy is continued until achieving a hemoglobin of 7 g per dL.

Absolute contraindications to HBO therapy include concurrent administration of chemotherapeutic agents (doxorubicin, bleomycin, and cisplatin), disulfiram therapy (blocks superoxide dismutase that is protective against oxygen toxicity), untreated pneumothorax, and premature infants susceptible to retrolental fibroplasias. Relative contraindications include a history of spontaneous pneumothorax, severe emphysema with CO_2 intoxication that increases the risk of pneumothorax, and congenital spherocytosis, where high PO_2 may cause severe hemolysis in fragile RBCs.

Adverse effects include oxygen-induced seizure when therapy is given at greater than 2 ATA, pulmonary oxygen toxicity, transient paresthesia of the fourth and fifth finger of the ulnar nerve distribution, serous otitis media, and progressive myopia. Major complications are extremely rare despite the potential adverse effects of HBO therapy.

Miller RD. *Miller's Anesthesia*. 7th ed. Philadelphia, PA: Elsevier, Churchill Livingstone; 2009:2485–2497.
Morgan GE, Mikhail MS, Murray MJ. *Clinical Anesthesiology*. 4th ed. New York, NY: McGraw-Hill; 2006:1028–1029.
Mortensen CR. Hyperbaric oxygen therapy. *Curr Anaesth Crit Care*. 2008;19:333–337.

SUGGESTED READINGS

Hypercalcemia: Acute Treatment
Organ-based Clinical: Endocrine/Metabolic

Juan Egas

Edited by Mamatha Punjala

KEY POINTS

1. Nearly 70% cases of hypercalcemic crisis are caused by malignancy and 20% secondary to primary hyperparathyroidism.
2. Hypercalcemic crisis is a life-threatening medical emergency and should be treated rapidly with rehydration followed by aggressive diuresis, particularly with loop diuretics because they aid in calcium excretion.
3. Bisphosphonates may also aid long term in reducing calcium serum levels, as they have a longer duration of action.

DISCUSSION

Calcium ion is involved in many physiologic processes such as cardiac function, enzymatic reactions, coagulation, and skeletal mechanical strength. Calcium homeostasis/balance is maintained by hormonal, renal, and dietary mechanisms. Up to 40% of the extracellular fluid calcium is protein bound; the rest of the total calcium is bound to phosphate or exists in an ionized form. Only the unbound ionized calcium is biologically active and is readily available for physiologic reactions. Calcium is acquired through the diet, and its intestinal absorption is mediated through the activated form of vitamin D (calcitriol). While calcitriol enhances bone absorption of calcium, the bones act as the main reservoirs of calcium in our system. Also, parathyroid hormone increases osteoclastic activity, inducing bone resorption, releasing calcium and its renal absorption while increasing the excretion of phosphate. Parathyroid hormone will also stimulate vitamin D activity through the activation of 1 alpha hydroxylase.

Hypercalcemic crisis is mainly caused by malignancy (up to 70% of the cases) and primary hyperparathyroidism (up to 20% of the cases). In hypercalcemia of malignancy, several mechanisms may be involved including the release of parathyroid hormone-related protein (PTHrP) and increased production of calcitriol or hypercalcemic cytokines such as interleukin 1 (IL-1), IL-6, tumor necrosis factor alpha, and prostaglandins. Other important causes are sarcoidosis and vitamin D toxicosis. Clinical findings are considered together as a hypercalcemic syndrome, and the severity is proportional to the calcium levels. Patients may be severely dehydrated with progression to acute renal failure presenting as oliguria/anuria, and azotemia. Other symptoms are nausea and vomiting with loss of appetite, mental status changes ranging from loss of initiative to somnolence and coma, cardiac dysrhythmias, hypotension with shortened QT time, cardiac arrest.

Independent of cause, hypercalcemic crisis is a life-threatening medical emergency, and prompt treatment should be immediately instituted. The first thing to determine in the management is kidney function, whether the patient is able to diurese efficiently. Hypercalcemia is always accompanied with hypercalciuria, which produces osmotic diuresis that leads to dehydration and hypovolemia. The management of hypercalcemia should focus on correcting hypovolemia and on facilitating urinary excretion of calcium. Intravenous fluid administration will not correct the hypercalcemia by itself and should be followed by intravenous loop diuretics, such as furosemide. Furosemide enhances urinary calcium excretion, but can be counterproductive in a patient who is severely dehydrated, and so close attention must be paid to intravascular volume status. It is pertinent that one avoids the use of thiazide diuretics and digitalis in hypercalcemic patients, as they are both associated with elevated serum calcium levels.

Although fluid repletion with effective diuresis to promote calcium excretion is the first line of treatment in the acute management of hypercalcemia, it does not treat the underlying cause. Calcitonin, which inhibits calcium resorption as mentioned previously, may be used and has a very rapid response, although it is not very efficient at decreasing serum calcium levels. For hypercalcemia of malignancy, corticosteroids have also been used. In addition, bisphosphonates, strong inhibitors of bone resorption, should be administered for long-term regulation of calcium levels because they have a longer duration of action, although they cannot be used in patients with renal failure. Finally, in patients with renal failure, dialysis is the first line of treatment.

SUGGESTED READINGS

Corvilain J. Calcium homeostasis and pathogenesis of hypercalcemia. *Horm Res.* 1984;20:8–12.
Costanzo L. *BRS Physiology.* 5th ed. Philadelphia, PA: Lippincott Williams & Wilkins; 2010.
Marino P. *The ICU Book.* 3rd ed. Philadelphia, PA: Lippincott Williams & Wilkins; 2006:644–647.

Hypercarbia: Alv Gas Equation
Generic Clinical Sciences: Anesthesia Procedures, Methods, Techniques

Jammie Ferrara

Edited by Shamsuddin Akhtar

H

1. The alveolar gas equation relates the alveolar concentration of oxygen (PAO_2) to inspired tension of oxygen (FiO_2), arterial CO_2 tension ($PaCO_2$), and respiratory quotient (RQ).
2. Alveolar CO_2 tension ($PaCO_2$) is the balance between total CO_2 production ($\dot{V}CO_2$) and alveolar ventilation ($\dot{V}A$).
3. Alveolar CO_2 tension is related more to CO_2 elimination than to CO_2 production.

In the assessment of the hypoxemic, hypercarbic patient, use of the alveolar gas equation may aid in determining the primary etiology of abnormal gas exchange. Such an abnormality may result secondary to hypoventilation, hypo-perfusion, increased dead space (e.g., pulmonary embolism), or increased intrapulmonary shunting (e.g., atelectasis). In order to understand where the primary disturbance lies, one must first understand the relationship between each variable as described by the alveolar gas equation.

Briefly, the inspired tension of oxygen (P_IO_2) in air at sea level is a product of barometric pressure (P_B) and the fraction of inspired oxygen (F_IO_2) or concentration of oxygen in air (i.e., 760 mm Hg × 0.21). However, when determining the inspired tension of oxygen in humidified air, one must factor in the pressure of water vapor ($PH_2O = 47$ mm Hg at 37° C). Therefore,

$$P_IO_2 = (P_B - PH_2O) \times F_IO_2$$

Furthermore, the alveolar tension of oxygen is dependent on the alveolar tension of CO_2 as with every breath, inspired gases are mixed in the alveoli from previously inspired breaths, whereby oxygen is absorbed and carbon dioxide is released. Arterial and alveolar tensions of CO_2 are essentially the same, and so $PaCO_2$ can be substituted. Therefore, the final alveolar gas equation is

$$PAO_2 = P_IO_2 - PaCO_2 / RQ$$

Or

$$[(P_B - PH_2O) \times F_IO_2] - PaCO_2 / RQ$$

where PAO_2 is the alveolar concentration of oxygen, P_IO_2 is the inspired tension of oxygen (P_IO_2), $PaCO_2$ is the arterial CO_2 tension, and RQ is the respiratory quotient. The RQ is the ratio of oxygen consumed (VO_2) to CO_2 produced (VCO_2);

$$RQ = \dot{V}CO_2 / \dot{V}O_2 = 200 \text{ mL/min} / 250 \text{ mL/min} = 0.8$$

Therefore, clinical situations of hypercarbia ($PaCO_2 > 75$ mm Hg) will result in hypoxia ($PaO_2 < 60$ mm Hg), particularly at room air, according to the equation. Alveolar CO_2 tension ($PACO_2$) relates the balance between total CO_2 production (VCO_2) and alveolar ventilation (VA).

$$PaCO_2 = \dot{V}CO_2/VA$$

$PACO_2$ is related more to CO_2 elimination/ventilation rather than production. This is evident during periods of hypoventilation or hypoperfusion, when the excess CO_2, increases total body CO_2 content. The actual production of CO_2, however, does not change significantly under most circumstances. In addition, the body has a large capacity to store CO_2 thereby buffering acute changes in the production of CO_2 (VCO_2). Per equation, if alveolar ventilation decreases, $PaCO_2$ is expected to increase by the same amount. During episodes of apnea, $PaCO_2$ may rise rapidly, roughly 6 mm Hg in the first minute, then more slowly at about 3 mm Hg per minute. Accordingly, hypercarbia may be overcome by increasing ventilation, thus improving alveolar tension of CO_2 and O_2.

SUGGESTED READINGS

Barash PG, Cullen BF, Stoelting RK, et al, eds. *Clinical Anesthesia*. 6th ed. Philadelphia, PA: Lippincott Williams & Wilkins; 2009:246.

Morgan GE, Mikhail MS, Murray MJ. *Clinical Anesthesiology*. 4th ed. New York, NY: McGraw Hill; 2006:558–561.

Stoelting RK, Miller RD. *Basics of Anesthesia*. 5th ed. Philadelphia, PA: Churchill Livingstone Elsevier; 2007:56–59.

Hypercarbia: O₂ Release to Tissues
Physiology

Laurie Yonemoto

Edited by Hossam Tantawy

H

1. The relationship between oxygen saturation and the partial pressure of oxygen in the blood is described by the oxygen–hemoglobin dissociation curve.
2. P50 is the partial pressure of oxygen at which 50% of hemoglobin is saturated and is normally 26 mm Hg.
3. Factors that shift the oxygen–hemoglobin dissociation curve to the left include hypothermia, alkalosis, and decreased 2,3-diphosphoglycerate (DPG).
4. Factors that shift the oxygen–hemoglobin dissociation curve to the right include hyperthermia, acidosis, and increased 2,3-DPG.
5. Hypercarbia shifts the oxygen–hemoglobin dissociation curve to the right by increasing hydrogen ion concentration.

The oxygen–hemoglobin dissociation curve is a sigmoid shaped curve that relates oxygen saturation and the partial pressure of oxygen in the blood, and is an important tool in understanding what factors influence the ability of hemoglobin to retain or release oxygen to tissues. The sigmoid shape of the curve is due to the increased ability of hemoglobin to bind oxygen as more and more oxygen molecules become attached. Each hemoglobin molecule can bind up to four oxygen molecules. As the partial pressure of oxygen increases, more molecules of oxygen bind up to a point where the hemoglobin molecules are completely saturated, giving the curve its characteristic sigmoid shape.

The partial pressure of oxygen in the blood at which 50% of hemoglobin is saturated, or the P50, is a conventional measure of hemoglobin affinity for oxygen, and is 26 mm Hg in a healthy person. Many factors influence the P50 of hemoglobin and subsequently shift

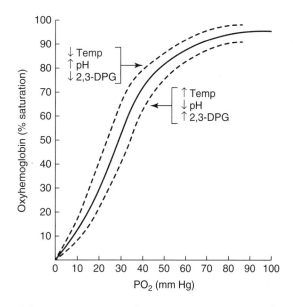

Figure 1. Oxygen-Hemoglobin Dissociation Curve (Images: www.rtmagazine.com.)

the oxygen–hemoglobin dissociation curve either to the left or to the right, increasing or decreasing the affinity of hemoglobin for oxygen, respectively.

Factors that shift the oxygen–hemoglobin dissociation curve to the left include hypothermia, alkalosis, and decreased 2,3-DPG. Factors that cause the oxygen–hemoglobin dissociation curve to shift to the right, thus decreasing the affinity of hemoglobin for oxygen, include acidosis, hyperthermia, and increased 2,3-DPG. These conditions allow for an increased amount of oxygen release to tissues (Fig. 1). Hypercarbia also leads to a rightward shift of the oxygen–hemoglobin dissociation curve, secondary to associated increases in hydrogen ion concentration. This is referred to as the Bohr effect. Eighty percent to 90% of carbon dioxide produced via metabolism is transported as bicarbonate ions and hydrogen ions in the blood by carbonic anhydrase. The increase in hydrogen ions results in a respiratory acidosis and a decrease in pH, thus shifting the curve and the P50 to the right. This ultimately makes oxygen more available to the tissues to accommodate increases in metabolism.

SUGGESTED READINGS

Barash PG, Cullen BF, Stoelting RK, et al. *Clinical Anesthesia*. 6th ed. Philadelphia, PA: Lippincott Williams & Wilkins; 2009:701–702.

Morgan GE, Mikhail MS, Murray MJ. *Clinical Anesthesiology*. 4th ed. New York, NY: McGraw Hill; 2006:562–563.

Stoelting RK, Miller RD. *Basics of Anesthesia*. 5th ed. Philadelphia, PA: Elsevier; 2007:55–56.

Hyperglycemia: Complications

Organ-based Clinical: Endocrine/Metabolic

Martha Zegarra

Edited by Mamatha Punjala

H

KEY POINTS

1. Hyperglycemia is commonly encountered in patients during the perioperative period and occurs both in diabetics and in nondiabetics.
2. Surgical stress, trauma, and infection lead to increases in glucose production and insulin resistance.
3. Hyperglycemia leads to poor outcomes in patients with acute myocardial infarction, critical illness, stroke, and traumatic brain injury.

DISCUSSION

Hyperglycemia is commonly encountered in patients during the perioperative period, and occurs both in diabetics and in nondiabetics. Many factors influence glucose levels in these patients, including surgical stress, trauma, and infection, all of which lead to a release of inflammatory and hormonal mediators. Release of these mediators increases both glucose production and insulin resistance. In addition, hyperglycemia may be caused or aggravated by therapeutic interventions, such as corticosteroid administration and total parenteral nutrition.

The complications of hyperglycemia in the perioperative period are many, and include diabetic ketoacidosis and hyperosmolar nonketotic coma. In addition, both diabetics and nondiabetic patients are at increased risk for post-op infections, immune suppression and poor wound healing. Furthermore, patients with acute myocardial infarction, stroke, and traumatic brain injury have been shown to have poor outcomes when they were concurrently hyperglycemic. Some studies have shown positive outcomes with decreased mortality in ICU patients whose glucose levels were aggressively managed; however, this also leads to an increased incidence of hypoglycemia, which can be severe. Management of glucose in the perioperative period remains controversial.

SUGGESTED READINGS

Barash PG, Cullen BF, Stoelting RK, et al, eds. *Clinical Anesthesia*. 6th ed. Philadelphia, PA: Lippincott Williams & Wilkins; 2009:1016, 1460–1461.

Marino PL. *The ICU Book*. 3rd ed. Philadelphia, PA: Lippincott Williams & Wilkins; 2007:239–240.

Hyperglycemia: Preop Rx

Organ-based Clinical: Endocrine/Metabolic

Gabriel Jacobs

Edited by Mamatha Punjala

H

1. Most recommendations include decreasing dose of administered insulin therapy before surgery; however, most studies support the goal of tight glycemic control to reduce the risk of postoperative complications secondary to hyperglycemia.
2. Hemoglobin A1C is a good indicator for *long-term* glycemic control. Preoperative hyperglycemia has been associated with poor perioperative outcomes.
3. Oral hypoglycemic should be held on the day of surgery and up to 24 hours before scheduled procedure, given the risk of hypoglycemia.
4. Metformin should be held for at least 24 hours before surgery, given its long half-life and propensity to severe lactic acidosis when associated with conditions creating poor tissue perfusion.

Preoperative Testing

Preoperative risk assessment of the diabetic patient should include a thorough history and physical assessing for complications of diabetes mellitus, including autonomic dysfunction, gastrointestinal (GI) dysmotility, and cardiovascular disease. ECG, electrolytes, creatinine, and hemoglobin A1C are utilized to stratify and assess patient compliance with diabetic control. Although preoperative blood glucose assessment is important, hemoglobin A1C can give insight into a patient's glucose control over the past several months. The goal hemoglobin A1C for patients younger than 5 years is 7% to 9%, whereas the goal hemoglobin A1C for patients older than 5 years is 6% to 8%. Higher levels suggest poorly controlled hyperglycemia. Often patients with uncontrolled diabetes present with hyperglycemia on the day of surgery. If blood glucose levels are greater than 270 mg per dL, it may be needed to delay surgery until tight control is achieved with intravenous (IV) insulin. With blood glucose less than 400 mg per dL, the surgery should be postponed until adequate control is achieved.

Preoperative Diabetes Medication Management

Oral hypoglycemic should be held the morning of surgery to avoid hypoglycemia in fasting patients. Metformin should be held for at least 24 hour before surgery, given its long half-life and propensity to severe lactic acidosis when associated with conditions creating poor tissue perfusion. Insulin should be continued in the perioperative period with different recommendations depending on the type of insulin used. Below are some *suggestions* for preoperative insulin use.

Regular → $^2/_3$ p.m. dose the night before, hold a.m. dose.

NPH → $^2/_3$ p.m. dose the night before, ½ a.m. dose.

Insulin pump → Decrease p.m. insulin rate to 70% of basal rate. In the morning of surgery, the basal rate can be reestablished. Patients on insulin pumps can continue to use them during the perioperative period for small surgeries; however, pumps should be discontinued and patients should be placed on an IV insulin continuous infusion for moderate/major surgery.

Lispro and aspart → Complete p.m. dose the night before and hold a.m. dose.

Glargine → ⅔ p.m. dose the night before, hold a.m. dose

Patients should be informed to use clear liquids/juices or a glucose tablet in case of hypoglycemia, before coming in for surgery. If possible, coordinate with the surgical team to schedule patients with hyperglycemia to be the first cases of the day. Whatever is the recommended advice followed, it is imperative to monitor the patient's blood glucose levels to maintain near euglycemic levels.

Many studies in critically ill patients have actually been conducted looking into the potential role of tight glycemic control perioperatively. It was found that morbidity, including renal dysfunction and need for dialysis, and mortality decreased with glucose levels controlled between 180 and 210 mg per dL. Further studies performed in postcardiac surgery patients have confirmed that mortality increased in patients with levels greater than 175 mg per dL. However, results regarding intraoperative control are much less clear, with many actually showing significant morbidity, including strokes, and mortality in tightly controlled patients.

Anesthetic Considerations
Patients with long-standing hyperglycemia come with a host of special anesthetic considerations. Diabetes can affect oxygen transport. Prolonged hyperglycemia can promote the covalent binding of glucose to the beta chains of hemoglobin, deleteriously affecting oxygen binding. In addition, diabetes can lead to GI dysmotility via damage to the ganglion cells of the GI tract. This can increase the risk of aspiration in diabetic patients. Autonomic dysfunction can be present in diabetic patients and can affect the body's ability to regulate heart rate and blood pressure. Autonomic dysfunction can lead to increased risk of intraoperative hypothermia due to circulatory dysregulation. Autonomic dysfunction can also affect the choice of induction agent. For example, etomidate may be a better choice over propofol or thiopental, given its lower incidence of cardiovascular side effects. Finally, diabetic patients are at greater risk for cardiovascular disease, which may influence preoperative cardiovascular risk assessment and testing.

SUGGESTED READINGS

Barash PG, Cullen BF, Stoelting RK, et al, eds. *Clinical Anesthesia*. 6th ed. Philadelphia, PA: Lippincott Williams & Wilkins; 2009:1296–1299.
Hines R. *Stoelting's Anesthesia and Co-existing Disease*. 5th ed. Philadelphia, PA: Saunders; 2008:375–376.
Miller RD. *Miller's Anesthesia*. 7th ed. Philadelphia, PA: Elsevier Churchill Livingstone; 2009.
Morgan GE Jr. *Clinical Anesthesiology*. 4th ed. New York, NY: McGraw Hill; 804–805.

Hyperkalemia: Drugs Causing

Pharmacology

Gregory Albert

Edited by Ala Haddadin

KEY POINTS

1. Improper administration of medications is a frequent cause of hyperkalemia.
2. Drugs that increase serum levels of potassium may be divided into those that shift potassium to the extracellular compartment, those that reduce renal elimination, and those that contain potassium.

DISCUSSION

Iatrogenic hyperkalemia from improper administration of medications is a major cause of patient morbidity and mortality. Knowledge of medications that increase serum potassium is vital to any competent practitioner, as this will reduce the incidence of life-threatening cardiac dysrhythmias such as ventricular fibrillation and asystole.

Drugs that stimulate the release of intracellular potassium into the blood stream are used ubiquitously in medicine. Beta-blockers, such as metoprolol, stimulate release of potassium. Succinylcholine, mannitol, and digoxin also cause increases in serum potassium. Drugs that reduce renal elimination of potassium also increase serum potassium levels. Examples of these medications include ACE-inhibitors, heparin, nonsteroidal anti-inflammatory drugs, amiloride, triamterene, spironolactone, trimethoprim, pentamidine, and calcineurin inhibitors. Some medications include potassium in their formulations and, when given, can increase serum potassium directly. These include certain penicillins and cardioplegic solutions.

SUGGESTED READING

Reilly R, Perazella M. *Nephrology in 30 Days*. Philadelphia, PA: McGraw-Hill Company; 2005:90–92.

Hypermagnesemia Rx

Generic Clinical Sciences: Anesthesia Procedures, Methods, Techniques

Rongjie Jiang

Edited by Lars Helgeson

KEY POINTS

1. Hypermagnesemia (>2.5 mEq per L) occurs primarily iatrogenically and rarely as a result of impaired renal function.
2. Signs and symptoms are directly related to the measured blood Mg^{2+} level, and mainly manifest as depression of the nervous, cardiovascular, and respiratory systems.
3. Normal magnesium balance includes elimination primarily via the kidneys, and the regulation is influenced by other factors including plasma calcium levels and volume and acid–base status.
4. Treatment of hypermagnesemia includes fluid administration followed by dieresis (particularly with loop diuretics) and dialysis for patients with renal failure. The use of intravenous (IV) calcium rapidly, but temporarily, decreases the serum Mg^{2+} level.

DISCUSSION

Hypermagnesemia (plasma levels >2.5 mg per dL) occurs mostly as a result of iatrogenic overdose such as parenteral nutrition, during treatment of torsades de pointes, and in obstetrics. Magnesium is commonly used in the management of premature labor and prevention of seizures in preeclamptic patients. The target Mg^{2+} level in obstetric practice is 5 to 7 mg per dL. It is occasionally seen with chronic use of antacids, laxatives, and enemas.

Normal magnesium balance is primarily maintained via the kidneys, with 25% being reabsorbed in the proximal tubule and approximately 50% in the thick ascending loop of Henle. Renal Mg^{2+} reabsorption is increased with hypocalcemia, hypomagnesemia, metabolic alkalosis, volume depletion, and increased parathyroid hormone levels. Increased renal excretion occurs with hypercalcemia, hypermagnesemia, volume expansion, diuretic use, phosphate depletion, ketoacidosis, and hyperaldosteronism. The signs and symptom of hypermagnesemia are directly related to the Mg^{2+} serum level and are summarized in Table 1. Since elevated magnesium levels impair both the release of acetylcholine and its effect at the neuromuscular junction, they can result in muscle weakness and accordingly potentiate the effect of neuromuscular blockers. Neuromuscular blocking doses should be reduced by 25% to 50%, if elevated magnesium levels are known.

Treatment of hypermagnesemia typically starts with volume expansion with administration of IV fluids, followed by diuresis. The definitive therapy is dialysis, particularly in patients with renal impairment. Temporary reversal of the effects of hypermagnesemia can be accomplished with calcium therapy (1 g or 5 to 10 mEq of calcium gluconate or

Table 1. Signs and Symptom of Hypermagnesemia

Symptoms	Magnesium Level (mg/dL)
Widened QRS, prolonged P-R, nausea	5–10 (supraphysiologic)
Complete heart block or cardiac arrest	>15 (severe hypermagnesemia)
Sedation, hypoventilation, decreased deep tendon reflexes, muscle weakness	20–34
Hypotension, bradycardia	24–48
Areflexia, coma, respiratory paralysis	48–72

10% calcium chloride 20 mg per kg IV [0.2 mL per kg—pediatric dosing, 5 to 10 mL—adult dosing]). Neonatal hypermagnesemia can occur immediately post partum, typically because of maternal Mg^{2+} therapy. Symptoms respond to intravascular volume expansion, dopamine, and calcium gluconate 100 to 200 mg per kg administered over a 5-minute period.

SUGGESTED READINGS

Barash P, Cullen BF, Stoelting RK, et al. *Clinical Anesthesia.* 6th ed. Philadelphia, PA: Lippincott Williams & Wilkins; 2009:14, 322.
Miller RD. *Miller's Anesthesia.* 7th ed. Philadelphia, PA: Elsevier, Churchill, and Livingstone; 2009:1713–1714, 2695, 2996.
Morgan GE Jr, Mikhail MS, Murray MJ. *Clinical Anesthesiology.* 4th ed. New York, NY: Lange Medical Books/ McGraw Hill; 2006:chap 28:686–687.

H

Hyperparathyroidism: Signs and Sx
Organ-based Clinical: Endocrine/Metabolic

Ashley Kelley and Kellie Park

Edited by Mamatha Punjala

H

KEY POINTS

1. Symptoms of hyperparathyroidism are secondary to the resultant hypercalcemia.
2. Early signs of hypercalcemia include vomiting and abdominal pain and sedation/somnolence, which may progress to symptoms including skeletal muscle weakness.
3. Patients with hypercalcemia can have polyuria and, if levels remain persistently elevated, are predisposed to the formation of kidney stones.

DISCUSSION

The parathyroid glands secrete parathyroid hormone (PTH), which is primarily responsible for the regulation of calcium. Normally, PTH functions by promoting bone resorption, limiting elimination by the kidneys, and indirectly increasing calcium absorption from the gastrointestinal (GI) tract, secondary to its effect on vitamin D. As a result, plasma calcium levels are increased, and so in clinical situations of excess PTH, hypercalcemia will ensue because of the symptoms mostly associated with hyperparathyroidism. Primary hyperparathyroidism can be caused by parathyroid carcinoma, adenoma or hyperplasia, whereas secondary hyperparathyroidism is a reactionary overproduction of PTH in response to hypocalcemia.

Hypercalcemia, defined as a serum calcium concentration of greater than 5.5 mEq per L (ionized [Ca^{2+}] of >2.5 mEq per L), has a wide range of effects on a number of organ systems. Early signs of hypercalcemia include GI symptoms, such as vomiting and abdominal pain, and central nervous system dysfunction like sedation/somnolence. Further neurologic sequelae include development of psychosis and decreased sensation of pain. Other GI symptoms include development of peptic ulcers secondary to increased secretion of gastric acid and pancreatitis. A common neuromuscular symptom is skeletal muscle weakness, which should be assessed pre-operatively because the response to administration of Neuromuscular Blocking Drugs (NMBDs) may be altered.

Hypercalcemia can lead to the development of polyuria and dehydration, and persistently elevated serum calcium levels can result in the formation of kidney stones and anemia. Secondary to increased bone resorption, patients may experience bone pain and develop osteopenia, with possible increased risk of osteoporosis vertebral compression and fractures. Hypercalcemia can also result in hypertension and ECG changes, including QT shortening and prolonged PR intervals, which can increase the risk of developing arrhythmias.

In assessing a patient preoperatively, close attention should be paid to the patient's intravascular volume status, as it may be made hypotensive on induction, secondary to dehydration and volume depletion. If calcium levels are too high, patients should be treated with aggressive fluid repletion and diuresis with loop diuretics, as they help increase excretion of calcium at the ascending loop of Henle and distal convoluted tubule.

SUGGESTED READINGS

Barash PG, Cullen BF, Stoelting RK, et al, eds. *Clinical Anesthesia.* 6th ed. Philadelphia, PA: Lippincott Williams & Wilkins; 2009:1284–1286.

Hines RL, Marschall KE. *Stoelting's Anesthesia and Co-existing Disease.* 5th ed. Philadelphia, PA: Churchill Livingstone; 2008:398–401.

Morgan GE Jr, Mikhail MS, Murray MJ. *Clinical Anesthesiology.* 4th ed. New York, NY: Lange Medical Books/McGraw Hill; 2006:809–810.

Hyperthyroidism: Signs
Organ-based Clinical: Endocrine/Metabolic

Terrence Coffey

Edited by Mamatha Punjala

H

KEY POINTS

1. Graves disease (toxic diffuse goiter) is the most common cause of hyperthyroidism.
2. Graves disease, toxic multinodular goiter, and toxic adenoma account for 99% of cases of hyperthyroidism.
3. Hyperthyroidism is characterized by a hypermetabolic state.
4. Signs and symptoms of hyperthyroidism include fatigue, anxiety, weight loss, diarrhea, heat intolerance, weakness, warm moist skin, tachycardia, and exophthalmos.
5. Thyroid storm is a life-threatening exacerbation of hyperthyroidism, and its presentation intraoperatively may be very similar to other life-threatening crises such as malignant hyperthermia and pheochromocytoma.

DISCUSSION

Hyperthyroidism is characterized by increasing T_4 and T_3 levels and normal or below normal levels of thyroid-stimulating hormone (TSH). Graves disease, toxic multinodular goiter, and toxic adenoma account for 99% of cases of hyperthyroidism. Hyperthyroidism is characterized by a hypermetabolic state. Signs and symptoms include anxiety, weight loss, diarrhea, heat intolerance, warm moist skin, skeletal muscle weakness, tachycardia, and restlessness. Graves disease is commonly associated with goiter, exophthalmos, and fine tremors. Wasting and fatigue are common. Patients may also have increased bone turnover secondary to hypermetabolic state, which can lead to osteoporosis. Hyperthyroidism may result in elevated systolic blood pressure and decreased diastolic blood pressure. In addition, hypocalcemia, thrombocytopenia, and mild anemia may be present. Elderly patients may present with atrial fibrillation, heart failure, and other cardiac arrhythmias.

It is desirable to make the hyperthyroid patient euthyroid before surgery. Intraoperative monitoring of patients with hyperthyroidism should be directed toward recognizing clinical signs of increased thyroid activity. These may include tachycardia, tachydysrhythmias, and hypertension.

Thyroid storm is a life-threatening condition sometimes recognized intraoperatively, often in patients with undiagnosed or undertreated hyperthyroidism. Thyroid storm may manifest intraoperatively as hyperthermia, tachycardia, dysrhythmias, myocardial infarction, or congestive heart failure. It may also manifest postoperatively with the same signs, but may also include confusion and agitation. Thyroid storm may be difficult to delineate from other life-threatening conditions such as pheochromocytoma and malignant hyperthermia. Free T_4 levels will be greatly elevated, but are not diagnostic.

SUGGESTED READINGS

Barash PG, Cullen BF, Stoelting RK, et al, eds. *Clinical Anesthesia*. 6th ed. Philadelphia, PA: Lippincott Williams & Wilkins; 2009:1131–1133.

Hines R, Marschall K. *Stoelting's Anesthesia and Co-existing Disease*. 5th ed. Philadelphia, PA: Churchill Livingstone; 2008:381–383.

Morgan GE, Mikhail MS, Murray MJ. *Clinical Anesthesiology*. 4th ed. New York, NY: McGraw-Hill; 2005:807–808.

Hypocalcemia: ECG Effects

Pharmacology

Dallen Mill

Edited by Qingbing Zhu

1. Calcium influx is responsible for phase 2, or the plateau phase, of the action potential of the myocardium.
2. Hypocalcemia results in delayed influx of calcium and therefore prolonged plateau phase, resulting in prolonged repolarization.
3. Hypocalcemia is manifested most commonly as prolonged QT interval on ECG.
4. T-wave inversions can occasionally be associated with hypocalcemia.

As in Figure 1, phase 1 of myocardial action potential is due to the efflux of potassium ions, which is eventually offset by the influx of calcium as manifested in phase 2, resulting in a plateau phase. Phase 3 is the result of calcium channels closing and the continued efflux of potassium out of cells, leading to cell repolarization.

A decrease in calcium concentration would therefore mean a slower influx, which would delay plateau formation, resulting in a prolonged action potential by prolonging

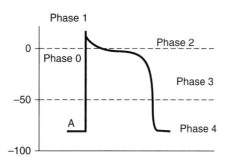

Figure 1. Cardiac myocyte action potential.

phase 2. This would delay repolarization, or phase 3, which is manifested by the T wave on an ECG tracing. Therefore, hypocalcemia primarily produces a prolonged QT interval in ECG.

As with other causes of QT interval prolongation, hypocalcemia may increase the risk of R-on-T phenomenon and the development of ventricular dysrhythmias such as torsades de pointe. Occasionally, T-wave inversions are also seen in patients with this electrolyte abnormality.

Calcium homeostasis is maintained by intestinal absorption, which is intricately associated with vitamin D metabolism, and renal reabsorption and excretion, which is highly dependent on the role of parathyroid hormone (PTH), which also serves to increase plasma calcium concentrations by increasing bone resorption. On the other hand, calcitonin works to increase calcium deposition in bones. The amount of biologically available (ionized) calcium is determined by this interplay and the percentage of protein-bound calcium, mostly with albumin.

Hypocalcemia may be caused by hypomagnesemia (inhibits PTH and tissue responsiveness to PTH), sepsis, multiple blood transfusions, alkalosis, pancreatitis, nutritional deficiencies, malabsorption, vitamin D deficiency, inflammatory bowel disease, short bowel syndrome, and hypoparathyroidism. Therefore, it is a risk after thyroidectomy, with inadvertent removal of some or all of the parathyroid glands, and patients should be monitored postoperatively for any or all signs and symptoms, including paresthesias, confusion, laryngeal stridor or laryngospasm, Trousseau sign (carpopedal spasm), Chvostek sign (masseter spasm), seizures, and cardiac arrhythmias. Decreased cardiac contractility resulting in hypotension or heart failure may also occur, and if it occurs intraoperatively, it may potentiate the effects of certain anesthetics and anesthetic adjuncts, such as volatiles and barbiturates, resulting in negative inotropy.

Management of hypocalcemia, particularly after thyroid surgery, is mostly directed at prevention with oral replacement therapy; however, if a patient begins experiencing symptoms, intravenous replacement therapy should be instituted immediately and on the basis of ionized (biologically active) calcium levels. Replacement is particularly important in avoiding the negative cardiac side effects as mentioned previously. Vigilance in monitoring patients on a telemetry unit may be necessary, as there are changes that can be seen on ECG before development of any deleterious consequences.

SUGGESTED READINGS

Foster DB. *Twelve-Lead Electrocardiology Theory and Interpretation*. New York, NY: Springer; 2007:11, 119.
Marino PL. *The ICU Book*. 3rd ed. Philadelphia, PA: Lippincott Williams & Wilkins; 2007:641–644.
Miller RD. Electrocardiography. In: *Miller's Anesthesia*. 7th ed. Philadelphia, PA: Elsevier; 2008:1362.
Morgan GE, Mikhail MS, Murray MJ. *Clinical Anesthesiology*. 4th ed. New York, NY: Lange Medical Books/ McGraw Hill; 2006:684–685.
Rosendorff C. *Essential Cardiology Principles and Practice*. Totowa, NJ: Humana Press; 2006:135.

Hypothermia: Infant vs. Toddler

Subspecialties: Pediatric Anesthesia

Kellie Park

Edited by Mamatha Punjala

KEY POINTS

1. Core temperature in humans is tightly regulated. Hypothermia is typically considered a core temperature below 36.1° C.
2. In neonates/infants and to a lesser degree in toddlers, the surface area of skin relative to body mass is great, and all forms of heat loss including radiant, convective, conductive, and evaporative mechanisms contribute severely to development of hypothermia.
3. Nonshivering thermogenesis is the primary means by which the infant generates heat to avoid hypothermia.
4. Shivering thermogenesis is not effective in neonates and early infancy, but becomes more important as the musculoskeletal system develops.

DISCUSSION

Core temperature in humans is tightly regulated. Temperature is usually preserved within ±0.2° C. Hypothermia is typically considered a core temperature below 36.1° C. Hypothermia is further categorized as "mild (33.9° to 36.0° C), moderate (32.2° to 33.8° C), or severe (below 32.2° C)." Although the site to measure core temperature is widely debated, typically esophageal or bladder temperatures are accepted as reliable gauges of core temperature.

In infants, the surface area of skin relative to body mass is greater than twice that compared with adults. Accordingly, convective forced air warmers are most effective in maintaining normothermia as most of the infants' body is in contact with the warmer. On the other hand, this method is essentially ineffective, as only a small portion of a toddlers' or adults' body is in contact with the warmer. Although surface area decreases from infants to toddlers, all forms of heat loss including radiant, convective, conductive, and evaporative mechanisms are much greater and contribute more severely to development of hypothermia. Also compared with toddlers, neonates and infants have less subcutaneous fat and less keratinized skin. The head of the infant is proportionally large compared with the body. The skull bones are thinner compared with toddlers, so heat loss is much greater from the head.

Nonshivering thermogenesis is the primary means by which the infant generates heat to avoid hypothermia. Neonates and infants rely primarily on the metabolism of brown fat to increase body temperature. Brown fat has an increased concentration of mitochondria. Mitochondria of brown fat have an uncoupled respiratory chain, and use oxidative phosphorylation to create heat rather than ATP. As blood flows to metabolically active brown fat, it is warmed as it returns to circulation and effectively regulates body temperature. Anesthetic agents including inhaled gases, fentanyl, and propofol inhibit the metabolism of brown fat, and therefore inhibit the thermogenesis to a greater degree in the infant.

It is not clear at which age thermogenesis shifts from nonshivering to shivering thermogenesis, but it does seem to occur later in infancy when the musculoskeletal system has matured and muscle mass has increased to a degree to be effective in thermoregulation. It is clear, however, that shivering thermogenesis is not effective in neonates and early infancy.

SUGGESTED READINGS

Cote CJ, Lerman J, Todres ID. *A Practice of Anesthesia for Infants and Children.* 4th ed. Philadelphia, PA: Saunders; 2009:25:557–564.

Ellis J. Neonatal hypothermia. *J Neonatal Nurs.* 2005;11(2):76–82.

Kurz A. Thermal care in the perioperative period. *Best Pract Res Clin Anaesthesiol.* 2008;22(1):39–48.

Hypothermia: pH Stat Management
Subspecialties: Critical Care

Thomas Gallen

Edited by Qingbing Zhu

H

KEY POINTS

1. Solubility of oxygen and carbon dioxide is temperature dependent. As temperature lowers, solubility increases.
2. pH-stat management uses arterial blood gas (ABG) measurements corrected to the actual patient temperature and uses the addition of carbon dioxide to the circuit to maintain a constant pH.
3. In alpha-stat strategy, blood gas measurements are not corrected to temperature.
4. In adults undergoing moderate hypothermic cardiopulmonary bypass, alpha-stat is the preferred strategy, as it may confer slightly better neurologic outcomes.
5. In deep hypothermic circulatory arrest (DHCA), pH-stat is the preferred strategy, as it appears to provide better protection against cerebral ischemia.

DISCUSSION

pH-stat and alpha-stat refer to methods of blood gas interpretation, and relate to the fact that the solubility of both oxygen and carbon dioxide is temperature dependent and can alter blood gas interpretation. The total quantity of molecules of oxygen or carbon dioxide is the sum of the number of molecules in the gas phase and the number of molecules in the liquid phase; however, the partial pressure measures only those molecules in the gas phase. At lower temperatures, there are relatively fewer molecules in the gas phase, and therefore a decreased partial pressure is measured. An example of this is as water boils, it begins bubbling as dissolved/liquid gas changes to a gaseous phase.

When an ABG is run in the laboratory, it is warmed to 37° C for analysis. If the patient temperature is less than 37° C, a second "temperature corrected" reading can be calculated on the basis of a normogram, which corrects for temperature-related changes. In alpha-stat strategy, the blood gas measurement is not corrected to temperature (i.e., laboratory values assume a patient temperature of 37° C regardless of actual temperature, and these are the values reported and used for management). This differs from pH-stat strategy, in which ABG measurements are reported with temperature correction or using actual body temperature (through the use of a normogram). To maintain a constant pH, carbon dioxide may be added to the system. In this case, the total body carbon dioxide level is increased, and the microcirculatory pH becomes increasingly acidic.

Hypothermia is a mainstay of perioperative surgical management in cardiac surgery patients, suppressing cerebral metabolism 6% to 7% per 1° C decline in temperature. Thus, it is important to understand its ramifications. In adults undergoing moderate hypothermic cardiopulmonary bypass, alpha-stat is the preferred strategy because it may confer slightly better neurologic outcomes. Alpha-stat strategy is based on the premise that by maintaining a neutral pH relative to the temperature, cellular function is best. This means that pH at 37° C is 7.4 and pH at 20° C is about 7.70. The theory is that histidine is an essential component of the protein buffer system, and in alpha-stat strategy, there is a constant ratio (alpha) of dissociated to nondissociated imidazole groups of histidine, yielding better enzyme action. The downside to this strategy is that it creates a leftward shift of the oxyhemoglobin dissociation curve, restricting tissue extraction at a potentially critical time. pH-stat uses the blood gas values to guide addition of carbon dioxide to maintain a temperature-corrected pH of 7.4. Resultant higher blood flows are seen, which may not only improve perfusion through cerebral vasodilation, but also put the patient at greater risk for cerebral edema, microemboli, and increased intracranial pressure. Furthermore, pH-stat may promote a "steal" phenomenon in patients with cerebrovascular disease, allowing blood to be directed away from marginally perfused areas. pH-stat may improve cerebral cooling, with increased cerebral blood flow to deep brain structures such as the brainstem, cerebellum, and thalamus. When performing DHCA, pH-stat is preferable. The improved cerebral protection seen may be multifactorial and includes improved oxygen delivery from a right-shifted oxyhemoglobin dissociation curve, improved homogeneity of brain cooling, decreased reperfusion injury due to more acidic blood, and more rapid recovery of cerebral high-energy phosphate stores. Therefore, pH-stat strategy during and immediately after DHCA probably provides better protection than alpha-stat.

SUGGESTED READINGS

Estafanous F. *Cardiac Anesthesia: Principles and Clinical Practice*. 2nd ed. Philadelphia, PA: Lippincott Williams & Wilkins; 2001:808–811.

Hensley FA, Martin DE, Gravlee GP. *A Practical Approach to Cardiac Anesthesia*. 4th ed. Philadelphia, PA: Lippincott Williams & Wilkins; 2008:393–394.

Kaplan JA, Grocott HP, Stafford-Smith M. *Kaplan's Cardiac Anesthesia*. 5th ed. Philadelphia, PA: Elsevier Saunders; 2006:991–992.

H

Hypovolemia Signs: Peds
Subspecialties: Pediatric Anesthesia

Kristin Richards

Edited by Mamatha Punjala

H

1. Physical examination should begin with weighing the child. Severity of hypovolemia is estimated using percent less of body weight (PLBW). PLBW = (Preillness weight − Illness weight)/Preillness weight × 100.
2. With a 5% to 10% (*mild*) loss of body weight, skin and mucous membranes become dry, but may continue to exhibit normal pulse, blood pressure, skin turgor, and fontanelle. There may be signs of increased thirst and reduced urine output.
3. *Moderate* (10% to 15%) dehydration results in tachycardia and orthostatic hypotension as the loss of fluid continues beyond the 5%. Tachypnea occurs as a result of acidosis. Dry buccal mucosa, sunken anterior fontanelle, reduced skin turgor, cool skin, markedly reduced urine output, listlessness, or irritability is noted as dehydration progresses.
4. *Severe* (>15%) hypovolemia manifests as rapid/weak pulse, shock (low BP), deep tachypneic respiration, markedly sunken fontanelle, parched buccal mucosa, mottled cool skin with tenting of skin noted on pinching. Anuria, lethargy, and coma ensue eventually.
5. Urine output is decreased, and an obtained specimen has a specific gravity rising above 1.020. Infants have a relative lack of renal concentrating ability, and the specific gravity in the first 3 months of life may not increase as significantly as it does in older children.

Dehydration/hypovolemia may result from a number of conditions including diarrhea, vomiting, poor oral intake, salt wasting (as may occur with congenital adrenal insufficiency), burns, or even heat stroke, and if left untreated or not corrected appropriately, it may develop into hypovolemic shock. Physical examination of a pediatric patient should include patient's weight, vital signs, and laboratory data including serum electrolytes, blood urea nitrogen, and creatinine.

The first sign of mild dehydration is tachycardia; however, this must be assessed on the basis of the difference from the normal/baseline heart rate. The normal heart rate of an infant is between 100 and 160, a toddler between 90 and 150, a 3 to 5 years old between 80 and 140, a 6 to 12 years old between 70 and 120, and an adolescent between 60 and 100. Tachycardia must also be taken into consideration with the child's clinical picture, in addition to a thorough history, as tachycardia may also present with fever, agitation, pain, or respiratory tract illnesses.

Also, palpation of the infant/child's pulse may be a good indicator of hypovolemia. If one is able to palpate the brachial pulse, tachycardia is unlikely secondary to hypovolemia; however, if one is unable to palpate peripheral pulses, or central pulses are weak (which would be a late sign), such as the femoral pulse, then the patient is likely hypovolemic and/or hypotensive. Of course, absent central pulses would be an indicator to initiate cardiopulmonary resuscitation. Hypotension is a late sign of severe dehydration. Once the child has lost more than 10% of body weight, signs of shock may start to appear. These signs include thready pulse, marked hypotension, and cold, clammy skin.

Dry mucous membranes are also an early sign of dehydration, but this clinical finding can be affected by rapid breathing and ingestion of fluids. However, the severely dehydrated infant may appear ill, lethargic, and irritable and have dry mouth, sunken fontanel, decreased urine output, and absent tears. The skin can be a reliable organ to assess circulation. Cool extremities or delayed capillary refill manifests secondary to a strong peripheral vasomotor response in reaction to decreased circulation and perfusion. In other words, to preserve perfusion of central critical organs, the peripheral vasculature vasoconstricts limiting peripheral perfusion, resulting in cool extremities. Assessment of capillary refill is also a measure of dehydration; however, capillary refill time may be affected by a cool ambient temperature, or naturally prolonged if checked on a child's foot. Compromise to an infant/child's circulation or perfusion can affect perfusion of the vital organs, which can subsequently manifest as hypotension or change in behavior, with decreased cerebral perfusion.

On laboratory evaluation, the initial electrolyte disturbance is often hypernatremia and hyperosmolality, which can result in triggering the renin–angiotensin system and subsequent release of vasopressin, thereby decreasing water excretion from the kidneys. As the child becomes more volume depleted, the patient may become more tachypneic and acidotic. Subsequently, further progression of hypovolemia, and therefore compromise to organ perfusion, can result in stupor, confusion, coma, respiratory compromise secondary to increased work of breathing, cyanotic extremities, and oliguria/anuria. If the patient's condition progresses to hypovolemic shock, the patient would experience a decrease in cardiac output, mean arterial pressure, wedge, and central venous pressure with an increase in systemic vascular resistance.

SUGGESTED READINGS

American Academy of Pediatrics, American College of Emergency Physicians. *APLS: The Pediatric Emergency Medicine Course*. 3rd ed. Washington, DC: American Academy of Pediatrics; 1998:32–43.

Fleisher GR, Ludwig S, eds. *Textbook of Pediatric Emergency Medicine*. Philadelphia, PA: Lippincott Williams & Wilkins; 2010:233–235.

Kliegman RM, Behrman RE, Jenson HB, et al. *Nelson Textbook of Pediatrics*. 18th ed. Philadelphia, PA: Saunders, an imprint of Elsevier; 2007:560, 413–414, 2301–2303.

Morgan GE, Mikhail MS, Murray MJ, eds. *Clinical Anesthesiology*. 4th ed. New York, NY: Lange Medical Books/McGraw-Hill Medical Publishing Division; 2006:937.

Hypox During Pneumonectomy: Rx
Organ-based Clinical: Respiratory

Kimberly Slininger

Edited by Shamsuddin Akhtar

KEY POINTS

1. In case of severe or abrupt onset of hypoxia, notify the surgeon and initiate two lung ventilation.
2. After confirming the correct position of the endotracheal tube (ETT), multiple maneuvers, including increasing the fraction of inspired oxygen and lung recruiting maneuvers (positive end-expiratory pressure [PEEP] and continuous positive airway pressure [CPAP]), can be applied to improve oxygenation when hypoxia is less severe or more gradual in onset.
3. Early clamping/ligation of the pulmonary artery is a treatment of hypoxia during one-lung ventilation (OLV) that is unique to pneumonectomies.

DISCUSSION

The incidence of hypoxia (O_2 sat $< 90\%$) during thoracic procedures is less than 1%. Part of the anesthetic management of patients undergoing pneumonectomy is determining which of those patients are at higher risk for developing intraoperative hypoxia. Patients undergoing right-sided procedures are more likely to develop hypoxia because the right lung receives a greater percentage of the cardiac output and thus creates a larger shunt during one lung ventilation of the left lung. Patient lung function appears to be paradoxically inversely correlated with likelihood of developing hypoxia during OLV. Patients undergoing procedures in the supine position are at higher risk of hypoxia than patients undergoing procedures in the lateral position. Patients undergoing thoracotomy in the lateral decubitus position will all require supplemental oxygen, since approximately 20% to 30% shunt is created. In lateral decubitus position, once the nondependent lung is isolated in preparation for surgical intervention, a shunt is created as it continues to receive a level of perfusion, which is not matched by ventilation.

Intraoperative management of hypoxia during pneumonectomy should be directed not only at treatment, but most importantly at determining the cause which aids in definitive management and resolution of said cause. In the case of severe or abrupt onset of hypoxia, the surgeon should be notified of the situation and two lung ventilation initiated, if feasible. Less severe and gradual onset of hypoxia can be treated through a series of maneuvers. First, the FiO_2 can be increased to 1.0 (100%). Second, placement of the ETT must be checked using fiberoptic bronchoscopy to confirm correct position of the double lumen tube. Also, one must auscultate the lungs to assess if there is wheezing, as bronchospasm may aggravate/initiate hypoxia.

The dependent lung in the lateral decubitus position will unfortunately have decreased compliance with subsequent atelectasis, dead space, and areas of shunt. Theoretically, hypoxic pulmonary vasoconstriction will help decrease the amount of shunt in the nondependent lung. Given the physiological changes, once a patient becomes hypoxic, lung-recruiting maneuvers can be applied to the ventilated lung to recruit atelectatic regions. The application of 5 to 10 cm H_2O of PEEP to the ventilated lung can improve oxygenation of the ventilated lung. In patients with underlying chronic obstructive pulmonary disease (COPD) or other lung diseases involving the ventilated lung, PEEP must be applied judiciously, to prevent shunting of blood away from ventilated areas. Finally, should hypoxia persist despite recruiting atelectatic regions of the dependent lung, one may apply 2 to 5 cm H_2O of CPAP with 100% oxygen. Accordingly, the combination of applying PEEP to the dependent lung, with CPAP to the nonventilated lung, could prove extremely successful in improving arterial oxygenation.

Finally, in patients undergoing pneumonectomy, the ipsilateral pulmonary artery can be clamped or ligated early in the procedure, as this will eliminate the shunt through the nonventilated/operative lung. However, this should really only be reserved for patients who are undergoing total pneumonectomy.

SUGGESTED READINGS

Barash P, Cullen B, Stoelting RK, et al, eds. *Clinical Anesthesia*. 6th ed. Philadelphia, PA: Lippincott Wilkins & Williams; 2009: chap 40:1052.

Hogue CW Jr. Effectiveness of low levels of non-ventilated lung continuous positive airway pressure in improving arterial oxygenation in one lung ventilation. *Anesth Analg*. 1994;79(2):364–367.

Miller RD, Eriksson LI, Fleisher LA, et al, eds. *Miller's Anesthesia*. 7th ed. Philadelphia, PA: Churchill Livingstone; 2009:1849–1853.

Rosenbaum SH, Ruskin KJ, eds. *Emergencies in Anesthesia*. 1st ed. New York, NY: Oxford University Press; 2011:378–380.

Slinger P, Suissa S, Adam J, et al. Predicting arterial oxygenation during one-lung ventilation with continuous positive airway pressure to the non-ventilated lung. *J Cardiothorac Anesth*. 1990;4(4):436–440.

Stoelting RK, Miller RD, eds. *Basics of Anesthesia*. 5th ed. Philadelphia, PA: Churchill Livingstone Elsevier; 2007:422–423.

H

Hypoxemia: Ventilator Management
Subspecialties: Critical Care

Nicholas Dalesio

Edited by Veronica Matei

KEY POINTS

1. Hypoxemia during mechanical ventilation is treated by increasing FIO_2, increasing mean airway pressure, and reducing V/Q mismatch.
2. An increase in FIO_2 increases the concentration of oxygen to the alveoli as determined by the alveolar gas equation.
3. Increasing mean airway pressure can be accomplished by using positive end-expiratory pressure (PEEP), increasing the inspiratory pressure, or increasing the inspiratory time by changing the inspiratory to expiratory ratio.
4. Improved oxygenation can be the result of a reduced V/Q mismatching as a function of a reduction in shunting, or reduced dead-space ventilation from improved alveolar ventilation.
5. V/Q mismatching from atelectasis, pneumonia, and pulmonary edema are causes of shunt.

DISCUSSION

Hypoxemia occurs when a patient's metabolic demands begin to outweigh oxygen supply. Hypoventilation, cardiac right-to-left shunt, and processes that cause a leftward shift in the oxygen–hemoglobin dissociation curve can lead to hypoxemia. Multiple lung diseases including acute lung injury (ALI), acute respiratory distress syndrome (ARDS), chronic obstructive pulmonary disease, V/Q mismatching (atelectasis, pneumonia, and pulmonary edema) can lead to hypoxemia.

Mechanical ventilation is often being performed concomitantly when hypoxemia occurs, otherwise, endotracheal intubation should be considered.

For initial treatment of hypoxemia, patients should be placed on an FIO_2 of 100%. Continuing patients on 100% for prolonged periods can lead to lung injury, and other methods of improving hypoxemia should be utilized. Hypoxemia related to certain medical conditions, such as ARDS, ALI, and right-to-left intracardiac shunts, may not improve with this maneuver.

Mechanical ventilation can be administered with or without endotracheal intubation. Continuous positive airway pressure (CPAP), which can be helpful in postoperative hypoventilation, acute congestive heart failure, and postpneumonectomy patients, acts to recruit alveoli by increasing airway pressure above closing capacity. CPAP differs from PEEP in that PEEP is assisted pressure only after expiration. In patients under positive pressure ventilation, PEEP is often used to recruit collapsed alveoli, leading to decreased dead space. Hypoxemia is improved secondary to increased surface area available for gas exchange. When hypoxemia is related to hypoventilation, increasing tidal volumes will improve hypoxemia. This also allows for alveoli recruitment in the same manner as CPAP and PEEP treatments.

Other maneuvers to improve hypoxemia and recruit alveoli include high-level pressure ventilation (such as airway pressure release ventilation [APRV]), inverse ratio ventilation (allowing for longer inspiratory times), and prone positioning. Studies evaluating these procedures have suggested improvement in hypoxemia; however, none have shown to have significant outcome differences when compared with standard therapies. If hypoxemia is related to disease processes leading to increased fluid within the lung, treatment with diuretics and fluid restriction have shown to be helpful.

Improving blood flow to areas being effectively ventilated can decrease V/Q mismatch, and can allow for more gas exchange. Inhaled nitric oxide is one such maneuver that increases blood flow within the lung and improves hypoxemia.

SUGGESTED
READINGS

Barash P, Cullen B, Stoelting R, et al, eds. *Clinical Anesthesia*. 6th ed. Philadelphia, PA: Lippincott Williams & Wilkins; 2009:1458–1459.

Dunn P. *Clinical Anesthesia Procedures of the Massachusetts General Hospital*. 7th ed. Philadelphia, PA: Lippincott Williams & Wilkins; 2007:311–312, 650.

H

IABP: Contraindications

Organ-based Clinical: Cardiovascular

Kevan Stanton

Edited by Benjamin Sherman

1. When considering placement of an intraaortic balloon pump (IABP), it is also important to consider contraindications to the placement.
2. IABPs can worsen aortic insufficiency and are thus relatively contraindicated in patients with this condition.
3. Severe vascular disease and aortic disease (dissections or aneurysms) can make placement of an IABP difficult and can increase the morbidity/mortality associated with the placement.
4. IABPs are indicated for bridge therapy and should not be placed in patients who are not expected to recover cardiac function, either spontaneously or by surgical intervention.

An IABP is an inflatable balloon on the end of a catheter that is placed percutaneously into the descending thoracic aorta just distal to the subclavian artery. Inflation of an IABP during diastole increases aortic diastolic pressure and thus the mean arterial pressure, improving systemic blood flow and coronary perfusion pressure because most of coronary blood flow occurs during diastole. During systole, balloon deflation results in afterload reduction, improving cardiac output and decreasing myocardial energy expenditure. Accordingly, this method for improving coronary and systemic perfusion is primarily employed in patients with acute myocardial infarction associated with cardiogenic shock, but most importantly in patients with likely reversible cardiac disease, either medically or surgically.

IABPs are sometimes used in the operative setting when multiple attempts at coming off cardiopulmonary bypass are unsuccessful. Left ventricular (LV) failure in the face of appropriate inotropic support that is likely to improve or resolve in 24 to 48 hours is the most common intraoperative indication for placement of an IABP. It may also be used for patients with unstable angina, acute mitral insufficiency, and planned heart transplantation.

Despite its level of usefulness, there are a number of scenarios in which an IABP is contraindicated. One relative contraindication to IABP placement is aortic insufficiency. The retrograde flow created in the ascending aorta by balloon inflation may worsen aortic regurgitation, leading to increased LV distention and decreased coronary artery perfusion. IABP placement is also contraindicated in septic/bacteremic patients because the IABP may become seeded with bacteria, making the infection nearly impossible to treat without removing the IABP.

Severe vascular disease is yet another contraindication to IABP placement. In patients with severe vascular disease, it may be technically difficult to even place the IABP. These patients also have a higher risk of thrombosis with IABP use. Other vascular contraindications include aortic dissection, recent (within 1 year) placement of a prosthetic graft in the thoracic aorta, and patients with aortic aneurysms.

Lastly, IABPs are indicated for bridge therapy; that is, it serves as a means to aid patients through a critical period, after which point improvement or resolution is likely. In patients who have irreversible cardiac disease and are not transplant candidates, IABPs are contraindicated because the likelihood that their cardiac status will improve to the point of being

283

able to remove the IABP is minimal, and an IABP is not a permanent solution. In the same regard, placement of IABP in patients with irreversible brain damage is also contraindicated because it is unlikely to improve their clinical outcome.

SUGGESTED READINGS

Barash PG, Cullen BF, Stoelting RK, et al, eds. *Clinical Anesthesia*. 6th ed. Philadelphia, PA: Lippincott Williams & Wilkins; 2009:1098–1100.
Hensley FA Jr, et al. *A Practical Approach to Cardiac Anesthesia*. 4th ed. Philadelphia, PA: Lippincott Williams & Wilkins; 2008:598–603.
Marino PL. *The ICU Book*. 3rd ed. Philadelphia, PA: Lippincott Williams & Wilkins; 2007:269–271.

Implantable Cardiac Defibrillator: Interventions

Organ-based Clinical: Cardiovascular

Dan Froicu

Edited by Qingbing Zhu

1. Involve consulting cardiologists for perioperative implantable cardiac defibrillator (ICD) management and surgical recommendations.
2. Pre- and postoperative device interrogation may be warranted to confirm ICD function.
3. Suggest usage of bipolar cautery and correct placement of devices with radiofrequency noise.
4. Monitor patient intra- and postoperatively for rhythm and rate changes and communicate cardiac events that occur during surgery.
5. Good communication with the surgical team is key in minimizing the impact of intraoperative electromagnetic and radiofrequency interference.
6. Restore the antitachyarrhythmia functions of the ICD as soon as possible. Have external cardioversion-defibrillation (ECD) available until device function is fully restored.

Patients with ICDs occasionally need surgical interventions similar to other patients. A focused history and examination are mandatory preoperatively. The history should elicit the type of ICD, the manufacturer, the last cardiology consult, and the available information from interrogation of the device and recommendations for the surgery. If electromagnetic interference is anticipated during the procedure, the antitachyarrhythmia functions should be suspended. The use of bipolar cautery, where possible, should be advised. An external cardioverter-defibrillator (ECD) should be available in the operating room.

Intraoperatively, the following interventions are advised: continue ASA standards in monitoring, and use of bipolar cautery and ultrasonic scalpel. The cautery should be used with short bursts at the lowest acceptable energy level. If radiofrequency catheter ablation is contemplated, the radiofrequency current path should be as far as possible from the ICD.

If an emergency defibrillation is needed intraoperatively, all interferences should be stopped. If the ICD was disabled using a magnet, the magnet should be removed to allow the unit to perform appropriately. If the ICD is programming disabled, it should be immediately reprogrammed. In either of these two situations (magnet or programming-disabled ICD), ECD should be available and ready to perform in the Operating Room (OR) in the event that a timely restoration of device function is not possible. The external defibrillator pads/paddles should be as far as possible from the ICD; the pads should be perpendicular to the axis/plane of the ICD leads.

Postoperatively, the patient should continue to have heart rate and rhythm monitored; a different (not the patient's ICD) defibrillator should be available in the patient's room at all times. The patient's ICD should be interrogated by a cardiologist where needed, and the antitachyarrhythmia functions should be restored as soon as possible. A postoperative cardiology/electrophysiology consult should be warranted.

Barash PG, Cullen BF, Stoelting RK, et al, eds. *Clinical Anesthesia*. 6th ed. Philadelphia, PA: Lippincott Williams & Wilkins; 2009:1546–1547.

Incompetent Exp Valve: Signs
Physics, Monitoring, and Anesthesia Delivery

Alexander Timchenko

Edited by Raj K. Modak

1. An incompetent expiratory valve that fails to close will result in rebreathing, manifested by an elevated $ETCO_2$.
2. An incompetent expiratory valve that fails to open will result in barotraumas, manifested by elevated peak airway pressures.

DISCUSSION

There are two unidirectional valves located in the anesthesia gas delivery circuit. The inspiratory valve allows the gas mixture from fresh gas inlet and gas from CO_2 canister into the inspiratory limb of the patient circuit. During the inspiration, the expiratory valve closes, thereby directing the gas through the inspiratory circuit.

There are two possible scenarios involved with an incompetent expiratory valve: when the valve is unable to close and when the valve is unable to open.

	Inspiration	Expiration
Normal valve function	Expiratory valve closes—exhaled gas from ventilator is directed through the CO_2 absorber, mixes with gas from the fresh gas inlet, and enters the inspiratory limb via open unidirectional inspiratory valve.	At the end of inspiration, inspiratory valve closes when pressure in the circuit becomes greater than the pressure in the circuit proximal to the inspiratory valve. Expiratory valve opens and exhaled gas leaves the patient circuit.
Valve remains open	Due to the path of least resistance, gas from ventilator goes in retrograde direction into the expiratory circuit through the incompetent valve. Small portion of the gas from ventilator is passing through the CO_2 canister. This will result in **Rebreathing** (elevation of CO_2 waveform).	At the end of inspiration, inspiratory valve closes when pressure in the circuit becomes greater than the pressure in the circuit proximal to the inspiratory valve. Expiratory valve opens, and exhaled gas leaves the patient circuit.
Valve remains closed	Expiratory valve closed—exhaled gas from ventilator is directed through the CO_2 absorber, mixes with gas from the fresh gas inlet, and enters the inspiratory limb via open unidirectional inspiratory valve.	Expiratory valve in the closed position prevents exhalation. Pressure builds up in the respiratory circuit. If the inspiratory valve is functional (i.e., closed on exhalation), **barotrauma** may occur, heralded by **peak airway pressures** with the potential to result in pneumothorax/ tension pneumothorax.

SUGGESTED READINGS

Morgan GE Jr, Mikhail MS, Murray MJ. *Clinical Anesthesiology.* 4th ed. New York, NY: Lange Medical books/ McGraw Hill; 2006:76–77.

Stoelting RK, Miller RD, eds. *Basics of Anesthesia.* 5th ed. Philadelphia, PA: Churchill Livingstone; 2007:194–196.

Increased ICP: Acute Rx
Organ-based Clinical: Neurologic and Neuromuscular

Ira Whitten

Edited by Ramachandran Ramani

1. Intracranial pressure (ICP) at or above 15 mm Hg is defined as an elevated ICP, also known as intracranial hypertension.
2. $PaCO_2$ and pH are the two important factors that influence cerebral blood flow (CBF) and ICP.
3. Elevations in ICP are initially compensated by displacement of cerebrospinal fluid (CSF) from cranium to spinal area, an increase in CSF absorption, a decrease in CSF production, or a decrease in total cerebral blood volume.
4. Treatment of acute elevations in ICP is directed against the cause of rise in ICP.
5. Loop diuretics, mannitol, and corticosteroids are also required in some cases.
6. Considering the effect of $PaCO_2$ on CBF, hyperventilation may be used as a maneuver for treatment of acute elevations in ICP.

DISCUSSION

Normal ICP is 10 to 15 mm Hg. Any perturbations in ICP, especially moderate-severe ICP (>30 mm Hg), can have a profound effect on cerebral perfusion pressure (CPP), although CPP is more dependent on mean arterial pressure (MAP).

$$CPP = MAP - ICP$$

A constant ICP at or above 15 mm Hg is defined as an elevated ICP, also known as intra-cranial hypertension. In the setting of intracranial hypertension, physiologic changes must occur to alter CPP and thereby maintain CBF. Respiratory gas tensions play a significant role in regulation of CBF and ICP and, in fact, are the most important extrinsic influence on CBF (Fig. 1). Acute changes in $PaCO_2$ have the highest influence, with approximately 1 to 2 mL/100 g/min change in CBF with every millimeter of mercury change in $PaCO_2$. CBF is also influenced by temperature and can also change approximately 5% to 7% for every 1° C change.

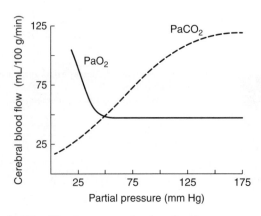

Figure 1. Response of cerebral blood flow to oxygen and carbon dioxide

ICP is also regulated by a variety of compensatory mechanisms, whereby initial increases in intracranial volume are mainly not associated with a rise in ICP. This may be accomplished by the displacement of CSF from the cranium to the spinal area, an increase in CSF absorption, a decrease in CSF production, or a decrease in total cerebral blood volume. Elevations in ICP may be secondary to a mass or fluid (hydrocephalus, intracranial hemorrhage, epidural or subdural hematomas) expanding in size, depressed skull fracture, or blockage of CSF drainage/absorption. With untreated persistent elevations in ICP, CBF is significantly decreased, and this can result in ischemia, which promotes brain edema, subsequently resulting in further increases in ICP. As a result, the cycle must be interrupted to prevent further elevations in ICP that could lead to potential cerebral herniation.

Accordingly, treatment of acute elevations in ICP is directed against the cause. In trauma situations or patients with an acute hemorrhagic event, surgical drainage of the blood/hematoma is definitive management. In cases of obstructing tumors or tumors with associated cerebral edema, primary treatment would be tumor resection if feasible, shunts for palliation for obstructing hydrocephalus if nonresectable, and corticosteroids, such as dexamethasone, for vasogenic tumors to aid decrease swelling. Corticosteroids are also supposed to restore the permeability of the blood–brain barrier in these instances.

Despite the cause, additional measures may be taken, including fluid restriction, diuresis with loop diuretics, or osmotic agents such as mannitol. Loop diuretics take approximately 30 minutes to take effect, and so for rapid decrease in ICP, mannitol (0.25 to 0.5 g per kg) is very effective. An osmotic agent, such as mannitol, works specifically to draw fluid out of a desired space, such as the cranium, by creating an osmotic gradient through which fluid will be drawn out of the parenchyma into the vasculature and, with the help of loop diuretics, excreted via the kidneys (assuming normal renal function). The goal is a serum osmolality of 300 to 315 mOsm per L. The downside of mannitol is that it draws fluid particularly out of normal areas of brain tissue, and can therefore cause rebound edema in areas of altered blood–brain barrier. Also, rapid diuresis has been known to cause subdural hematomas in elderly patients secondary to rupture of bridging veins. Finally, as evidenced by Figure 1, hyperventilation of patients by keeping $PaCO_2$ between 30 and 33 mm Hg will reduce CBF and therefore reduce ICP.

SUGGESTED READINGS

Barash P, Cullen BF, Stoelting RK, et al. *Clinical Anesthesia*. 6th ed. Philadelphia, PA: Lippincott Williams & Wilkins; 2009:222–229.

Morgan GE Jr, Mikhail MS, Murray MJ. *Clinical Anesthesiology*. 4th ed. New York, NY: Lange Medical Books/ McGraw-Hill; 2006:614–618, 631–632.

Inhalational Anesthesia: Resp Effects and Ventilatory Effects

Pharmacology

Brooke Albright and Xing Fu

Edited by Raj K. Modak

1. The use of volatile anesthetics usually results in only a mild reduction of minute ventilation through a decrease in tidal volume and a concomitant increase in respiratory rate.
2. The ventilatory effects of volatile agents are Minimum alveolar concentration (MAC) dependent, and one will see a greater decrease in tidal volume and a greater rise in respiratory rate with higher concentrations. The exception to this is isoflurane at concentrations above 1 MAC.
3. Nitrous oxide is also known to increase respiratory rate and decrease tidal volume. This effect is secondary to central nervous system simulation and, perhaps, the activation of pulmonary stretch receptors.
4. Hypoxic drive, the ventilatory response to arterial hypoxia that is mediated by peripheral chemoreceptors in the carotid bodies, is markedly depressed by even small amounts of inhalational agents, but has minimal effect on hypercapnic respiratory drive.

The use of volatile anesthetics usually results in only a mild reduction of minute ventilation through a decrease in tidal volume and a concomitant increase in respiratory rate. These effects are MAC dependent, and one will see a greater decrease in tidal volume and a greater rise in respiratory rate with higher concentrations of volatile inhaled agents. Isoflurane is the one exception to this rule, as at concentrations above 1 MAC, it does not continue to increase respiratory rate. As the overall change is a mild decrease in minute ventilation, there is also an associated increase in resting $PaCO_2$. However, the stimulation associated with surgery may offset the depressive effects of inhaled agents and cause increases in both respiratory rate and tidal volume and, therefore, cause a reduction in resting $PaCO_2$ instead.

Nitrous oxide is also known to increase respiratory rate and decrease tidal volume. This effect is secondary to central nervous system simulation and, perhaps, the activation of pulmonary stretch receptors. The net effect is nominal change in minute ventilation and resting $PaCO_2$ level. Nitrous oxide used in conjunction with volatile agents, desflurane and sevoflurane, results in a decreased $PaCO_2$ when compared with equal MAC concentrations of those inhaled agents in oxygen.

Hypoxic drive, the ventilatory response to arterial hypoxia that is mediated by peripheral chemoreceptors in the carotid bodies, is markedly depressed by even small amounts of inhalational agents, but has minimal effect on hypercapnic respiratory drive.

Barash PG, Cullen BF, Stoelting RK, et al, eds. *Clinical Anesthesia*. 5th ed. Philadelphia, PA: Lippincott Williams & Wilkins; 2006:432.

Hines RL, Marschall KE, eds. *Stoelting's Anesthesia and Co-existing Disease*. 5th ed. Philadelphia, PA: Saunders Elsevier; 2002:127–128.

Morgan GE, Mikhail MS, Murray MJ. *Clinical Anesthesiology*. 4th ed. New York, NY: McGraw-Hill; 2005:164, 169, 172–173.

Intravascular: Extracellular Volume Ratio
Physiology

Jorge Galvez

Edited by Ala Haddadin

1. Total body water is distributed among three compartments: intravascular, interstitial, and intracellular.
2. Intravascular volume only accounts for 4% to 6% of total body water.
3. Osmotic pressure gradients influence the distribution of total body water.

DISCUSSION

Total body water is distributed between two compartments: intracellular and extracellular, the latter is subdivided into intravascular and interstitial. The distribution of water among the three compartments is influenced by osmotic forces, solute concentrations, and the permeability of the membranes between the compartments to the solutes present. The relationship between the three compartments also varies with age and sex (Table 1).

Table 1. Body Water Distribution Relative to Lean Body Weight

	Men (%)	Women (%)	Term Infant (%)
Intracellular compartment	40	33	50
Extracellular compartment	20	17	25
Intravascular space	5	4	6
Interstitial space	15	12	19
Total body water	60	50	70–75

The effective intravascular volume is subject to regulation by:

- baroreceptors in the aortic arch and carotid sinus, which regulate sympathetic activity;
- atria and ventricles, which release natriuretic peptides if increased wall tension is sensed;
- baroreceptors in the juxtaglomerular apparatus, which regulate the renin–angiotensin pathway;
- hypothalamus, which regulates serum osmolarity (275 to 295 mOsm per kg) by stimulating thirst or extraction to regulate plasma Na^+ concentration.

Assessment of fluid balance must take all factors into account, including medical history, perioperative history, preoperative volume status, fluid loss (evaporative, blood loss, urine output, gastric suctioning), third-space losses, duration of surgery, type of anesthesia, and fluid replacement therapy (crystalloid, colloid, blood products).

Monitoring of intravascular volume may be achieved with noninvasive or invasive monitors. Noninvasive monitoring includes physical examination findings such as jugular venous filling, orthostatic hypotension, tachycardia, skin turgor, and the appearance of mucous membranes. Hypovolemia leads to reduced tissue perfusion, which results in reduced urine output, confusion, and somnolence/coma. Hypervolemia results in hypertension, pulmonary edema, arrhythmias (atrial fibrillation secondary to atrial stretch), increased urine output, jugular venous distention. Advanced hemodynamic and invasive monitors include arterial blood pressure, blood gas analysis, central venous pressure, pulmonary artery wedge pressure, cardiac index, systemic vascular resistance, stroke volume, mixed venous oxygen saturation, and echocardiography (transthoracic or transesophageal).

SUGGESTED READING

Miller RD. *Miller's Anesthesia*. 7th ed. (online edition). Philadelphia, PA: Churchill Livingstone Elsevier; 2009:2783–2804.

Intubation in Pierre-Robin
Subspecialties: Pediatrics

Christina Biello

Edited by Mamatha Punjala

KEY POINTS

1. Pierre-Robin syndrome is characterized by micrognathia, a hypoplastic mandible and pseudomacroglossia.
2. Anesthetic management involves preparation for a difficult airway.
3. Difficulty in intubating these patients with a standard direct laryngoscopy is due to the hypoplastic mandible and difficulty pushing the posteriorly located tongue and other tissue into that limited space.

DISCUSSION

Pierre-Robin sequence is defined as micrognathia due to a hypoplastic mandible, glossoptosis with a caudally displaced insertion of the tongue, and therefore a pseudomacroglossia. Patients with Pierre-Robin sequence can also have high-arched cleft palates. The pathology begins in the 9th week of in utero development, when mandibular hypoplasia causes a posteriorly located tongue and impairment of the closure of the posterior soft palate.

The safest approach to the management of the difficult airway of Pierre-Robin or any other known difficult or challenging airway is to have a plan formulating the steps and having special equipment readily available in the event of failed mask ventilation or endotracheal intubation. Having surgical colleagues skilled in bronchoscopy and tracheostomy in the room is advisable. Some steps that may need to be performed to alleviate the airway obstruction include prone positioning, nasal pharyngeal airway, suturing the tongue to the bottom lip, and jaw thrust. If these maneuvers fail to relieve the obstruction and endotracheal intubation is impossible, a tracheostomy should be performed.

SUGGESTED READINGS

Cote CJ, Lerman J, Todres ID. *A Practice of Anesthesia for Infants and Children.* 4th ed. Philadelphia, PA: Saunders-Elsevier; 2009:276, 709.
Smith D. *Smith's Recognizable Patterns of Human Malformation.* 4th ed. Philadelphia, PA: Saunders-Elsevier; 2006:262.

Isoflurane: CMRO$_2$ Effect

Pharmacology

Amit Mirchandani

Edited by Ramachandran Ramani

KEY POINTS

1. At concentrations greater than 1 MAC, isoflurane is a cerebrovasodilator that increases cerebral blood flow (CBF) and intracranial pressure (ICP).
2. Of the volatile anesthetics, isoflurane is the least powerful cerebrovasodilator, but the most potent depressant of CMRO$_2$.

DISCUSSION

Halothane, enflurane, sevoflurane, desflurane, and isoflurane all have direct vasodilatory effects, which increase CBF. At equal anesthetic potency, isoflurane causes the smallest increase in CBF. The significance of increased CBF comes into play with a patient who has increased ICP. Since volatile anesthetics increase CBF, they would subsequently increase ICP under conditions of abnormal intracranial elastance. Thus, in the case of a patient with a high ICP, it would be important to use the volatile agent that would have the least increase in CBF, such as isoflurane.

Although isoflurane is one of the least powerful vasodilators, it is the most powerful depressant of cerebral metabolic requirement of oxygen consumption (CMRO$_2$). Isoflurane decreases cerebral metabolic oxygen requirements in a dose-dependent fashion, and at 2 MAC, it may produce an electrically silent electroencephalogram (EEG). There is no additional decrease in cerebral metabolic rate once an isoelectric EEG is achieved. This metabolic effect of isoflurane helps in minimizing its effect on CBF.

SUGGESTED READINGS

Barash PG, Cullen BF, Stoelting RK, eds. *Clinical Anesthesia*. 5th ed. Philadelphia, PA: Lippincott Williams & Wilkins; 2006:752.

Morgan GE, Mikhail MS, Murray MJ. *Clinical Anesthesiology*. 4th ed. Philadelphia, PA: McGraw-Hill Professional; 2005:169.

Newfield P, Cottrell JE, eds. *Handbook of Neuroanesthesia*. 4th ed. Philadelphia, PA: Lippincott Williams and Wilkins; 2007:30–31.

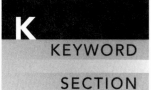

Ketamine: Pharmacodynamics

Pharmacology

Trevor Banack

Edited by Thomas Halaszynski

KEY POINTS

1. Ketamine binds noncompetitively to the *N*-methyl-D-aspartate (NMDA) receptor.
2. The analgesic effects of ketamine are primarily due to its activity in the thalamic and limbic systems of the central nervous system.
3. Cardiovascular effects of ketamine resemble sympathetic nervous system stimulation.
4. Ketamine has minimal respiratory depression effects and causes no change in the ventilatory response to carbon dioxide.
5. One of the major drawbacks of using ketamine is the increased incidence of emergence delirium.

DISCUSSION

Ketamine is a derivative of phencyclidine that causes a "dissociative anesthesia" witnessed on electroencephalogram (EEG) as the dissociation between the thalamocortical system and the limbic system. There are two optical isomers of ketamine: S(+)-ketamine and R(–)-ketamine. Ketamine binds noncompetitively to the NMDA receptor. It has also been recognized that ketamine may exert effects at other sites including opioid receptors, monoaminergic receptors, muscarinic receptors, voltage-sensitive sodium channels, and L-type calcium channels. The analgesic effects of ketamine are primarily due to its activity in the thalamic and limbic systems. The thalamic and cortical systems are important in processing painful stimuli. In the spinal cord, NMDA receptor activation results in spinal cord sensitization. NMDA receptor antagonism with the use of ketamine can decrease spinal cord sensitization and reduce postoperative pain.

Ketamine is reported to be a potent cerebral vasodilator capable of increasing cerebral blood flow by 60% in the presence of normocapnia. However, it was shown in mechanically ventilated animals with increased ICP that there was no further increase in ICP after ketamine was given. The use of ketamine results in decreased alpha rhythm and increased theta activity on EEG. Onset of delta activity coincides with loss of consciousness.

Cardiovascular effects of ketamine resemble sympathetic nervous system, stimulation. Systemic and pulmonary arterial blood pressure, heart rate, cardiac output, cardiac work, and myocardial oxygen requirements are increased after intravenous ketamine administration. The direct stimulation of the central nervous system, leading to increased sympathetic nervous system outflow, seems to be the most important mechanism for cardiovascular stimulation.

Ketamine has minimal respiratory depression effects and causes no change in the ventilatory response to carbon dioxide. Ketamine causes bronchodilation and has been used to treat bronchospasm. Antisialagogues are often used before ketamine administration because of increased salivary and tracheobronchial gland secretions.

One of the major drawbacks of using ketamine is the increased incidence of emergence delirium. Other possible postoperative ketamine side effects include auditory, proprioceptive, and visual illusions. Incidence of ketamine-induced emergence delirium ranges from 5% to 30%. The most effective prevention of emergence delirium is with the use of benzodiazepines or opioids. It has been reported that having a preoperative discussion with the patient about potential ketamine side effects has also decreased the incidence of emergence delirium.

294

SUGGESTED READINGS

Hirota K, Lambert DG. Ketamine: its mechanism(s) of action and unusual clinical uses. *Br J Anaesth.* 1996;77:441–444.

Kohrs R, Durieux ME. Ketamine: teaching an old drug new tricks. *Anesth Analg.* 1998;87:1186–1193.

Pfenninger E, Dick W, Ahnefeld FW. The influence of ketamine on both normal and raised intracranial pressure of artificially ventilated animals. *Eur J Anaesthesiol.* 1985;2:297–307.

Reich DL, Silvay G. Ketamine: an update on the first twenty-five years of clinical experience. *Can J Anaesth.* 1989;36:186–197.

Stoetling RK, Hiller SC, eds. *Pharmacology and Physiology in Anesthetic Practice.* 4th ed. Philadelphia, PA: Lippincott Williams & Wilkins; 2006.

Takeshita H, Okuda Y, Sari A. The effects of ketamine on cerebral circulation and metabolism in man. *Anesthesiology.* 1972;36:69–75.

Wagner LE, Gingrich KJ, Kulli JG, et al. Ketamine blockade of voltage gated sodium channels: evidence for a shared receptor site with local anesthetics. *Anesthesiology.* 2001;95:1406–1413.

White PF, Way WL, Trevor AJ. Ketamine: its pharmacology and therapeutic uses. *Anesthesiolgy.* 1982;56:119–136.

Wong DH, Jenkins LC. An experimental study of the mechanism of action of ketamine on the central nervous system. *Can Anaesth Soc J.* 1974;21:57–67.

Ketamine Analgesic Mechanism
Subspecialties: Pain

Emilio Andrade

Edited by Thomas Halaszynski

K

KEY POINTS

1. Ketamine is a water-soluble phencyclidine derivative that produces dissociative anesthesia.
2. Dissociative anesthesia is produced by interrupting the transmission of impulses from the thalamus to the limbic system.
3. Ketamine binds noncompetitively at *N*-methyl-D-aspartate (NMDA) receptors, blocking activation by glutamate.
4. Analgesia can be achieved with ketamine doses of 0.2 to 0.5 mg per kg intravenously (IV), but the standard dose for induction of anesthesia is 1 to 2 mg per kg IV.

DISCUSSION

Ketamine is a water-soluble phencyclidine derivative that exists as two optical isomers: S(+)-ketamine and R(–)-ketamine, where the S(+) isomer is more potent than the R(–) isomer. In the United States, a racemic mixture of ketamine is the only available form. The S(+) isomer of ketamine racemic solutions produces more analgesia than the R(–) isomer.

Ketamine produces a dissociative anesthesia by interrupting the transmission of impulses from the thalamus to the limbic system. The thalamus is involved in the transmission of sensory impulses, whereas the limbic system is involved with the processing and interpretation of these stimuli. Ketamine is also an antagonist at NMDA receptors. NMDA receptors are located in the spinal cord dorsal horn and are crucial in pain modulation and processing. NMDA receptors are activated by the excitatory neurotransmitter glutamate, which is abundant in the central nervous system. Ketamine binds noncompetitively to the NMDA receptor, and therefore blocks activation of NMDA receptors by glutamate. Ketamine potentiates the effects of gamma aminobutyric acid (GABA) as well, and there is a mild local anesthetic effect of ketamine secondary to binding with voltage-gated sodium channels.

Ketamine is used for induction of anesthesia at higher doses than those required for analgesia. Analgesia can be achieved with 0.2 to 0.5 mg per kg IV of ketamine, whereas anesthesia can be achieved only with an induction dose of 1 to 2 mg per kg IV or 5 to 10 mg per kg IM of ketamine. Ketamine can be a useful adjuvant to reduce narcotic requirements while managing postoperative pain or chronic pain. Ketamine increases blood pressure, heart rate, and cardiac output, but has minimal effects on respiratory drive.

SUGGESTED READINGS

Morgan G, Mikhail M, Murray M, eds. *Clinical Anesthesiology*. 4th ed. New York, NY: Lange Medical Books/McGraw-Hill; 2006:197–199.
Stoelting RK, Hillier SC, eds. *Pharmacology & Physiology in Anesthetic Practice*. 4th ed. Philadelphia, PA: Lippincott Williams & Wilkins; 2006:167–170.
Stoelting R, Miller R. *Basics of Anesthesia*. 5th ed. Philadelphia, PA: Churchill Livingstone; 2007:106–108.

Ketamine Receptor Effects

Pharmacology

Tori Myslajek

Edited by Jodi Sherman

KEY POINTS

1. Ketamine is an anesthetic drug that produces both amnesia and analgesia.
2. The effects of ketamine are thought to occur primarily via inhibitory actions at N-methyl-D-aspartate (NMDA) receptors, thereby decreasing presynaptic release of glutamate and potentiating the inhibitory effects of gamma aminobutyric acid.
3. It is thought that some of the effects of ketamine also come from actions at opioid receptors, monoaminergic receptors, muscarinic receptors, and voltage-sensitive sodium and L-type calcium channels.

DISCUSSION

Ketamine is a phencyclidine derivative that produces amnesia and intense analgesia, unlike other anesthetics. It produces a phenomenon termed *dissociative anesthesia* that is characterized by electroencephalogram evidence of thalamocortical and limbic system dissociation. Clinically, the patient appears to be cataleptic and noncommunicative, but wakeful with a nystagmic gaze. Frequently, there are hypertonic and purposeful movements that do not correlate with surgical stimulation. Favorable characteristics include high lipid solubility with rapid onset, minimal respiratory depression, and bronchodilation. Unfavorable characteristics include emergence delirium, hallucinations, and distorted visual and auditory sensation.

Ketamine acts primarily via NMDA receptors, where it participates in noncompetitive binding to the phencyclidine site. These receptors are ligand-gated ion channels that bind glutamate with glycine as a coagonist. By inhibiting NMDA receptors, ketamine decreases presynaptic release of glutamate, thereby potentiating the inhibitory effects of gamma aminobutyric acid. This appears to be the source of its general anesthetic effects, in addition to some of the analgesic effects.

Ketamine is thought to exert effects via several additional receptors including opioid receptors (mu, delta, and kappa in both the brain and the spinal cord), monoaminergic receptors, muscarinic receptors, and voltage-sensitive sodium and L-type calcium channels. Furthermore, it is thought that ketamine suppresses the production of inflammatory mediators by neutrophils and directly inhibits cytokines, possibly contributing to its analgesic properties.

Anesthesia by ketamine is antagonized by anticholinesterase drugs. It is suggested that the anticholinergic symptoms of ketamine, such as emergence delirium and bronchodilation, result from antagonist effects at muscarinic receptors.

Ketamine shares a binding site with local anesthetics at voltage-gated sodium channels. Although ketamine is noted to have mild local anesthetic–like properties, this does not appear to be the source of its anesthetic effects. Finally, unlike other intravenous anesthetics such as propofol and etomidate, ketamine has a weak action at $GABA_A$ receptors.

SUGGESTED READINGS

Miller RD, Eriksson LI, Fleisher LA, et al. *Miller's Anesthesia*. 6th ed. Philadelphia, PA: Churchill Livingstone; 2005:345–350.

Stoelting RK, Hillier SC. *Pharmacology & Physiology in Anesthetic Practice*. 4th ed. Philadelphia, PA: Lippincott Williams & Wilkins; 2006:167–168.

K

Ketorolac: Renal Function and Dysfunction

Pharmacology and Organ-based Clinical: Renal Urinary/Electrolytes

Holly Barth and Donald Neirink

Edited by Thomas Halaszynski

KEY POINTS

1. Ketorolac is a cyclooxygenase (COX) inhibitor that leads to inhibition of prostaglandin synthesis, and is an excellent choice for postoperative pain (can be used alone or in conjunction with opioids).
2. Ketorolac inhibits the cyclooxygenase-1 (COX-1) enzyme, thereby leading to the inhibition of prostaglandin synthesis and renal protection.
3. Impaired prostaglandin activity can result in a decreased glomerular filtration rate, decreased renal blood flow, and increased renal vascular resistance.
4. Inhibition of prostaglandin synthesis secondary to ketorolac in a patient with renal impairment may result in hyperkalemia.

DISCUSSION

Ketorolac is a nonsteroidal anti-inflammatory agent (NSAID) that can be used for the control and pain management of mild-to-moderate pain (postoperative) and/or as part of a multimodal approach in severe pain management. The primary mechanism that NSAIDs have for analgesia is through the inhibition of COX, which results in the inhibition of prostaglandin synthesis. NSAIDs can be used in conjunction with opioids to create a multimodal approach to the control of postoperative pain.

Ketorolac inhibits the COX-1 enzyme, and therefore inhibits prostaglandin synthesis for approximately 8 to 24 hours. As a result, the renal protective function of prostaglandins is inhibited as well. Impaired prostaglandin activity may result in a decreased glomerular filtration rate, decreased renal blood flow, increased renal vascular resistance, and hyperkalemia (secondary to the reduced excretion of potassium). Inhibiting prostaglandin synthesis can also cause renal medullary ischemia.

Nephrotoxicity can be initiated in the ischemic kidneys, but not necessarily in the normal kidneys. In addition, ketorolac is eliminated by the kidneys and should be avoided in patients with renal failure. Additional adverse effects of NSAIDs in patients with underlying kidney disease include increased venous pressure, low cardiac output, and endotoxemia.

In young, healthy patients, the use of ketorolac as the sole drug for postoperative analgesia is unlikely to cause renal toxicity. However, such a risk increases greatly in the event that other nephrotoxic agents, such as aminoglycosides or intravenous contrast dye, are administered together. The risk for nephrotoxicity may also be increased in patients with underlying hypovolemia, congestive heart failure, sepsis, and preexisting renal dysfunction.

SUGGESTED READINGS

Barash PG, Cullen BF, Stoelting RK, et al, eds. *Clinical Anesthesia.* 6th ed. Philadelphia, PA: Lippincott Williams & Wilkins; 2009:1484–1485.

Miller RD, ed. *Miller's Anesthesia.* 6th ed. Philadelphia, PA: Elsevier, Churchill, and Livingstone; 2006:803, 2719–2720.

Stoelting RK, Hillier SC, eds. *Pharmacology & Physiology in Anesthetic Practice.* 4th ed. Philadelphia, PA: Lippincott Williams & Wilkins; 2006:281.

Lambert–Eaton Syndrome: Physiology
Physiology

Meredith Brown

Edited by Jodi Sherman

KEY POINTS

1. Lambert–Eaton syndrome is an autoimmune condition that is commonly associated with neoplasms such as small cell lung cancer.
2. Antibodies are produced against presynaptic voltage-gated calcium channels, resulting in a decrease in the amount of acetylcholine released with nerve stimulation.
3. Manifestations of Lambert–Eaton syndrome include proximal muscle weakness and autonomic dysfunction.
4. Improvement of the symptoms of Lambert–Eaton syndrome may occur with treatment of the underlying neoplasms, 3,4-diaminopyridine, immunosuppression, plasmapheresis, and intravenous immunoglobulin (IVIG).
5. The symptoms of Lambert–Eaton syndrome resemble those of myasthenia gravis, but there are many key differences between the disorders.

DISCUSSION

Lambert–Eaton syndrome is a myasthenic syndrome that is associated with carcinomas, most notably small cell lung cancer and lymphoproliferative diseases; however, the syndrome has also been described in patients without evidence of neoplasms. Lambert–Eaton syndrome results from autoimmune production of antibodies against voltage-gated calcium ion channels that are located at the motor endplate. When depolarization occurs at these endplates, the amount of calcium released is decreased, resulting in muscle weakness.

The hallmark symptom occurring in Lambert–Eaton syndrome is proximal extremity weakness that improves with exercise. Autonomic dysfunction including orthostatic hypotension, impotence, constipation, xerostomia, and altered sweating may also occur. Treatment of the underlying neoplasm may improve the manifestations of the syndrome. 3,4-Diaminopyridine, which prolongs the action potential and increases acetylcholine release, as well as immunosuppression, plasmapheresis, and IVIG, may aid in treatment of the symptoms of Lambert–Eaton syndrome. Patients with this syndrome may demonstrate increased sensitivity to succinylcholine and nondepolarizing muscle relaxants.

Lambert–Eaton syndrome resembles myasthenia gravis, but there are many differences between them. Lambert–Eaton syndrome more commonly affects males, whereas myasthenia gravis is more common in female patients. Muscle groups most commonly affected differ between the disorders, with proximal limb weakness most prominent in Lambert–Eaton syndrome, and extraocular and facial muscle weakness most prominent in myasthenia gravis. Patients with myasthenia gravis respond well to therapy with anticholinesterase drugs, whereas patients with Lambert–Eaton syndrome will not see an improvement in symptoms with this therapy.

SUGGESTED READINGS

Barash PG, Cullen BF, Stoelting RK, et al. *Clinical Anesthesia*. 6th ed. Philadelphia, PA: Lippincott Williams & Wilkins; 2009:627–628.

Hines RL, Marschall KE, eds. *Stoelting's Anesthesia and Co-existing Disease*. 5th ed. Philadelphia, PA: Churchill Livingstone; 2008:454–455.

Laparoscopy: Increased PaCO$_2$

Generic, Clinical Sciences: Anesthesia Procedures, Methods, Techniques

Adrianna Oprea

Edited by Lars Helgeson

KEY POINTS

1. During laparoscopy, the increase in PaCO$_2$ is due to carbon dioxide (CO$_2$) absorption across the peritoneal mucosa.
2. Elevated intraabdominal pressure and procedure duration both increase the rate of CO$_2$ absorption.
3. Hypoventilation due to smaller tidal volumes, coupled with decreased mobility of the diaphragm, worsens the ventilation–perfusion (V/Q) mismatch, which contributes to increased PaCO$_2$.

DISCUSSION

Laparoscopic pneumoperitoneum is accomplished with pressurized CO$_2$. This insufflation leads to hemodynamic, pulmonary, renal, splanchnic, and endocrine pathophysiologic changes, most of which are not clinically significant. In some situations, complications can develop depending on the intraabdominal pressure, amount of CO$_2$ absorbed, circulatory volume of the patient, ventilation technique used, underlying pathologic conditions, and type of anesthesia.

Hypercarbia occurs when CO$_2$ production and absorption exceeds its elimination. CO$_2$ is highly soluble and very rapidly absorbed from the peritoneal cavity into the circulation. This absorption, combined with smaller tidal volumes and increased V/Q mismatch, leads to increased arterial CO$_2$ levels and decreased pH. The amount of CO$_2$ absorbed from the peritoneal cavity during pneumoperitoneum at typical pressures is equivalent to adding 5% to 25% to the body's baseline metabolic CO$_2$ production. Subcutaneous emphysema, elevated intraabdominal pressure, and increased duration of insufflation increase the amount of CO$_2$ absorbed.

Hypercarbia may develop as a result of increased peritoneal absorption of CO$_2$ and/or decreased elimination of CO$_2$. Absorption of CO$_2$ is increased particularly during prolonged surgery using high intraabdominal pressure. Elimination of CO$_2$ is reduced in patients with compromised cardiopulmonary function and decreased minute ventilation. In addition, ventilation is impeded by Trendelenburg position and high intraabdominal pressure, which causes a cephalad displacement of the diaphragm and worsening V/Q mismatch. Severe hypercarbia may develop despite aggressive hyperventilation.

Moderate hypercarbia has a stimulatory effect by direct action on the cardiovascular system and by an indirect action through sympathoadrenal stimulation. However, when PaCO$_2$ exceeds 60 mm Hg, cardiodepressive effects develop, resulting in decreased cardiac contractility, increased sensitivity of the myocardium to the arrhythmogenic effects of catecholamines, and systemic vasodilatation. Cardiovascular collapse, acidosis, and fatal dysrhythmias may occur.

PaCO$_2$ is estimated intraoperatively by the capnographic measurement of the partial pressure of end-tidal CO$_2$, which is generally 3 to 5 mm Hg lower than PaCO$_2$ during general anesthesia. Because absorbed CO$_2$ can be effectively eliminated only via the lungs, hypercarbia can be minimized by adjusting the ventilator settings (hyperventilation, positive end-expiratory pressure [PEEP]).

SUGGESTED READINGS

Barash PG, Cullen BF, Stoelting RK. *Clinical Anesthesia.* 5th ed. Philadelphia, PA: Lippincott Williams & Wilkins; 2006:1064–1068.

Morgan GE, Mikhail MS, Murray MJ. *Clinical Anesthesiology.* 4th ed. New York, NY: McGraw-Hill; 2005:582–583.

Laryngospasm Mechanism

Anatomy

Anna Clebone

Edited by Jodi Sherman

1. Any stimulation of the airway can cause laryngospasm, an involuntary and sudden closure of the vocal cords.
2. Sensory innervation to the pharynx is provided by the glossopharyngeal nerve (CN IX), and sensory innervation to the larynx is provided by branches of the vagus nerve (CN X).
3. Motor innervation to most of the pharynx and larynx, including the muscles responsible for laryngospasm, is via the accessory nerve (CN XI).
4. Initial treatment of laryngospasm is undertaken by the application of positive pressure to the airway with 100% oxygen.

Laryngospasm is a sudden closing of the vocal cords, resulting in the inability to ventilate. The negative intrathoracic pressure generated by the patient while attempting to breathe against the closed vocal cords can cause negative pressure pulmonary edema. Any stimulation of the airway above or including the vocal cords can cause laryngospasm.

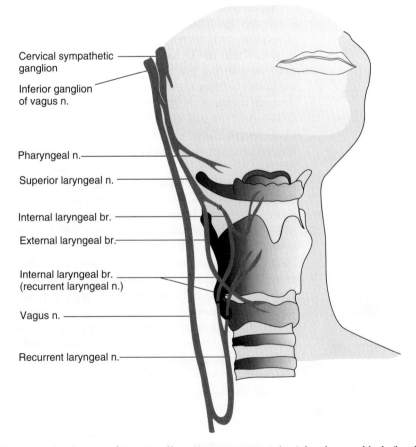

Cervical sympathetic ganglion

Inferior ganglion of vagus n.

Pharyngeal n.

Superior laryngeal n.

Internal laryngeal br.

External laryngeal br.

Internal laryngeal br. (recurrent laryngeal n.)

Vagus n.

Recurrent laryngeal n.

Figure 1. Laryngeal innervation. (Courtesy of http://www.nysora.com/peripheral_nerve_blocks/head_and_neck_block/3049-regional-topical-anesthesia-endotracheal-intubation.html.)

Sensory innervation to the pharynx is provided by the glossopharyngeal nerve (CN IX), and sensory innervation to the larynx is provided by branches of the vagus nerve (CN X) (Fig. 1). Above the vocal cords, the internal branch of the superior laryngeal nerve innervates the larynx, whereas below (and inclusive of) the vocal cords, the recurrent laryngeal nerve innervates the larynx. The superior laryngeal nerve (a branch of CN X) divides into the external laryngeal nerve and the internal laryngeal nerve. The inferior laryngeal nerve is also known as the recurrent laryngeal nerve.

Potential instigators of laryngospasm during induction and emergence of anesthesia include blood, secretions, in situ airway devices, or manipulations such as oropharyngeal suctioning and deflation–inflation of the endotracheal tube cuff. These can trigger the motor activation of the lateral cricoarytenoids, the thyroarytenoid, and the cricothyroid muscles, closing the vocal cords. Motor innervation of most of the pharynx and larynx, including the muscles responsible for laryngospasm, is via CN XI, the accessory nerve. The exception to motor innervation of the pharynx and larynx by CN XI is the stylopharyngeus muscle, which is innervated by the glossopharyngeal nerve. Anesthesiologists can attempt to prevent laryngospasm by performing extubations when patients are deeply anesthetized or fully awake; however, it may still occur. Treatment of laryngospasm is undertaken by the application of positive pressure to the airway with 100% oxygen. If this fails to break the laryngospasm, the patient can be treated with intravenous lidocaine or propofol to deepen sedation, or succinylcholine to quickly relax muscles.

SUGGESTED READINGS

Barash PG, Cullen BF, Stoelting RK, et al, eds. *Clinical Anesthesia*. 6th ed. Philadelphia, PA: Lippincott Williams & Wilkins; 2009:669–770, 1428–1429.

Moore K, Agur AMR. *Essential Clinical Anatomy*. 2nd ed. Philadelphia, PA: Lippincott Williams & Wilkins; 2002:606–642.

Morgan GE, Mikhail MS, Murray MJ. *Clinical Anesthesiology*. 4th ed. New York, NY: Lange/McGraw-Hill; 2006:111.

Laryngospasm Treatment Options
Generic Clinical Sciences: Anesthesia Procedures, Methods, Techniques

Frederick Conlin

Edited by Mamatha Punjala

1. Laryngospasm is a potentially disastrous complication of general anesthesia that the clinician must be prepared to diagnose and treat rapidly.
2. Attempting to "break" the laryngospasm with continuous 10 to 20 cm of H_2O positive pressure ventilation is usually the first step in treatment.
3. Laryngospasm that does not respond to continuous positive pressure ventilation may be treated with intravenous or subcutaneous succinylcholine, intravenous lidocaine, increasing the depth of anesthesia, or tracheal reintubation (to stent open the vocal cords).

Laryngospasm is a brief spasm of the vocal cords that temporarily makes it difficult to speak or breathe. Laryngospasm is a potentially disastrous complication of general anesthesia seen in the perioperative period, especially during intubation and extubation. The clinician must anticipate and be prepared to rapidly diagnose and treat. It occurs when the superior laryngeal nerve is irritated by the presence of blood, saliva, a foreign body, or reactive airway, as seen in cases of upper respiratory tract infection, while the patient is in the second stage of anesthesia; however, there are case reports of laryngospasm occurring in awake patients, usually associated with gastroesophageal reflux disease. The stimulation results in spasm and closure of the glottis, prohibiting air movement and gas exchange. Possible sequelae include negative pressure pulmonary edema, hypoxia, and cardiac arrest. For this reason, patients should be extubated either after demonstrating that they are fully awake or while they are deeply anesthetized.

The first step in the treatment of laryngospasm is gentle continuous positive pressure ventilation with 100% oxygen. This may be augmented with chin lift, jaw thrust, and an oral or nasal airway if necessary. Should positive pressure ventilation fail to achieve air movement, then either intravenous lidocaine or succinylcholine (intramuscularly or intravenously) may be administered. In addition, establishing a deeper level of anesthesia with intravenous induction agents or inhalational agents may also be helpful to relieve laryngospasm. The definitive treatment is reintubation and extubation with the patient fully awake. Finally, case reports of bilateral laryngeal nerve blocks for refractory laryngospasm exist in the literature.

Barash PG, Cullen BF, Stoelting RK. *Clinical Anesthesia.* 6th ed. Philadelphia, PA: Lippincott Williams & Wilkins; 2009:1428–1429.

Mevorach DL. The management and treatment of recurrent postoperative laryngospasm. *Anesth Analg.* 1996;83(5):1110–1111.

Morgan GE, Mikhail MS, Murray MJ. *Clinical Anesthesiology.* 4th ed. New York, NY: McGraw Hill; 2005:938–939.

Laser-safe Endotracheal Tubes

Generic Clinical Sciences: Anesthesia Procedures, Methods, Techniques

Thomas Gallen

Edited by Raj K. Modak

KEY POINTS

1. When performing laser surgery in or around the airway, laser safe tubes should be used.
2. Before activating the laser, delivered oxygen concentration should be reduced to a minimum and nitrous oxide should be discontinued.
3. Laser ETT cuffs should be inflated with colored saline to enable identification of cuff rupture.
4. Endotracheal tubes made of polyvinylchloride may be ignited in as little as 26% oxygen concentrations.
5. The LaserFlex, a flexible metal tube with two cuffs, is contraindicated in neodymium-doped yttrium aluminum garnet (Nd:YAG) laser cases because the laser may damage the endotracheal tube and injure the patient.

DISCUSSION

Laser is an acronym standing for Light Amplification by Stimulated Emission of Radiation. Surgical lasers include the argon, potassium titanyl phosphate (KTP), frequency-doubled yttrium aluminum garnet (YAG), Nd:YAG, CO_2, and helium–neon (He–Ne). He–Ne are low power lasers commonly used to aim other lasers such as the CO_2 and Nd:YAG. The CO_2 laser has minimal tissue penetration and is absorbed by water allowing for precision lasering, commonly used when performing surgery on the oropharynx and around the vocal cords. Argon is typically used in ophthalmic or dermatologic procedures due to substantial absorption by hemoglobin and resultant minimal tissue penetration (0.05–2.0 mm). KTP and YAG lasers also have substantial absorption by hemoglobin without substantial tissue penetration. The Nd:YAG is by far the most powerful, with tissue penetration between 2 and 6 mm. It is used in tumor-debulking procedures, particularly in the trachea, mainstem bronchi, and upper airway.

In the past, endotracheal tubes made of red rubber, silicone, or polyvinylchloride tubes and used during laser procedures, were susceptible to ignition with as little as 26% FiO_2. To limit their flammability, they were wrapped with reflective tape. Problems arose with tubes kinking, gaps in tape coverage, and inadvertent use of nonreflective tape. Presently, there are several laser-resistant endotracheal tubes in the market. LaserFlex (Mallinckrodt) consists of a flexible metal tube with two cuffs that is a good choice for CO_2 lasers but is contraindicated in Nd:YAG laser cases. The Lasertubus (Rüsch) offers resistance to all types of medical lasers including Nd:YAG. It is a soft white rubber tube covered by merocel sponge and microcorrugated silver foil; the outer merocel layer must be kept wet during use.

Regarding operating room (OR) fires in general, in 2008, the American Society of Anesthesiologists released the "Practice Advisory for the Prevention and Management of Operating Room Fires" in which they advocate education of OR personnel on procedures in the event of a fire, conducting fire drills, and general preparation in the event of a fire. In any fire, there must be an oxidizer and ignition source (commonly a laser or electrocautery unit; other sources include heated probes, drills and burrs, argon beam coagulators, fiberoptic light cables and defibrillator pads/paddles) and a fuel (tracheal tube, sponge, alcohol containing prep solutions, and oxygen masks). Specifically regarding laser surgery, it is strongly agreed upon that laser-resistant endotracheal tubes should be used and that the tube should be appropriate for both the procedure and the laser that is to be used.

The endotracheal tube cuff should be inflated with colored saline rather than air whenever possible; the colored saline will serve as a marker for cuff perforation. Before activating the laser, the surgeon should notify the anesthesiologist and grant adequate time to reduce delivered oxygen concentration to the minimum required level, to avoid hypoxia (preferably <30%), stop the use of nitrous oxide, and wait a few minutes for the oxidizer-enriched atmosphere to dissipate.

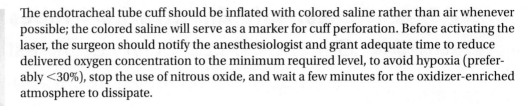

SUGGESTED READINGS

Barash PG, Cullen BF, Stoelting RK, et al, eds. *Clinical Anesthesia.* 6th ed. Philadelphia, PA: Lippincott Williams & Wilkins; 2009:185–190.

Caplan RA, Barker SJ, Connis RT, et al. Practice advisory for the prevention and management of operating room fires. *Anesthesiology.* 2008;108:786–801.

Lobato EB, Gravenstein N, Kirby RR. *Complications in Anesthesiology.* 1st ed. Philadelphia, PA: Lippincott Williams & Wilkins; 2008:772–773, 777–778.

Latex Allergy: Foods

Generic Clinical Sciences: Anesthesia Procedures, Methods, Techniques

Nehal Gatha

Edited by Raj K. Modak

KEY POINTS

1. While undergoing anesthesia, latex allergy is the second most common cause of anaphylaxis in patients.
2. A history of allergies to certain foods should be identified in patients preoperatively, as it has been shown that latex allergens can cross-react with certain food allergens.
3. The most common foods that cross-react with latex include avocadoes, bananas, chestnuts, mangoes, kiwis, passion fruit, but this cross-reactivity has also been seen with turnips, zucchini, and others.

DISCUSSION

Latex allergy can be a very serious allergy in the health care setting, causing symptoms ranging from pruritis and rash to anaphylaxis, cardiovascular collapse, and death. While undergoing anesthesia, latex allergy is the second most common cause of anaphylaxis in patients, causing approximately 15% of allergic reactions. As latex is so prevalent in the operating room, this allergy should be identified early on. Most true allergies to latex likely involve an IgE-mediated hypersensitivity response to proteins in latex. It has also been shown that many of the latex allergens cross-react with allergens in certain foods. Specifically, class 1 chitinases, which are plant proteins in certain foods, cross-react with hevein, a major latex allergen, causing the majority of cross-reactivity. This cross-reactivity has been seen in chestnuts, avocadoes, bananas, and passion fruits, while also being relatively common in mangoes and kiwis. There have also been reports of this cross-reactivity with turnips and zucchini, among other foods.

This cross-reactivity is important, as many patients may not know if they are allergic to latex; however, if they have a severe reaction to any of these foods, latex precautions should be considered. Most often, this cross-reactivity can cause a reaction in people who have repeated exposures to latex and then develop a severe allergy to one of the foods listed above.

A feature that distinguishes an allergic reaction to latex from a drug allergy is the time of onset of the reaction after exposure. Allergic reactions to drugs typically manifest within 5 to 10 minutes of exposure, whereas allergic reactions to latex are relatively delayed, manifesting more than 30 minutes after exposure.

SUGGESTED READINGS

Blanco C. Latex-fruit syndrome. *Curr Allergy Asthma Rep.* 2003;3(1):47–53. doi:10.1007/s11882-003-0012-y.

Hines RL, Marschall KE, eds. *Stoelting's Anesthesia and Co-existing Disease.* 5th ed. Philadelphia, PA: Churchill Livingstone; 2008:527, 529–530.

Morgan GE, Mikhail MS, Murray MJ. *Clinical Anesthesiology.* 4th ed. New York, NY: Lange Medical Books/McGraw-Hill; 2006:973–974.

Pereira C, Tavares B, Loureiro G, et al. Turnip and zucchini: new foods in the latex-fruit syndrome. *Allergy.* 2007;62:452–453.

Leukoreduction: Viral Transmission
Organ-based Clinical: Hematologic

Jinlei Li

Edited by Ala Haddadin

KEY POINTS

1. Leukoreduction has been demonstrated to reduce, but not to eliminate, the transmission of viruses that are almost exclusively transmitted through leukocytes, such as cytomegalovirus (CMV), human T-cell leukemia virus (HTLV-I/II), and Epstein–Barr virus (EBV).
2. Leukocytes may be involved in the reactivation and dissemination of other viruses that are not exclusively transmitted by leukocytes.
3. Leukoreduction can be performed by blood centers either before or after storage, before blood product administration.

DISCUSSION

Leukoreduction has been demonstrated to reduce, but not to eliminate, the transmission of viruses that are almost exclusively transmitted through leukocytes, such as CMV, HTLV-I/II, and EBV. Blood donors are first screened to exclude transmissible medical conditions and preexisting conditions that may be exacerbated by blood donation. Once the blood is collected, it is routinely tested for hepatitis B, hepatitis C, syphilis, HTLV-I/II, and HIV-1 and HIV-2. Most centers employ extremely sensitive nucleic acid testing for viral RNA according to U.S. Food and Drug Administration requirements. This has significantly reduced the window period, and the current false-negative rate is exceedingly low.

The current estimated transmission rates of common viral diseases in North America are as follows: hepatitis B, 1 in 269,000; hepatitis C, 1 in 1,600,000; HIV, 1 in 1,781,000; HTLV, 1 in 2,900,000; and West Nile virus, intermediate/very low. The transmission rate of CMV varies; for example, in nonleukoreduced donor blood, the rate is 7%; in leukoreduced donor blood, it is 2% to 4%; and in seronegative donor blood, it is 1% to 2%. The transmission of rate of EBV is 0% to 5%. Rates of transmission have significantly dropped since the application of molecular testing techniques. Leukoreduction can be performed by blood centers either before storage or after storage, before blood product administration.

CMV, HTLV-I/II, and EBV are transmitted almost exclusively through leukocytes. CMV typically causes asymptomatic or mild systemic diseases; however, in immunocompromised patients, it can cause severe infections. In these patients, transfusion of seronegative blood product would be ideal. The prevalence of CMV seropositivity among blood donors is close to 40% to 60%. Current screening tests cannot detect newly infected donors during window periods; however, studies have shown that the risk of transmission of CMV with leukocyte-reduced and CMV-negative blood products are comparable. Leukocytes may also be involved in the reactivation and dissemination of other viruses that are not exclusively transmitted by leukocytes. Another proven benefit of leukoreduction is the prevention of febrile reactions to blood transfusion.

SUGGESTED READINGS

Blaichman MA. The clinical benefits of the leukoreduction of blood products. *J Trauma.* 2006;60(6 suppl):S83–S90.

Drummond JC, Petrovitch CT, Lane TA. *Clinical Anesthesia.* 6th ed. Philadelphia, PA: Lippincott Williams & Wilkins; 2009:369–376.

Morgan GE, Mikhail MS, Murray M. *Clinical Anesthesiology.* 4th ed. New York, NY: Lange/McGraw-Hill; 2006:697–703.

Lithotomy Position: Nerve Injury

Generic Clinical Sciences: Anesthesia Procedures, Methods, Techniques

Archer Martin

Edited by Raj K. Modak

KEY POINTS

1. Lithotomy position is the second most commonly used position for urologic and gynecologic procedures.
2. Lithotomy position is associated with multiple comorbidities, including physiologic effects on the cardiovascular system, respiratory mechanics, and neurological injury.
3. Nerve injury can occur in the lower or upper extremities, with the most common injury involving the brachial plexus.
4. Pressure to the patient's lateral leg, near the knee, may result in damage to the common peroneal nerve, resulting in inability to dorsiflex the foot on the affected side.

DISCUSSION

Lithotomy position is the second most commonly used position for urologic and gynecologic procedures. The supine position is the most common. Lithotomy position involves placing the patient supine, with legs placed in the flexed position, supported by foot straps, leg supports, or both.

The lithotomy position is associated with multiple comorbidities, including physiological changes in the cardiovascular and respiratory systems. Injury to one or multiple nerves can be seen with the lithotomy position. Nerves that can be injured include the following: common peroneal nerve, saphenous nerve, obturator nerve, femoral nerve, and sciatic nerve. The most common nerve injury associated with the lithotomy position, however, involves the brachial plexus. The particular nerve injured depends on the exact inappropriate positioning of a patient in the lithotomy position.

If the patient's lateral thigh is resting on a support strap used for lithotomy positioning, pressure near the knee may result in damage to the common peroneal nerve (Fig. 1). The patient will be unable to dorsiflex the foot on the affected side. Pressure on the medial side of the thigh can damage the saphenous nerve. Flexion of the thigh during lithotomy positioning may damage the femoral, sciatic, and obturator nerves. As several nerves are at risk for potential injury in the lithotomy position, it is important to carefully position the patient and check and pad potential areas of pressure.

SUGGESTED READING

Morgan GE, Mikhail MS, Murray MJ. *Clinical Anesthesiology*. 4th ed. New York, NY: Lange/McGraw-Hill; 2006:758–759.

308

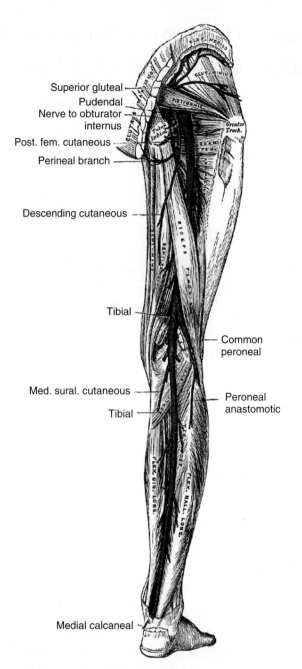

Superior gluteal
Pudendal
Nerve to obturator internus
Post. fem. cutaneous
Perineal branch

Descending cutaneous

Tibial

Common peroneal

Med. sural. cutaneous

Tibial

Peroneal anastomotic

Medial calcaneal

Figure 1. Peroneal nerve, Gray's anatomy.

Local Anesthesia: Methemoglobinemia

Pharmacology

Roberto Rappa

Edited by Jodi Sherman

KEY POINTS

1. Methemoglobinemia is associated with the administration of large doses of prilocaine and benzocaine.
2. Methemoglobin is an oxidized form of hemoglobin.
3. Methemoglobinemia is normally spontaneously reversible, but can be readily reversed with the intravenous administration of methylene blue 1 to 2 mg per kg.
4. A variety of drugs and disease states can result in the formation of clinically significant methemoglobinemia

DISCUSSION

Methemoglobinemia is a unique side effect associated with the administration of large doses of the amide-type local anesthetic prilocaine and the ester-type local anesthetic benzocaine. The formation of methemoglobin is proportional to the dose of local anesthetic administered. For example, administration of greater than 600 mg of prilocaine will result in clinically significant methemoglobin formation in adults.

Methemoglobin is an oxidized form of hemoglobin (oxidation of the ferrous ion [Fe^{2+}] on the heme group of the hemoglobin molecule into the ferric [Fe^{3+}] state). This process results in a hemoglobin molecule that has very little affinity for oxygen. With elevated red blood cell concentrations of methemoglobin, little oxygen is delivered to peripheral tissues, resulting in clinically significant tissue hypoxia.

Methemoglobin concentrations can be measured by co-oximetry, and under normal circumstances, the concentration is less than 1%. Methemoglobin has the same absorption coefficient at both red and infrared wavelengths. This identical absorption pattern corresponds to a measured SpO_2 of 85%. Therefore, in the setting of methemoglobin toxicity, when the SpO_2 is greater than 85%, this corresponds to a falsely high saturation. When the SpO_2 is less than 85%, this corresponds to a falsely low reading.

Methemoglobin is formed from the metabolism of prilocaine. Prilocaine readily undergoes hepatic metabolism to form O-toluidine. O-toluidine subsequently causes oxidation of hemoglobin to methemoglobin. Prilocaine is found in a number of topical local anesthetic solutions. It is commonly combined with lidocaine and is utilized as a eutectic mixture in EMLA (eutectic mixture of local anesthetics) cream. EMLA is a popular dermal anesthetic used in the pediatric patient population, to facilitate the placement of intravenous catheters.

Caution is advised when using prilocaine in infants younger than 12 months, especially if already receiving treatment with methemoglobinemia-inducing agents (Table 1).

Table 1. Drugs That Increase Formation of Methemoglobin

Acetanilid	Acetaminophen
Benzocaine	Aniline dyes
Dapsone	Chloroquine
Nitrates and nitrites	Naphthalene
Nitroglycerin	Nitrofurantoin
Pamaquine	Nitroprusside
Phenacetin	Paraaminosalicylic acid
Phenytoin	Phenobarbital
Quinine	Primaquine
Sulfonamides	

Prilocaine is also contraindicated rarely in patients with congenital or idiopathic methemoglobinemia. Caution is also advised in infants younger than 3 months, who physiologically may not have fully mature hepatic enzyme systems.

Benzocaine is commonly found in over-the-counter topical local anesthetic ointments. It is also found as a 20% formulation in Hurricane spray. Hurricane spray is commonly utilized as a topical oral mucosal anesthetic in preparation for bronchoscopy, fiberoptic intubation, and upper endoscopy.

Methemoglobinemia is spontaneously reversible. There exist a variety of enzymatic systems in the body that minimize the degree of oxidative stress. These systems can counteract the formation of methemoglobin and help restore the oxygen carrying (ferrous) state of hemoglobin. In disease states or drug therapy, however, these protective systems can soon become overwhelmed, resulting in the formation of clinically significant methemoglobinemia. This condition can be readily reversed with the intravenous administration of methylene blue 1 to 2 mg per kg.

SUGGESTED READINGS

Hines RL, Marschall KE, eds. *Stoelting's Anesthesia and Co-existing Disease.* 5th ed. Philadelphia, PA: Churchill Livingstone; 2008:415.

Morgan GE, Mikhail MS, Murray MJ. *Clinical Anesthesiology.* 4th ed. New York, NY: Lange Medical Books/ McGraw-Hill; 2006:140–141.

Local Anesthetic: Trans Neurol Sx

Generic Clinical Sciences: Anesthesia Procedures, Methods, Techniques

Marianne Saleeb

Edited by Thomas Halaszynski

KEY POINTS

1. Transient neurologic symptoms (TNSs) are characterized by postoperative pain or dysesthesia in the buttocks or lower extremity(s) that may occur after resolution of spinal anesthesia.
2. Studies have shown that this syndrome is mostly associated with higher concentrations of lidocaine spinal anesthesia as well as patient lithotomy position and ambulatory surgery.
3. All forms of lidocaine, including isobaric, hypobaric, and diluted, have been implicated, but the actual mechanism and cause of the syndrome is unknown.
4. The relative risk of developing TNS after intrathecal lidocaine anesthesia is seven times greater compared with bupivacaine, prilocaine, or procaine, although cases of TNS have been reported with the use of these local anesthetics as well.

DISCUSSION

TNS are characterized by postoperative pain or dysesthesia in the buttocks and/or lower extremities, usually after the resolution of spinal anesthesia (most often when lidocaine has been used). In theory, TNS are a manifestation of neurotoxicity of some local anesthetics, but most commonly occurring with hyperbaric lidocaine. All forms of lidocaine, including isobaric, hypobaric, and even diluted, have been implicated, but the actual mechanism and cause of the syndrome remains unknown. Many studies have shown that this syndrome is most often associated with lidocaine spinal anesthesia as well as the lithotomy position and/or ambulatory surgery. There have also been case reports of TNS occurring after resolution of epidural anesthesia. Patients usually complain of pain in the buttocks and lower extremity(s) that spontaneously resolves after several days. A number of clinical conditions may mimic TNS. Paraspinal muscle spasm caused by trauma could potentially mimic TNS, but usually occurs early in the recovery period. Degenerative disk disease and postdural puncture headache can confound the clinical course of TNS, and diagnosis of TNS seems to be one of exclusion.

However, the exact mechanism of injury remains unknown, but recent findings show that intrathecal administration of local anesthetics is known to increase glutamate concentration in cerebrospinal fluid and histopathologic changes of motor neurons in the lumbar spinal cord. These are the potential mechanisms suggesting damage of dorsal and ventral roots. In vitro studies of cultured neurons exposed to different concentrations of local anesthetics have shown changes in growth of cones and neurites, which may be related to TNS. The relative risk of developing TNS after intrathecal lidocaine anesthesia is seven times greater when compared with other local anesthetics such as bupivacaine, prilocaine, or procaine, although cases of TNS have been reported with the use of these other local anesthetics as well.

SUGGESTED READINGS

Aguilar JL, Peláez R. Transient neurological syndrome: does it really exist? *Curr Opin Anaesthesiol.* 2004;17(5):423–426.

Morgan GE, Mikhail MS, Murray MJ. *Clinical Anesthesiology.* 4th ed. New York, NY: Lange/McGraw-Hill; 2006:321.

Evron S, Gurstieva V, Ezri T, et al. Transient neurological symptoms after isobaric subarachnoid anesthesia with 2% lidocaine: the impact of needle type. *Anesth Analg.* 2007;105:1494–1499.

Lumbar Nerve Roots: Innervation

Pain

Garth Skoropowski

Edited by Jodi Sherman

KEY POINTS

1. Six nerves arise from the lumbar plexus, including the iliohypogastric, ilioinguinal, genitofemoral, lateral femoral cutaneous, femoral, and obturator.
2. Regional blocks of these nerves are indicated for surgery of the thigh and knee.
3. The sciatic nerve encompasses the L4 through S3 nerve roots and innervates most of the lower leg and ankle, except for a medial strip of skin innervated by the saphenous nerve, a branch of the femoral nerve.
4. Obturator reflex from electrocautery through bladder wall causes external rotation and adduction and may cause bladder perforation.

DISCUSSION

The lumbar nerve roots coalesce to form the lumbar plexus. Six nerves arise from this plexus, including the iliohypogastric, ilioinguinal, genitofemoral, lateral femoral cutaneous, femoral, and obturator (Table 1).

Table 1. Lumbar Nerve Roots

Nerve	Root	Motor	Sensory
Iliohypogastric	L1	Internal oblique, transversus abdominis	Posterolateral gluteal skin
Ilioinguinal	L1	Internal oblique, transversus abdominis	Medial thigh and genital area
Genitofemoral	L1, L2	Cremasteric muscle	Anterior thigh and genital area
Lateral femoral cutaneous	L2, L3	No motor	Anterior and lateral thigh
Femoral	L2, L3, L4	Anterior thigh	Anterior and medial leg
Obturator	L2, L3, L4	Medial thigh	Medial thigh

The lumbar plexus contains three of the four major nerves that innervate the lower extremities, including the femoral, obturator, and lateral femoral cutaneous. Regional blocks of these nerves are indicated for surgery of the thigh and knee. The other nerve is the sciatic nerve, which contains L4 through S3 nerve roots and innervates most of the lower leg and ankle, except for a medial strip of skin innervated by the saphenous nerve, a branch of the femoral nerve.

During transurethral resections of bladder tumors, the obturator reflex triggered by electrocautery can cause bladder rupture. This injury has been reported with regional anesthesia. Muscle paralysis is the only definitive way to prevent this injury.

SUGGESTED READINGS

Benzon HT, Rathmel JP, Wu CL, et al, eds. *Raj's Practical Management of Pain.* 4th ed. Philadelphia, PA: Mosby Elsevier; 2008:889.

Drake RL, Vogl AW, Mitchell AWM. *Gray's Anatomy for Students.* Philadelphia, PA: Churchill Livingstone Elsevier; 2010:378–381.

Morgan GE, Mikhail MS, Murray MJ. *Clinical Anesthesiology.* 4th ed. New York, NY: McGraw-Hill; 2006:759, 342–344.

Lung Protect Vent: Pressure Goal
Organ-based Clinical: Respiratory

Anjali Vira

Edited by Veronica Matei

1. Mechanical ventilation should be instituted with the goal of maintaining peak inflation pressures less than or equal to 35 to 40 cm H_2O.
2. There is no evidence that shows superiority of volume control ventilation versus pressure control ventilation.
3. Patients with acute lung injury (ALI) or acute respiratory distress syndrome (ARDS) are not able to tolerate the same tidal volumes as healthy patients, and high tidal volumes in this subset of patients have been associated with further deterioration of pulmonary disease and increased mortality.

Mechanical ventilation is most commonly used in the ICU to manage respiratory failure, and in the operating department, when muscle relaxation has been administered to a patient, in order to facilitate a surgical procedure. Mechanical ventilation can be used as partial or full ventilatory support, and settings are decided depending on the patient's pulmonary condition. For full ventilatory support, there has been no evidence to show a benefit of volume control versus pressure control mechanical ventilation.

When volume control ventilation is used, an initial tidal volume (V_t) of 8 to 10 mL per kg is common at a rate of 10 to 12 breaths each minute. This initial setting may be altered in the setting of pulmonary disease to maintain peak inflation pressures less than or equal to 35 to 40 cm H_2O. At peak inflation pressures of greater than 35 to 40 cm H_2O, mechanical ventilation has been shown to cause barotrauma and volutrauma by overdistention of alveoli. Overdistention has been shown to promote lung injury.

An example of the need for adjustment of initial ventilatory settings is in the management of patients with ALI and ARDS. In the setting of sepsis and trauma, ALI and ARDS can occur. They are defined by an inflammatory cascade leading to increased pulmonary capillary permeability, alveolar epithelial cell destruction, and pulmonary vasoconstriction. These patients often require ventilatory support, and the appropriate management of their ventilator settings can directly affect their outcome. In these patients, it has been shown that an FiO_2 greater than 0.5, high peak inflation pressures greater than 35 cm H_2O, and high tidal volumes greater than 8 to 10 mL per kg can lead to iatrogenic deterioration of pulmonary status. Furthermore, tidal greater than 10 mL per kg in these patients has been associated with an increase in mortality; therefore, tidal volumes of 5 to 6 mL per kg are preferred.

Barash PG, Cullen BF, Stoelting RK, et al, eds. *Clinical Anesthesia*. 6th ed. Philadelphia, PA: Lippincott Williams & Wilkins; 2009:1455–1458.
Morgan GE, Mikhail MS, Murray MJ. *Clinical Anesthesiology*. 4th ed. New York, NY: Lange/McGraw-Hill; 2006:1035, 1036, 1042.

Lung Resection Outcome: PFTs
Organ-based Clinical: Respiratory

Gabriel Pitta

Edited by Shamsuddin Akhtar

KEY POINTS

1. The main goals of pulmonary function tests (PFTs) in patients undergoing lung resection is to determine the chance of postoperative ventilator dependence.
2. PFTs used for predicting lung resection outcome need to consider three basic ideas: respiratory mechanics, gas exchange, and cardiorespiratory interaction.
3. Split-lung function tests also provide an insight into the amount of tissue resection that can be tolerated by the patient.

DISCUSSION

Most of the patients who undergo lung resection are smokers with a certain degree of COPD. They are prone to postoperative complications based on their preoperative lung disease and the amount of lung resected. Preoperative evaluation should include assessment for exertional dyspnea, chronic cough, and hemoptysis (which may be indicative of a tumor invading the respiratory tract and possibly complicating intubation/ventilation) and cigarette smoking history in pack-years.

PFTs, encompass three basic themes: respiratory mechanics, gas exchange, and cardiorespiratory interactions. The most valid test for respiratory mechanics is the predicted postoperative FEV_1 (ppoFEV1%), which is calculated as **ppoFEV1% = preoperative FEV1% × [(1−% functional lung tissue removed) / 100]**. The percentage of functional lung tissue removed is calculated by dividing the number of subsegments of each lobe removed by 42 total subsegments and expressing it as a percentage. Patients with a ppoFEV1% greater than 40% are at reduced risk, while those less than 30% are at an increased risk of ventilator dependence. Preoperative assessment of RV/TLC finds high risk for postoperative mortality with a ratio greater than 40%. Although maximum voluntary ventilation (MVV) is a nonspecific test that has not been systematically evaluated as a predictor of morbidity, it is generally accepted that an MVV less than 50% of predicted value is an indication of high risk.

Lung parenchymal function is assessed with the diffusing capacity of carbon monoxide (DLCO), which correlates with the total functioning surface area of the alveolar–capillary interface. A DLCO of less than 40% correlates with both increased respiratory and cardiac complications and is to a large degree independent of the FEV_1.

Cardiopulmonary interaction is best assessed using maximal oxygen consumption (VO_2max). The risk of morbidity and mortality is unacceptably high if preoperative VO_2max is less than 15 mL/kg/min, whereas few patients with a VO_2max greater than 20 mL/kg/min have respiratory complications. The ability to climb five flights of stairs correlates with a VO_2max of greater than 20 mL/kg/min, and climbing two flights corresponds to a VO_2max of approximately 12 mL/kg/min. The distance walked in a 6-minute test also correlates well to VO_2max, with a 6MWT less than 2,000 ft correlating to less than 15 mL/kg/min. Postresection exercise capacity can be calculated in a similar manner as ppoFEV1%, with a ppoVO2max less than 10 mL/kg/min, reflecting an absolute contraindication to pulmonary resection.

SUGGESTED READINGS

Barash PG, Cullen BF, Stoelting RK, et al, eds. *Clinical Anesthesia*. 5th ed. Philadelphia, PA: Lippincott Williams & Wilkins; 2006:816.

Miller RD, Eriksson LI, Fleisher LA, et al, eds. *Miller's Anesthesia*. 7th ed. Philadelphia, PA: Churchill Livingstone Elsevier; 2009:1820–1822.

LV Failure Dx/Rx Post-CPB

Organ-based Clinical: Cardiovascular

Chi Wong

Edited by Benjamin Sherman

1. The differential diagnosis of left ventricular (LV) failure post-cardiopulmonary bypass (post-CPB) includes inadequate preload, ischemia, valvular dysfunction, pulmonary problems, metabolic abnormalities, reperfusion injury, and preexisting LV failure.
2. LV failure is diagnosed by the inability to wean off CPB, with persistently low cardiac output (CO), ECG signs of myocardial ischemia, and cardiac dysrhythmias.
3. Treatments include correcting the underlying disorder and providing support with inotropes, inodilators, vasopressors, and/or use of a mechanical assisted device.

DISCUSSION

The differential diagnosis of LV failure post-CPB includes inadequate preload, ischemic injury, cardiac conduction problems, valvular dysfunction, postperfusion lung syndrome, metabolic abnormalities, medications, and preexisting LV failure. Ischemic injury includes graft failure or inadequate coronary blood flow secondary to incomplete revascularization, coronary vasospasm, coronary embolism, tachycardia causing inadequate diastolic filling time, incomplete myocardial preservation during CPB, and evolving myocardial infarction. Ischemia and reperfusion injury post-CPB cause myocardial stunning, resulting in systolic and/or diastolic dysfunction that is reversible. Calcium may worsen reperfusion injury and should be avoided. Post-CPB myocardial injury most commonly occurs as a result of suboptimal myocardial preservation during CPB.

LV failure is diagnosed by the inability to wean off CPB, with persistently low CO, ECG signs of myocardial ischemia, and cardiac dysrhythmias. Transesophageal ECG may demonstrate LV wall motion abnormalities and/or valvular dysfunction. Left atrial filling pressures are elevated and systemic blood pressure is decreased.

Treatments include correcting the underlying disorder and providing inotrope, inodilator, and/or vasopressor support. First-line inotropes include epinephrine, dopamine, or dobutamine. Initial temporizing measures include intravenous boluses of ephedrine (5 to 20 mg) or epinephrine (4 to 10 μg) to increase contractility and BP. Infusions are selected on the basis of the current clinical situation. If heart rate (HR) is normal and systemic vascular resistance (SVR) is low or normal, provide vasopressor support with epinephrine or dopamine. If SVR is elevated, dobutamine or milrinone may be used. Provide hemodynamic support with norepinephrine or phenylephrine if SVR is low and CO is normal or elevated. If HR is elevated, low-dose epinephrine or milrinone may be used. If HR is low without pacing, dobutamine or dopamine may be used. The use of milrinone significantly reduces SVR and may require concurrent use of an arterial vasoconstrictor such as phenylephrine or norepinephrine. Administer nitroglycerin if there is evidence of ischemia to maximize coronary blood flow as long as systemic blood pressure is adequate. Once medical treatments have been exhausted, mechanical surgical support device such as intraaortic balloon pump or LV-assisted device may be necessary.

SUGGESTED READINGS

Barash PG, Cullen BF, Stoelting RK, et al, eds. *Clinical Anesthesia*. 6th ed. Philadelphia, PA: Lippincott Williams & Wilkins; 2009:1095–1098.

Hensley FA Jr, Martin DE, Gravlee GP. *A Practical Approach to Cardiac Anesthesia*. 4th ed. Philadelphia, PA: Lippincott Williams & Wilkins; 2008:241–243.

Morgan GE, Mikhail MS, Murray MJ. Anesthesia for cardiovascular surgery. In: *Clinical Anesthesiology*. 4th ed. New York, NY: McGraw Hill; 2006:494–495.

Magnesium Complications

Pharmacology

Margaret Rose

Edited by Lars Helgeson

KEY POINTS

1. Magnesium is an essential component of calcium and potassium homeostasis, as well as a cofactor for many membranous ion pumps and enzymatic reactions.
2. It helps maintain normal vascular tone and stabilize cardiac and neuronal membranes.
3. In addition to hypomagnesemia and hypokalemia, therapeutic indications for magnesium include cardiac arrhythmias (especially torsades de pointes), premature labor, preeclampsia, and eclampsia.
4. Symptoms of toxicity include central nervous system (CNS) depression, decreased muscle tone, and ECG changes. Severe toxicity can result in apnea, paralysis, coma, complete heart block, and cardiac arrest.
5. Interventions for hypermagnesemia include administration of saline to increase extracellular volume, diuresis, calcium administration (temporizing measure), and hemodialysis.

DISCUSSION

Magnesium is found mainly intracellularly, with less than 1% located in the serum. Of this portion, 50% is the active ionized divalent cation, with the remaining being protein bound or chelated. Ionized magnesium is an essential cofactor for many enzymatic reactions (i.e., DNA synthesis, glucose utilization, and adenyl cyclase) and helps regulate various membranous ion pumps (i.e., Na-K ATPase pump, Ca-ATPase pump, slow calcium channels).

Clinically, magnesium's importance often relates to its role in calcium and potassium homeostasis, as well as its property in stabilizing cellular membranes. Its regulation of slow calcium channels help maintain normal vascular tone and prevent vasospasm. It also interacts with the parathyroid hormone regulatory system, and thus abnormal magnesium levels can lead to aberrant calcium metabolism. Through the regulation of Na-K ATPase pumps and the reabsorption of potassium by the renal tubule, magnesium levels can also affect potassium plasma levels. Furthermore, magnesium stabilizes the cellular membranes of axons and myocardial cells and can influence the release of neurotransmitters at the neuromuscular junction as well as the rate of calcium release by the sarcoplasmic reticulum.

In addition to hypomagnesemia and hypokalemia, therapeutic indications for magnesium include cardiac arrhythmias (especially torsades de pointes), premature labor, preeclampsia, and eclampsia. It has also been used clinically to treat patients with tetanus as well as pheochromocytoma. In cardiac anesthesia, it is a common adjuvant, giving when coming off of cardiopulmonary bypass. Not only does it stabilize myocardial cell membranes, but it also improves myocardial oxygen supply/demand ratio by preventing vasospasm and by antagonizing catecholamine activity. Furthermore, it can attenuate the increase of action potential duration and membrane repolarization associated with ischemic myocardium. Magnesium is also a common component of over-the-counter antacids and enemas.

Complications

Magnesium may prolong the action of nondepolarizing muscle blockers. It may also decrease the levels of tetracycline and doxycycline.

Hypermagnesemia is typically iatrogenic, resulting from overuse of antacids or enemas, but can also occur during the use of parenteral nutrition or tocolysis in obstetric patients, especially in the setting of decreased renal function. It has rarely been associated with hypothyroidism, Addison disease, and lithium toxicity.

Clinically, hypermagnesemia is characterized by progressively worsening CNS depression and decreasing muscular tone. Severe hypermagnesemia can result in decreased ventilation, apnea, paralysis, coma, complete heart block, and cardiac arrest (see Table 1).

Table 1. Manifestations of Elevated Magnesium Concentration

Magnesium Level (mg/dL)	Manifestation
2.5–5.0	Typically asymptomatic
5.0–7.0	Lethargy Drowsiness Flushing Nausea and vomiting Diminished deep tendon reflex
7.0–12	Somnolence Loss of deep tendon reflexes Hypotension ECG changes
>12	Complete heart block Cardiac arrest Apnea Paralysis Coma

Adapted from Barash PG, Cullen BF, Stoelting RK, et al, eds. *Clinical Anesthesia*. Philadelphia, PA: Lippincott Williams & Wilkins; 2006:202–204, with permission.

The use of magnesium infusions for preeclampsia and tocolysis in obstetrics is common, and is generally considered to be safe for the fetus. The neonates of these pregnancies are often found to be somewhat hypermagnesemic, which may last for several days, generally requiring no specific intervention, however. Although neonatal hypotonia and depression has been reported after maternal magnesium therapy, intrauterine hypoxia and other factors may have likely contributed.

Treatment

Symptomatic hypermagnesemia is difficult to treat. Any magnesium containing therapeutics must be stopped. Acutely expanding the extracellular volume with the administration of intravenous saline can help dilute the concentration of magnesium as well as increase urine output, which should be augmented with furosemide. The administration of intravenous calcium can transiently antagonize cardiac toxicity while other interventions are initiated. In urgent situations or in patients with renal failure, hemodialysis may be required.

Barash PG, Cullen BF, Stoelting RK, et al, eds. *Clinical Anesthesia*. Philadelphia, PA: Lippincott Williams & Wilkins; 2006:202–204.
Briggs GG, Freeman RK, Yaffe SJ. *Drugs in Pregnancy and Lactation*. Philadelphia, PA: Lippincott Williams & Wilkins; 2005:956–961.

SUGGESTED READINGS

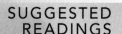

Malig Hypertherm: Assoc Disorders
Pharmacology

Martha Zegarra

Edited by Thomas Halaszynski

KEY POINTS

1. Disorders associated with malignant hyperthermia (MH) include the following:
   a. Duchenne muscular dystrophy
   b. Central core disease
   c. Osteogenesis imperfecta
   d. Evans myopathy
   e. King-Denborough syndrome
2. Only central core disease, an inborn disorder causing chronic muscle weakness, appears to be truly linked to MH.
3. The effect of inhalational anesthetics on patients with Duchenne muscular dystrophy is now thought to be a form of anesthesia-induced rhabdomyolysis.
4. More than 80% of patients with trismus, along with flaccidity of other muscles, do not prove to be susceptible to MH by muscle testing.

DISCUSSION

MH is a rare myopathy characterized by an acute hypermetabolic state within muscle tissue. Thus, it is not unexpected that MH patients may react adversely to conditions that alter muscle permeability or metabolism; conversely, several other diseases that affect muscle tissue show a relatively high-associated incidence of MH. Of these disorders, Duchenne muscular dystrophy, central core disease, osteogenesis imperfecta, Evan myopathy, and King-Denborough syndrome are most commonly cited.

Clear linkage or association of MH to other disease processes has been somewhat confusing and problematic. Only central core disease, an inborn disorder causing chronic muscle weakness, appears to be truly linked to MH. Most families with central core disease have a mutation at the calcium release channel of skeletal muscle (*ryr 1*) locus. The effect of inhalational anesthetics on patients with Duchenne muscular dystrophy is now thought to be a form of anesthesia-induced rhabdomyolysis. It still shares common clinical and biochemical characteristics, but the underlying mechanism for rhabdomyolysis is different. In addition, dantrolene does not treat anesthesia-induced rhabdomyolysis. Dantrolene side effects (muscular weakness) are undesirable in this patient population, and may detract from appropriate management.

Masseter spasm, another condition commonly associated with MH, is defined as jaw muscle rigidity in conjunction with limb muscle weakness after dosing succinylcholine. If there is rigidity of other muscles in addition to trismus, the association with MH is absolute, and inhalational anesthetics should be halted as soon as possible and treatment of MH begun. However, more than 80% of patients with trismus, along with flaccidity of other muscles, do not prove to be susceptible to MH by muscle testing. Finally, extremely rare phenomena of stress-induced MH have been described; they do not require exposure to anesthetic agents, but are thought to be triggered by trauma, vigorous exercise, or high environmental temperature.

SUGGESTED READINGS

Hines RL, Marschall KE, eds. *Stoelting's Anesthesia and Coexisting Disease.* 5th ed. Philadelphia, PA: Churchill-Livingstone/Elsevier; 2010:623–624.

Miller RD, Eriksson LI, Fleisher LA, et al. *Miller's Anesthesia.* 7th ed. Philadelphia, PA: Churchill-Livingstone/Elsevier; 2010:1182, 1188–1189.

Morgan GE, Mikhail MS, Murray MJ. *Clinical Anesthesiology.* 4th ed. New York, NY: Lange Medical Books/McGraw Hill; 2006:170–171, 945, 948.

Management: Lumbosacral Radiculopathy
Subspecialties: Pain

Robert Schonberger
Edited by Thomas Halaszynski

KEY POINTS

1. Radicular symptoms must first be assessed for clinical severity to assess for the presence of a neurosurgical emergency, as cauda equina syndrome or severe or progressive motor impairment may be indications for urgent surgical nerve decompression.
2. For less urgent cases of lumbosacral radiculopathy, first-line conservative treatment commonly includes rest and oral nonsteroidal anti-inflammatory medications to assist with reducing nerve swelling.
3. Epidural steroid injections will also help to reduce nerve swelling, potentially providing a therapeutic level of nerve decompression.
4. Physical therapy and massage may also provide relief to some patients with lumbosacral radiculopathy.

M

DISCUSSION

First-line conservative treatment for lumbosacral radiculopathy commonly includes medications to reduce nerve swelling and inflammation that may be achieved with rest and oral nonsteroidal anti-inflammatory drugs. Physical therapy to strengthen the core muscles supporting the back may also be helpful along with massage, which can be a useful component in releasing any myofascial component to the pain. Epidural steroid injections may provide relief by reducing tissue inflammation in the area(s) of nerve root impingement.

Surgical interventions have shown varying efficacy in controlled trials. In the presence of severe or progressive motor impairment or cauda equina syndrome, urgent attempts at surgical decompression of nerve roots may prove to be essential. In more indolent and chronic situations, surgery may still be offered to decompress the relevant nerve root or roots. Surgical decompression generally consists of discectomy, or discectomy with fusion.

SUGGESTED READING

Miller RD, ed. *Miller's Anesthesia*. 6th ed. Philadelphia, PA: Elsevier/Churchill Livingstone; 2005:2773–2774.

Mannitol Osmolarity Effects

Pharmacology

James Shull

Edited by Ramachandran Ramani

KEY POINTS

1. Mannitol is an osmotic diuretic.
2. The principle site of action is the proximal convoluted tubule.
3. The osmotic effect of mannitol causes high urine flow, which has several useful clinical applications.

DISCUSSION

Mannitol is an osmotic diuretic. As a six-carbon sugar, it is readily filtered at the glomerulus, but it is not reabsorbed in the tubule. This poor reabsorption in the tubule is what allows mannitol to have a diuretic effect. As mannitol remains in the tubule it retains water through an osmotic effect, which then causes the retained water to be excreted.

The principle site of action is the proximal convoluted tubule, where the majority of isotonic reabsorption occurs. Mannitol also causes, to a lesser degree, the retention of water in the descending limb of the loop of Henle and the collecting tubule.

Mannitol's osmotic diuretic effect causes a high urine output, which makes it useful for several clinical applications, including the dilution of nephrotoxic substances within the tubule to prevent kidney injury, reduction of intraocular pressure during ophthalmic surgery, conversion of oliguric renal failure to nonoliguric renal failure, and reduction of the intracranial pressure.

SUGGESTED READING

Morgan GE, Mikhail MS, Murray MJ, eds. Renal physiology & anesthesia. In: *Clinical Anesthesiology*. 4th ed. New York, NY: McGraw-Hill; 2005:736–737.

M

MAO Inhibitor: Meperidine Toxicity

Pharmacology

Dmitri Souzdalnitski

Edited by Jodi Sherman

KEY POINTS

1. Potentially fatal excess of serotonin in the central nervous system (CNS) synapses may be produced by a combination of meperidine and monoamine oxidase inhibitors (MAOIs).
2. The condition termed *serotonin syndrome (SS)* is manifested as a triad of somatic, autonomic, and neuropsychiatric derangements. It should not be confused with meperidine toxicity.
3. The treatment of SS is symptomatic. In cases of this syndrome or meperidine neurotoxicity, naloxone should not be used.

M

DISCUSSION

Meperidine was first described in 1939 and is currently used extensively for acute pain control and postoperative shivering. The interactions of meperidine with MAOIs and multiple other SSRI medications can cause SS. Meperidine belongs to a phenylpiperidine derivatives group, one of the four synthetic groups of opioids. Other similar synthetic opioids are not known to cause SS, unless they are also members of the phenylpiperidine group such as tramadol and methadone.

Meperidine blocks opioid receptors, as well as sodium channels, in a similar fashion to lidocaine, and is additionally a weak serotonin reuptake inhibitor. When combined with MAOIs or other medications that increase CNS serotonin levels, meperidine is thought to produce SS by increasing the availability of serotonin at the 5-HT1A receptor.

SS is characterized by somatic, autonomic, and neuropsychiatric derangements, including hyperreflexia and hypertonia, and is more pronounced in the lower extremities as compared with the upper. Finally, mydriasis and pronounced diaphoresis are also seen. The development of this syndrome is dose dependent on the various etiologic drugs, but can also be facilitated by patient factors, including inherited and acquired deficits in peripheral serotonin metabolism, hypertension, atherosclerosis, and dyslipidemias. These disease processes are all associated with a reduction in endothelial monoamine oxidase activity, and thus with a reduced capacity to metabolize serotonin.

Finally, SS should not be confused with meperidine toxicity. Meperidine toxicity causes CNS excitation, largely from normeperidine, a major metabolite of the drug. This toxicity is characterized by mental status changes and seizures, and is often seen in patients with underlying renal disease and liver cirrhosis. Treatment of these disorders should include immediate discontinuation of the offending drug, as well as supportive therapy for the various symptoms that arise from this disorder.

SUGGESTED READINGS

Boyer EW, Shannon M. The serotonin syndrome. *N Engl J Med.* 2005;352:1112–1120.

Guo SL, Wu TJ, Liu CC, et al. Meperidine-induced serotonin syndrome in a susceptible patient. *Br J Anaesth.* 2009;103(3):369–370.

Latta KS, Ginsberg BS, Barkin RL. Meperidine, a critical review. *Am J Ther.* 2002;9:53–68.

Morgan GE, Maged SM, Murray MJ. *Clinical Anesthesiology.* 4th ed. New York, NY: McGraw-Hill; 2006:745.

Rosow C, Dershwitz M. Pharmacology of opioid analgesics. In: Longnecker DE, Brown DL, Newman MF, et al, eds. *Anesthesiology.* New York, NY: McGraw-Hill Companies; 2008:869–897.

Mapleson D: Rebreathing
Subspecialties: Pediatric Anesthesia

Michael Archambault

Edited by Mamatha Punjala

M

KEY POINTS

1. The Mapleson classification of breathing systems distinguished each of the systems on the basis of the location of the fresh gas inflow and adjustable pressure-limiting (APL) valves in relation to the patient.
2. During spontaneous ventilation, Mapleson D requires high fresh gas flow to prevent rebreathing.
3. When high fresh gas flows are used (>100 mL/kg/min), minute ventilation best determines the alveolar carbon dioxide. With low fresh gas flows, alveolar carbon dioxide levels are dependent on the fresh gas flow and are independent of minute ventilation.
4. The Bain modification has the same rebreathing characteristics as the Mapleson D circuit.

DISCUSSION

In 1954, Mapleson classified a series of breathing apparatus that can be used for ventilation. His classifications distinguished each of the systems on the basis of the location of the fresh gas inflow and APL valve in relation to the patient. Mapleson classified six separate configurations (see Table 1). Fresh gas flow for the Mapleson D is located proximally with a distal APL valve. During spontaneous ventilation, the Mapleson D requires high fresh gas flow to prevent rebreathing. Rebreathing can be nearly eliminated if fresh gas flow is equal to mean inspiratory flow rate. Using an inspiratory to expiratory ratio of 1:1 or 1:2, the mean inspiratory flow rate is two to three times the minute ventilation.

Table 1. Classification and Characteristics of Mapleson Circuits

Mapleson Class	Other Names	Configuration	Required Fresh Gas Flows	
			Spontaneous	Controlled
A	Magill attachment		Equal to minute ventilation (≈80 mL/kg/min)	Very high and difficult to predict
B			2 × minute ventilation	2–2½ × minute ventilation
C	Waters' to-and-fro		2 × minute ventilation	2–2½ × minute ventilation

(continued)

Table 1. Classification and Characteristics of Mapleson Circuits *(continued)*

Mapleson Class	Other Names	Configuration	Required Fresh Gas Flows Spontaneous	Controlled
D	Bain circuit		2–3 × minute ventilation	1–2 × minute ventilation
E	Ayre's T-piece		2–3 × minute ventilation	3 × minute ventilation (I:E =1:2)
F	Jackson-Rees' modification		2–3 × minute ventilation	2 × minute ventilation

FGI, fresh gas inlet; APL, adjustable pressure-limiting (valve).
Modified from Morgan GE, Mikhail MS, Murray MJ. *Clinical Anesthesiology.* 4th ed. New York, NY: Lange/McGraw-Hill; 2006:35, with permission.

M

When high fresh gas flows are used (>100 mL/kg/min), minute ventilation best determines the alveolar carbon dioxide. With low fresh gas flows, alveolar carbon dioxide levels are dependent on the fresh gas flow and are independent of minute ventilation. With slow inspiratory time or low inspiratory flow, fresh gas flow can make up a larger percentage of the inspired air mixture, thus reducing rebreathing. With long expiratory pauses or a slow respiratory rate, there is greater time for mixing of expired air with fresh gas, further limiting rebreathing.

In 1972, Bain and Spoerel proposed a modification of the Mapleson D circuit. They incorporated the fresh gas flow in a coaxial configuration within the circuit. This configuration allows warming on the fresh gas by the countercurrent of warmed expired air. The Bain modification has the same rebreathing characteristics as the Mapleson D circuit.

SUGGESTED READINGS

Morgan GE, Mikhail MS, Murray MJ. *Clinical Anesthesiology.* 4th ed. New York, NY: Lange/McGraw-Hill; 2006:35.
Motoyama EK, Davis PJ, eds. *Smith's Anesthesia for Infants and Children.* 7th ed. Philadelphia, PA: Mosby Elsevier; 2006:276–278.

Mask CPAP: Physiol Effect
Organ-based Clinical: Respiratory

Suzana Zorca

Edited by Veronica Matei

KEY POINTS

1. Mask continuous positive airway pressure (CPAP) acts as a pneumatic stent for the upper airways, preventing collapse of floppy pharyngeal structures, especially during sleep. For the lower airways, CPAP provides continuous pressure to help recruit small airways prone to atelectasis/collapse.
2. CPAP is indicated for treatment of obstructive sleep apnea (OSA) and acute hypoxemic respiratory failure, in patients with good mental status and few secretions, and during weaning trials after prolonged intubation.
3. Contraindications to the use of CPAP include altered mental status, inability to cooperate with treatment, poor anatomic fit, copious secretions, and impaired ventilation.

DISCUSSION

Mask CPAP was initially described in the early 1980's by Colin Sullivan as a "pneumatic splint" for the upper airways. Since then, CPAP has been shown to act as a pneumatic air column that keeps floppy pharyngeal airways open while at the same time providing continuous pressure to smaller airways prone to collapse. A mechanical traction effect on the trachea occurs when lower airways collapse and lung volume decreases. This tends to increase upper airway resistance and collapsibility, contributing to nocturnal airway obstruction in patients with OSA. By opening collapsed alveoli and increasing functional lung volume, CPAP provides additional support for the upper airways by relieving caudal traction on the trachea. CPAP thus robustly improves upper airway patency and is the treatment of choice for OSA.

CPAP is also useful in treating other acute respiratory disorders. By providing positive pressure to recruit alveoli in the lower airways, it significantly improves oxygenation in conditions of severe atelectasis or lower airway collapse. By stenting open small airways, CPAP also compresses the pulmonary interstitium, which can help force fluid into negatively pressured lymphatics and decrease pulmonary edema. Of note, CPAP should be distinguished from noninvasive positive pressure ventilation (bilevel PAP), which can provide a pressure differential to assist in ventilation and alleviate the work of breathing. Continuous airways pressure does not provide ventilator support, and is therefore not useful in conditions of hypoventilation or respiratory muscle fatigue. Furthermore, although recruiting collapsed alveoli generally improves oxygenation, this recruitment maneuver can have adverse effects if too much CPAP is used; the ensuing compression of alveolar capillaries and increased shunt physiology can paradoxically worsen oxygenation in patients with significant V/Q mismatch.

In terms of cardiovascular effects, CPAP decreases preload by compressing the inferior vena cava and superior vena cava, impeding venous return. The increased intrathoracic pressure also effectively reduces cardiac afterload. Because of these effects, relatively hypovolemic patients may suffer from hypotension on initiation of CPAP, whereas patients in heart failure often see improvement in cardiac output. In patients with pulmonary artery hypertension, the increased oxygenation relieves hypoxic vasoconstriction, lowering PA pressures. This unburdens the RV, improving contractility.

In summary, given these physiologic considerations, indications for CPAP include the following:

1. OSA—CPAP is the treatment of choice for relief of upper airway collapse during sleep.
2. Acute pulmonary edema—short-term use of CPAP can have an excellent effect on oxygenation and improve cardiac output.
3. Hypoxemia from atelectasis—CPAP can be used as a temporizing measure in patients with inadequate oxygenation due to bilateral effusions, surgical insufflations, or splinting/incisional pain, provided the patient has good mental status and adequate respiratory drive.
4. Mild acute respiratory distress syndrome (ARDS)/transfusion-related acute lung injury (TRALI)—temporary use of CPAP can improve oxygenation and avoid mechanical ventilation in patients whose disease is expected to reverse in less than 48 hours.
5. Periextubation—CPAP can be used to prevent airway collapse in patients undergoing weaning or in the immediate postextubation period.

Conversely, contraindications to CPAP include the following:

1. Poor mental status, due to inability to protect airway/decreased airway reflexes, or inability to comply with treatment.
2. Poor anatomic fit/facial hair/facial trauma/ENT surgery/surgery on the upper airways or the esophagus.
3. Secretions and chronic risk of aspiration—concern for aspiration in pneumonia or reflux due to impaired lung-protective mechanisms of clearing secretions.
4. Impending muscle fatigue or concern for hypercapnic respiratory failure, in which case, BiPAP or invasive mechanical ventilation would be required.

SUGGESTED READINGS

Sullivan CE. Remission of severe obesity-hypoventilation syndrome after short-term treatment during sleep with nasal continuous positive airway pressure. *Am Rev Respir Dis.* 1983;128(1):177–81.

Barash PG, Cullen BF, Stoelting RK, et al, eds. Anesthesia for cardiac surgery. In: *Clinical Anesthesia.* 6th ed. Philadelphia, PA: Lippincott Williams & Wilkins; 2009:237.

Liesching T, Kwok H, Hill NS. Acute applications of noninvasive positive pressure ventilation. *Chest.* 2003;124(2):699–713.

Randerath WJ, Sanner BM, Somers VK, eds. CPAP: sleep apnea: current diagnosis and treatment. In: *Progress of Respiratory Research.* Vol 35. Basel, Switzerland: S. Karger AG; 2006:126–139.

M

Maternal Mortality Causes

Subspecialties: Obstetric

Michael Tom

Edited by Lars Helgeson

1. Maternal mortality is about 11.8 deaths per 100,000 live births in the United States.
2. Mortality rates are higher in patients older than 35 years, African American patients, and patients without prenatal care.
3. Leading causes of death include pulmonary embolism and pregnancy-induced hypertension (PIH).
4. 2–3% of maternal deaths are due to anesthesia-related causes.

Pregnancy-related death is calculated as the number of pregnancy-related deaths divided by the number of live births. In the period between 1991 and 1999, mortality was 11.8 deaths per 100,000 live births in the United States. Mortality was higher in women older than 35 years, African American patients, and patients without prenatal care. Pulmonary embolism and PIH were leading causes of maternal mortality associated with live births, whereas hemorrhage, PIH, and sepsis were the leading causes of death associated with stillbirths. Other important causes of death were amniotic fluid embolism and intracranial hemorrhage. Over 50% of patient deaths occurred between 1 and 42 days post partum, and one-third died within 24 hours.

Maternal mortality due to anesthesia-related causes is 2% to 3% (Fig. 1). Between 1985 and 1990, maternal mortality was 32 deaths per 1,000,000 live births because of general anesthesia, and 1.9 deaths per 1,000,000 live births because of regional anesthesia. Most deaths occur during or after emergency cesarean section and uncommonly during elective cesarean section.

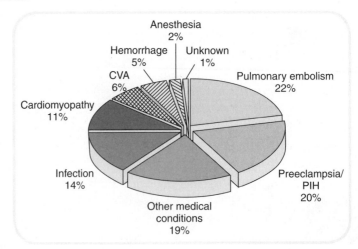

Figure 1. Causes of pregnancy-related mortality on the basis of data from the Centers for Disease Control and Prevention (deaths associated with undelivered, ectopic, and molar pregnancies as well as abortions are excluded). (Taken from Morgan G, Mikhail M, Murray M. *Clinical Anesthesiology.* 4th ed. New York, NY: McGraw-Hill; 2006:892, with permission.)

Morgan G, Mikhail M, Murray M. *Clinical Anesthesiology.* 4th ed. New York, NY: McGraw-Hill; 2006:891–893.

Maximum ABL Calculation

Subspecialties: Pediatric Anesthesia

Margo Vallee

Edited by Mamatha Punjala

1. Estimated circulating blood volume varies with age, and is critical to understand, when providing care for pediatric patients.
2. Red blood cell mass in the infant is highly variable.
3. Maximal allowable blood loss (ABL) can be estimated using a simple formula: $ABL = EBV \times [H_O - H_L]/[H_A]$.
4. In general, transfusion can easily be avoided in healthy patients with a hemoglobin of 10 g per dL or above, whereas transfusion is frequently necessary in healthy patients with a hemoglobin of less than 7 g per dL.

M

Knowledge of blood volumes is of key importance in pediatric surgical patients. It is necessary for the proper assessment of intravascular volume status as well as for decision making regarding replacement of losses with crystalloid or colloid versus red cells. Estimates of circulating blood volumes in pediatric patients differ by patient age and can be found in Table 1.

Table 1. Estimated Circulating Blood Volume

Patient	Blood Volume (mL/kg)
Premature newborn	90–100
Full-term newborn	80–90
3 mo to 1 y	75–80
3–6 y	70–75
>6 y	65–70

Smith M. Anesthesia for Infants and Children, 7th ed. Philadelphia: *Mosby Elsevier*, 2006: 367–368.

Red blood cell mass in the infant is highly variable. Despite the increased oxygen-binding capacity of fetal hemoglobin, the intrauterine environment is relatively hypoxic. This results in a relatively high hemoglobin level in term infants. After birth, there is a dramatic decrease in erythropoiesis. This decrease is due to the increase in tissue oxygen level that occurs at birth, and this leads to a decrease in erythropoietin production. This is commonly referred to as *physiologic anemia of infancy*. The nadir occurs between 8 and 12 weeks. Other factors that contribute to this anemia include a dilutional effect due to increased plasma volume and shortened red blood cell survival of 80 to 100 days in term infants and 60 to 80 days in premature infants. In premature infants, the nadir is typically seen at 6 weeks, and can often be more dramatic than that of term infants. Values can be found in Table 2.

Table 2. Normal Pediatric Hemoglobin Values

Age	Value (g/dL)
Birth	18–22.0
8–14 d	17
3 mo	10–11
2 y	11

328

Table 2. Normal Pediatric Hemoglobin
(continued)

Age	Value (g/dL)
3–5 y	12.5–13.0
5–10 y	13–13.5
10+ y	14.5

Modified from Gregory GA. *Pediatric Anesthesia.* 3rd ed. Philadelphia, PA: Churchill Livingstone Inc.; 1994:127–130, with permission.

Maximal ABL can be estimated using a simple formula:

$$ABL = EBV \times [H_O - H_L]/[H_A],$$

where EBV is estimated blood volume, H_O is initial hematocrit, H_L is lowest acceptable hematocrit, and H_A is the average of the initial and lowest hematocrit.

For example, if a 1-year-old weighing 10 kg had a starting hematocrit of 36 and a lowest acceptable hematocrit of 30, then the ABL would be 750 mL × [36–30]/33 = 136 mL. The decision to transfuse must be made on the basis of the starting hemoglobin level, intraoperative blood loss, and the cardiovascular status. In general, transfusion can easily be avoided in healthy patients with a hemoglobin of 10 g per dL or above, whereas transfusion is frequently necessary in healthy patients with a hemoglobin of less than 7 g per dL. When the decision to transfuse is made, it is important to know how much to transfuse. A simple equation can be used to estimate the amount of blood needed to transfuse to obtain a target hematocrit. The typical hematocrit of a unit of packed PBCs is between 60% and 80%.

$$Packed\ RBCs\ (mL) = [(Blood\ loss - ABL) \times Desired\ hematocrit]/Hematocrit\ of\ packed\ RBCs.$$

For example, if blood loss was 200 mL with an ABL as above of 136 mL and a desired hematocrit of 30%, one would transfuse [(200–136) × 30%]/75% = 25.6 mL.

Gregory GA. *Pediatric Anesthesia.* 3rd ed. Philadelphia, PA: Churchill Livingstone Inc; 1994:127–130.
Lerman J, Cote C, Steward D. *Manual of Pediatric Anesthesia.* 6th ed. Philadelphia, PA: Churchill Livingstone Inc; 2010:133–134.
Motoyama E, Davis P, eds. *Smith's Anesthesia for Infants and Children.* 7th ed. Philadelphia, PA: Mosby Inc; 2006:367–368, 397.

SUGGESTED READINGS

Meconium: Tracheal Suctioning
Subspecialties: Obstetric Anesthesia

Sharif Al-Ruzzeh

Edited by Lars Helgeson

KEY POINTS

1. Endotracheal intubation in newborns with meconium staining is recommended and practiced, but has not improved outcome.
2. Vigilant and continuous suctioning and cleansing of the airway in meconium-stained babies appears to provide a better outcome, without the need for intubation.
3. Routine endotracheal intubation at birth, in vigorous meconium-stained term babies, has not been shown to be superior to routine resuscitation, including oropharyngeal suction.
4. Routine endotracheal intubation in babies with meconium aspiration may be associated with increased mortality.

M

DISCUSSION

Due to the risks associated with meconium aspiration, anesthesiologists, pediatricians, and obstetricians have recommended immediate endotracheal intubation in all depressed newborns with meconium staining. The endotracheal tube facilitates ventilation and also direct access for tracheal and bronchial suctioning. Supporters of this technique rightly defend it, because the meconium contains particulate material that is not amenable to oropharyngeal suctioning, even with the widest available suction catheters.

On the basis of the evidence from nonrandomized studies, it has been recommended that all babies born through thick meconium should have their tracheas intubated, so that suctioning of their airways can be performed. The aim is to reduce the incidence and severity of meconium aspiration syndrome. However, for term babies who are vigorous at birth, endotracheal intubation may be both difficult and unnecessary.

Several randomized controlled trials of endotracheal intubation at birth, in vigorous term meconium-stained babies, did not support routine use of endotracheal intubation at birth in this subset. Endotracheal intubation did not reduce mortality, meconium aspiration syndrome, other respiratory symptoms and disorders, pneumothorax, oxygen need, stridor, or convulsions. It has not been shown to be superior to routine resuscitation, including oropharyngeal suction. Interestingly, there is some evidence indicating increased mortality with routine intubation of this subset.

However, intubation of depressed babies born through meconium remains the intervention of choice.

SUGGESTED READINGS

Al Takroni AM, Parvathi CK, Mendis KB, et al. Selective tracheal suctioning to prevent meconium aspiration syndrome. *Int J Gynaecol Obstet.* 1998;63(3):259–263.

Halliday HL, Sweet DG. Endotracheal intubation at birth for preventing morbidity and mortality in vigorous, meconium-stained infants born at term. *Cochrane Database of Systematic Reviews.* 2001; (1): CD000500. doi:10.1002/14651858.

Stoelting R, Miller R. *Basics of Anesthesia.* 5th ed. Philadelphia, PA: Churchill Livingstone; 2007:502.

Mediastinal Tumor: Airway Obstr
Organ-based Clinical: Respiratory

Stephanie Cheng

Edited by Shamsuddin Akhtar

1. Anterior mediastinal masses may cause superior vena cava syndrome, airway compression, and cardiac compression.
2. Airway obstruction may occur during induction and on emergence of anesthesia.
3. Preoperative radiation therapy could potentially decrease the dangers of general anesthesia.
4. Awake fiberoptic intubation with preservation of spontaneous ventilation during general anesthesia may minimize cardiorespiratory complications in patients with anterior mediastinal masses.

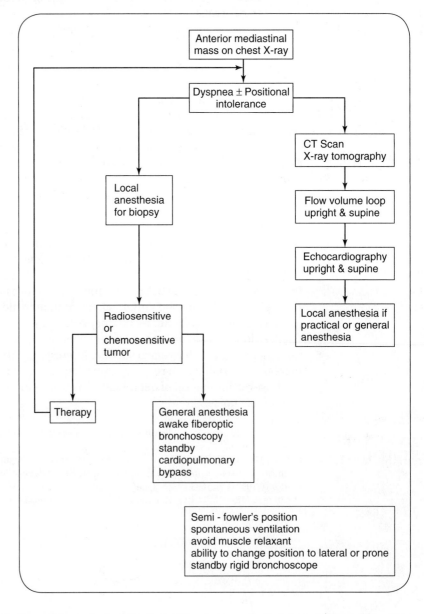

Figure 1. Preoperative evaluation of patients with anterior mediastinal masses. (Adapted from Neuman GG, Weingarten AE, Abramowitz RM, et al. The anesthetic management of the patient with an anterior mediastinal mass. *Anesthesiology.* 1984;60:144–147, with permission.)

M

DISCUSSION

Anterior mediastinal masses can cause several problems in patients requiring anesthesia, especially during induction of anesthesia. These tumors may cause superior vena cava obstruction (SVC syndrome), airway compression, and cardiac compression. Cases of airway obstruction have been reported both during induction and on emergence of anesthesia. It was found that forced expiratory volume in one second (FEV1) and peak expiratory flow test values were much lower when patients with mediastinal tumors were lying supine than upright. In this patient population, it was suggested that induction of anesthesia can be associated with airway obstuction. Preoperative radiation therapy or carrying out the planned surgical procedure with local anesthesia may avoid potential cardiorespiratory complications during anesthesia. In patients found with mediastinal masses, further investigation must be pursued (see Fig. 1).

In some studies, the incidence of cardiorespiratory complications among patients with anterior mediastinal masses during anesthesia can be as high as 38%. Factors that have been associated with increased perioperative cardiorespiratory complications include (1) signs and symptoms suggestive of cardiorespiratory dysfunction, (2) obstructive or restrictive pulmonary mechanics as indicated by pulmonary function tests (PFTs), and (3) greater than 50% tracheal compression as demonstrated on preoperative radiographic studies. In cases where there is increased concern for cardiorespiratory complications during induction of anesthesia, femoral vessels may be cannulated in anticipation of urgent cardiopulmonary bypass.

Preoperative radiation therapy could potentially shrink the mass and decrease the dangers of general anesthesia, but, at the same time, treatment may make it more difficult to diagnose the tumor. Thus, it is necessary to weigh the benefit of decreased airway compromise with possibility of inaccurate diagnosis.

In the event general anesthesia must be administered in patients with significant tumor bulk, awake fiberoptic intubation with spontaneous ventilation during general anesthesia should be considered. This technique avoids the changes in lung and chest wall physiology during muscle paralysis. This technique preserves the normal transpulmonary pressure gradient, thereby maintaining patent airways, even in the face of extrinsic airway compression.

M

SUGGESTED READINGS

Barash PG, Cullen BF, Stoelting RK, et al, eds. *Clinical Anesthesia*. 6th ed. Philadelphia, PA: Lippincott Williams & Wilkins; 2009:1058–1059.
Neuman GG, Weingarten AE, Abramowitz RM, et al. The anesthetic management of the patient with an anterior mediastinal mass. *Anesthesiology*. 1984;60:144–147.

Mediastinoscopy: Vascular Compression
Organ-based Clinical: Cardiovascular

Francis vanWisse

Edited by Veronica Matei

KEY POINTS

1. Mediastinoscopy is typically performed for tissue diagnosis and possible resection of mediastinal masses.
2. Due to the many structures within the mediastinum, there is potential for hemorrhage, nerve damage, and vascular compression.
3. The other major complication is cardiovascular collapse secondary to compression of the heart or major vessels.

DISCUSSION

The mediastinum is divided into three compartments: anterior, middle, and posterior. The anterior compartment contains the thymus, pericardium, lymph nodes, and extensions of the thyroid and parathyroid glands. The middle compartment contains the heart, great vessels, trachea, main bronchi, nodes, and phrenic and vagus nerves. The posterior compartment contains the descending aorta, esophagus, thoracic duct, azygous and hemizygous veins, part of the vagus nerve, sympathetic chains, and lymph nodes. Tumors are usually one of the four T's (thymomas, terrible lymphomas, teratomas, or thyroid masses).

Mediastinal masses may cause obstruction of major airways, main pulmonary arteries, atria, and the superior vena cava. The other major complication is cardiovascular collapse secondary to compression of the heart or major vessels. Symptoms of supine presyncope suggest vascular compression. Transthoracic echocardiography is indicated for patients with vascular compressive symptoms.

Mediastinoscopy is commonly performed for tissue diagnosis and possible resection of the mass. During the procedure, vascular compression could be the result of the mediastinal mass or surgical manipulation. Blood pressure should be measured on the left arm since the right subclavian and right carotid arteries may be compressed during this procedure. Pulse oximetry on bilateral extremities can be used for comparison and detection of vascular compromise.

Intraoperative vascular compression caused by the mediastinal mass usually responds to repositioning of the patient. It must be determined before induction if there is a position that causes less compression and fewer symptoms. In severe cases, bifemoral cannulation before induction for standby cardiopulmonary bypass can be considered. If the vascular compression is the result of surgical manipulation, retraction of surgical scope/instrument relieves the compression.

Miller RD. *Miller's Anesthesia*. 7th ed. Orlando, FL: Churchill Livingstone; 2009: chap 59: 1874–1876.

SUGGESTED READING

M

Metabolic Alk: Resp Compensation

Generic Clinical Sciences: Anesthesia Procedures, Methods, Techniques

Milaurise Cortes

Edited by Hossam Tantawy

KEY POINTS

1. Metabolic alkalosis is defined by pH levels greater than 7.4 and bicarbonate levels greater than 27 mEq per L.
2. Causes of metabolic alkalosis include states of extracellular fluid depletion, excessive acid loss, and excessive bicarbonate administration.
3. Treatment options include correcting the underlying cause, dialysis, renal bicarbonate wasting, or hydrogen administration.
4. Respiratory compensation occurs by hypoventilation/hypercarbia.

M

DISCUSSION

Metabolic alkalosis is defined by pH levels greater than 7.4 and bicarbonate levels greater than 27 mEq per L. Causes of metabolic alkalosis include factors that lead to hypovolemia and loss of acid, such as vomiting, dehydration, continuous nasogastric suction, and diuretic use. In addition, excessive administration of bicarbonate either orally or parentally can be a culprit, that is, lactate or citrate administration. Inadvertent excessive citrate or lactate administration can occur during the administration of blood products in renally impaired patients.

Electrolytes play a role in metabolic alkalosis during hypovolemia, when the body attempts to correct this state of extracellular fluid depletion by reabsorbing sodium along with chloride. However, this in turn can lead to the secretion of potassium, therefore causing hypokalemia, and can also promote the secretion of hydrogen ions, thereby worsening the metabolic alkalosis.

Side effects of metabolic alkalosis include decreased cardiac output, which then results in decreased tissue perfusion. This alkalemic state can be worsened during anesthetic management with inadvertent hyperventilation (respiratory alkalosis).

Treatment of metabolic alkalosis includes correction of the underlying cause, that is, intravascular volume repletion and electrolyte repletion. More aggressive treatment options include acetazolamide administration, which causes renal bicarbonate wasting, dialysis, or the administration of hydrogen in the form of 0.1 N hydrochloric acid (100 mmol per L).

In the setting of metabolic alkalosis, one may see respiratory compensation. The respiratory centers sense the elevated blood pH levels, and this results in hypoventilation/hypercarbia. For every increase in bicarbonate by 1 mEq per L, one may see an increase in $PaCO_2$ of 0.5 to 0.6 mm Hg. However, this respiratory compensation can be limited when oxygen chemoreceptors sense hypoxemia, and this in turn would trigger an increase in ventilation. As a result, it is rare to see the $PaCO_2$ go above 55 mm Hg.

During anesthetic management where ventilation is controlled, one can decrease the minute ventilation to create a state of hypercarbia.

SUGGESTED READINGS

Barash PG, Cullen BF, Stoelting RK, et al, eds. *Clinical Anesthesia.* 6th ed. Philadelphia, PA: Lippincott Williams & Wilkins; 2009:291–292.

Morgan G, Mikhail M, Murray M. *Clinical Anesthesiology.* 4th ed. New York, NY: McGraw-Hill Medical; 2005:712, 720–721.

Stoelting RK, Dierdorf SF. *Anesthesia and Co-existing Disease.* 3rd ed. New York, NY: Churchill Livingstone; 1993:337.

Metformin: Contrast Dye Interaction
Pharmacology

Jeffrey Widelitz

Edited by Mamatha Punjala

KEY POINTS

1. Metformin is a biguanide class medication for the treatment of type II diabetes mellitus.
2. A serious side effect of metformin is lactic acidosis, most commonly in patients with some renal or hepatic dysfunction.
3. Contrast dye can cause contrast-induced nephropathy (CIN), impairing clearance of metformin and placing patients at an increased risk for developing lactic acidosis.

M

DISCUSSION

Metformin belongs to the biguanide class of antidiabetic medications. Its main role is in the treatment of diabetes mellitus type II, especially when accompanied by obesity and insulin resistance. The most serious complication associated with its use is lactic acidosis. This complication is seen in most people having impaired liver or kidney function. Patients undergoing radiographic treatments that require contrast dyes are at risk for developing CIN.

CIN could temporarily impair renal clearance of metformin, placing these patients at a much higher risk for developing lactic acidosis. Therefore, it is recommended that patients with normal renal function temporarily stop taking metformin before these procedures and return to taking metformin 2 days after the test.

SUGGESTED READING

Parra D, Legreid AM, Beckey NP, et al. Metformin monitoring and change in serum creatinine levels in patients undergoing radiologic procedures involving administration of intravenous contrast media. *Pharmacotherapy.* 2004;24(8):987–993.

Methadone Treatment Management

Pharmacology

Caroline Al Haddadin

Edited by Thomas Halaszynski

KEY POINTS

1. Methadone is a synthetic mu- and delta-opioid receptor agonist with properties similar to morphine.
2. Methadone binds to the glutamatergic *N*-methyl-D-aspartate (NMDA) receptors, resulting in antagonism to glutamate, and causes monoamine uptake inhibition.
3. Methadone is most often used for long-term pain management and for treatment of opioid abstinence syndromes because of its long half-life.
4. Methadone (Dolophine) has a plasma half-life of 15 to 30 hours (average 24 hours), an onset of 0.5 to 1 hours, and a duration of action of 4 to 6 hours (analgesic half-life), and its bioavailability is 90% after oral dosing.

M

DISCUSSION

Methadone (Dolophine) is a synthetic opioid used in clinical practice for analgesia, has an antitussive effect, and is used for treatment of opioid abstinence. Methadone (Dolophine) has a plasma half-life of 15 to 30 hours, an onset of 0.5 to 1 hours, and a duration of action of 4 to 6 hours, and bioavailability is 90% after oral dosing.

The side effects of methadone include nausea and vomiting (which may be treated with antiemetics), respiratory depression, and decreased intestinal motility. In addition, methadone may affect the cardiac system by causing arrhythmias (associated with blocking the delayed rectifier potassium channel and prolonging repolarization), bradycardia, syncope, flushing, and QT-interval prolongation.

Before the initiation of methadone therapy, clinicians should obtain ECG to measure the QTc interval, and a subsequent ECG should be checked within 30 days of continued methadone therapy (ECG should be checked annually if methadone therapy continues). If the QTc is greater than or equal to 500 milliseconds, the clinician should consider discontinuing the drug, reducing the dose, or switching to another narcotic for pain control.

During administration of anesthesia for the opioid-naïve patient, the initial dose of methadone should be 20 mg (typically in divided doses), which will not usually produce respiratory depression. Initially, 8 to 12 mg of methadone should be administered before induction of general anesthesia (titrating to a respiratory rate to 6 to 8 per minute), and the remaining portion of the initial dose can be given immediately before surgical incision. Postoperatively, the doses of methadone should be administered in smaller increments (over multiple intervals) along with continuous monitoring of respiratory status, pain scores, and mental status.

Chart 1. Conversion from oral morphine to oral methadone.
- For total oral morphine dose <100 mg/24 h, the estimated daily oral methadone dose is 20%–30% of the morphine dose.
- For total oral morphine dose of 100–300 mg/24 h, the total estimated daily oral methadone dose is 10%–20% of the morphine dose.
- For total oral morphine dose of 300–600 mg/24 h, the total estimated oral methadone is 8%–12% of the morphine dose.
- For total oral morphine dose of 600–1,000 mg/24 h, the total estimated oral methadone is 5%–10% of the morphine dose.
- For total oral morphine dose of >1,000 mg/24 h, the estimated oral methadone dose is 5% of the morphine dose.

336

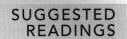

SUGGESTED
READINGS

M

From the National Comprehensive Cancer Network, Practice Guidelines; Adult Cancer Pain; and Lexicomp Drug Database (January 23, 2008).

Barash PG, Cullen BF, Stoelting RK, et al, eds. Opioids. In: *Clinical Anesthesia*. 6th ed. Philadelphia, PA: Lippincott Williams & Wilkins; 2009:chap 14.

Krantz MJ, Martin J, Stimmel B, et al. QTc interval screening in methadone treatment. *Ann Intern Med.* 2009;150(6):387–395.

Morgan GE Jr, Mikhail MS, Murray MJ. Nonvolatile anesthetic agents. In: *Clinical Anesthesiology*. 4th ed. New York, NY: McGraw-Hill Medical; 2005:chap 8.

Methemoglobinemia: SpO$_2$ Effects and Treatment

Generic Clinical Sciences: Anesthesia Procedures, Methods, Techniques

Lisbeysi Calo and Mary DiMiceli

Edited by Ala Haddadin

M

KEY POINTS

1. Methemoglobin is formed by the oxidation of ferrous iron (Fe^{2+}) to ferric iron (Fe^{3+}).
2. Methemoglobinemia can be acquired or congenital.
3. Methemoglobin has a higher affinity for oxygen than does normal Hb, thus preventing release of oxygen to tissues, and is also unable to bind oxygen, thus decreasing oxygen-carrying capacity.
4. The presence of MetHb may be detected by pulse oximetry.
5. Goal of treatment of MetHb is reduction of ferric iron back to ferrous iron, which can be accomplished using methylene blue (1 mg per kg).

DISCUSSION

Methemoglobinemia may either be congenital or acquired. Methemoglobin is formed when ferrous iron (Fe^{2+}) form is oxidized to ferric iron (Fe^{3+}), which can occur naturally in small amounts in vivo. This process is regulated by MetHb NADH reductase (or NADPH MetHb reductase is minor pathway), which aids in donating an electron to the ferric iron form, thus reducing it to ferrous iron and reestablishing normal Hb. Thus, congenital methemoglobinemia is a result of low levels of MetHb NADH reductase or an abnormal variant of hemoglobin (HgM), which is not amenable to reduction despite adequate levels of the enzyme. Acquired methemoglobinemia can be a direct result of certain medications, of which local anesthetics have been implicated in many case studies, particularly benzocaine.

In the oxidized state, MetHb has a higher affinity for oxygen, thus shifting the hemoglobin–oxygen dissociation curve to the left and rendering oxygen incapable of being released to tissues. In addition, oxygen cannot be taken up by MetHb, thus decreasing oxygen-carrying capacity.

The presence of MetHb may be detected by decreased arterial oxygen saturations as measured by pulse oximetry; however, it is not always sensitive. Conventional pulse oximetry is based on the fact that the absorption of red and infrared light differs between oxygenated and reduced Hb. In addition, it uses plethysmography to identify arterial pulsations because it is the ratio of absorption of both light spectrums during arterial pulsation that is calculated to be the arterial oxygen saturation. Oxygenated Hb (HbO$_2$) absorbs more infrared light, whereas deoxyhemoglobin absorbs more red light. Carboxyhemoglobin, due to its high affinity for oxygen, absorbs light identically to HbO$_2$, thereby causing a falsely elevated oxygen saturation. MetHb has high absorbance of both red and infrared light, thus resulting in a 1:1 absorption ratio and an SpO$_2$ of 85%, regardless of the percentage of MetHb. In other words, pulse oximetry is falsely low when patients really have oxygen saturations greater than 85% and is falsely elevated in patients with actual oxygen saturations less than 85%. Case reports have documented normal oxygen tension measured on arterial blood gas analysis in patients with an SpO$_2$ of 85%, but with increased MetHb levels. Because it is difficult to detect via the conventional two-wavelength pulse oximeter, one case study proposes the use of more discriminate pulse oximeters that use eight wavelengths of light. In this study, they were able to diagnose methemoglobinemia more than an hour before results from a blood sample and CO-oximetry analysis were available.

The goal of treatment is to reduce ferric iron to ferrous iron, which can be accomplished by the intravenous administration of methylene blue (1 mg per kg as a 1% solution). Methylene blue acts as a cofactor for NADPH MetHb reductase. Since hemoglobin M does not respond to normal levels of the reductase enzymes, administration of methylene blue will not aid in the treatment of this form of congenital methemoglobinemia.

In 2005, the Rainbow (C) technology rad 57 and Masimo (C) rad 7 were introduced. The rad 57 device uses eight wavelengths of light to measure SpO_2 as well as $SpCO_2$. These devices are used to noninvasively measure methemoglobin level via a finger sensor along with pulse oximeter reading. They can also provide other physiologic data. A built-in valgorithm allows these devices to automatically monitor the respiratory variations of the pulse oximeter curve.

SUGGESTED READINGS

Anderson S, Hajduczek J, Barker S. Benzocaine-induced methemoglobinemia in an adult: accuracy of pulse oximetry with methemoglobinemia. *Anesth Analg.* 1988;67:1099–1101.

Annabi EH, Barker SJ. Severe methemoglobinemia detected by pulse oximetry. *Anesth Analg.* 2009;108:898–899.

Morgan GE Jr, Mikhail MS, Murray MJ. *Clinical Anesthesiology.* 4th ed. New York, NY: Lange Medical Books/ McGraw Hill; 2006:140–141.

M

Methods: Uterine Relaxation

Subspecialties: Obstetrics

Lisbeysi Calo

Edited by Lars Helgeson

KEY POINTS

1. The regulation of uterine relaxation is poorly understood. Research into myometrial and regulatory proteins is ongoing.
2. Intentional uterine relaxation is used to prevent placental separation, abruptio placentae, premature labor, spontaneous abortion, and decreased fetal perfusion. It is also necessary during fetal surgery.
3. Opiates, benzodiazepines, neuromuscular blockers, and propofol do not significantly affect uterine tone. Barbiturates decrease uterine tone in a dose-dependent fashion.
4. Potent inhalational anesthetics provide good uterine relaxation, whereas nitrous oxide does not.
5. Nitroglycerin produces excellent uterine relaxation. Beta-mimetics are effective in delaying delivery in preterm labor for about 48 hours. Magnesium infusion may also be used to accomplish tocolysis. Progesterone decreases the incidence of preterm labor. None of these agents show benefit in terms of improving perinatal morbidity and mortality.
6. Oxytocin receptor blockers such as atosiban and barusiban provide a relatively selective pharmacologic target. These drugs are used in Europe, but not in the United States at this time.

M

DISCUSSION

Uterine activity should be evaluated for both intensity and frequency. The force is usually expressed in Montevideo units, which is the product of the uterine pressure above baseline tone and the number of contractions in a 10-minute period. Uterine relaxation is defined as a decrease in contraction strength or uterine tone.

Uterine relaxation is required when performing fetal surgery and the EXIT procedure. It is important to avoid uterine tetanus (hyperstimulation caused by oxytocin infusion) and its detrimental effects on fetal perfusion. In addition, pregnant patients undergoing non-obstetric or obstetric surgery are at increased risk for premature labor or postoperative loss of the fetus; uterine relaxation is of value in these cases. Terbutaline can be used as 0.25-mg subcutaneous administration every 1 to 6 hours to achieve uterine relaxation. Side effects of terbutaline therapy include hypertension, tachycardia, and pulmonary edema.

Equipotent doses of the halogenated agents produce equal uterine relaxation. None of the volatile agents have a particular advantage regarding fetal effects or in decreasing uterine tone. Drugs that relax the uterus may increase blood loss after vaginal delivery or C-section. Inhalational agents at a minimal alveolar concentration (MAC) of less than 1.5 during anesthesia have minimal effects on blood loss if the agent is blown off rapidly on delivery. Oxytocin may also be administered to increase uterine tone to lessen bleeding from the placental implant site. An alternative to reduce blood loss is to decrease the volatile agent to less than 0.5 MAC by adding nitrous oxide, a propofol infusion, and/or narcotics. Inhalational anesthesia for vaginal delivery with very low doses of halogenated agents (maintaining consciousness) appears to have minimal effect on uterine activity, duration of labor, or postpartum blood loss. At high concentration, halogenated agents will block the response to oxytocin. Intravenous (IV) nitroglycerine infusion or sevoflurane at 2 MAC may be used for the fetal EXIT procedure and transuterine surgery. Hypotension is often a consequence of these methods, which can be corrected with a phenylephrine infusion.

Ritodrine and terbutaline were introduced as selective adrenergic beta-2 receptor (ADRB2) agonists in the 1980s. These two agents, along with calcium channel blockers (magnesium sulfate and indomethacin), have been used to produce uterine relaxation. More commonly, however, they are used during the pre- or postpartum period.

The effect of labor pain on uterine activity is unclear. Although multiple studies suggest that increased sympathetic activity predisposes to dysfunctional labor, other studies indicate that stress response peptides (neuropeptide Y, atrial natriuretic peptide) may affect uterine activity. Some earlier studies suggested that epidural analgesia results in decreased uterine activity. Recent evidence suggests that this is instead due to IV fluid administration.

The high density of oxytocin receptors in the pregnant uterus provides a relatively selective pharmacologic target. In 2000, atosiban became the first oxytocin receptor antagonist for the management of preterm labor, which is used in Europe. The newer oxytocin receptor antagonist barusiban is more potent and selective.

SUGGESTED READINGS

Bernal AL. The regulation of uterine relaxation. *Semin Cell Dev Biol*. 2007;18(3):340–347.

Chestnut DH, ed. *Obstetric Anesthesia: Principles and Practice*. 2nd ed. St Louis, MO: Mosby; 1999:331–332.

Hughes SC, Levinson G, Rosen MA, eds. *Shnider and Levinson's Anesthesia for Obstetrics*. 4th ed. Philadelphia, PA: Lippincott Williams & Wilkins; 2001:41–54.

Morgan G, Mikhail M, Murray M. *Clinical Anesthesiology*. 4th ed. New York, NY: McGraw-Hill Medical; 2005:912–913.

M

Metoclopramide: Esoph Sphincter Tone

Pharmacology

Tiffany Denepitiya-Balicki

Edited by Lars Helgeson

KEY POINTS

1. Metoclopramide is a dopamine receptor antagonist that is both a weak antiemetic and a prokinetic agent.
2. Metoclopramide's mechanism of action is multifactorial consisting of
   - vagal antagonism, central 5-hydroxytryptamine type 3 ($5HT_3$) antagonism, and dopamine receptor antagonism
   - $5HT_4$ agonism
3. Most of its effect is within the upper gastrointestinal (GI) tract, resulting in increased lower esophageal sphincter tone and gastric motility.

M

DISCUSSION

Metoclopramide is a dopamine receptor antagonist that serves as an antiemetic and a prokinetic agent. Dopamine acts as an inhibitor of the GI tract, lowering both intragastric pressure and pyloric sphincter tone. The activation of the D_2 dopamine receptor in the GI tract prevents the release of acetylcholine (which is largely responsible for motility in the GI tract), thereby decreasing motility. Metoclopramide allows for the release of acetylcholine in the GI tract, thereby increasing GI motility. Metoclopramide may also act on the vagal system as a central $5HT_3$ antagonist, and as a $5HT_4$ agonist, which will increase lower esophageal sphincter tone and induces small intestine contraction.

Although metoclopramide is available in oral formulation, preoperatively and intraoperatively, it is often administered intravascularly or intramuscularly (IM). The onset of action for an IM dose is approximately 15 minutes, whereas IV onset of action is approximately 3 minutes. When given IV, it must be administered slowly over 5 to 10 minutes or longer to avoid extrapyramidal side effects.

Acutely, patients clinically may exhibit anxiety, dysphoria, and dystonia (continuous muscle contraction), or subacutely may demonstrate parkinsonian-type symptoms. These side effects are usually reversible via treatment with antihistamine and/or anticholinergics. On rare occasions, metoclopramide may be associated with galactorrhea and methemoglobinemia.

The weak antiemetic property of metoclopramide results from its influence in the chemoreceptor trigger zone.

SUGGESTED READING

Pasricha PJ. Treatment of disorder of bowel motility and water flux; antiemetics; agents used in biliary and pancreatic disease. In: Brunton LL, Lazo J, Parker K, eds. *Goodman and Gilman's Pharmacological Basis of Therapeutics*. 11th ed. New York, NY: McGraw-Hill; 2006:chap 37.

Metoclopramide: Gastric Effects
Pharmacology

Jennifer Dominguez
Edited by Lars Helgeson

M

KEY POINTS

1. Metoclopramide is a dopamine receptor antagonist that has a complex range of peripheral and central effects.
2. It is used primarily in clinical practice for its prokinetic effects on the upper gastrointestinal system and as an antiemetic.
3. Metoclopramide stimulates peristalsis and contractility of the gastric fundus and antrum, relaxes the pyloric sphincter, and increases the tone of the lower esophageal sphincter.
4. Metoclopramide can produce extrapyramidal side effects and dystonias, particularly with rapid administration or extremes of age.

DISCUSSION

Metoclopramide is used for prevention and treatment of postoperative nausea and vomiting, as well as to enhance gastric motility and promote emptying in the preoperative period. It was developed almost 50 years ago as a derivative of para-aminobenzoic acid. Structurally, it resembles procainamide.

The underlying mechanism by which metoclopramide stimulates gastric motility and emptying is related to its antagonism of dopamine at the D_2 receptors in the upper gastrointestinal tract. Dopamine is an inhibitory neurochemical in the gastrointestinal tract. It may decrease the release of acetylcholine from the synapses of myenteric motor neurons by binding to D_2 receptors in the gut. Thus, by interfering with the binding of dopamine to D_2 receptors, metoclopramide stimulates peristalsis and contractility of the gastric fundus and antrum, relaxes the pyloric sphincter, and increases the tone of the lower esophageal sphincter. Although D_2 receptors are found throughout the gastrointestinal tract, they have been found to have little clinical effect on large bowel motility.

As an antiemetic, metoclopramide may be most useful in treating nausea and vomiting associated with gastric dysmotility, such as diabetic gastroparesis. It should not be used in patients with bowel obstruction. In general, newer antiemetics are more effective, with fewer adverse effects. Metoclopramide has also been used in clinical practice as an adjunct for prevention of aspiration pneumonitis with H_2 blockers. Some studies have not shown any additional benefit compared with H_2-blocker monotherapy. In theory, it may be beneficial by increasing tone at the gastroesophageal sphincter.

Metoclopramide has a number of complex actions on the central nervous system that are not completely understood. It works centrally to treat/prevent nausea and vomiting by inhibiting dopamine in chemoreceptor trigger zone of the fourth ventricle. The drug also antagonizes 5-HT_4 receptors and vagal and central 5-HT_3 receptors. Metoclopramide can produce extrapyramidal effects, particularly in children, young people, and the elderly. Dystonias can occur acutely after rapid intravenous administration, and patients can develop parkinsonian symptoms after several weeks of therapy. These adverse effects are usually reversible with discontinuation of the drug, and can be treated with anticholinergic or antihistaminic drugs.

Metoclopramide is generally given in doses of 10 mg intravenously or intramuscularly. Adverse effects tend to be seen at higher doses. Its onset of action is 1 to 3 minutes, and its duration of action is 1 to 2 hours. It has a half-life of 4 to 6 hours. With oral administration, metoclopramide is absorbed quickly and reaches peak concentrations in about 1 hour.

SUGGESTED READINGS

Brunton LL, Lazo JS, Parker KL, eds. *Goodman and Gilman's: The Pharmacological Basis of Therapeutics.* 11th ed. New York, NY: McGraw-Hill; 2006:985–986.

Calvey N, Williams N, eds. *Principles and Practice of Pharmacology for Anaesthetists.* 5th ed. New York, NY: Blackwell Publishing; 2008:240–241.

Miller RD, ed. *Miller's Anesthesia.* 6th ed. Philadelphia, PA: Churchill Livingstone; 2004:2598.

M

Midazolam: Bioavail versus Route
Subspecialties: Pediatric Anesthesia

Alexey Dyachkov

Edited by Mamatha Punjala

KEY POINTS

1. The bioavailability of midazolam depends on its route of administration.
2. Bioavailability is defined as the fraction of an administered drug that reaches the systemic circulation.
3. The oral dose of midazolam must be about twice as high as intravenous (IV) dose to achieve comparable clinical effects secondary to a high degree of first-pass metabolism.
4. The rate of elimination of midazolam, as compared with its bioavailability, is independent of the route of administration.

M

DISCUSSION

Midazolam is a short-acting benzodiazepine class drug, producing dose-dependent anxiolytic, anterograde amnestic, sedative, hypnotic, anticonvulsant, and spinally mediated muscle relaxant effects.

Bioavailability is the fraction of an administered drug that reaches the systemic circulation. By definition, when a medication is administered IV, its bioavailability is 100%; however, when a medication is administered via other routes, its bioavailability decreases (due to incomplete *absorption* and *first-pass metabolism*).

Absorption is the rate at which a drug leaves its site of administration.

Factors increasing absorption: large particle size, high lipid solubility (low ionization), high concentration, state (liquids, crystalloids), high area of absorption, good blood supply, application of heat, or local vasodilation.

First-pass metabolism of midazolam: hepatic microsomal oxidation of the imidazole ring with formation of 1-hydroxymidazolam (main metabolite), 4-hydroxymidazolam (smaller amounts), and 1,4-dihydroxymidazloam (even smaller amounts). Two metabolites of midazolam, 1-hydroxymidazolam and 4-hydroxymidazolam, have their own pharmacologic activity.

Possible routes of midazolam administration and bioavailability:

- IV: 100%.
- IM: 85%.
- SQ: 96%.
- PO: Only 36% to 52%, due to high hepatic clearance. Thus, the oral dose must be about twice as high as IV to achieve comparable clinical effects. The elimination half-life of oral midazolam, on the other hand, is similar or identical to that observed after IV administration, indicating that the rate of elimination is independent of the route of administration.
- Intranasal: 78%. Recommended dose is 0.2 mg per kg. Although it may be suitable for children, it is not convenient in adults because this dose translates into 3 mL of solution. Other data report variation from 50% to 83%.
- Rectal: 52%
- Buccal: 74.5%. 0.5 mL (2.5 mg) was delivered on the right and the left buccal mucosa (total of 5 mg). It may be assumed that patient acceptance of the buccal mode of midazolam administration will be higher than that of the intranasal route. After intranasal midazolam, owing to its bitter taste, children develop a distrust of further management.

345

SUGGESTED
READINGS

Allonen H, Ziegler G, Klotz U. Midazolam kinetics. *Clin Pharmacol Ther.* 1981;30:653–661.

Björkman S, Rigemar G, Idvall J. Pharmacokinetics of midazolam given as an intranasal spray to adult surgical patients. *Br J Anaesth.* 1997;79:575–580.

Burstein AH, Modica R, Hatton M, et al. Pharmacokinetics and pharmacodynamics of midazolam after intranasal administration. *J Clin Pharmacol.* 1997;37:711–718.

Clausen TG, Wolff J, Hansen PB, et al. Pharmacokinetics of midazolam and alpha-hydroxy-midazolam following rectal and intravenous administration. *Br J Clin Pharmacol.* 1988;25:457–463.

Crevoisier C, Eckert M, Heizmann P, et al. Relation entre l'efflet clinique et la pharmacocinétique du midazolam aprés administration i.v. et i.m. 2ème communcation: Aspects pharmacocinétiques. *Arzneimittelforschung.* 1981;31:2211–2215.

Greenblatt DJ, Abernethy DR, Locniskar A, et al. Effects of age, gender and obesity on midazolam kinetics. *Anesthesiology.* 1984;61:27–35.

Heizmann P, Eckert M, Ziegler WH. Pharmacokinetics and bioavailability of midazolam in man. *Br J Clin Pharmacol.* 1983;16:43s–49s.

Klotz U, Ziegler G. Physiologic and temporal variation in hepatic elimination of midazolam. *Clin Pharmacol Ther.* 1982;32:107–112.

Pecking M, Montestruc F, Marquet P, et al. Absolute bioavailability of midazolam after subcutaneous administration to healthy volunteers. *Br J Clin Pharmacol.* 2002;54(4):357–362.

Reves JG, Fragen RJ, Vinik HR, et al. Midazolam: pharmacology and uses. *Anesthesiology.* 1985;62:310–324.

Schwagmeier R, Alincic S, Striebel HW. Midazolam pharmacokinetics following intravenous and buccal administration. *Br J Clin Pharmacol.* 1998;46:203–206.

Smith MT, Eadie MJ, Brophy TO. The pharmacokinetics of midazolam in man. *Eur J Clin Pharmacol.* 1981;19:271–278.

Tolksdorf W, Eick C. Rektale, orale and nasale pramedikation mit Midazolambei Kindernim Alter von 1–6 Jahren. *Anaesthesist.* 1991;40:661–667.

Walberg EJ, Wills RJ, Eckhert J. Plasma concentrations of midazolam in children following intranasal administration. *Anesthesiology.* 1991;74:233–235.

M

Milrinone: Pharmacology and CV Effects

Pharmacology

Juan Egas and Johnny Garriga

Edited by Qingbing Zhu

M

1. Milrinone is an analogue of amrinone.
2. It exerts its effects by inhibition of phosphodiesterase III, which leads to increased levels of cyclic AMP.
3. It increases the dynamic efficacy of cytoplasmic calcium concentration.
4. It indirectly increases the myocardial contractility and the acceleration of myocardial relaxation.
5. It can cause vasodilatory effect in vascular smooth muscle mediated by phosphorylation of myosin light chain kinase or activation of KATP channels.
6. It has potential fatal side effects, including ventricular arrhythmias and increase of myocardial oxygen consumption.
7. It has been associated with increased mortality when used as chronic treatment, but not in the case of short-term treatment after cardiac surgery.
8. It does not cause thrombocytopenia and liver toxicity, which may be seen with amrinone use.

Milrinone is a bipyridine methyl carbonitrile analogue of amrinone that exhibits prominent inotropic and vasodilator activity devoid of amrinone's adverse effects such as thrombocytopenia and liver toxicity.

To understand the pharmacodynamics of milrinone, we have to review the signal transduction pathway of catecholamines. It begins with the release of norepinephrine (NE) from sympathetic autonomic nerve terminals. NE interacts with beta receptors on the cell surface and induces a conformational change in the receptor. The conformational change enables an interaction between the beta receptor and the G protein (guanine nucleotide binding protein) subtype S (S indicates that it causes stimulation and not inhibition of adenylyl cyclase). The Gs protein transduces the signal to a third component of this system, namely, the adenylyl cyclase enzyme, which acts as amplifier of the signal. Adenylyl cyclase converts intracellular ATP to the second messenger cAMP (increasing its intracellular concentration), which in turn activates protein kinase A that will phosphorylate enzymes, leading to cellular responsiveness. The biologic signal produced by cAMP is terminated by phosphodiesterase enzyme activity, cleaving the cyclic form to a linear 5-AMP, which is devoid of biologic activity.

Milrinone selectively inhibits peak III phosphodiesterase, which is the predominant form of this enzyme in the heart and vascular smooth muscle, and therefore leads to increased levels of cAMP.

In the heart, increased levels of cAMP raise the inward conductance of Ca^{2+} via voltage-dependent channels during depolarization, and this results in larger contractile force (increases inotropism, dp/dt, EF, CI). During diastole, higher levels of cAMP lead to increased reuptake of cytosolic Ca^{2+}, which allows for greater myocardial cell relaxation. In vascular smooth muscle, vasodilatory effect is independent of the endothelium and is presumably mediated by phosphorylation of myosin light chain kinase or activation KATP channels.

Hemodynamic effects of milrinone have been studied extensively. The positive inotropism and decreased vascular resistance are reflected in an increased stroke volume, stroke work, and CI and decreased left ventricular end-diastolic pressure (LVEDP), afterload (systemic vascular resistance), and pulmonary vascular resistance. Compared with dobutamine, milrinone does not increase myocardial oxygen consumption and may be better tolerated in congestive heart failure (CHF) patients in whom afterload reduction therapy may be limited by hypotension, especially 48 hours after cardiac surgery. Both drugs increase the CI to the same extent, but milrinone causes a significantly greater reduction in right atrial pressure, pulmonary capillary wedge pressure, and LVEDP. Milroinone is also less arrhythmogenic and is not associated with tolerance or tachyphylaxis after prolonged use. Milrinone infusions may be linked to an overall decrease in the MAP, but this decrease has not been associated to a clinical deterioration of the hemodynamic status. Milrinone has been associated with increased mortality when used as chronic treatment for New York Heart Association class IV (NYHA IV) patients, but not in the case of short term post-op use in treating CHF after cardiac surgery.

Heart failure is the leading cause of hospitalization in people older than 65 years. Pharmacologic agents such as oral loop diuretics, beta-blockers, ACE inhibitors, angiotensin receptor blockers, vasodilators, and aldosterone receptor antagonists have been used in the treatment of heart failure. In decompensated heart failure, treatment with these drugs may not stabilize the patient. Milrinone may be used as one of the last pharmacologic agents in the management of decompensated heart failure, in particular in diastolic heart failure.

Diastolic heart failure occurs as a consequence of excessive preload (i.e., renal failure), excessive afterload (i.e., hypertension), or structural and functional abnormalities of the ventricle. Furthermore, diastolic heart failure results in impaired ventricular relaxation and impaired compliance with increased chamber stiffness. This dysfunction manifests an increase in the left ventricular pressure for a given volume during diastole (see Fig. 1). As a consequence of the impaired relaxation, the left ventricle is unable to fill to a sufficient volume to support normal cardiac output. Milrinone is used in the management of heart failure only when conventional treatment with vasodilators and diuretics proves to be inadequate.

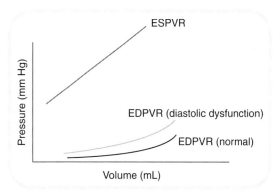

Figure 1. End-diastolic pressure–volume relation in diastolic dysfunction.

A milrinone infusion is usually initiated with a loading dose of 50 μg per kg followed by a continuous infusion of 0.25 to 1.0 μg/kg/minute. The elimination half-life of milrinone is 0.5 to 1 hour; because of such a short half-life, stopping milrinone rapidly may result in adverse outcomes.

Milrinone is often saved as one of the last resort agents in the treatment of heart failure because of potential fatal side effects including ventricular arrhythmias and increase of myocardial oxygen consumption. Multiple studies, however, have demonstrated that milrinone therapy has significantly decreased the NYHA functional class status in patients with heart failure (see Fig. 2).

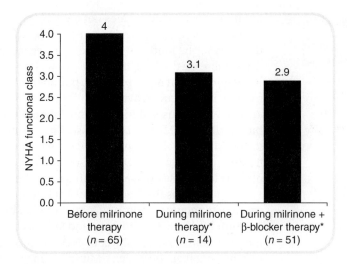

Figure 2. The effect of milrinone therapy on NYHA functional class.

SUGGESTED READINGS

Colucci WS, Wright RF, Braunwald E. New positive inotropic agents in the treatment of congestive heart failure. Mechanisms of action and recent clinical developments. *N Engl J Med.* 1986;314:290–299.

Colucci WS. Myocardial and vascular actions of milrinone. *Eur Heart J.* 1989;10(suppl C):32–38.

Lambert DG. Signal transduction: G proteins and second messengers. *Br J Anaesth.* 1993;71(1):86–95.

Liu JJ, Doolan LA, Xie B, et al. Direct vasodilator effect of milrinone, an inotropic drug, on arterial coronary bypass grafts. *J Thorac Cardiovasc Surg.* 1997;113(1):108–113.

McMurray JJ, Pfeffer MA. Heart failure. *Lancet.* 2005;365:1877–1889.

Rettig GF, Schieffer HJ. Acute effects of intravenous milrinone in heart failure. *Eur Heart J.* 1989; 10(suppl C):39–43.

Vroom MB, Pfaffendorf M, van Wezel HB, et al. Effect of phosphodiesterase inhibitors on human arteries in vitro. *Br J Anaesth.* 1996;76:122–129.

Wright EM, Sherry KM. Clinical and haemodynamic effects of milrinone in the treatment of low cardiac output after cardiac surgery. *Br J Anaesth.* 1991;67:585–590.

M

MOCA Requirements

Generic, Clinical Sciences: Anesthesia Procedures, Methods, Techniques

Jammie Ferrara

Edited by Raj K. Modak

1. The American Board of Anesthesiologists (ABAs) has instilled a time-limited (10 years) certification: Maintenance of Certification in Anesthesiology (MOCA).
2. The MOCA program allows ABA diplomats with a time-limited certificate in the specialty of anesthesiology to maintain their certification.
3. There are four requirements to MOCA: professional standing, lifelong learning and self-assessment, cognitive examination, and practice performance, assessment, and improvement.

M

With no age-specific conditions placed on state medical licensure or on the practice of anesthesiology, practice limitation and retirement remains at the discretion of the individual anesthesiologist. Since 2000, members of the American Board of Anesthesiology (ABA) have instilled time-limited certification. The MOCA program allows ABA diplomats with a time-limited certificate in the specialty of anesthesiology to maintain their certification.

The MOCA cycle is a 10-year period of four key components (Fig. 1):

The American Board of Anesthesiology (ABA)
Maintenance of Certification in Anesthesiology (MOCA) Program
Certification End Year 2019

REQUIREMENTS	ACTION ITEMS	TIMING
Part I – Professional Standing (PS)		
Hold an active, unrestricted medical license in the United States (US) or Canada. All US and Canadian medical licenses must be unrestricted.	Review and update your medical license information via your portal account through the ABA website at www.theABA.org.	Continuous
Part II – Lifelong Learning and Self-Assessment (LLSA)		
Continually seek to improve the quality of your clinical practice and patient care through self-directed professional development. This should be done through self-assessment and learning opportunities related to your practice. Your LLSA requirement for maintenance of certification is 350 credits of continuing medical education (CME) activities. Of the 350 credit total: • At least 250 credits must be Category 1 credits (ACCME/AMA PRA-approved). • At most 100 credits may be for programs and activities for which Category 1 credit is not awarded. • Beginning with 2006, no more than 70 credits per calendar year will be credited toward LLSA requirement. • At least 60 credits earned through completion of either the ASA's ACE or SEE programs. • At least 20 credits of Patient Safety CME available through the ASA and ABMS.	Submit your LLSA (CME) activities to the ABA via your portal account for any activities completed since the day after you were certified. Instructions can be found at: http://www.theaba.org/pdf/How_to_Submit_CME_for_MOCA.PDF	Continuous
Part III – Cognitive Examination (CE)		
Demonstrate your cognitive expertise by passing an ABA examination administered via computer under secure, proctored, standardized testing conditions. The examination is comprised of 200 questions, of which approximately one-half of the questions are in General Anesthesia and approximately one-twelfth of the questions are in each of the following areas: Pediatric Anesthesia, Cardiothoracic Anesthesia, Neuroanesthesia, Critical Care Medicine, Obstetrical/Gynecologic Anesthesia, and Pain Medicine.	In years 7 to 10, pass the examination. Examination prerequisites: • Satisfactory Professional Standing (PS). • One satisfactory Practice Performance Assessment and Improvement (PPAI) Attestation. • At least 200 LLSA credits granted toward the total of 350.	2016-2019 two exams offered per year
Part IV – Practice Performance Assessment and Improvement (PPAI)		
<u>Case Evaluation</u>: A four-step process where you assess your practice and implement changes that improve patient outcomes. <u>Simulation</u>: A hands-on opportunity to learn and perform valuable crisis management techniques in a simulation setting at an ASA-endorsed center.	Complete both a Case Evaluation and Simulation Course during your 10-year MOCA cycle. One PPAI activity must be completed between years 1 to 5, and the second between years 6 to 10.	2010-2014 2015-2019

Figure 1. Summary of 2009 MOCA requirements. (From Warner MA. *Certification and Maintenance of Certification.* Raleigh, NC: The American Board of Anesthesiology; 2009. http://www.theaba.org, with permission.)

1. Professional standing
2. Lifelong learning and self-assessment
3. Cognitive examination
4. Practice performance, assessment, and improvement

MOCA is an opportunity for physicians to document competency in patient care, medical knowledge, practice-based learning and improvement, interpersonal and communication skills, professionalism, and systems-based practice. An anesthesiologist's MOCA cycle starts the day after the ABA awards the initial certification. When an anesthesiologist has completed all MOCA program requirements within the 10-year program, the ABA awards a MOCA certificate. At the time of MOCA completion, the candidate must be capable of performing independently, without accommodation, or with reasonable accommodation. The board reserves the right to make the final determination of whether each candidate meets all of the requirements for MOCA according to the four components.

Barash PG, Cullen BF, Stoelting RK, et al, eds. *Clinical Anesthesia*. 6th ed. Philadelphia, PA: Lippincott Williams & Wilkins; 2009:78.
Warner MA. *Certification and Maintenance of Certification*. Raleigh, NC: The American Board of Anesthesiology; 2009. http://www.theaba.org.

Monitoring for Residual NMB

Generic, Clinical Sciences: Anesthesia Procedures, Methods, Techniques

Gabriel Jacobs

Edited by Raj K. Modak

1. Peripheral nerve stimulation is a very common method of monitoring the depth of neuromuscular blockade (NMB).
2. Five seconds sustained head lift and hand grip are some of the clinical signs that one can use to assess neuromuscular recovery.
3. Optimal patient relaxation should be maintained to the level of one to two twitches, with reversal agents given only when at least two (ideally three or four) twitches are observed with train-of-four (TOF) monitoring.

M

DISCUSSION

While the best way to monitor a patient's muscle strength is through voluntary muscle contraction, this is not possible in the anesthetized patient. Electrical and mechanical stimulation are the primary means to evaluate the level of muscle relaxation in the anesthetized patient. Electrical nerve stimulation is the most common practice in clinical anesthesia. Single twitch, TOF, tetanic stimulation, posttetanic count stimulation, and double burst stimulation are just some of the different types of electrical stimulation monitoring. A peripheral nerve stimulator should be used on all patients who receive intermediate or long acting NMB agents. Ulnar nerve (adductor pollicis) and facial nerve stimulation are the most common sites of monitoring.

TOF is one of the most common methods of electrical stimulation monitoring. TOF involves four supramaximal stimuli given in intervals of 0.5 second. TOF is best used to monitor nondepolarizing blockade, and it is less painful than other methods of electrical monitoring (tetanic) and generally does not affect the degree of NMB in the muscle group being tested. In a nonparalyzed patient, one can observe four muscle contractions of equal strength. In a patient who has received nondepolarizing NMB, zero to four twitches can be observed with decreasing intensity. Loss of the fourth twitch represents a 75% block, loss of the third twitch reflects an 80% block, and loss of the second twitch reflects a 90% block.

Tetany is a very rapid delivery of electrical stimulation to a muscle group (usually 50 Hz) applied for 5 seconds. As with TOF, fade can be observed in tetany. Fade is due to depletion of presynaptic acetylcholine. At the beginning of tetany, large amounts of acetylcholine are released. As the stores are depleted, fade ensues. Muscle contraction is sustained in a non-neuromuscular blocked muscle because even though much of the presynaptic terminal's acetylcholine is depleted, there is still enough to evoke a muscle response. In patients who have received nondepolarizing muscle relaxants, the amount of acetylcholine needed is increased due to a decrease in the number of effective postsynaptic acetylcholine receptors, thus leading to fade. Tetany can be very painful, and should not be used in awake patients.

Different muscle groups have different sensitivities to paralytics. The diaphragm, rectus abdominis, laryngeal adductors, and orbicularis oculi muscles recover from blockade faster than the adductor pollicis does. The diaphragm is very resistant to both depolarizing and nondepolarizing NMB agents, though the time of onset is very fast compared with other muscle groups. The diaphragm requires 1.4 to 2 times as much muscle relaxation to have the same response you might see in the adductor pollicis.

Posttetanic Count Stimulation is a method of electrical stimulation that can be used to assess the depth of intense NMB, when nondepolarizing NMBs are used. In this method, a tetanic stimulus of 50 Hz for 5 seconds is applied, a single twitch is elicited 3 seconds later at 1 Hz.

Some common clinical signs of recovery from NMB include 5-seconds hand grip, sustained 5-seconds head lift, sustained 5-seconds leg lift, and a maximum inspiratory pressure of 40 to 50 cc H_2O or greater.

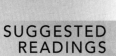

Barash PG, Cullen BF, Stoelting RK, et al, eds. *Clinical Anesthesia*. 6th ed. Philadelphia, PA: Lippincott Williams & Wilkins; 2009:1301–1302.

Miller RD, Ericksson LI, Fleisher LA, et al, eds. *Miller's Anesthesia*. 7th ed. Philadelphia, PA: Churchill Livingstone; 2010:861–862.

Morgan GE Jr, Mikhail MS, Murray MJ. *Lange Clinical Anesthesiology*. 4th ed. New York, NY: Lange Medical Books/McGraw-Hill; 2006:670.

M

Morbid Obesity: Post-op Complications

Generic, Clinical Sciences: Anesthesia Procedures, Methods, Techniques

Ervin Jakab

Edited by Lars Helgeson

M

KEY POINTS

1. Morbidly obese patients have comorbidities with significant effect on postoperative complications.
2. Postoperative hypoxia is the most frequent postoperative complication, and is often due to hypoventilation, apneic episodes, and ventilation/perfusion (V-Q) mismatch resulting from atelectasis. Proper monitoring, management of sleep apnea, postoperative pain, timing of extubation, supplemental oxygen, and pulmonary toilet are of paramount importance.
3. Sudden death may occur from acute postoperative pulmonary embolism or arrhythmias in the context of hypoxia/sympathetic surge related to apneic episodes.
4. Deep venous thrombosis and pulmonary embolism are more frequent in morbidly obese patients, especially in the context of chronic venous stasis. Prophylaxis for thrombotic complications should be instituted in all morbidly obese patients.
5. Other postoperative considerations in morbidly obese patients are related to difficulty during cardiopulmonary resuscitation, wound infections, specific complications in bariatric surgery, and positioning problems (e.g., peripheral nerve injury and rhabdomyolysis).

DISCUSSION

In the context of the current obesity epidemic, anesthesiologists face difficult challenges in terms of perioperative care of morbidly obese patients. Many of these patients undergo a full spectrum of surgical procedures related to treating complications of obesity (e.g., orthopedic, coronary artery disease, peripheral vascular disease, varicose veins, and cholelithiasis) as well as independent situations (pregnancy, cancer, trauma, etc.)

Obesity is defined as body mass index (BMI) greater than 30, and is further classified into three levels: obesity class I (BMI 30 to 34.9), obesity class II (BMI 35 to 39.9), and obesity class III, or morbid obesity (BMI > 40). The postoperative complications in these patients are influenced by the medical consequences of obesity (see Table 1). In addition, surgical, nursing, and hospital expertise in caring for morbidly obese patients have a considerable effect on postoperative morbidity and mortality.

Table 1. Medical Consequences of Obesity with Impact in the Perioperative Care

System	Pathology
Respiratory	OSA, hypoventilation, asthma, pulmonary hypertension
Cardiovascular	Atherosclerosis, coronary artery disease, arrhythmias, sudden cardiac death, cardiac failure, systemic hypertension, peripheral vascular disease, thromboembolism
Gastrointestinal	Gastroesophageal reflux disease, gallbladder disease, nonalcoholic fatty liver disease, hernias
Metabolic	Diabetes mellitus, hypothyroidism

Table 1. Medical Consequences of Obesity with Impact in the Perioperative Care *(continued)*

System	Pathology
Renal	End-stage renal disease
Neurologic	Stroke
Hematologic	Hypercoagulability, polycythemia

Adapted from Barash PG, Cullen BF, Stoelting RK, et al, eds. *Clinical Anesthesia.* 6th ed. Philadelphia, PA: Lippincott Williams & Wilkins; 2009:1230–1245.

There are several respiratory considerations specific to morbidly obese patients. Preoperative hypoxia and surgery involving the thorax or upper abdomen (vertical incisions) increase the risk of postoperative hypoxia. This added risk extends for several days into the postoperative period. Obese patients should be monitored with pulse oximetry and possibly arterial blood gases. Supplemental oxygen should be routinely provided. A 45° modified sitting position will unload the diaphragm, resulting in decreased intrathoracic pressure and improved V-Q ratio.

The incidence of atelectasis is increased after general anesthesia and further worsened by postoperative pain. Consequently, adequate analgesia, use of binder for abdominal support, early ambulation, deep breathing exercises, and incentive spirometry should be implemented. Continuous positive airway pressure or bilevel positive airway pressure has been advocated.

During apneic spells, arterial hypoxemia can be rapid and profound. Awakening in response to apnea is associated with significant sympathetic discharge, which in the presence of hypoxemia may induce lethal arrhythmias and death in the absence of coronary artery disease. Given the high incidence of obstructive sleep apnea (OSA) in morbidly obese patients, preoperative assessment of OSA risk and implementing appropriate therapy are of paramount importance, especially when intravenous narcotics are used.

Prompt extubation in patients with underlying cardiopulmonary disease reduces the likelihood of ventilator dependency. This requires complete reversal of neuromuscular blocking agents and a fully awake patient to ensure that an adequate airway and tidal volume can be maintained.

There are several cardiac considerations specific to morbidly obese patients. Arrhythmias may be related more to apneic episodes rather than to ischemia (see above). Although there is a higher prevalence of coronary artery disease in morbidly obese patients, the postoperative mortality related to myocardial infarction is low. During cardiac resuscitation, the higher transthoracic impedance from the fat may obligate several attempts of electric shock; chest compressions may not be effective and mechanical compression devices may be required. Thrombotic complications such as deep venous thrombosis and pulmonary embolism are increased in patients with a history of venous stasis disease (chronic leg edema, venous insufficiency, stasis dermatitis). Mechanical devices (sequential alternating compressive devices on the lower extremities), low-dose anticoagulation therapy (unfractionated or low-molecular weight heparin), and early ambulation should all be utilized. Placement of a vena caval filter before surgery may be also considered in high-risk patients.

Another major complication seen in this population is poor wound healing and increased incidence of wound infection. Large subcutaneous fat with poor blood supply predisposes to wound infections that could lead to incisional hernia and fascial dehiscence with considerable morbidity. Nerve injuries are also more common in the obese patients. Ulnar neuropathy related to intraoperative positioning has been found to occur more frequently in obese male patients. On the other hand, postoperative polyneuropathies may be related to malnutrition and vitamin deficiencies. Rhabdomyolysis may be seen in morbidly obese patients undergoing prolonged operative procedures. It manifests as myalgias in the postoperative period and elevated creatine phosphokinase (CPK).

Sudden death may occur secondary to arrhythmias (see above) or acute postoperative pulmonary embolism.

SUGGESTED READINGS

Barash PG, Cullen BF, Stoelting RK, et al, eds. *Clinical Anesthesia.* 6th ed. Philadelphia, PA: Lippincott Williams & Wilkins; 2009:1230–1245.

McGlinch BP, Que FG, Nelson JL, et al. Perioperative care of patients undergoing bariatric surgery [review]. *Mayo Clin Proc.* 2006;81(10)(suppl):S25–S33. PMID: 17036576.

Morgan GE Jr, Mikhail MS, Murray MJ. *Clinical Anesthesiology.* 4th ed. New York, NY: McGraw Hill, Lange Medical Books; 2006:813–815.

Morbid Obesity: Rapid Desaturation and Hypoxemia Physiology

Generic Clinical Sciences: Anesthesia Procedures, Methods, Techniques

Zhaodi Gong and Rongjie Jiang

Edited by Lars Helgeson

1. Morbidly obese patients desaturate more rapidly than patients with a normal body mass index (BMI).
2. The main cause for the rapid oxygen desaturation in morbidly obese patients is reduced functional residual capacity (FRC).
3. Some degree of hypoxemia is common in morbid obesity; conventional respiratory function tests are only mildly affected by obesity, but much more so in morbid obesity.
4. Morbid obesity results in a decreased FRC and expiratory reserve volume, and an increase in closing volume to FRC ratio. This is associated with the closure of peripheral lung alveoli, ventilation/perfusion (V/Q) ratio mismatch, and hypoxemia. This is accentuated in the supine and, especially, Trendelenburg positions.
5. Physiologic changes responsible for hypoxemia in the morbidly obese population include reduced lung volumes with normal lung compliance, decreased chest wall compliance, a heightened demand for ventilation, elevated work of breathing, respiratory muscle inefficiency, and increased respiratory resistance.
6. Application of continuous positive airway pressure (CPAP) during preoxygenation helps decrease rapid desaturation associated with obese patients.

Respiratory complications of obesity impact general health, quality of life, and longevity. Whereas morbidly obese patients are commonly slightly hypoxemic, mildly obese patients have the capacity to maintain SpO_2 and eliminate rising levels of CO_2 in the blood by increasing minute ventilation. However, morbidly obese patients are usually unable to adequately increase their minute ventilation when stressed, acutely resulting in significant hypercarbia and hypoxemia.

It is a well-known phenomenon that obese patients become hypoxemic much faster than normal adults. This is primarily due to decreased FRC and the resulting ventilation/perfusion (V/Q) mismatch. Excessive adipose tissue over the thorax decreases chest wall compliance, with lung compliance remaining normal. In addition, increased abdominal mass forces the diaphragm cephalad, resulting in a restrictive lung disease pattern. FRC may fall below closing capacity, causing some alveoli to close during normal tidal volume ventilation, resulting in a significant V/Q mismatch. Supine and Trendelenburg positions accentuate the reduction in lung volume.

Nocturnal sleep apnea commonly develops in patients with obesity, leading to remodeling and restructuring of the walls of the pulmonary tree, including the arterioles. Rarely, this can lead to pulmonary hypertension. Subsequently, these patients may develop resting hypoxia, hypercarbia, polycythemia, and cardiac failure—the obesity hypoventilation syndrome (OHS).

These abnormalities were initially attributed to mechanical limitations and decreased chest wall compliance preventing adequate ventilation. However, the decreased thoracic compliance did not improve in patients with OHS who underwent significant weight reduction, suggesting abnormal pulmonary architecture and mechanics.

Respiratory muscle weakness, impaired central drive, increased inspiratory threshold or abnormal ventilatory load compensation, and increased work of breathing may also contribute to the development of hypoxemia in morbidly obese patients.

Use of CPAP before induction recruits collapsed alveoli, thereby improving the V/Q ratio, which in turn prolongs the time until desaturation begins.

SUGGESTED
READINGS

Bady E, Achkar A, Pascal S, et al. Pulmonary arterial hypertension in patients with sleep apnoea syndrome. *Thorax*. 2000;55(11):934–939.

Koenig SM. Pulmonary complications of obesity. *Am J Med Sci*. 2001;321(4):249–279.

Miller RD. *Miller's Anesthesia*. 7th ed. Philadelphia, PA: Elsevier, Churchill, and Livingstone; 2009:386, 2092, 2098.

Sharp JT, Henry JP, Sweany SK, et al. The total work of breathing in normal and obese men. *J Clin Invest*. 1964;43(4):728–739.

M

MRI Monitoring Hazards

Physics, Monitoring, and Anesthesia Delivery Devices

Ashley Kelley

Edited by Raj K. Modak

M

KEY POINTS

1. Anesthesiologists may be called upon to provide general anesthesia or sedation to patients undergoing MRI studies.
2. Anesthesia care in the setting of an MRI is subject to a special set of challenges secondary to loss of access to the patient and the inability to use any ferromagnetic objects.
3. Anesthesia monitoring standards must be upheld while taking special care to avoid harm to the patient and caregiver.
4. Ferromagnetic items are a "missile threat" and can be lethal if brought within the range of the MRI magnet.

DISCUSSION

General anesthesia or monitored sedation is sometimes used during MRI studies, primarily when patient immobility is desired. This is especially applicable to pediatric patients and patients who are critically ill. Patients who are experiencing pain or are claustrophobic may also require general anesthesia or sedation to facilitate the completion of the imaging study.

There are many safety factors to consider when providing anesthesia or sedation in the setting of an MRI machine. Patients must be properly screened prior to the exam to ensure that they do not have any metal in their body that would be a contraindication to an MRI, such as pacemakers, aneurysm clips, or hardware from orthopedic procedures. These same requirements apply to anesthesiologists providing care for patients undergoing MRI studies. Patients must also not have pulmonary artery (PA) catheters with pacing wires or thermistors in place. Only MRI-compatible metals that are nonferromagnetic can be used for room equipment, as magnetic metal–containing objects pose a "missile threat" to the patient because of the magnetic field created by the MRI magnet. Standard pulse oximeters and electrocardiogram (EKG) electrodes cannot be used and must be replaced by monitors that are MRI compatible. The anesthesiologist must take care to avoid "looping" the leads of EKG electrodes and pulse oximeters, as this can induce currents and cause burns and monitor interference artifact. The ferrous connectors on blood pressure cuffs must be replaced. In addition, there must be a nonferromagnetic anesthesia machine in the room. The noise inside of the scanner can be very loud and cause hearing loss, and so patients should be protected with earplugs or headphones.

Additional safety issues arise secondary to the loss of access to the patient during an MRI. Access to the airway is usually limited, and thus airway protection, or maintenance of a patent airway, and monitoring via $ETco_2$, must be assured. The anesthesiologist must have long connections, or wireless capability, available for standard patient monitors as well as for invasive monitors like arterial lines that may be in place in critically ill patients. A fully functional anesthesia machine must be present outside of the MRI room in case of emergency. It must be possible to quickly remove the patient from the MRI and transfer him/her to this "primary station" so that the optimal care can be provided.

SUGGESTED READINGS

Jaffe RA, Samuels SI. *Anesthesiologist's Manual of Surgical Procedures.* 4th ed. Philadelphia, PA: Lippincott Williams & Wilkins; 2009:1467–1473.

Morgan GE, Mikhail MS, Murray MJ. *Clinical Anesthesiology.* 4th ed. New York, NY: McGraw-Hill; 2006:152–154.

Stoelting RK, Miller RD, eds. *Basics of Anesthesia.* 5th ed. Philadelphia, PA: Churchill Livingstone; 2007:553–554.

Multiple Sclerosis: Exacerbation of Symptoms

Physiology

Shaun Gruenbaum

Edited by Thomas Halaszynski

1. Although the risk of surgery and/or anesthesia toward exacerbation of multiple sclerosis (MS) is controversial, complications of surgery (especially hyperthermia and infection) are associated with an increased risk of MS exacerbations.
2. Severity of the disease is an important risk factor for MS exacerbation.
3. The rate of relapse of MS decreases during pregnancy, especially during the third trimester, and increases during the first 3 months post partum.
4. Although local anesthetics may slightly increase the risk of MS exacerbation, their use is not contraindicated in patients with MS.
5. Spinal anesthesia, but not epidural anesthesia or peripheral nerve blocks, has been associated with an increased risk of MS exacerbation.

M

The risk of surgery and anesthesia creating exacerbation of symptoms in MS is controversial. Although there have been case reports in the literature describing MS exacerbation after general and regional anesthesia, no correlation has been demonstrated between the anesthesia and the disease course of MS. Nevertheless, before surgery, patients with MS should be counseled of the potential risk of relapse despite appropriate anesthesia. MS exacerbation after surgery, when it does occur, is more likely to occur during the postoperative period.

There have been no studies that demonstrate any individual anesthetic agent as the causative entity leading to a relapse in MS; as a result, both inhaled and intravenous anesthetics may be used in the MS patient population. However, complications of surgery, particularly infection and hyperthermia, may exacerbate MS. Even a 0.5° C increase in temperature can block the conduction of demyelinated nerves, leading to deterioration of nerve tissue at the site of demyelination. Therefore, all patients with MS undergoing surgery should have temperature closely monitored, and hyperthermia should be avoided. The stress response of surgery has not been shown to exacerbate symptoms of MS and the National Multiple Sclerosis Society (NMSS) echoes this sentiment.

The severity of MS is an important risk factor assessing for symptom exacerbation. Severely debilitated patients or those with significant respiratory compromise may have difficulties recovering from surgery, increasing the risk of postoperative relapse. Therefore, a thorough history and physical examination should be performed on *all* patients with MS, with particular attention paid to neurologic and respiratory systems. In addition, comparing preoperative and postoperative conditions/states of MS patients may help identify potential relapse. Patients with MS are often administered steroids as part of their maintenance regimen and/or for the treatment of relapses, and stress dose steroids may be indicated during the perioperative period.

The prevalence of MS is highest in women of childbearing age. Although pregnancy is thought to be protective because the incidence of MS relapse declines during pregnancy, especially during the third trimester, the postpartum period is associated with an increased rate of MS relapse. Nevertheless, there are concerns about the optimal anesthetic management for this MS population group. Epidural anesthesia has not been shown to further increase the rate of MS relapse in pregnancy. Analgesia and anesthetic management for this patient population should be made on an individualized basis.

The risk of regional anesthesia for relapse of MS symptoms is controversial. In one study by the NMSS, 98 patients received a total of more than 1,000 doses of local anesthetics, and only 4 cases of MS exacerbations followed the administration of local anesthetics during regional techniques. Despite this small risk, the NMSS asserts that the use of local anesthetics need not be avoided in patients with MS.

Although epidural anesthesia and peripheral nerve blocks have not been implicated in MS exacerbations, the use of spinal anesthesia has been associated with MS relapse. Although the exact pathophysiology is unknown, it is hypothesized that demyelination that occurs with MS results in a lack of a protective sheath around the spinal cord, resulting in increased risk from neurotoxic effects of local anesthetics. Thus, spinal anesthesia is generally not recommended in patients with MS. However, epidural anesthesia typically requires a lower concentration of local anesthetic and may be better tolerated by patients with MS.

SUGGESTED READINGS

Barash PG, Cullen BF, Stoelting RK. *Clinical Anesthesia*. 5th ed. Philadelphia, PA: Lippincott Williams & Wilkins; 2009:628–629.
Confavreux C, Hutchinson M, Hours MM, et al. Rate of pregnancy-related relapse in multiple sclerosis. *N Engl J Med*. 1998;339:285–291.
Stoelting RK, Dierdorf SF. *Handbook for Anesthesia and Co-existing Disease*. 2nd ed. New York, NY: Churchill Livingstone; 2002:201.

Multiple Sclerosis Exacerbation

Generic, Clinical Sciences: Anesthesia Procedures, Methods, Techniques

Dallen Mill

Edited by Ramachandran Ramani

KEY POINTS

1. Controversy exists concerning the impact of general, neuraxial, and regional anesthesia on the natural history of multiple sclerosis (MS).
2. Many authorities do not recommend spinal anesthesia in patients with MS.
3. A recent study suggests that the complications of neuraxial anesthesia in the setting of preexisting central nervous system (CNS) disorders may not be as frequent as previously thought.

M

DISCUSSION

MS is a T-cell–mediated demyelination of neurons in both the central nervous system and the peripheral nervous system, resulting in a multitude of neurologic symptoms. The impact of anesthesia on MS is unclear. This is in part due to the exacerbating effects of issues commonly associated with surgical procedures, but not necessarily related to anesthesia, including infection, elevated temperature, and physical and emotional stress. Regional anesthesia is preferred in patients with MS. Some of these patients may have specific indications for regional or neuraxial anesthetic techniques, such as those with respiratory compromise or cognitive dysfunction. A recent case report described a severe brachial plexopathy after single-injection nerve block in a patient with MS. Worsening symptoms have also been reported with spinal anesthesia, resulting in its use not traditionally being recommended.

In a recent retrospective study comprising 139 patients with preexisting CNS disorders who received neuraxial anesthesia, it was concluded that the risks commonly associated with neuraxial anesthesia in this population may not be as frequent as previously thought. The study did not identify any patients with new or worsening postoperative neurologic deficits when compared with preoperative findings, including those patients (54%) who received spinal anesthesia.

Depolarizing neuromuscular blocking agents should be avoided in patients with MS because of the potential for hyperkalemia with subsequent cardiac arrhythmias secondary to upregulation of extrajunctional nicotinic receptors. Nondepolarizing agents appear to be safe.

Neurologic derangements associated with MS require consideration before the administration of anesthesia. For example, exaggerated hypotension can result from autonomic dysfunction, and prolonged mechanical ventilation may be required as a result of respiratory muscle weakness.

SUGGESTED READINGS

Barash PG, Cullen BF, Stoelting RK, et al, eds. *Clinical Anesthesia.* 6th ed. Philadelphia, PA: Lippincott Williams & Wilkins; 2009:628–629.

Hebl JR, Horlocker TT, Schroeder DR. Neuraxial anesthesia and analgesia in patients with preexisting central nervous system disorders. *Anesth Analg.* 2006;103:223–228.

Koff M, Cohen J, McIntyre JJ, et al. Severe brachial plexopathy after an ultrasound-guided single-injection nerve block for total shoulder arthroplasty in a patient with multiple sclerosis. *Anesthesiology.* 2008;108:325–328.

Miller R. Preoperative evaluation. In: *Miller's Anesthesia.* 7th ed. Philadelphia, PA: Churchill Livingstone; 2009:927–950.

Myasthenia: Muscle Relaxant Effects
Physiology

Christina Mack

Edited by Jodi Sherman

KEY POINTS

1. Myasthenia gravis (MG) is an autoimmune disorder that results in a decrease in functional acetylcholine receptors.
2. The cardinal symptom of this disorder is muscle fatigue that worsens with repetitive use and improves with rest.
3. Patients with MG are resistant to the effects of depolarizing neuromuscular blockers and extremely sensitive to the effects of nondepolarizing neuromuscular blockers.
4. Patients with MG are commonly treated with anticholinesterase inhibitors for relief of muscle fatigue symptoms.

DISCUSSION

MG is an autoimmune disorder in which circulating antibodies to nicotinic acetylcholine receptors and other muscle membrane proteins result in a decrease in the number of post-synaptic receptors and a decrease in the number of folds in the postsynaptic membrane. The cardinal symptom of this disorder is muscle fatigue that worsens with repetitive use and improves with rest. MG affects skeletal muscles and is classified on the basis of the type and severity of muscles involved (see Table 1).

Table 1. Classification of MG Severity

Class	Description
I	Ocular muscle weakness
II	Mild nonocular muscle weakness ± ocular muscle weakness
III	Moderate nonocular muscle weakness (except in the perioperative period)
IV	Severe nonocular muscle weakness ± ocular muscle weakness
V	Tracheal intubation (except in the perioperative period) or tracheostomy to protect the airway with or without mechanical ventilation

Adapted from Morgan E, et al. Anesthesia for patients with neuromuscular disease—myasthenia gravis. In: *Clinical Anesthesiology*. 4th ed. New York, NY: McGraw-Hill; 2006:818.

MG affects the actions of both depolarizing and nondepolarizing neuromuscular blocking agents. These patients are typically resistant to the effects of succinylcholine and have increased sensitivity to the effects of nondepolarizing neuromuscular blockers. The dose of succinylcholine may have to be increased to 2 mg per kg to achieve adequate muscle relaxation for direct laryngoscopy; at this dose, however, a phase II block can occur. Nondepolarizing muscular blockers will have a faster onset and more prolonged duration of action in MG patients. Short- or intermediate-acting nondepolarizing agents are preferred, starting at one-tenth of the standard dose and slowly titrating until the desired effect is observed.

Patients with MG are commonly treated with anticholinesterase inhibitors for relief of muscle fatigue symptoms. These drugs should be held on the day of surgery to avoid interference with neuromuscular blocking agents. The exception to this precaution is patients with class IV (severe disease), as they deteriorate significantly without anticholinesterase inhibitor treatment. Monitoring of neuromuscular function is critical for MG patients. The

effect of reversal agents may be less than anticipated for patients already taking anticholinesterase inhibitors. Consequently, mechanical ventilations should be continued until
neuromuscular function has spontaneously recovered.

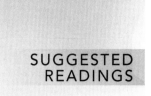

**SUGGESTED
READINGS**

Dierdorf S, Walton S. Rare and coexisting diseases—myasthenia gravis. In: Barash PG, Cullen BF, Stoelting RK,
et al, eds. *Clinical Anesthesia*. 6th ed. Philadelphia, PA: Lippincott Williams & Williams; 2009:626–627.
Neustein S, et al. Anesthesia for thoracic surgery—myasthenia gravis. In: Barash PG, Cullen BF, Stoelting RK, et al,
eds. *Clinical Anesthesia*. 6th ed. Philadelphia, PA: Lippincott Williams & Williams; 2009:1064–1066.

M

Myasthenia Gravis: Postop Management

SECTION
Generic, Clinical Sciences: Anesthesia Procedures, Methods, Techniques

Bijal Patel and Kellie Park

Edited by Ramachandran Ramani

M

KEY POINTS

1. Myasthenia gravis (MG) is an autoimmune disease in which acetylcholine receptors at the neuromuscular junction are the site of pathology, resulting in muscle weakness.
2. Patients with MG are at increased risk for postoperative respiratory failure.
3. Duration of MG greater than 6 years, a history of chronic respiratory disease unrelated to MG, pyridostigmine dose greater than 750 mg per day, and a preoperative vital capacity less than 2.9 L may indicate the need for postoperative ventilation in patients undergoing transsternal thymectomy.
4. Postoperative doses of opioids should be decreased by 33% for patients taking anticholinesterase medications, as it is believed that they increase the analgesic effect of opioids.

DISCUSSION

MG is an autoimmune disease in which acetylcholine receptors at the neuromuscular junction are targeted, resulting in muscle weakness. Patients with this condition are at an increased risk for postoperative respiratory failure. Although a patient may appear to have adequate respiration immediately after surgery, his or her condition may deteriorate several hours later. There are certain criteria that may indicate the need for prolonged ventilation after surgery, specifically after transsternal thymectomy. These include duration of MG greater than 6 years, a history of chronic respiratory disease unrelated to MG, pyridostigmine dose greater than 750 mg per day, and a preoperative vital capacity less than 2.9 L. The predictive value of these criteria does not necessarily apply to transcervical thymectomy or other surgical procedures. Treatment with oral anticholinesterase or plasmapheresis before surgery or perioperative steroids may decrease the incidence of postoperative respiratory failure.

Monitoring patients for respiratory failure is of utmost concern, with pulse oximetry often not being enough, but instead regular measurements of vital capacity, tidal volume, and negative inspiratory force being beneficial.

Opioids are used for postoperative pain management, but it is important to note that reduced doses must be used in patients taking anticholinesterases. These medications are believed to increase the analgesic effect of opioids, and as such, doses should be decreased by approximately 33%.

An important part of managing MG patients postoperatively is to look for myasthenic crisis and cholinergic crisis. When a patient has been dosed with anticholinesterases, especially if neuromuscular blockade was used, underdosing of anticholinesterase can lead to myasthenic crisis. These patients will be very weak and often unable to breathe, and their pupils will appear to be large. These patients can be treated with edrophonium. If too much anticholinesterase is administered intraoperatively, weakness can again ensue in a cholinergic crisis. These patients will be weak and have constricted pupils. Atropine can be used to treat these patients. Prompt recognition and treatment is important to avoid respiratory failure.

SUGGESTED READINGS

Barash PG, Cullen BF, Stoelting RK, et al, eds. *Clinical Anesthesia.* 6th ed. New York, NY: Lippincott Williams & Wilkins; 2009:1064–1067.

Hines RL, Marschall KE. *Anesthesia and Co-existing Disease.* 5th ed. Philadelphia, PA: Churchill Livingstone; 2008:450–454.

Kumar V, Abbas AK, Fausto N. *Robbins and Cotran Pathologic Basis of Disease.* 7th ed. Philadelphia, PA: Elsevier Saunders; 2005:1344.

M

Myocardial Ischemia: Acute MR
Organ-based Clinical: Cardiovascular

Adnan Malik

Edited by Benjamin Sherman

M

KEY POINTS

1. Myocardial ischemia may cause acute mitral regurgitation (MR) secondary to papillary muscle dysfunction, with tethering of the mitral valve in the open position or due to the rupture of the papillary muscle or chordae tendineae with flail or prolapse of the leaflet.
2. Bacterial endocarditis and chest trauma are two other causes of acute MR.
3. Acute MR causes elevation in left atrial pressures and pulmonary edema.
4. Pulmonary capillary wedge waveform will demonstrate a large *v* waves in acute MR.
5. The intraoperative management of acute MR involves afterload reduction with anesthetic agents and vasodilators, preload reduction with diuretics, and utilization of inotropes to increase contractility and heart rate.

DISCUSSION

Acute MR is usually due to myocardial ischemia, leading to papillary muscle dysfunction with subsequent shortening and tethering of the valve into the open position. Myocardial infarction can cause rupture of the papillary muscle or chordae tendineae with flail or prolapse of the mitral leaflets. Other causes of acute MR are infection of the leaflet with valve destruction/perforation or possibly acute chest trauma.

Myocardial ischemia with MR results in a holosystolic murmur radiating to the axilla. Approximately 40% of patients who suffer a posterior-septal myocardial infarction, and 20% of who suffer an anterior-septal infarction develop papillary muscle dysfunction. The posterior-medial papillary muscle is more prone to ischemia because it is usually perfused by one coronary arterial vessel, whereas the anterior-lateral papillary muscle is perfused by two.

Acute MR may cause an elevation in left atrial volume and pressure, which, in turn, is transmitted to the pulmonary circulation, causing pulmonary edema. As a compensatory mechanism for an acute decrease in cardiac output, the sympathetic system responds with tachycardia and increased contractility. This response, however, requires an increase in myocardial oxygen demand in an already ischemic myocardium, potentially increasing the severity of ischemia.

Echocardiography is the diagnostic tool of choice in the detection of acute MR. Besides grading the severity of MR, echocardiography can frequently differentiate the etiology of MR and direct appropriate treatment (ischemia induced, bacterial endocarditis, papillary or chordae rupture). Pulmonary capillary wedge tracings are also useful in the diagnosis of acute MR. In acute MR, a relatively noncompliant left atrium will often result in large *v* waves, also known as cannon *v*-waves (see Fig. 1).

Intraoperative management depends on the etiology. If papillary dysfunction is suspected, treating the ischemia may improve valvular function. If bacterial endocarditis is suspected, appropriate antibiotic therapy may halt the destructive process, yet surgical repair is likely required if symptomatic regurgitation is present. If the MR is due to papillary apparatus rupture, afterload reduction with anesthetic agents and vasodilators, preload reduction with diuretics, and utilization of inotropes to increase contractility, surgical repair planning is warranted.

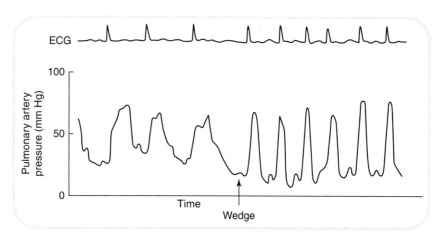

Figure 1. Pulmonary Artery tracing in acute Mitral Regurgitation. (From Morgan GE, Mikhail MS, Murray MJ. *Clinical Anesthesiology.* 4th ed. New York, NY: McGraw-Hill http://www.accessmedicine.com, with permission.)

SUGGESTED READINGS

Barash PG, Cullen BF, Stoelting RK, et al, eds. *Clinical Anesthesia.* 6th ed. Philadelphia, PA: Lippincott Williams & Wilkins; 2009:1084–1085.

Hensley FA, Martin DE. *A Practical Approach to Cardiac Anesthesia.* 2nd ed. Boston, MA: Little, Brown and Company; 1995:311–315.

Morgan GE, Mikhail MS, Murray MJ. *Clinical Anesthesiology.* 4th ed. New York, NY: Lange McGraw-Hill; 2006:469–471.

Voci P, Bilotta F, Caretta Q, et al. Papillary muscle perfusion pattern. A hypothesis for ischemic papillary muscle dysfunction. *Circulation.* 1995;91(6):1714–1718.

M

Myocardial O$_2$ Consumption: Determinants

Physiology

Kristin Richards

Edited by Qingbing Zhu

KEY POINTS

1. A determinant of myocardial oxygen consumption (MVO$_2$) is myocardial wall tension.
2. The following factors could change myocardial wall tension, resulting in increased MVCO$_2$:
   - Increased preload
   - Increased afterload
   - Increased contractility

DISCUSSION

The law of LaPlace states that wall tension (T) is proportional to the product of intraventricular pressure (P) and ventricular radius (r):

$$T \propto P \cdot r$$

Myocardial wall tension is the tension generated by myocytes that results in intraventricular pressure at a particular ventricular radius. When the ventricle needs to generate greater pressure, for example, with increased afterload or inotropic stimulation, the wall tension is increased. This relationship also explains why a dilated ventricle with an increased preload has to generate increased wall tension to produce the same intraventricular pressure.

Factors that result in increased tension development by the cardiac myocytes, the rate of tension development, or the number of tension generating cycles per unit time will increase MVO$_2$. For instance, if the heart rate is doubled, the MVO$_2$ will be doubled because ventricular myocytes are generating twice the number of tension cycles per minute.

Myocyte contraction is the primary factor determining MVO$_2$ above basal levels. Increasing contractility also increases MVO$_2$ because of increase in the rate of tension development, as well as in the magnitude of tension, both of which result in increased ATP hydrolysis and oxygen consumption.

Increased tension, and therefore an increased MVO$_2$, is also seen with an increase in afterload. Increasing preload, increasing ventricular end-diastolic volume, also increases MVO$_2$ by increase of tension from the enlarged left ventricle radius. However, the increase is much less than what might be expected because of the law of LaPlace.

SUGGESTED READING

Klabunde RE. *Cardiovascular Physiology Concepts*. 1st ed. Philadelphia, PA: Lippincott Williams & Wilkins; 2005:116. http://cvphysiology.com/index.html.

Myotonic Dyst: Aspiration Risk
Physiology

Jordan Martin

Edited by Thomas Halaszynski

1. Myotonic dystrophy, delayed relaxation of skeletal muscle, may cause an increased risk of aspiration secondary to ineffective coughing and pharyngeal muscle weakness.
2. Myotonic dystrophy may cause a prolonged response to muscle relaxants and an increased risk of aspiration secondary to delayed gastric emptying and impaired swallowing.
3. Patients with myotonic dystrophy should not receive preoperative opioids or sedatives.
4. Patients with myotonic dystrophy have progressive involvement and deterioration of function with skeletal, cardiac, and smooth muscle.

M

DISCUSSION

Myotonia or delayed relaxation after contraction of musculature is the key characteristic of myotonic dystrophy. This condition affects multiple organ systems throughout the body. From an anesthesiologist's perspective, this can result in atypical responses to medications (especially muscle relaxants) and situations that require extra vigilance, such as pharyngeal muscle weakness in conjunction with delayed gastric emptying that increases the risk of aspiration of gastric contents.

The abnormal muscle physiology, normally protective of the airway, can result in an increased risk of pulmonary aspiration. This risk arises from a combination of abnormalities of the muscles in both the pulmonary system and the gastrointestinal system. Involvement of smooth muscles in the gastrointestinal tract can result in intestinal hypomotility, delayed gastric emptying, gastroparesis, and impaired swallowing. Furthermore, in the respiratory tract, diminished musculature leads to ineffective coughing, pharyngeal muscle weakness, and secretion retention. This combination of increased gastric contents and decreased pulmonary protection amplifies the risk of pulmonary aspiration (can lead to pulmonary infections and even death).

Consequently, avoidance or careful use of preoperative opioids or sedatives is recommended. Unfortunately, some patients may be presymptomatic or even undiagnosed. Because myotonic dystrophy is inherited as an autosomal dominant trait, family history can be extremely important. These undiagnosed patients and those experiencing severe weakness or proximal weakness or undergoing upper abdominal surgery are at particular risk for complications secondary to the aspiration potential.

SUGGESTED READINGS

Barash PG, Cullen BF, Stoelting RK, et al, eds. *Clinical Anesthesia*. 6th ed. Philadelphia, PA: Lippincott Williams & Wilkins; 2009:622–625.

Miller RD. *Miller's Anesthesia*. 6th ed. Philadelphia, PA: Elsevier; 2005:536–537, 1099.

Morgan GE, Mikhail MS, Murray MJ. *Clinical Anesthesiology*. 4th ed. New York, NY: McGraw-Hill; 2006:817–823.

N$_2$O: CBF and CMRO$_2$

Organ-based Clinical: Neurologic and Neuromuscular

Harika Nagavelli

Edited by Ramachandran Ramani

KEY POINTS

1. Cerebral blood flow (CBF) is dependent on arterial CO$_2$ tension, cerebral autoregulation of cerebral perfusion pressure (CPP), and metabolic activity of the brain.
2. Cerebral metabolic rate (CMR) is often measured as cerebral metabolic rate of oxygen consumption (CMRO$_2$).
3. Volatile anesthetics decrease CBF at lower doses and increase CBF at higher doses.
4. Although nitrous oxide may increase CBF to a lesser extent compared with other volatile anesthetics, it does have properties that are detrimental to protecting the brain.

DISCUSSION

Inhalational anesthetics have a dose-dependent effect on the CBF. At lower doses, volatile anesthetics such a halothane, desflurane, sevoflurane, and isoflurane induce a CMRO$_2$-mediated decrease in CBF (decrease in CMRO$_2$ causes a decrease in CBF); at higher doses, however, the vasodilatory effects of the inhalational anesthetic overcome the CMRO$_2$-mediated decrease, causing an increase in CBF. Cerebral autoregulation of blood pressure involves adjustments made by the cerebral resistance to maintain stable CBF. These affects are seen with changes in mean arterial pressure (MAP) and intracranial pressure (ICP) to maintain a stable CPP.

Nitrous oxide causes an increase in CBF, but does not affect cerebral blood volume (CBV). The net effect of the increase in CBF is magnified when nitrous oxide is used in conjunction with volatile anesthetics at greater than 1 MAC. In contrast, CBF remains largely unaffected when nitrous oxide is administered with intravenous (IV) anesthetics such as opioids, benzodiazepines, barbiturates, propofol, or etomidate. These IV anesthetics, in general, appear to cause vasoconstriction and a decrease in CMRO$_2$. Currently, there is no consensus on the effect of nitrous oxide on CMRO$_2$. By itself, it can cause a rise in CMRO$_2$. In clinical practice, N$_2$O is always administered in combination with other anesthetics. The impact of arterial carbon dioxide tension on CBF remains unchanged under the influence of anesthetics including nitrous oxide, whereas the autoregulation of cerebral resistance to changes in MAP is lost with the use of volatile anesthetics.

Although there is no absolute contraindication against the use of nitrous oxide in neurosurgical patients, in the clinical setting of unresolved and elevated ICP, nitrous oxide may not be the choice for volatile anesthetic agent. Furthermore, nitrous oxide is contraindicated when nitrous oxide may be able to enter a closed gas space, potentially causing pneumocephalus or even tension pneumocephalus.

SUGGESTED READINGS

Barash PG, Cullen BF, Stoelting RK, et al, eds. *Clinical Anesthesia*. 6th ed. Philadelphia, PA: Lippincott Williams & Wilkins; 2009:423, 1005–1009.

Miller RD, Eriksson LI, Fleisher LA, et al, eds. *Miller's Anesthesia*. 7th ed. Philadelphia, PA: Elsevier, Churchill Livingstone; 2009:chap 13:320–321.

Nalbuphine: Plateau Effect Mechanism

Pharmacology

Soumya Nyshadham

Edited by Jodi Sherman

N

KEY POINTS

1. Nalbuphine is a partial agonist-antagonist, effecting opioid mu and kappa receptors.
2. Partial agonists of a specific drug have affinity to a receptor site, but with decreased efficacy, compared with a full agonist drug. In the presence of increasing levels of full agonist, a partial agonist can serve as an antagonist, and is thereby termed a *partial agonist-antagonist*.
3. Nalbuphine, like other opioid agonist-antagonists, exhibits a plateau effect, whereby giving higher doses beyond a fixed point will not produce further effects.
4. As with other opioid agonists, nalbuphine may cause respiratory depression. However, it exhibits a plateau effect that is roughly equal to that produced by 0.4 mg per kg of morphine.
5. Nalbuphine's partial antagonist effects can blunt the respiratory depression produced by full mu agonists; unlike naloxone, it does not fully reverse analgesia.

DISCUSSION

An agonist is a drug that produces a particular effect at the receptor site with an associated affinity and efficacy. Antagonists, on the other hand, bind to the same site as agonists with similar affinity, but poor efficacy. A partial agonist binds with similar or lesser affinity as a full agonist but with decreased efficacy. In the presence of an antagonist, full agonists must be in higher dosages to reach maximum efficacy (see Fig. 1). In the presence of increasing levels of full agonist, a partial agonist can serve as an antagonist at its receptor site.

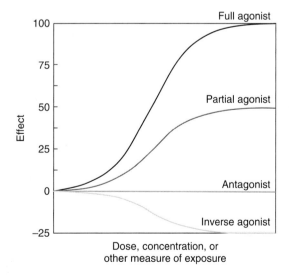

Figure 1. The dose-dependent effect of agonist, partial agonist, antagonist, and inverse agonist. (From Miller RD, Stoelting RK. *Basics of Anesthesia*. 5th ed. Philadelphia, PA: Churchill Livingstone; 2007:45.)

Opioid agonist-antagonists bind to mu receptors as either a partial agonists or antagonists. These drugs also often function as partial agonists at kappa and delta receptors. The primary role of these drugs has been the tempering of postoperative analgesia, but at times, they can be used intraoperatively as sedative adjuncts. Nalbuphine is a partial agonist at mu and kappa receptors, and like most opioids, respiratory depression results. However, this effect of nalbuphine exhibits a plateau effect that is roughly equal to that produced by 0.4 mg per kg of morphine. Consequently, beyond this specific "ceiling dose," the respiratory depression resulting from nalbuphine will reach a distinct end point. This peak maximum effect is secondary to the partial agonism and antagonism at receptor sites. Hence, in the presence of a pure agonist, nalbuphine is an antagonist to full agonists at opioid receptors, blunting respiratory depression; unlike naloxone, nalbuphine does not fully reverse analgesia. This is useful particularly in labor and delivery when compared with fentanyl, whose respiratory depression outlasts its relatively short period of analgesic effect (roughly 60 minutes).

SUGGESTED READING

Barash PG, Cullen BF, Stoelting RK, et al, eds. *Clinical Anesthesia*. 6th ed. New York, NY: Lippincott Williams & Wilkins; 2009:488–489.
Miller RD, Stoelting RK. *Basics of Anesthesia*. 5th ed. Philadelphia, PA: Churchill Livingstone; 2007:44–46, 120.
Morgan GE, Mikhail MS, Murray MJ. *Clinical Anesthesiology*. 4th ed. Philadelphia, PA: McGraw-Hill Professional; 2006:894–895.

N

Nasal Fiberoptic Intubation

Generic, Clinical Sciences: Anesthesia Procedures, Methods, Techniques

Kimberly Slininger

Edited by Lars Helgeson

KEY POINTS

1. Indications for nasal fiberoptic intubation include surgeries in which having an oral endotracheal tube (ETT) would interfere with the surgical field or cases in which there is mechanical obstruction of the oropharynx.
2. Technique for fiberoptic placement of nasal ETT is similar to the technique for oral fiberoptic intubation.

DISCUSSION

Specific indications for nasal intubation include oral, mandibular, or facial surgeries where an oral endotracheal tube (ETT) would interfere with the surgical field. Other indications include cases where there is a mechanical obstruction in the oropharynx that would preclude the placement of a tube orally. Lastly, any condition that renders the patient unable to open his or her mouth, which includes severe temporomandibular joint (TMJ) or mandibular fractures, also requires nasal intubation.

Contraindications to nasal fiberoptic intubations are the same as those for a regular nasal intubation, and include basilar skull fractures, coagulopathies, and mechanical obstruction. Basilar skull fractures pose the risk of accidental entry into the cranium. Nasal intubations have a high risk of epistaxis, which can be made worse by coagulopathies. Stopping the bleeding is difficult because of the inability to directly compress the bleeding site.

The technique for doing a nasal fiberoptic intubation is similar to that of a standard oral fiberoptic intubation. The ETT should be large enough to easily slide over the fiberoptic bronchoscope. This means that the ETT inner diameter should be at least 1.5 mm greater than the diameter of the fiberoptic bronchoscope. It is important to carefully size the ETT ahead of time to ensure that it will pass through the nasal passage. Both nostrils should be prepared with topical anesthesia and a vasoconstrictor. Warming the ETT to soften it and lubricating it will help its passage through the nasopharynx. Once the ETT is placed into the nasopharynx, the fiberoptic bronchoscope can be threaded through the ETT. The nasal passage tends to keep the fiberoptic scope in a midline position and tends to direct the scope toward the trachea. The bronchoscope and ETT can be manipulated as needed to direct the bronchoscope into the trachea. Once the trachea has been successfully entered, the ETT can carefully be threaded over the bronchoscope and placed into the trachea. Final position of the ETT should be confirmed by visualizing the carina and tracheal rings with the nasotracheal tube in place using the fiberoptic bronchoscope.

SUGGESTED READINGS

Dorsch JA, Dorsch SA. *Understanding Anesthesia Equipment.* 5th ed. Philadelphia, PA: Lippincott Williams & Wilkins; 2008:585–586.
Stoelting RK, Miller RD. *Basics of Anesthesia.* 5th ed. Philadelphia, PA: Churchill Livingstone; 2005:224.

Negative Pressure Pulmonary Edema: Physiology

Generic Clinical Sciences: Anesthesia Procedures, Methods, Techniques

Tara Paulose

Edited by Veronica Matei

KEY POINTS

1. Negative pressure pulmonary edema is an acute process that results from excessive negative inspiratory forces in the setting of relieved airway obstruction.
2. The presence of bilateral, fluffy infiltrates on chest X-ray can help make the diagnosis.
3. Treatment of negative pressure pulmonary edema is largely supportive.

N

DISCUSSION

Negative pressure pulmonary edema (also known as postobstructive pulmonary edema) is an acute process that results after removal of an airway obstruction (such as laryngospasm). In this setting, the negative pulmonary pressure created during inspiration, exceeds that of a patient without such obstruction. This increase in negative pressure precipitates an increase in venous return. Increased blood volume in the pulmonary circuit disrupts the pulmonary capillary walls resulting in acute pulmonary edema.

The clinical signs of negative pressure pulmonary edema include pink froth within an endotrachael tube and abrupt oxygen desaturation in an extubated patient. This diagnosis can be confirmed with a chest X-ray showing bilateral interstitial infiltrates.

Treatment of negative pressure pulmonary edema should begin preemptively, with the administration of continuous positive pressure (as appropriate) in the operating room and supportively thereafter. Therapies postextubation should include maintenance of airway patency, oxygen supplementation as appropriate, diuresis, and reintubation with mechanical ventilation if necessary. Most cases resolve within 24 hours of the initial insult.

SUGGESTED READINGS

Barash PG, Cullen BF, Stoelting RK, et al, eds. *Clinical Anesthesia*. 6th ed. Philadelphia, PA: Lippincott Williams & Wilkins; 2009:1308–1309.

Miller RD, Steeling RK. *Basics of Anesthesia*. 5th ed. Philadelphia, PA: Churchill Livingstone; 2007:569.

Morgan G, Mikhail M, Murray M. *Clinical Anesthesiology*. 4th ed. New York, NY: McGraw-Hill Medical; 2006:1040–1043.

Neonatal Bradycardia: Rx

Subspecialties: Obstetric Anesthesia

Hyacinth Ruiter

Edited by Lars Helgeson

1. The risk factors for neonatal bradycardia include prematurity, multiple congenital anomalies, and maternal narcotic use.
2. Positive-pressure ventilation should be initiated if the heart rate is less than 100 beats per minute, persistent cyanosis despite 100% oxygen, and shallow, gasping breaths.
3. When the heart rate is less than 60 beats per minute or is between 60 and 80 beats per minute and not improving, the neonate should be intubated and chest compressions should be started.
4. Epinephrine at a dose of 0.01 to 0.03 mg per kg should be given for asystole or a heart rate of less than 60 beats per minute after attempts at chest compressions and adequate ventilation demonstrate no clinical improvement.
5. Naloxone, 0.1 μg per kg intravenously or 0.2 μg per kg intramuscularly, should be administered to reverse a maternal history of narcotics less than 4 hours before delivery if there are signs of neonatal depression.

N

Neonatal bradycardia is a serious and well-known complication that calls for urgent attention and action. Risk factors for neonatal bradycardia include maternal narcotic use, prematurity, and multiple congenital anomalies. The etiology of neonatal apnea includes respiratory muscle fatigue, decreased ventilatory drive, decreased responsiveness to hypoxia, and hypercarbia. The treatment of neonatal bradycardia begins with tactile stimulation, and mask ventilation will be necessary if breathing efforts remain poor. Positive-pressure ventilation should be initiated if the heart rate is less than 100 beats per minute, cyanosis persists despite 100% oxygen availability, and shallow gasping breaths are taken. After providing effective breaths at a rate of 40 to 60 breaths per minutes for 15 to 30 seconds, the heart rate should be reassessed.

If the heart rate remains between 60 and 80 beats per minute and is improving, assisted ventilation is continued. Chest compressions are initiated when the heart rate does not rise above 80 beats per minute. The neonate should be intubated and chest compressions started when the heart rate is less than 60 beats per minute or is between 60 and 80 beats per minute and not improving. The indications for intubation include inadequate respiratory effort, prolonged positive-pressure ventilation, and ineffective mask ventilation.

Neonates with significant bradycardia may receive caffeine and theophylline. These central nervous system (CNS) stimulants decrease the threshold for the ventilatory response to hypercarbia, thereby increasing central respiratory drive. High-risk neonates may benefit from spinal anesthesia with a decreased incidence of postoperative apnea and bradycardia. Epinephrine, 0.01 to 0.03 mg per kg, should be given for asystole or a heart rate of less than 60 beats per minute, along with chest compressions and adequate ventilation. Naloxone, 0.1 μg per kg intravenously or 0.2 μg per kg intramuscularly, is given to reverse a maternal history of narcotics less than 4 hours before delivery if there are signs of neonatal respiratory depression. Sodium bicarbonate, 2 mEq per kg of a 0.5 mEq per mL 4.2% solution, can be given for a severe metabolic acidosis.

Barash PG, Cullen BF, Stoelting RK, et al, eds. *Clinical Anesthesia.* 6th ed. Philadelphia, PA: Lippincott Williams & Wilkins, a Wolters Kluwer Business; 2009:1191.

Miller RD. *Miller's Anesthesia.* 6th ed. Philadelphia, PA: Churchill Livingstone; 2005:2348–2363.

Neonatal vs. Adult Cardiac Phys
Subspecialties: Pediatric Anesthesia

Michael Archambault

Edited by Mamatha Punjala

KEY POINTS

1. In utero, the fetus relies on a parallel circulation that converts to a series system after birth.
2. The increase in left atrial pressure causes closure of the foramen ovale, and the ductus arteriosus closes due to decreasing prostaglandin levels and increasing oxygen tension.
3. Because of decreased contractility, the neonate is unable to increase stroke volume, and cardiac output is dependent on heart rate.
4. The immature cardiac tissue also handles periods of ischemia better than adult cardiac tissue.
5. It is thought that sympathetic innervation of the neonatal heart is incomplete, and thus the neonate will have decreased uptake of catecholamines.

DISCUSSION

The neonatal heart and the adult heart differ substantially. Immediately after birth, the neonatal circulation begins its transition from fetal circulation to adult circulation. In utero, the fetus relies on a parallel circulation that converts to a series system after birth. With clamping of the umbilical cord, the low-resistance placenta is separated from the neonatal circulation, and the systemic vascular resistance of the neonate increases. The pulmonary vasculature changes from high resistance to low resistance with the initiation of breathing. This increases blood flow through the pulmonary vasculature and increases left atrial pressure. The increase in left atrial pressure causes closure of the foramen ovale. After birth, the ductus arteriosus closes due to decreasing prostaglandin levels and increasing oxygen tension. Though both the foramen ovale and ductus arteriosus functionally close, they are not anatomically closed. During the first 2 weeks of life for the term infant (or the first several weeks of extrauterine life for the preterm infant), the neonate may revert back to fetal circulation during periods of hypoxia, acidosis, or decreases in temperature.

In addition to circulatory differences, the neonatal heart also has important structural differences from the adult heart. The neonatal heart has decreased myocardial cellular mass resulting in decreased contractility. In addition to lower cell mass, differences in the contractile proteins within the cellular mass produce a less compliant ventricle. Because of decreased contractility, the neonate is unable to increase stroke volume, and cardiac output is dependent on heart rate.

When stressed, the neonatal heart responds differently than the adult heart. The neonatal heart is more resistant to hypoxia. Hypoxia decreases contractility markedly in the adult heart, whereas the neonatal heart withstands hypoxia better. Transient hypoxia is tolerated because immature myocardium has higher rates of anaerobic glycolysis and greater myocardial glycogen stores. With prolonged hypoxia, myocardial contractility decreases and the neonate reverts back to fetal circulation.

The immature cardiac tissue also handles periods of ischemia better than adult cardiac tissue. The neonatal heart following the reversal of ischemia can work almost as efficiently, whereas the adult heart usually has compromised function following an ischemic insult. In addition, the neonatal cardiac tissue is more resistant to acidosis with less depression in contractility than the adult heart.

Last, the neonate responds differently to catecholamines than do adults. It is thought that sympathetic innervation of the neonatal heart is incomplete, and thus the neonate will have decreased uptake of catecholamines. In animal studies, epinephrine infusions cause increase in cardiac output through increased heart rate, not increased contractility.

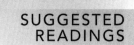

Lake CL. *Pediatric Cardiac Anesthesia*. 3rd ed. Stamford, CT: Appleton and Lange; 1998:37–48.

Miller RD, ed. *Miller's Anesthesia*. 6th ed. Philadelphia, PA: Elsevier; 2005:2368–2369.

Motoyama EK, Davis PJ, ed. *Smith's Anesthesia for Infants and Children*. 7th ed. Philadelphia, PA: Mosby Elsevier; 2006:70–86.

N

Nerve AP Termination Mechanism
Physiology

K. Karisa Walker

Edited by Ramachandran Ramani

1. Action potentials (APs) are transmitted along axons via depolarization of voltage-gated ion channels.
2. APs will propagate until they reach a synapse or neuromuscular junction, or are halted.
3. Local anesthetics (LAs) bind to voltage-gated sodium channels, rendering them nonfunctional and blocking transmission of the AP.
4. Sufficient length of nerve must be affected by the LA to block AP transmission.

N

APs originate from presynaptic nerve impulses and propagate down the length of the nerve by sequential depolarization of the cell membrane through the opening and closing of voltage-gated sodium and potassium channels (see Fig. 1). The termination of transmission of the AP occurs when an endpoint (synapse or neuromuscular junction) is reached or terminated by another influence, such as an LA.

The LAs work by binding to voltage-gated sodium channels. The sodium channel is a transmembrane protein consisting of an alpha subunit and two beta subunits. The alpha subunit is both the site of ion conduction and LA binding. Reversible binding of the drug to the receptor occurs on the axoplasmic surface, preventing the influx of sodium ions into the nerve cell.

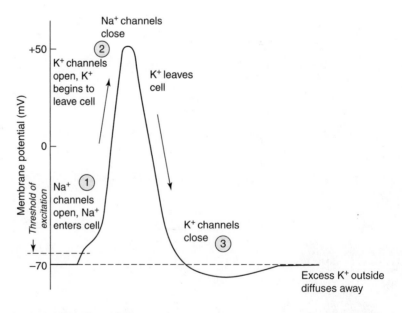

Figure 1. Neuronal action potential. (From Carlson NA. *Foundations of Physiological Psychology*. Needham Heights, MA: Simon & Schuster; 1992:53.)

For termination of the action potential and clinical effect of the LA to occur, a defined length of nerve needs to be rendered nonexcitable, preventing the impulse from bypassing the small blocked segment to continue transmission. Predictably, this length is reduced with high concentration of LA or myelination of the nerve. The length of nerve affected by the LA is determined by the volume administered. In a myelenated axon, 84% of sodium conductance at three successive nodes of Ranvier must be blocked to successfully terminate AP transmission.

SUGGESTED READINGS

Barash PG, Cullen BF, Stoelting RK, et al, eds. *Clinical Anesthesia*. 6th ed. Philadelphia, PA: Lippincott Williams & Wilkins; 2009:534–535.

Carlson NA. *Foundations of Physiological Psychology*. Needham Heights, MA: Simon & Schuster; 1992:53.

Hadzic A. *The Textbook of Regional Anesthesia and Acute Pain Management*. New York, NY: McGraw-Hill Medical; 2007:chap 6.

Nerve Block Landmarks
Anatomy

Kevan Stanton

Edited by Thomas Halaszynski

1. Anatomical landmarks are an important aide in determining the location for peripheral nerve block placement.
2. During peripheral nerve blockade procedures, the needle entry site(s) can be aided by defining/outlining anatomical landmarks.
3. Body habitus may make these landmarks difficult to distinguish.
4. Proper understanding of anatomy is a prerequisite prior to performing regional anesthesia.

The following is a list of landmarks for nerve blockade of upper and lower extremities:

Upper Extremity Peripheral Nerve Block Landmarks	
Interscalene block	The interscalene groove at the level of the cricoid cartilage (C6)
Supraclavicular block	1.5–2 cm posterior to midpoint of superior border of the clavicle in the interscalene groove
Infraclavicular block	2 cm below the midpoint of the inferior clavicular border
Axillary block	A line is drawn tracing the course of the axillary artery at the axillary skin crease from the lower axilla as proximally as possible, and the needle entry site is marked over the artery at the axillary skin crease
Musculocutaneous nerve block	(A) Body of proximal biceps, 2–5 cm below deltoid muscle
	(B) At the elbow, 1 cm proximal to intercondylar line, lateral to the biceps tendon
Median nerve block at the elbow	Medial to the brachial artery at the intercondylar line
Median nerve block at the wrist	Below the flexor carpi radialis and palmaris longus tendons, 2–3 cm proximal to the wrist crease
Radial nerve block at the elbow	2 cm lateral to the biceps tendon on the intercondylar line
Radial nerve block at the wrist	Over the extensor pollicis tendon at the base of the first metacarpal
Ulnar nerve block at the elbow	(A) Posterior to the medial epicondyle
	(B) Posterior to the medial epicondyle and 3–5 cm below the elbow
Ulnar nerve block at the wrist	Beneath the flexor carpi ulnaris tendon between the pisiform bone and the ulnar artery. May be approached medially or laterally to the carpi ulnaris tendon

Lower Extremity Peripheral Nerve Block Landmarks

Psoas compartment block (posterior approach to lumbar plexus)	(A) Classic: 3 cm caudal and 5 cm lateral from intersection of intercristal and spinal midline. (B) Modified: 1 cm cephalad to intercristal line at two-third the distance from the midline to the posterior superior iliac spine (PSIS) line (a line at the PSIS parallel to the midline)
Perivascular three-in-one femoral nerve block	Lateral to the intersection of the femoral artery and inguinal ligament line (from anterior superior iliac spine to the pubic tubercle)
Modified femoral (fascia iliaca) block	1 cm caudal to inguinal ligament at two-third the distance from the line connecting the pubic tubercle to the anterior-superior iliac spine (ASIS)
Lateral femoral cutaneous nerve block	2 cm medial and 2 cm caudal to the ASIS
Obturator nerve block	1–2 cm lateral and 1–2 cm caudal to the pubic tubercle
Parasacral block	6 cm inferior to the PSIS on the line connecting the PSIS and the ischial tuberosity
Sciatic nerve block—classic posterior approach of labat	3–4 cm along the line of the greater trochanter and sacral hiatus. Line is drawn between PSIS and the greater trochanter, then a perpendicular line is drawn bisecting this line 5 cm caudad. Then a line is drawn between the greater trochanter and the sacral hiatus. Entry point is marked at the intersection of this line with the perpendicular line
Sciatic nerve block—subgluteal approach	Midpoint of the line connecting the greater trochanter and ischial tuberosity. Draw a line between greater trochanter and ischial tuberosity. Second line is drawn perpendicular to first and bisecting it to extend 4–6 cm caudad. The entry site is found at the intersection of the lines. Adjustment of insertion site may be up to 4–6 cm distally from intersection of lines
Sciatic nerve block—anterior approach	Draw a line between ASIS and the pubic tubercle. A parallel line is then drawn starting at the greater trochanter. A perpendicular line is made starting from one-third between pubic tubercle and ASIS, and entry site is marked where this line intersects the second line (usually located at level of the lesser trochanter)
Popliteal fossa block—posterior approach	5–10 cm superior to the popliteal skin fold, 1 cm lateral to the midline of the popliteal triangle. Outline the popliteal triangle: Popliteal skin fold, edge of semimembranous, and edge of biceps femoris. Vertical line is drawn bisecting the triangle, and entry site is marked 5–10 cm superior to the base of triangle and 1 cm lateral to bisecting line
Popliteal fossa block—lateral approach	The groove between the vastus lateralis and biceps femoris at the level of the superior border of the patella
Posterior tibial nerve block	Postero-lateral to the tibial artery at the level of the medial malleolus
Sural nerve block	Between the lateral malleolus and the Achilles tendon
Deep peroneal, superficial peroneal, and saphenous nerve block	Lateral to the anterior tibial artery at the intermalleolar line. The anterior tibial artery is palpated between the extensor hallucis longus tendon and the extensor digitorum longus tendon at the intermalleolar line. The entry site is lateral to the artery, between the tendons

N

SUGGESTED READING

Miller RD, Eriksson LI, Fleisher LA, et al, eds. *Miller's Anesthesia.* 7th ed. Philadelphia, PA: Churchill Livingstone; 2010:1640–1661.

Neuraxial Anesth: Cardiovascular Effects
Subspecialties: Regional Anesthesia

Alexander Timchenko

Edited by Thomas Halaszynski

KEY POINTS

1. Neuraxial anesthesia can be associated with cardiovascular disturbances such as hypotension, bradycardia, and tachycardia, alone or in combination.
2. Neuraxial anesthesia of preganglionic sympathetic fibers from the thoracic-5 (T5) to lumbar-1 (L1) can produce peripheral vasodilation with venous pooling and decreased venous return to the heart.
3. Risk factors for hypotension from neuraxial anesthesia include age greater than 40, combination of neuraxial anesthesia with general anesthesia, use of angiotensin-converting enzyme (ACE) inhibitors/angiotensin II receptor blockers (ARBs), obesity, and hypovolemia.
4. Bradycardia associated with neuraxial anesthesia is mediated by sympathetic blockade at the thoracic 1 to 4 (T1–4) level.
5. Sympathetic blockade at T1–4 from neuraxial anesthesia may lead to unopposed vagal tone that leads to bradycardia, worsening heart block, or asystole.

DISCUSSION

Neuraxial anesthesia by administration of local anesthetic medications into the epidural space or cerebral spinal fluid (CSF) can be achieved by various techniques. Local anesthetics from either the amino amide or ester family of drugs are commonly chosen for this purpose. Cardiovascular effects common after administration of local anesthetics for neuraxial anesthesia include hypotension, bradycardia, or tachycardia.

The hypotensive response from neuraxial anesthesia is mediated by the T5–L1 preganglionic sympathetic efferent fibers that define the vasomotor constrictor tone in arteries and veins. Local anesthetics used in neuraxial anesthesia blockade at these spinal levels can lead to vasodilation below the level of the block along with decreased venous return to the heart. There is a greater decrease in venous vessel tone than arterial tone with subsequent reduced systemic vascular resistance, but the venous pooling is a greater contributor to the resultant hypotension than effect on the arterial side of the circulation. Arterial vasodilation may be minimized by compensatory vasoconstriction above the level of the block achieved with neuraxial anesthesia. However, in situations of a high sympathetic block from neuraxial anesthesia, the compensatory vasoconstriction may not be functional. Additional factors contributing to hypotension include reverse-Trendelenberg patient positioning and intra-abdominal compression of the inferior vena cava, such as by a gravid uterus. It is imperative to ensure left-lateral displacement of the uterus to improve adequate venous return at optimal levels in the pregnant patient. The hypotensive effects of neuraxial anesthesia may be compensated by the renin-angiotensin system. Therefore, patients undergoing therapy with ACE inhibitors or ARBs are at an increased risk for developing hypotension secondary to neuraxial anesthesia.

Risk factors for the development of hypotension after neuraxial anesthesia include the following:

- Combination of neuraxial anesthesia with general anesthesia
- Hypovolemia
- Obesity
- Age greater than 40 years
- Patients taking ACE inhibitors or ARBs.

The cardio-accelerator fibers are typically found at the T1–4 level. Involvement of these fibers by local anesthetics used in neuraxial anesthesia may lead to bradycardia, complete heart block, or asystole. When adverse effects on heart rate occurs in combination with decreased venous return, patients may become quite hypotensive. The level of local anesthesia achieved with neuraxial anesthesia at the T1–4 dermatome can result in unopposed parasympathetic stimulation of the vagus nerve. Presence of a first-degree heart block prior to neuraxial anesthesia may be a risk factor for progression to an even higher grade of heart block. An additional mechanism for bradycardia during neuraxial anesthesia involves the intracardiac stretch receptors, which decrease heart rate by the vagus nerve–mediated reflex that results when intracardiac filling pressures begin to fall. Risk factors for bradycardia include high sympathetic block, age younger than 50, ASA I patients, and use of beta-blocker therapy.

SUGGESTED READINGS

Barash PG, Cullen BF, Stoelting RK, et al, eds. *Clinical Anesthesia*. 6th ed. Philadelphia, PA: Lippincott Williams & Wilkins; 2009:995–996.

Miller RD. *Miller's Anesthesia*. 6th ed. Philadelphia, PA: Elsevier Churchill Livingstone; 2005:573–603.

Morgan GE, Mikhail MS, Murray MJ. *Clinical Anesthesiology*. 4th ed. New York, NY: McGraw-Hill; 2006:263–275.

Neuraxial Opioids Action Site

Subspecialties: Pain

Suzana Zorca

Edited by Jodi Sherman

KEY POINTS

1. Neuraxial opioids such as morphine, fentanyl, and sufentanil act directly at mu receptors (MOR or OPR1) within the substantia gelatinosa of the spinal cord. They also reach cerebral opioid receptors through cephalad spread via the cerebrospinal fluid (CSF), as well as central and peripheral effector targets after local absorption by the vasculature.
2. The onset and duration of action, as well as the spread of segmental analgesia and propensity for delayed side effects, depends on the physicochemical properties of the opioid, especially molecular weight and lipid solubility.
3. Neuraxial opioids, unlike local anesthetics, do not typically cause sympathetic denervation, motor loss, or loss of proprioception. Their most commonly encountered side effects including respiratory depression, nausea and vomiting (N/V), pruritus, and urinary retention are caused primarily by rostral migration via CSF.

DISCUSSION

Opioids are the second most commonly administered group of drugs after local anesthetics for neuraxial anesthesia. They can be used alone or in combination with local anesthetic drugs for spinal, epidural, or combined spinal–epidural techniques to provide intra- or postoperative analgesia. Neuraxial opioids can reduce local anesthetic requirements and its subsequent side effects such as motor blockade. The effects of neuraxial opioids are complex and occur by at least three different following mechanisms:

1. Direct regional effect on opioid receptors in the substantia gelatinosa of the dorsal horn of the spinal cord
2. Effects on cerebral opioid receptors after cephalad spread through the CSF
3. Central and peripheral effects after vascular uptake

Neuraxial opioid analgesia involves at least three distinct anatomic areas of the central nervous system (CNS): the substantia gelatinosa of the spinal cord (terminal axons of primary afferents within laminae I and II, which inhibit nociceptive stimuli from C- and A-delta fibers), the ventromedial medulla, and the periaqueductal-periventricular gray matter. The relative contribution by each of these mechanisms depends on the physico-chemical properties of the opioid and dose administered.

Hydrophilic opioids such as morphine take longer to penetrate tissues and therefore have a slower onset and longer duration of action than lipophilic agents such as fentanyl and sufentanil. Slow penetration into tissues also allows more time for cephalad spread of the agent, increasing the spread of segmental analgesia. Hydrophilic compounds such as morphine and hydromorphone are therefore likely to have contributions from all the three mechanisms above. In contrast, lipophilic opioids such as fentanyl and sufentanil have faster tissue penetration, allowing faster onset and shorter duration of action. In addition, this decreases cephalad spread and potential for delayed side effects such as respiratory depression.

On a molecular level, neuraxial opioids bind to opioid receptors (G-protein–coupled receptors modulating the effect of inhibitory G-proteins) present pre- and postsynaptically on nociceptive cells. They reduce neuronal excitation and decrease the release of nociceptive neurotransmitters. Mu, delta, and kappa receptors are present in the dorsal horn of the spinal cord. Mu-1 and delta receptor activations decrease somatic pain; Mu-2 receptor activation results in commonly seen side effects such as respiratory depression, bradycardia, euphoria, and ileus. Mu-1 and kappa receptors inhibit visceral pain. Neuraxial opioids are relatively specific agonists of Mu receptors (also known as OPR1). This explains the "selective" blockade of pain sensation, without attendant loss of motor, sensory, and sympathetic function.

The main side effects of neuraxial opioids are similar to those encountered after systemic administration: pruritus (most common in obstetric patients resulting from interaction with mu receptors in the trigeminal nucleus and a posited cross-reactivity of opioids at estrogen receptors), N/V, respiratory depression (biphasic—early and late, especially with the increased systemic absorption of lipid-soluble opioids, activating receptors in the ventral medulla after rostral spread through CSF). Naloxone is effective at relieving pruritus, from sedating effects primarily and not due to inhibition from histamine release live antihistamines. Urinary retention is also seen, and is postulated to occur as a result of activation of opioid receptors in the sacral spinal cord that inhibits sacral parasympathetic outflow. This increases detrusor muscle relaxation and bladder capacity, and can predictably be reversed with naloxone.

Other side effects of neuraxial opioids include dose-dependent sedation (especially with neuraxial sufentanil), or alternatively CNS excitation, that is, tonic skeletal muscle rigidity due to cephalad migration and action at nonopioid receptors in the brainstem or basal ganglia. Viral reactivation can occur (e.g., herpes simplex virus labialis due to action of neuraxial opioids at receptors in the trigeminal nucleus). Ocular dysfunction (miosis, nystagmus, vertigo), delayed gastric emptying, thermoregulatory dysfunction, and oliguria secondary to antidiuretic hormone release stimulated by cephalad migration of opioids can also be seen.

SUGGESTED READINGS

Axelsson K, Gupta A. Local anaesthetic adjuvants: neuraxial versus peripheral nerve block. *Curr Opin Anaesthesiol.* 2009;22(5):649–654.

Coda BA. Opioids. In: Barash PG, Cullen BF, Stoelting RK, et al, eds. *Clinical Anesthesia.* 6th ed. Philadelphia, PA: Lippincott Williams & Wilkins; 2009:465–492.

Sinatra RS. Opioids and opioid receptors. In: Sinatra RS, Jahr JS, Watkins-Pitchford JM, eds. *The Essence of Analgesia and Analgesics.* Cambridge: Cambridge University Press; 2011:73–81.

Yaksh TL, Wallace MS. Opioids, analgesia, and pain management. In: Brunton L, Chabner B, Knollman B, eds. *Goodman & Gilman's the Pharmacological Basis of Therapeutics.* 12th ed. New York, NY: McGraw-Hill; 2011:481–526.

N

Neuromusc Disease: Sux Hyperkalemia

Pharmacology

Caroline Al Haddadin

Edited by Thomas Halaszynski

KEY POINTS

1. Succinylcholine (sux) is a depolarizing muscle relaxant that works at the neuromuscular junction, depolarizing both presynaptic and extrajunctional receptors.
2. Sux increases serum potassium concentrations by approximately 0.5 to 1.0 mEq per L, which is usually insignificant in persons with normal baseline potassium levels.
3. In patients with preexisting hyperkalemia, burns, massive trauma, stroke, neuromuscular disorders, and Duchenne muscular dystrophy, the potassium release secondary to sux administration can cause cardiac arrest that is resistant to traditional cardiopulmonary resuscitation measures.
4. Severe hyperkalemia after sux resulting in cardiac arrest has also been seen in acidotic hypovolemic patients.

DISCUSSION

Sux is a depolarizing muscle relaxant that works at the neuromuscular junction, depolarizing both presynaptic and extrajunctional receptors. Depolarization of the muscle by sux releases potassium by intracellular to extracellular shift and by increasing serum potassium concentrations by approximately 0.5 to 1.0 mEq per L. This potassium increase is usually insignificant in persons with normal baseline potassium levels. However, sux administration can result in life-threatening elevated potassium levels in patients with preexisting hyperkalemia and certain conditions like burns, massive trauma, and neuromuscular disorders. The risk of sux-induced hyperkalemia appears to be highest 7 to 10 days after an injury, such as from extensive burns, major degenerative injuries, spinal cord transection, and trauma.

Following denervation injuries, there is an upregulation of extrajunctional immature acetylcholine receptors. Thus, when sux is administered and binds to these receptors, potassium can be released in a widespread and extensive manner. The resulting hyperkalemia can lead to cardiac arrest that is often refractory to cardiopulmonary resuscitation measures. Cardiac arrest refractory to resuscitation will require administration of calcium, bicarbonate, insulin and glucose, dantrolene, and even initiation of cardiopulmonary bypass to treat. Of note, the release of potassium by sux is not prevented reliably by precurarization, as only large doses of nondepolarizing blockers can abolish this effect.

Multiple reports of cardiac arrest have been documented after administration of sux to children with Duchenne muscular dystrophy. The condition is associated with a weakened muscular structure, rhabdomyolysis, and preexisting hyperkalemia. Sux is thought to destroy the muscle membrane, causing a release of its intracellular contents (including potassium).

SUGGESTED READINGS

Barash PG, Cullen BF, Stoelting RK. *Clinical Anesthesia*. 5th ed. Philadelphia, PA: Lippincott Williams & Wilkins; 2009:506, 624.

Morgan GE, Mikhail MS, Murray MJ. *Clinical Anesthesiology*. 4th ed. New York, NY: McGraw-Hill; 2006:214.

Neuromuscular Block: Vecuronium

Pharmacology

Ira Whitten

Edited by Jodi Sherman

KEY POINTS

1. Vecuronium is an intermediate-acting ammonio steroid, nondepolarizing muscle relaxant.
2. Vecuronium is useful for tracheal intubation and maintenance of muscle paralysis during short to intermediate duration surgical procedures.
3. Vecuronium has no cardiovascular effects and does not trigger the release of histamine at clinical doses.
4. As vecuronium is partially excreted by the kidneys, extended duration of action may be seen in renal failure.
5. Vecuronium is heavily excreted in the bile; prolonged block is sometimes seen in liver failure.

N

DISCUSSION

Vecuronium acts as a competitive antagonist of nicotinic acetylcholine receptors at the motor end plate, thus preventing muscle fiber depolarization. The standard dose of vecuronium for tracheal intubation is 0.1 to 0.2 mg per kg, and its onset time is approximately 3 to 4 minutes. To maintain muscle paralysis, vecuronium may be redosed in boluses of 0.01 to 0.02 mg per kg or run as a continuous infusion of 1 to 2 μg/kg/min. The duration to 25% recovery, or one muscle twitch, is 35 to 45 minutes.

Approximately 30% to 40% of vecuronium undergoes deacetylation in the liver to produce 3-OH, 17-OH, and 17-(OH)2 vecuronium metabolites. The 3-OH vecuronium metabolite is the most potent and has 60% to 80% of the activity of its parent compound, with a clearance rate of 3.5 mL/kg/min. A large portion, roughly 30% to 40%, of a vecuronium dose is excreted into the bile unchanged. The kidney also accounts for 25% of elimination, and renal failure can lead to accumulation of vecuronium and its metabolites. The overall elimination rate of vecuronium is 3 to 6 mL/kg/min.

Similar in structure to pancuronium, vecuronium lacks an *N*-methyl group and it is this structural change that gives vecuronium its pharmacologic properties and relatively benign side-effect profile. Unlike pancuronium, vecuronium has little to no cardiovascular effects at standard clinical doses and does not cause histamine release. Vecuronium's structure makes it unstable in solution; therefore, it is manufactured as a powder that must be reconstituted for clinical use.

SUGGESTED READINGS

Barash PG, Cullen BF, Stoelting RK, et al, eds. *Clinical Anesthesia*. 6th ed. Philadelphia, PA: Lippincott Williams & Wilkins; 2009:504–514.

Miller RD. *Miller's Anesthesia*. 7th ed. Philadelphia, PA: Churchill Livingstone; 2009:1180–1185.

Neuromuscular Diseases: Muscle Pain

Organ-based Clinical: Neurologic and Neuromuscular

Emilio Andrade

Edited by Ramachandran Ramani

KEY POINTS

1. Muscle pain is a side effect from the administration of succinylcholine.
2. The incidence is higher in women, younger patients, muscular individuals, and patients having ambulatory surgery.
3. Differential diagnosis must rule out other possible causes such as position-related muscle injuries due to excessive pressure or stretch, as well as causes associated with a specific procedure.
4. Therapy includes reassurance, rest, hydration, and anti-inflammatory medications.

N

DISCUSSION

Muscle pain has been described as one of the side effects from the administration of succinylcholine. The incidence of postoperative myalgia is increased, most commonly in women, muscular individuals, young patients, and patients having ambulatory surgery. It is seen less in pregnancy and in extremes of age. The administration of rocuronium 0.06 to 0.1 mg per kg before the administration of succinylcholine has been used to prevent postoperative myalgia. Differential diagnosis must rule out other causes of muscle pain, such as pressure injury from prolonged operation, stretch, or other position-related injuries as well as pain associated with the procedure itself.

Although the exact mechanism for succinylcholine-induced myalgias remains unknown, possible causes could be unsynchronized contractions of muscle groups, myoglobinemia, and increases in serum creatinine kinase. The pain can be quite severe and can result in gross limitation of function. Communication with the patients and follow-up can be of great value in reducing anxiety and providing explanations for the symptoms. Rest as well as hydration and anti-inflammatory medications, if not contraindicated, is the therapeutic option for management of succinylcholine-induced myalgias.

SUGGESTED READING

Morgan GE, Mikhail MS, Murray MJ. *Clinical Anesthesiology*. 4th ed. New York, NY: Lange Medical Books/ McGraw-Hill Medical Publishing Division; 2006:254.

Nitroglycerin: Uterine Relax

Subspecialties: Obstetric Anesthesia

Lisbeysi Calo

Edited by Lars Helgeson

KEY POINTS

1. The safety, predictability, and convenient use of intravenous (IV) nitroglycerin (NTG) make it a useful agent to produce uterine relaxation.
2. NTG can be used safely in awake patients, offering advantages over traditional methods of uterine relaxation requiring general anesthesia.
3. NTG rapidly affects hemodynamics and should only be used when hemodynamic monitoring, IV fluids, and vasopressors are readily available.
4. NTG can be useful when rapid and transient uterine relaxation is emergently needed during vaginal and cesarean deliveries for extraction of a retained placenta and to aid in the replacement of a prolapsed or inverted uterus.

DISCUSSION

NTG was first synthesized in 1846, and has many uses in medicine. Its safety, efficacy, predictability, and convenient use make it a useful agent to produce uterine relaxation.

Intravenous NTG, at a dose of 50 to 100 μg, is an effective smooth muscle relaxant with a very brief duration of action. NTG relaxes the uterine smooth muscle by increasing intracellular production of cyclic guanosine monosphosphate (cGMP), which acts as a mediator for the dephosphorylation of the myosin light chain. NTG is metabolized in the uterus to its active compound nitric oxide (NO). NTG is also useful with cervical spasm; smooth muscle constitutes approximately 10% to 15% of the cervical tissue.

Although general anesthesia may also be used to provide uterine relaxation, NTG can be used in awake patients, thus offering advantages in the full-stomach obstetric population. Similarly, uterine relaxation with NTG avoids potential cardiovascular depression associated with inhalation anesthetic agents. However, IV NTG can affect hemodynamics and is also contraindicated in patients with hypovolemia. Hemodynamic monitoring, IV fluids, and vasopressors should be readily available when using NTG. Typically, a phenylephrine infusion is started at the same time as the NTG and is titrated to adequate blood pressure.

During obstetric emergencies, there is often the need for rapid and transient relaxation of the cervix and uterus to allow obstetric maneuvers during both vaginal and cesarean deliveries (such as difficult breech and twin deliveries). The traditional anesthetic management in this context has been rapid sequence induction of general anesthesia and maintenance with a halogenated agent, which can be time consuming and carries several potential complications. Intravenous NTG is useful in this setting.

In addition, NTG can be useful in causing the uterine relaxation needed for extraction of a retained placenta. It can also be used to aid in the replacement of a prolapsed or inverted uterus after normal vaginal delivery.

SUGGESTED READINGS

Alfabet KM, Spencer JT, Zinberg S. Intravenous nitroglycerin for uterine relaxation for an inverted uterus. *Am J Obstet Gynecol.* 1992;166:1237–1238.

Chestnut D, Polley LS, Tsen LC, et al. *Chestnut's Obstetric Anesthesia, Principles and Practice.* 4th ed. Philadelphia, PA: Mosby Elsevier; 2009:368.

Peng ATC, Gorman RS, Shulman SM, et al. Intravenous nitroglycerin for uterine relaxation in the postpartum patient with retained placenta. *Anesthesiology.* 1989;71:172–173.

Nitroprusside Toxicity: Dx

Pharmacology

Tiffany Denepitiya-Balicki

Edited by Benjamin Sherman

KEY POINTS

1. Nitroprusside is a potent antihypertensive agent whose mechanism of action is directed at both arteriolar and venous smooth muscle relaxation.
2. With high concentrations of nitroprusside, cyanide toxicity can result, clinically demonstrated by tachyphylaxis to nitroprusside, cardiac dysrhythmias, metabolic acidosis, and increased venous oxygen content.
3. Treatment of nitroprusside toxicity includes 100% oxygen via mechanical ventilation and administration of amyl nitrate, 3% sodium nitrate, sodium thiosulfate, and/or hydroxocobalamin.

DISCUSSION

Nitroprusside is a potent antihypertensive agent whose mechanism of action is directed at both arteriolar and venous smooth muscle relaxation. One nitric oxide and five cyanide molecules are released during the degradation of nitroprusside (Fig. 1). Nitric oxide stimulates an increase in intracellular cyclic guanosine 3′-5′-monophosphate (cGMP), which then decreases intracellular calcium levels, triggering vascular smooth muscle relaxation.

As illustrated in Figure 2, within an erythrocyte, an electron is donated to nitroprusside, creating two entities: an unstable nitroprusside compound and methemoglobin. The unstable nitroprusside spontaneously converts to five cyanide ions, which can follow one of three pathways: (a) it can combine with the methemoglobin and create cyanmethemoglobin, (b) it can bind to thiosulfate and create thiocyanate, or (c) it can bind to cytochrome oxidase. The final pathway can result in interference with electron transport and result in cellular hypoxia.

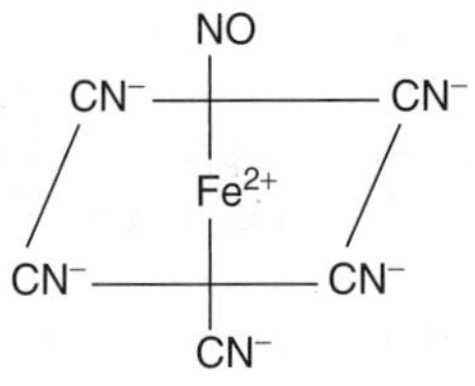

$$CN^- \underset{\displaystyle CN^-}{\overset{\displaystyle NO}{\underset{\displaystyle Fe^{2+}}{\big|}}} CN^-$$

$$CN^- \qquad CN^-$$

Nitroprusside

Figure 1. Molecular structure of nitroprusside. (Adapted from Morgan GE, Mikhail MS, Murray MJ. *Clinical Anesthesiology*. 5th ed. New York, NY: McGraw-Hill; 2006:256–258.)

SNP + Oxyhemoglobin $\longrightarrow$ (SNP)⁻ + Methemoglobin
(SNP)⁻ $\longrightarrow$ 5CN⁻

CN⁻ + Methemoglobin $\longrightarrow$ Cyanmethemoglobin

or

Rhodanase, vitamin B₁₂
CN⁻ + Thiosulfate $\xrightarrow{\hspace{3cm}}$ Thiocyanate

or

CN⁻ + Cytochrome oxidase $\longrightarrow$ Cyanide toxicity

Figure 2. Mechanism of nitroprusside metabolism. (Adapted from Morgan GE, Mikhail MS, Murray MJ. *Clinical Anesthesiology*. 5th ed. New York, NY: McGraw-Hill; 2006:256–258.)

Cyanide toxicity is clinically demonstrated by tachyphylaxis to nitroprusside (as increasing doses are required to create the desired hypotensive effect), cardiac dysrhythmias, metabolic acidosis, and increased venous oxygen content. Cyanide toxicity is not typically observed when nitroprusside is infused at rates less than 0.5 mg/kg/h. It is generally recommended that the total dose of nitroprusside not exceed 1.5 to 2 mg per kg over a 24-hour period (in patients with normal hepatic and renal function).

After identifying toxicity, patients should receive 100% oxygen with a low threshold to institute mechanical ventilation, as this will increase the amount of oxygen available. Pharmacologic treatment is aimed at reducing the amount of cyanide bound to cytochrome oxidase, thereby improving cellular oxygen utilization. This is accomplished in several ways.

1. Administration of amyl nitrite (either by direct inhalation or via the anesthesia circuit) or 3% sodium nitrate increases the amount of methemoglobin and then forms more cyanmethemoglobin. These treatments should be used with caution because they do shift the oxygen–hemoglobin curve to the left and potentially worsen oxygen delivery to the tissues. In patients with concomitant carbon monoxide poisoning or severe anemia, these therapies should be used with *extreme caution.*

2. Sodium thiosulfate, a sulfur donor, can decrease cyanide levels by binding to cyanide and forming thiocyanate, which is excreted renally. In patients with renal failure however, thiocyanate may accumulate and cause nausea, hypoxia, thyroid abnormalities, muscle weakness, and psychosis.

3. Hydroxocobalamin, a precursor of B_{12}, has a strong affinity for cyanide molecules and forms cyanocobalamin, which is renally excreted. This intravenous treatment was approved by the U.S. Food and Drug Administration in 2006 and marketed as the "Cyanokit."

In many institutions where hydroxocobalamin is available, the initial treatment for cyanide toxicity is hydroxocobalamin and sodium thiosulfate because they do not form methemoglobin with possible decreases in oxygen delivery.

SUGGESTED READINGS

Barash PG, Cullen BF, Stoelting RK. *Clinical Anesthesia.* 5th ed. Philadelphia, PA: Lippincott Williams & Wilkins; 2009:365.

Desai S, Su M. Cyanide poisoning. UpToDate. 2011. http://www.uptodate.com/contents/cyanide-poisoning. Accessed May 22, 2012.

Kaplan JA, Finlayson DC, Woodward S. Vasodilator therapy after cardiac surgery: a review of the efficacy and toxicity of nitroglycerin and nitroprusside. *Can Anaesth Soc J.* 1980;27:254–259.

Morgan GE, Mikhail MS, Murray MJ. *Clinical Anesthesiology.* 5th ed. New York, NY: McGraw-Hill; 2006:256–258.

NMB: Volatile Agent Interaction

Pharmacology

Holly Barth

Edited by Jodi Sherman

KEY POINTS

1. Neuromuscular blockade is enhanced by volatile anesthetics.
2. Decreasing the minimum alveolar concentration of volatile anesthetic leads to greater recovery of neuromuscular blockade.
3. At deep levels of anesthesia, duration of action and recovery from neuromuscular blockade may be prolonged.
4. Proposed mechanism of action is decreased synaptic transmission at neuromuscular junction at levels of deep anesthesia.

DISCUSSION

Volatile anesthetics enhance the activity of neuromuscular blocking drugs in a dose-related fashion. However, not all volatile anesthetics are equal in their effects. The order of potentiation of neuromuscular blockade by the anesthetics is as follows:

Desflurane > Sevoflurane > Isoflurane > Halothane > Barbiturate-opioid or Propofol anesthesia. Nitrous oxide has no effect.

Inducing deep anesthesia with volatile agents may result in decreased synaptic transmission at the neuromuscular junction, thus potentiating the antagonistic effect of nondepolarizing neuromuscular blockade. This effect results in prolonged action of neuromuscular blockade at deep anesthesia as well as recovery from the neuromuscular blockade. Proposed mechanisms are (a) volatile agent effect on central interneuron synapses and alpha-motor neurons, (b) inhibition of postsynaptic nicotinic acetylcholine receptors, and (c) increased receptor binding by the neuromuscular blockade at the receptor site.

Because all the volatile anesthetics enhance the activity of neuromuscular drugs, it is important to remember that the decreasing depth leads to greater recovery of the neuromuscular blockade.

SUGGESTED READINGS

Barash PG, Cullen BF, Stoelting RK, et al, eds. *Clinical Anesthesia.* 6th ed. Philadelphia, PA: Lippincott Williams & Wilkins; 2009:514.

Miller RD, Fleisher LA, Johns RA, et al. *Miller's Anesthesia.* 6th ed. Philadelphia, PA: Elsevier, Churchill and Livingstone; 2005:515–516.

NMB Drug Interactions

Pharmacology

Trevor Banack

Edited by Thomas Halaszynski

KEY POINTS

1. Volatile anesthetics produce dose-dependent enhancement of the magnitude and duration of neuromuscular blockade produced by nondepolarizing neuromuscular-blocking drugs.
2. Aminoglycoside antibiotics are well known for enhancing the neuromuscular blockade produced by nondepolarizing neuromuscular-blocking drugs.
3. Local anesthetics, in small doses, can enhance neuromuscular blockade produced by nondepolarizing neuromuscular-blocking drugs.
4. Furosemide, 1 mg per kg intravenously (IV), enhances neuromuscular blockade produced by nondepolarizing neuromuscular-blocking drugs.
5. Magnesium enhances neuromuscular blockade produced by nondepolarizing neuromuscular-blocking drugs, and to a lesser extent, enhances neuromuscular blockade produced by succinylcholine.
6. Patients chronically taking phenytoin and carbamazepine are relatively resistant to pancuronium, cisatracurium, rocuronium, vecuronium, pipecuronium, but not to mivacurium and atracurium nondepolarizing neuromuscular-blocking drugs.

N

DISCUSSION

There are many drugs that interact with nondepolarizing neuromuscular-blocking. Volatile anesthetics produce dose-dependent enhancement of the magnitude and duration of neuromuscular blockade produced by nondepolarizing neuromuscular-blocking drugs. The greatest enhancement of neuromuscular blockade has been observed with desflurane, enflurane, isoflurane, and sevoflurane, and least with the combination of nitrous oxide and opioids. Interestingly, the decrease in dose requirements as a result of volatile anesthetics is less for intermediate-acting than for long-acting nondepolarizing neuromuscular-blocking drugs.

Aminoglycoside antibiotics are well known for enhancing the neuromuscular blockade produced by nondepolarizing neuromuscular-clocking drugs. Antibiotics may exert effects on the prejunctional membranes similar to those exerted by magnesium, resulting in decreased release of acetylcholine.

Local anesthetics in small doses can enhance neuromuscular blockade. Large doses of local anesthetics can block neuromuscular transmission. Ester local anesthetics compete with other drugs for plasma cholinesterase, which may prolong the effect of succinylcholine.

Quinidine potentiates neuromuscular blockade produced by nondepolarizing and depolarizing neuromuscular-blocking drugs, presumably by interfering with the prejunctional release of acetylcholine.

Furosemide, 1 mg per kg IV, enhances neuromuscular blockade produced by nondepolarizing neuromuscular-blocking drugs. This effect most likely reflects furosemide-induced inhibition of cAMP production, leading to decreased prejunctional output of acetylcholine. One of the side effects of diuretic use is chronic hypokalemia, which decreases the amount of pancuronium needed and increases the required dose of neostigmine needed for reversal.

Magnesium enhances neuromuscular blockade produced by nondepolarizing neuromuscular-blocking drugs, and to a lesser extent, enhances neuromuscular blockade produced by succinylcholine. The effect of magnesium has been thought to be the result of decreased prejunctional release of acetylcholine and decreased stabilization of postjunctional membranes to acetylcholine.

Lithium may enhance the neuromuscular-blocking effects of depolarizing and nondepolarizing neuromuscular-blocking drugs.

Patients chronically taking phenytoin and carbamazepine are relatively resistant to pancuronium, cisatracurium, rocuronium, vecuronium, pipecuronium, but not to mivacurium and atracurium nondepolarizing neuromuscular-blocking drugs. The possible mechanism to the resistance is an increased hepatic clearance and decreased elimination halftime. However, acute treatment with phenytoin has resulted in augmentation of neuromuscular blockade produced by rocuronium.

SUGGESTED READINGS

Caldwell JE, Laster MJ, Magorian T, et al. The neuromuscular effects of desflurane, alone and combined with pancuronium or succinylcholine in humans. *Anesthesiology.* 1991;74:412–418.

Chapple DJ, Clark JS, Hughes R. Interaction between atracurium and drugs used in anaesthesia. *Br J Anaesth.* 1983;55:S17–S22.

Dotan ZA, Hana R, Simon D, et al. The effect of vecuronium is enhanced by a large rather than a modest dose of gentamicin as compared with no preoperative gentamicin. *Anesth Analg.* 2003;96:750–754.

Fogdall RP, Miller RD. Neuromuscular effects of enflurane, alone and combined with d-tubocurarine, pancuronium, and succinylcholine, in man. *Anesthesiology.* 1975;42:173–177.

Ghoneim MM, Long JP. The interaction between magnesium and other neuromuscular blocking agents. *Anesthesiology.* 1970;32:23–27.

Havdala HS, Borison RL, Diamond BI. Potential hazards and applications of lithium in anesthesiology. *Anesthesiology.* 1979;50:535–537.

Miller RD, Roderick LL. Diuretic-induced hypokalaemia, pancuronium neuromuscular blockade and its antagonism by neostigmine. *Br J Anaesth.* 1978;50:541–544.

Miller RD, Sohn YJ, Matteo RS. Enhancement of d-tubocurarine neuromuscular blockade by diuretics in man. *Anesthesiology.* 1976;45:442–445.

Miller RD, Way WL, Dolan WM, et al. Comparative neuromuscular effects of pancuronium, gallamine, and succinylcholine during forane and halothane anesthesia in man. *Anesthesiology.* 1971;35:509–514.

Miller RD, Way WL, Katzung BG. The potentiation of neuromuscular blocking agents by quinidine. *Anesthesiology.* 1967;28:1036–1041.

Richard A, Girard F, Girard DC, et al. Cisatracurium-induced neuromuscular blockade is affected by chronic phenytoin or carbamazepine treatment in neurosurgical patients. *Anesth Analg.* 2005;100:538–544.

Rupp SM, McChristian JW, Miller RD. Neuromuscular effects of atracurium during halothane-nitrous oxide and enflurane-nitrous oxide anesthesia in humans. *Anesthesiology.* 1985;63:16–19.

Rupp SM, Miller RD, Gencarelli PJ. Vecuronium-induced neuromuscular blockade during enflurane, isoflurane, and halothane anesthesia in humans. *Anesthesiology.* 1984;60:102–105.

Sokoll MD, Gergis SD. Antibiotics and neuromuscular function. *Anesthesiology.* 1981;55:148–159.

Soriano SG, Sullivan LJ, Venkatakrishnan K, et al. Pharmacokinetics and pharmacodynamics of vecuronium in children receiving phenytoin or carbamazepine for chronic anticonvulsant therapy. *Br J Anaesth.* 2001;86:223–229.

Spacek A, Nickl S, Neiger FX, et al. Augmentation of the rocuronium-induced neuromuscular block by the acutely administered phenytoin. *Anesthesiology.* 1999;90:1551–1555.

Stoelting RK, Hillier SC. *Pharmacology and Physiology in Anesthetic Practice.* 4th ed. Philadelphia, PA: Lippincott Williams & Wilkins; 2006:224–227.

N

NMB Reversal: Assessment

Physics, Monitoring, and Anesthesia Delivery

Jennifer Dominguez

Edited by Thomas Halaszynski

1. Clinical measures of residual neuromuscular blockade are insensitive and are subjective methods for assessing reversal of blockade.
2. Clinically significant residual neuromuscular blockade, train-of-four (TOF) ratio less than 0.9, can exist in the absence of visual or tactile fade in response to TOF, tetanic, and double-burst stimulation (DBS).
3. Objective measurement of neuromuscular block recovery (spontaneous and drug assisted) has recently been advocated to help prevent clinically significant postoperative weakness.
4. Intravenous administration of an anticholinesterase provides drug-assisted antagonism (TOF ratio >0.7) at the neuromuscular junction produced by nondepolarizing muscle relaxants.

N

Neuromuscular function after the administration of neuromuscular blocking drugs can be monitored clinically by objective and subjective measures of block recovery. Clinical assessment, such as sustained head lift for 5 seconds, is a measure of block recovery and requires patient cooperation (Table 1). Subjective measures include evaluating the muscular response to either electrical or magnetic stimulation of a peripheral motor nerve (commonly used), but have been called into question for lack of sensitivity. Objective methods of recording muscle responses to stimulation include measurement of evoked mechanical response of the muscle (mechanomyography [MMG]), evoked electrical response of the muscle (electromyography [EMG]), acceleration of the muscle response (acceleromyography [AMG]), and evoked electrical response in a piezoelectric film sensor attached to the muscle (piezoelectric neuromuscular monitor [P_ZEMG] and phonomyography [PMG]). These measures may provide more accurate assessment of block recovery by quantitative measurements.

There are a number of clinical assessments commonly used to monitor recovery from neuromuscular blockade (Table 1); however, evidence suggests that these may be unreliable measures of block recovery. In one study, unanesthetized volunteers were given mivacurium and asked to perform specific tasks at various points during block recovery.

Table 1. Clinical Tests of Postoperative Neuromuscular Recovery

Unreliable

Sustained eye opening

Protrusion of the tongue

Arm lift to the opposite shoulder

Normal tidal volume

Normal or nearly normal vital capacity

Maximum inspiratory pressure < 40 to 50 cm H_2O

Most Reliable

Sustained head lift for 5 s

Sustained leg lift for 5 s

Sustained handgrip for 5 s

Sustained "tongue depressor test"

Maximum inspiratory pressure >40 to 50 cm H_2

Adapted from Miller RD, Eriksson LI, Fleisher LA, et al. *Miller's Anesthesia.* 7th ed. Philadelphia, PA: Churchill Livingstone; 2009:1515–1531.

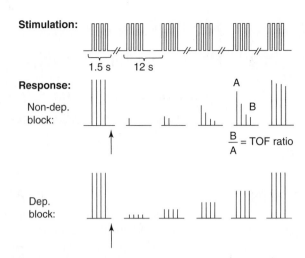

Figure 1. Train of four stimulation. (Adapted from Miller RD, Eriksson LI, Fleisher LA, et al. *Miller's Anesthesia.* 7th ed. Philadelphia, PA: Churchill Livingstone; 2009:1515–1531.)

They were able to perform the head-lift test when the TOF ratio at the adductor pollicis muscle was greater than 0.62, but needed a TOF ratio of at least 0.86 to hold a tongue depressor between their teeth. Thus, patients who are able to sustain head lift may still have clinically significant weakness. This study also showed that the upper airway muscles used to retain a tongue depressor are very sensitive to neuromuscular blockade.

Subjective assessment by visual or tactile evaluation of muscle response to nerve stimulation is commonly used in clinical practice to evaluate neuromuscular blockade. This can be accomplished by either electrical or magnetic nerve stimulation, although electrical stimulation is more common and practical. Any peripheral nerve can theoretically be stimulated; however, the ulnar and facial nerves are often monitored in clinical practice. To achieve assessment of neuromuscular function, application of an electrical stimulus 20% to 25% greater than necessary for maximal response (supramaximal stimulation) is required. A number of different patterns of electrical nerve stimulation are available, including single-twitch, TOF, tetanus, posttetanic count (PTC), and DBS.

In TOF nerve stimulation, four supramaximal electrical stimuli are administered every 0.5 second (2 Hz). Each stimulus produces a muscle contraction, and assessment of the amplitude of the fourth response relative to the first response provides the basis for assessment of block recovery. The TOF ratio is calculated by dividing the amplitude of the fourth response by the amplitude of the first response. Before administration of a muscle relaxant, all four responses are the same, and the TOF ratio is 1.0. A "fade" TOF response is characteristic of nondepolarizing neuromuscular blockade, but is not seen in phase I blocks with depolarizing neuromuscular blockers (Fig. 1). When large doses or infusions of depolarizing neuromuscular blockers are given, fade or phase II block can occur.

Visual and tactile evaluation of neuromuscular blockade by TOF or 50-Hz tetanic stimulation may not detect fade. Studies have shown that it is not possible to quantify the degree of block recovery manually or visually when the TOF ratio is greater than 0.40. DBS is somewhat more sensitive, but becomes unreliable at TOF ratios from 0.6 to 0.9. Sustained tetany for 5 seconds after a 100-Hz tetanus is the most sensitive measure, and may be detected when the TOF ratio is as high as 0.8 to 0.9. However, tetanic stimulation can be painful, and patients should be well anesthetized to tolerate this stimulus. Thus, it may be impractical in the perioperative setting, with an awake or semiawake patient.

Because these subjective measures of TOF or tetanic stimulation can be unreliable, some have advocated the use of objective measures of neuromuscular blockade in routine clinical practice. The current literature recommends a target TOF ratio greater than 0.9 to safely predict block recovery since upper airway function does not recover completely until the TOF ratio at the adductor pollicis muscle is at least 0.9.

SUGGESTED READINGS

Barash PG, Cullen BF, Stoelting RK. *Clinical Anesthesia*. 5th ed. Philadelphia, PA: Lippincott Williams & Wilkins; 2009:517–523.

Brull SJ, Murphy GS. Residual neuromuscular block: lessons unlearned. Part II: methods to reduce the risk of residual weakness. *Anesth Analg*. 2010;111:129–140.

Kopman AF, Yee PS, Neuman GG. Relationship of the train-of-four fade ratio to clinical signs and symptoms of residual paralysis in awake volunteers. *Anesthesiology*. 1997;86:765.

Miller RD, Eriksson LI, Fleisher LA, et al. *Miller's Anesthesia*. 7th ed. Philadelphia, PA: Churchill Livingstone; 2009:1515–1531.

Murphy GS, Brull SJ. Residual neuromuscular block: lessons unlearned. Part I: definitions, incidence, and adverse physiologic effects of residual neuromuscular block. *Anesth Analg*. 2010;111:120–128.

Viby-Mogensen J, Claudius C. Evidence-based management of neuromuscular block. *Anesth Analg*. 2010;111:1–2.

N

NO Hemodynamic Effect
Pharmacology

Juan Egas

Edited by Qingbing Zhu

1. After being synthesized in endothelial cells, nitric oxide (NO) causes vasodilation by activating a second messenger system on vascular smooth muscle cells.
2. The administration of NO synthase inhibitors results in unopposed vasoconstriction, causing increases in blood pressure by more than 30%.
3. Pathologic activation of NO synthase, as seen in cirrhosis and other conditions, leads to vasodilation and hypotension that is largely refractory to vasopressors.

Although NO serves many roles in various organ systems, its ability to cause vasodilation and regulate blood pressure is one of its most important functions. NO is synthesized from the terminal guanidino nitrogenof L-arginine by the enzyme NO synthase, an inducible enzyme present in endothelial cells. NO subsequently activates soluble guanylate cyclase (sGC) in vascular smooth muscle cells, resulting in the production of 3′5′-monophosphate (cGMP) and vasodilation (Fig. 1).

There is evidence that NO-dependent vasodilation is maintained through the physical activation of endothelial cells by mechanical forces such as pulsatile flow and sheer stress, as well as by chemical mediators including acetylcholine, bradykinin, substance P, and calcium. In addition, studies have demonstrated that there is continuous release of NO in the arterial circulation to maintain a basal vasodilatory tone that opposes the physiologic basal vasoconstriction mediated by neurohumoral mechanisms.

The significance of NO role in vasodilation and blood pressure regulation has been demonstrated by the administration of NO synthase inhibitors. Studies have shown that NO synthase inhibitors will cause intense vasoconstriction secondary to an unopposed

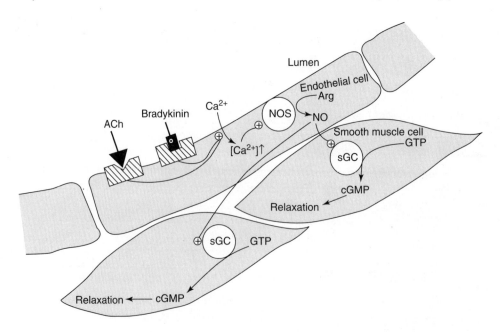

Figure 1. The mechanism of vascular smooth muscle relaxation by NO. (Adapted from Knowles RG, Moncada S. Nitric oxide as a signal in blood vessels. *Trends Biochem Sci.* 1992;17:399–402.)

basal constrictive tone. It has been observed in many species that blood pressure increases by more than 30% in the presence of NO synthase inhibitors. Similarly, disruptions at various other steps in the NO-regulated vasodilation cascade have been shown to result in hypertension. The endogenous NO-dependent vasodilator cascade can be exploited by the administration of nitroglycerin or sodium nitroprusside, which get converted to NO and cause vasodilation. The actions of NO are short-lived; within a few seconds of causing vasodilation, NO is quickly oxidized by hemoglobin and other oxidants and converted to the stable end products nitrite and nitrate.

In certain pathologic states, the myocardial inducible isoform of NO synthase can be activated by inflammatory cytokines and endotoxin lipopolysaccharides. These states of shock are associated with venous pooling, myocardial depression, and hypotension that tend to be resistant to vasopressors. However, these effects can be prevented by the treatment of glucocorticoids and NO synthase inhibitors. Similarly, the hyperdynamic state observed in patients with cirrhosis has also been shown to be associated with an increased activity of an inducible isoform of NO synthase, resulting in vasodilation and refractory hypotension. The expression of NO synthase has been shown to be reduced in the pulmonary arteries of patients with chronic primary and secondary pulmonary hypertension, suggesting a possible therapeutic role of inhaled NO for the treatment of these conditions.

SUGGESTED READINGS

Barash PG, Cullen BF, Stoelting RK, et al, eds. *Clinical Anesthesia*. 6th ed. Philadelphia, PA: Lippincott Williams & Wilkins; 2009:228.
Griffiths MJ, Evans TW. Inhaled nitric oxide therapy in adults. *N Engl J Med*. 2005;353:2683–2695.
Knowles RG, Moncada S. Nitric oxide as a signal in blood vessels. *Trends Biochem Sci*. 1992;17:399–402.
Moncada S, Higgs A. The L-arginine nitric oxide pathway. *N Engl J Med*. 1993;329:2002–2010.

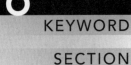

O$_2$ Release

Physiology

Jammie Ferrara

Edited by Hossam Tantawy

KEY POINTS

1. Oxygen is carried in the blood in two forms: dissolved and bound to hemoglobin.
2. The oxygen–hemoglobin dissociation curve describes the relationship between oxygen saturation (SO$_2$) and the partial pressure of oxygen in the blood (PO$_2$).
3. The P50, or oxygen tension at which hemoglobin is 50% saturated, is 26 mm Hg.
4. Factors that shift the curve to the right (increased temperature, acidosis, and increased 2,3-diphosphoglycerate [2,3-DPG]) lower oxygen affinity and displace oxygen from hemoglobin, making oxygen more readily available to bind to tissues.
5. Factors that shift the curve to the left (decreased temperature, alkalosis, and decreased 2,3-DPG) increase hemoglobin's affinity for oxygen, thereby reducing its availability to tissues.

DISCUSSION

Oxygen is transported in the body either by dissolving in blood or by binding to hemoglobin. Henry's law describes gas concentration as proportional to its partial pressure.

$$\text{Henry's law: Gas concentration} = \alpha \times \text{Partial pressure}$$

In Henry's law, α is the gas solubility coefficient for a given solution at a given temperature. In the human body, with a PaO$_2$ of 100 mm Hg, the amount of O$_2$ dissolved in blood is

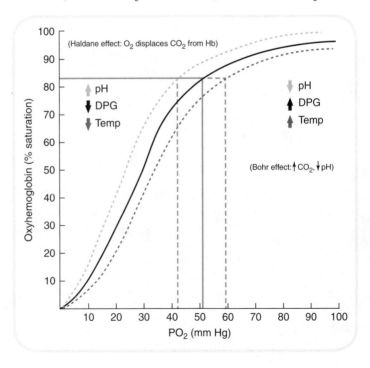

Figure 1. Hemoglobin dissociation curve.

very small compared with that bound to hemoglobin. Each hemoglobin protein can bind up to four oxygen molecules. The oxygen–hemoglobin dissociation curve describes the relationship between oxygen saturation and the partial pressure of oxygen. As the partial pressure of oxygen increases, the hemoglobin molecule saturation of oxygen increases to a point in which it is completely saturated, giving the curve its characteristic sigmoid shape.

The P50 in adults, or partial pressure of oxygen at which 50% of hemoglobin is saturated, is 26 mm Hg. P50 is affected by hydrogen ion, temperature, and 2,3-DPG. These factors shift the curve either to the left or to the right, thereby increasing or decreasing the affinity of hemoglobin for oxygen, respectively. Hyperthermia, acidosis, and increased 2,3-DPG shift the curve to the right, thereby lowering oxygen affinity and displacing oxygen from hemoglobin, which makes oxygen more readily available to bind to tissues. Hypothermia, alkalosis, and decreased 2,3-DPG shift the curve to the left and increase hemoglobin's affinity for oxygen, thereby reducing its availability to tissues.

Hydrogen ion reduces the binding of oxygen to hemoglobin, which is referred to as the Bohr effect. As CO_2 tension increases, there is an associated increase in hydrogen ion concentration, thus shifting the curve to the right. Therefore, CO_2-rich capillaries help to facilitate the release of oxygen to tissues by decreasing hemoglobin's affinity for oxygen. The lower CO_2 in pulmonary capillaries help facilitate the uptake of oxygen from alveoli onto hemoglobin.

SUGGESTED READINGS

Barash PG, Cullen BF, Stoelting RK, et al, eds. *Clinical Anesthesia*. 6th ed. Philadelphia, PA: Lippincott Williams & Wilkins; 2009:701–702.

Morgan GE, Mikhail MS, Murray MJ. *Clinical Anesthesiology*. 4th ed. New York, NY: McGraw Hill; 2006:561–563.

Stoelting RK, Miller RD. *Basics of Anesthesia*. 5th ed. Philadelphia, PA: Elsevier; 2007:55–56.

Obesity: Airway Evaluation

Generic, Clinical Sciences: Anesthesia
Procedures, Methods, Techniques

Anna Clebone

Edited by Lars Helgeson

KEYWORD

SECTION

KEY POINTS

1. A thorough airway examination is necessary in all patients, including obese patients. An awake intubation should be considered in any patient who is liable to present difficulties with mask ventilation and/or intubation.
2. A neck circumference of at least 40 cm is predictive of a difficult intubation; however, obesity alone is an independent risk factor for intubation difficulty.
3. A body mass index (BMI) of greater than 30 kg per m² is associated with difficult mask ventilation.
4. Correct positioning is more important in obese patients. Use of a ramp for positioning should be considered. Placing the patient into an ideal sniffing position should be accomplished before induction.

DISCUSSION

A thorough airway examination is necessary in all patients, particularly the obese. This includes Mallampati score, thyromental distance, neck range of motion, evaluation of dentition, and the upper lip bite test. The American Society of Anesthesiologists (ASA) difficult airway algorithm provides preoperative guidance in how to approach a potential difficult intubation (see Fig. 1).

One factor shown to be predictive of difficult intubation in obese patients is neck circumference. In a study by Brodsky et al., patients with a BMI of 40 or greater, neck

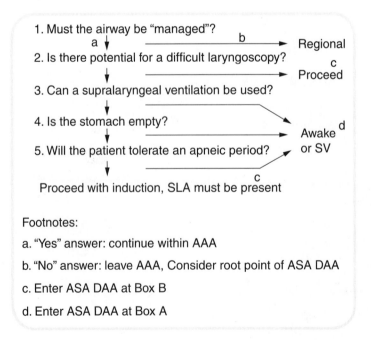

Figure 1. The Airway Approach Algorithm. (Rosenblatt W. The Airway Approach Algorithm: a decision tree for organizing preoperative airway information. *J Clin Anesth.* 2004;16(4):312–316.)

circumference proved to be a statistically significant factor in predicting "problematic" intubation (defined as: graded laryngoscopy view $\times$ number of intubation attempts $\geq$3). The probability of a difficult intubation by direct laryngoscopy was 5% in patients with a neck circumference of 40 cm and 35% in patients with a neck circumference of 60 cm.

Kheterpal et al. looked at factors predictive of difficult mask ventilation (MV). A BMI greater than or equal to 30 kg per m² was an independent predictor of mask ventilation, which was inadequate, unstable, or requiring two providers. Other independent predictors of grade 3 mask ventilation were Mallampati classification III or IV, age 57 years or older, presence of a beard, severely limited jaw protrusion, and snoring. Independent predictors of grade 4 mask ventilation, classified in this study as "impossible to ventilate" (which occurred in 0.16% of cases), were snoring and a thyromental distance of less than 6 cm.

Whether the decision is made for an awake or asleep intubation in a particular obese patient, special care must be taken to optimally position the patient before induction. In obese patients, elevating the chest and shoulders with a ramp is helpful in achieving proper airway alignment.

SUGGESTED READINGS

Barash PG, Cullen BF, Stoelting RK, ed. *Clinical Anesthesia*. 6th ed. Philadelphia, PA: Lippincott Williams & Wilkins; 2009:1230–1245.

Brodsky JB, Lemmens HJM, Brock-Utne JG, et al. Morbid obesity and tracheal intubation. *Anesth Analg*. 2002;94(3):732–736.

Kheterpal S, Han R, Tremper K, et al. Incidence and predictors of difficult and impossible mask ventilation. *Anesthesiology*. 2006;105(5):885–891.

Practice guidelines for the management of the difficult airway: an updated report by the American Society of Anesthesiologists Task Force on Management of the Difficult Airway. *Anesthesiology*. 2003;98:1269–1277.

Rosenblatt W. The Airway Approach Algorithm: a decision tree for organizing preoperative airway information. *J Clin Anesth*. 2004;16(4):312–316.

Obstructive Sleep Apnea: Dx

Generic, Clinical Sciences: Anesthesia Procedures, Methods, Techniques and Organ-based Clinical: Respiratory

Frederick Conlin

Edited by Veronica Matei

KEY POINTS

1. Obstructive sleep apnea (OSA) is a very common disease, and occurs in up to 5% of obese patients.
2. OSA should be suspected in patients reporting daytime sleepiness or partner descriptions of sleeping patterns, but diagnosis should be confirmed with a polysomnography sleep study.
3. Polysomnography is the standard test used to determine the presence of OSA and incorporates monitoring of respirations, ECG, electroencephalography (EEG), electromyography (EMG), vital signs, pulse oximetry, and snoring to make the diagnosis.
4. Patients who suffer from OSA present a challenge for anesthesiologists, as they frequently possess multiple medical comorbidities. In addition, mask ventilation, direct laryngoscopy, and intubation of these patients can be difficult.
5. Managing postoperative pain with respiratory depressants such as opioids in patients with OSA requires careful titration and close observation because of their inclination to obstruct.

DISCUSSION

OSA is a common disease that occurs in up to 5% of obese patients and between 1% and 4% of the adult male population. Although most patients with OSA note daytime sleepiness as their primary complaint, the sufferers are at increased risk for hypertension, myocardial infarction, dysrhythmias, stroke, vascular disease, diabetes mellitus, and hepatic dysfunction.

Risk factors for OSA include obesity, increasing age, male gender, current smoking, and ethanol use. During preoperative evaluation, the anesthesiologist should evaluate the patient for history of daytime sleepiness, lack of restful sleep, and partner reports of characteristic sleep patterns. Hypertension, macroglossia, and large tonsils may be present on physical examination. Patients suspected to have OSA should be treated as at high risk for these comorbid conditions, and further evaluation or optimization may be considered before elective surgery.

Polysomnography is the standard test used to determine the presence of OSA, and incorporates monitoring of respirations, ECG, EEG, EMG, vital signs, pulse oximetry, and snoring to make the diagnosis. Severity of disease is estimated by the number of events per total sleep time, with mild being 5 to 15 events per hour and severe being more than 30 events per hour. Although other methods of evaluating OSA exist, they are not considered the gold standard. Treatment of OSA involves continuous positive airway pressure (CPAP), oral appliances, and in some cases surgery.

The anesthetic implications of OSA include the risk of difficult mask ventilation, direct laryngoscopy, and intubation, as well as comorbid conditions. Postoperatively, adequate control of pain can be challenging because of the risk of airway obstruction and hypoventilation with even modest doses of opiates. These patients should be monitored closely while pain medications are slowly titrated to comfort. Patients using CPAP at home should have it available at bedside and use it while sleeping.

SUGGESTED READINGS

Barash PG, Cullen BF, Stoelting RK, et al, eds. *Clinical Anesthesia.* 6th ed. Philadelphia, PA: Lippincott Williams & Wilkins; 2006:1425–1426.

Crapo JD Karlinsky JB, Glassroth J, et al, eds. *Baum's Textbook of Pulmonary Disease.* 7th ed. Philadelphia, PA: Lippincott Williams & Wilkins; 2004:1425–1438.

Miller RD, ed. *Miller's Anesthesia.* 7th ed. Philadelphia, PA: Churchill Livingstone; 2009: chap 34: 2089–2104.

Oculocardiac Reflex Management

Generic, Clinical Sciences: Anesthesia Procedures, Methods, Techniques

Thomas Gallen

Edited by Ramachandran Ramani

KEY POINTS

1. The oculocardiac reflex (OCR) is caused by pressure or stretch on the globe or its muscles/nerves that results in dysrhythmias, most often bradycardia.
2. The severity of the OCR determines management and ranges from discontinuation of stimulus and continuous monitoring to the administering of atropine (7 to 10 μg per kg); in the gravest of circumstances, cardiopulmonary resuscitation may be required.
3. Hypoxia, hypercarbia, and light anesthesia can decrease the threshold for the OCR.
4. It is more common in children because of their increased vagal tone.

DISCUSSION

The oculocardiac reflex is a trigeminal–vagal reflex elicited by traction on extraocular muscles, pressure on the globe of the eye, or increased intraocular pressure. OCR may occur with eye muscle surgery, retinal detachment repair, enucleation, ocular pain, and ocular trauma. The occurrence of OCR is more frequent with regional anesthetic techniques. The reflex manifests most commonly as bradycardia, but can also be seen as bigeminy, nodal rhythms, ectopic beats, atrioventricular block, and asystole. The manifestations may continue as long as the inciting stimulus is present. OCR may demonstrate fatigue, in which the reflex fades despite ongoing or repeat stimulation. Hypoxia, hypercarbia, and light anesthesia can decrease the threshold for the OCR.

The afferent limb transmits the stimulus from the ciliary ganglion through the ophthalmic division of the trigeminal nerve (V1) to the Gasserian ganglion and to the trigeminal nucleus adjacent to the fourth ventricle. The efferent pathway transmits via the vagus nerve, affecting parasympathetic outflow to the heart. A fully successful retrobulbar block (blocking all nerves from the globe except the superior oblique motor nerve) can block the reflex, although OCR may occur during the placement of the block.

The severity of the reflex can be determined by continuous ECG monitoring, and this will in turn determine the management. No action is warranted if the manifestation is bradycardia or ectopic beats with a stable blood pressure and if the symptoms resolve within 20 seconds. If dysrhythmias are significant, persistent, or symptomatic, the inciting stimulus should be discontinued immediately and the patient assessed for hypoxemia, hypercarbia, and light plane of anesthesia. If the initial steps fail, atropine 7 to 10 μg per kg can be administered intravenously to effect. In the rare event of asystole, chest compressions may be necessary to temporize the situation and circulate the atropine.

In adults, the low likelihood of adverse outcomes secondary to OCR does not justify the inherent risk of prophylactic atropine administration. However, in children, significant OCR may occur as a result of their high vagal tone, and prophylactic administration of atropine, 0.02 mg per kg, or glycopyrrolate, 0.01 mg per kg, has become common practice, particularly for strabismus surgery.

SUGGESTED READINGS

Barash PG, Cullen BF, Stoelting RK, et al, eds. *Clinical Anesthesia.* 6th ed. Philadelphia, PA: Lippincott Williams & Wilkins; 2009:1327.

Longnecker DE, Brown DL, Newman MF, et al, eds. *Anesthesiology.* New York, NY: McGraw-Hill; 2008:1558–1561.

Old MI: Preoperative Risk Assessment

Generic Clinical Sciences: Anesthesia Procedures, Methods, Techniques

Gabriel Jacobs

Edited by Qingbing Zhu

KEY POINTS

1. Studies have shown that after a myocardial infarction (MI), the highest risk of perioperative events is within the subsequent 30 days; however, with the advent of percutaneous transluminal coronary angioplasty (PTCA), coronary artery bypass grafting (CABG), and thrombolysis, the time period is now likely less significant.
2. Depending on the treatment of the previous MI, elective surgeries may have to be delayed from 4 to 6 weeks (after angioplasty or bare metal stents) or for as long as 12 months (after drug-eluting stents).
3. The type of procedure is important to consider when determining perioperative risk in a patient with a history of MI.
4. Certain physical examination findings and poor exercise tolerance may suggest sequelae of a prior MI or ongoing ischemia, respectively, and may help determine perioperative risk.

DISCUSSION

Special considerations are taken into account when providing anesthesia to patients with a known or suspected history of previous MI. The goals of the preoperative evaluation for these patients include risk assessment, determination of whether patients will benefit from additional preoperative testing, and the formation of an appropriate anesthetic plan.

The time since the MI, subsequent interventions and therapies, and the patient current functional status must be considered when determining the risk of patients with a history of MI. Several epidemiologic studies have shown that patients who undergo surgery within 6 months of suffering an MI have a variable rate of perioperative events, ranging from 5% to 86%. According to the American Heart Association/American College of Cardiology Task Force on Perioperative Evaluation of the Cardiac Patient Undergoing Non-cardiac Surgery, an MI within 30 days places patients in the highest risk group, whereas after 30 days, patients are in the intermediate risk group. This emphasizes the importance of a judicious perioperative risk assessment in this specific patient population. In recent years, with the routine use of PTCA, CABG, and thrombolysis, the time period is likely less significant than that in the past.

Elective surgical procedures should be delayed to varying degrees depending on the treatment of previous MI. For instance, patients treated with angioplasty only should delay elective surgery for 4 to 6 weeks after the intervention, because of an increased risk of ischemic complications. Similarly, patients treated with a bare metal stent should delay elective surgery for 4 to 6 weeks. Patients treated with a drug-eluting stent should have elective surgeries delayed for up to 12 months to allow for adequate endothelialization.

In a patient with a past MI, the type of surgery the patient will undergo is an important predictor of risk. The American Heart Association/American College of Cardiology Guidelines risk stratification for noncardiac surgery is displayed in Table 1. Surgeries with high cardiac risk (reported risk as often as >5%) include prolonged surgery with large fluid shifts and blood loss, emergency surgery, major vascular surgery, and thoracic surgery. Surgeries with intermediate cardiac risk (risk generally around 1% to 5%) include carotid endarterectomy, orthopedic surgery, prostate surgery, intraperitoneal and intrathoracic

Table 1. Cardiac Risk[a] Stratification for Noncardiac Surgical Procedures in Patients with Known Coronary Artery Disease

High	Reported cardiac risk often >5% • Emergent major operations, particularly in the elderly • Aortic and other major vascular • Peripheral vascular • Anticipated prolonged surgical procedures associated with large fluid shifts and/or blood loss
Intermediate	Reported cardiac risk generally <5% • Carotid endarterectomy • Head and neck • Intraperitoneal and intrathoracic • Orthopedic • Prostate
Low[b]	Reported cardiac risk generally <1% • Endoscopic procedures • Superficial procedures • Cataract • Breast

[a]Combined incidence of cardiac death and nonfatal MI.
[b]Do not generally require further preoperative cardiac testing.
Adapted from Barash PG, Cullen BF, Stoelting RK, et al, eds. *Clinical Anesthesia*. 5th ed. Philadelphia, PA: Lippincott Williams & Wilkins; 2009:573–575, with permission.

surgery, and surgery to the head and neck. Endoscopic procedures, superficial procedures, cataract surgery, and breast surgery pose low cardiac risk (risk < 1%).

Although the physical examination in patients with ischemic heart disease may be unremarkable, there are several findings that can help the anesthesiologist determine whether further testing is needed. In patients with a previous MI, increased jugular venous distention (JVD) and peripheral edema can point to right-sided heart failure, and rales and a S3 gallop can indicate left ventricular dysfunction. The importance of a detailed history cannot be underestimated, as exercise tolerance (particularly the ability to walk four flat blocks and climb two flights of stairs) is an important predictor of ongoing ischemia and high perioperative risk.

SUGGESTED READINGS

Barash PG, Cullen BF, Stoelting RK, et al, eds. *Clinical Anesthesia*. 5th ed. Philadelphia, PA: Lippincott Williams & Wilkins; 2009:573–575.
Hines RL, Marschall KE, eds. *Stoelting's Anesthesia and Co-existing Disease*. 5th ed. Philadelphia, PA: Saunders Elsevier; 2008:11–13.
Miller RD, Fleisher LA, Johns RA, et al. *Miller's Anesthesia*. 6th ed. New York, NY: Elsevier Churchill Livingstone; 2005:1061–1062, 1071.

Opioid Neurotoxicity: Rx
Subspecialties: Pain

Ervin Jakab

Edited by Thomas Halaszynski

KEY POINTS

1. Opioid-induced neurotoxicity is often seen in patients receiving high doses of opiates for long periods, especially after accumulation in the body, secondary to dehydration, reduced metabolism, or reduced excretion.
2. Opioid rotation, changing actual opioid to a different drug, and reducing the equianalgesic dose by 20% to 50%, is a safe and reliable method of decreasing the incidence of toxicity while retaining analgesia.
3. Symptoms of neurotoxicity may resolve within a few days of opioid reduction or discontinuation, but this should be done with caution and not usually at the expense of achieving adequate analgesia.
4. Circadian modulation, hydration, and other medications (amphetamines, naloxone, neuroleptics, corticosteroids, benzodiazepines, and clonidine) may be useful adjuncts in the treatment of opioid neurotoxicity.

DISCUSSION

Opioid-induced neurotoxicity (OIN) is a recently recognized syndrome that follows long periods of administration with high doses of opioids. Studies have suggested that OIN occurs by N-methyl-D-aspartate receptor activation and subsequent activation of intracellular positive apoptosis regulators such as Bax and caspases. OIN is a multifactorial syndrome that causes a spectrum of symptoms including confusion or drowsiness, cognitive impairment, severe sedation, hallucinosis, delirium, myoclonus, seizures hyperalgesia, and allodynia. OIN is often associated with psychoactive medications and fluid depletion, and frequent renal failure can also be present. OIN can occur with any opioid, but is more likely to occur when using opioids with active metabolites, such as meperidine, codeine, morphine, and (to a lesser degree) hydromorphone. Oxycodone has active metabolites, but whether they are clinically significant is debatable; however, there are no active metabolites of fentanyl or methadone.

OIN typically develops within a few days to a week of initiating an opioid or reaching a dose of opioid that causes metabolite buildup. Several strategies have been proposed and successfully used in the management of OIN. If symptoms are mild and are not particularly bothersome to the patient, simply monitoring for signs of progression of OIN may be appropriate. Circadian modulation of opioid administration may be helpful in the treatment of OIN. Factors such as dehydration, infection, or adding drugs that depress the central nervous system can tip a frail older adult into opioid toxicity. In frail older adults who have any signs of OIN, it is best to rotate to another opioid, preferably one with no active metabolites. Patients who have severe renal failure or are frail should start with an opioid that has few or no active metabolites.

Opioid rotation can be a safe and reliable method to decrease toxicity, but can retain analgesia. The ideal alternate opioid has yet to be determined. If a patient develops OIN while on morphine, a trial of hydromorphone or oxycodone is usually effective, and vice versa. It is generally recommended to decrease the new opioid by at least 20% to 50% of the equianalgesic dose. If OIN develops after rotation of first-line agonists, methadone or parenteral fentanyl may be used.

Symptoms of OIN may resolve within a few days of lowering the dose, which in itself demonstrates that opioids play a causative role in the neurotoxicity syndrome. Dose reduction or discontinuation of opioids should be done in a stepwise manner to prevent symptoms of opioid withdrawal. Given the profile of the typical chronic pain patient, dose reduction is often difficult and should not be done at the expense of achieving adequate pain control during acute pain inducing situations.

The active metabolites of opioid agonists are water soluble and are likely to accumulate in patients with renal failure or volume depletion. Therefore, adequate hydration is often a useful adjunct in the treatment of OIN.

In some patients, even a minimal analgesic dose may produce significant sedation. These patients can benefit from stimulant treatment with amphetamine and its derivatives. In addition, these amphetamine medications may have multiple effects as adjuvant drugs for pain management.

Naloxone can be used in cases of massive opioid overdose, but with extreme caution, as it can precipitate an opioid withdrawal syndrome or produce tonic–clonic seizures. Neuroleptics, such as haloperidol, can be used for the temporary management of hallucinations and agitated delirium, while the previously discussed long-term strategies take effect. A number of other medications, such as corticosteroids, barbiturates, benzodiazepines, and clonidine, have been suggested for the symptomatic management of OIN. Although the above medications may help to reduce symptoms or allow for opioid rotation, it is important to note that they do not address the underlying cause.

SUGGESTED READINGS

Broadbent A, Glare P. Neurotoxicity from chronic opioid therapy after successful palliative treatment for painful bone metastases. *J Pain Symptom Manage.* 2005;29:520–524.

Daeninck PJ, Bruera E. Opioid use in cancer pain. Is a more liberal approach enhancing toxicity? *Acta Anaesthesiol Scand.* 1999;43:924–938.

Sweeny C, Bogan C. *Textbook of Palliative Medicine.* London, UK: Hodder Arnold; 2006:390–401.

Opioid Reversal

Pharmacology

Nehal Gatha

Edited by Thomas Halaszynski

1. Opioid reversal is most often accomplished using naloxone, which is a competitive antagonist functioning at opioid receptors.
2. Opioid receptor antagonist is used to treat opioid-induced toxicity (especially respiratory depression).
3. Small doses of opioid reversal should be titrated to effect. Rapid or abrupt reversal of opioids can result in significant sympathetic stimulation and other significant side effects, especially in those who are opioid dependent or having acute pain.
4. Nalmefene and naltrexone are pure opioid antagonists, currently with little clinical use.

DISCUSSION

Endogenous and exogenous opioids act on the mu (μ), delta (δ), and kappa (κ) receptors. Exogenous opioids may cause side effects when used for treatment of pain (μ, δ, and κ mediated) or sedation including muscle rigidity, constipation, hallucinations, physical dependence, and respiratory depression (μ mediated). The indication for opioid reversal is primarily respiratory depression or acute overdose.

The most commonly used opioid reversal agent is naloxone. Naloxone is a pure competitive antagonist at opioid receptors. It has a much greater affinity for μ receptors than the other opioid receptors, and this enables it to reverse respiratory depression at low doses while not completely reversing pain control. However, abrupt reversal of opioids can result in sympathetic stimulation observed by a patient's acute perception of pain, or in opioid-dependent patients, acute opioid withdrawal. The effects of acute opioid withdrawal can be combativeness, dangerous tachycardia, ventricular irritability, hypertension, and pulmonary edema. To prevent these complications, naloxone should be titrated to achieve adequate ventilation and alertness. The administration of 0.1 to 0.4 mg of intravenous (IV) naloxone every few minutes for a controlled opiate reversal is recommended. Naloxone can be given IV, intramuscularly (IM), or via an endotracheal tube.

The clinical half-life of naloxone is 20 to 60 minutes, and is due to rapid redistribution from the central nervous system. The half-life of many opioids extends beyond this 20- to 60-minute period, creating the possibility for respiratory depression to recur, necessitating the need to re-bolus naloxone. Therefore, IM or continuous administration of naloxone is advisable if long-acting opioids have been used and adverse side effects (respiratory depression) should occur. Given IM, a 2-mg dose of naloxone will show opioid reversal onset within 5 to 10 minutes. Infusion of naloxone is typically administered at 4 to 5 μg/kg/hr. Neonatal respiratory depression due to maternal opioid use will also respond to naloxone in doses of 10 μg per kg.

Nalmefene and naltrexone are newer pure opioid antagonists, also with a high affinity for the μ receptor. Because these drugs have substantially longer half-lives than naloxone, they have the theoretical use for outpatients who will be unmonitored. However, to overcome the resulting antagonized pain control from these medications, patients may then take excessive doses of oral pain medications (causing sedation and respiratory depression) that could peak after the antagonist has worn off. Similarly, these drugs should not be used in unconscious patients.

Morgan GE, Mikhail MS, Murray MJ. *Clinical Anesthesiology.* 4th ed. New York, NY: McGraw-Hill; 2006:190–196, 283–288.

SUGGESTED READING

Oral Clonidine: MAC Effect

Pharmacology

Rongjie Jiang

Edited by Jodi Sherman

KEY POINTS

1. Clonidine is a selective partial agonist of α-2 receptors (α-2 to α-1 ratio approximately 200:1).
2. In addition to its antihypertensive effects, clonidine's analgesic, anxiolytic, and hypnotic properties make it a potentially useful premedication and anesthetic adjuvant.
3. Chronic administration of clonidine decreases anesthetic requirements by 10% to 20%, and acute premedication (90 minutes before induction at a dose of 4.5 to 5 μg per kg) decreases anesthetic requirements by 35% to 45%.
4. There is a synergetic effect between clonidine and benzodiazepines, opioids, and volatile agents.

DISCUSSION

Clonidine is a selective partial agonist of α-2 receptors (α-2 to α-1 ratio approximately 200:1). The main effect of clonidine is sympatholysis by stimulating prejunctional α-2 receptors, thereby reducing norepinephrine release. Studies have also demonstrated a synergetic effect between α-2 agonists and benzodiazepines, opioids, and volatile agents.

In addition to its antihypertensive effects, clonidine's analgesic, anxiolytic, and hypnotic properties make it a potentially useful premedication and anesthetic adjuvant. In general, the anesthetic potency of a volatile general anesthetic is measured by its minimum alveolar concentration (MAC), and the MAC is useful in determining the effects of a medication on anesthetic requirements. Oral clonidine, when given as a premedication, has been shown to reduce the MAC in animal and human studies while maintaining hemodynamic stability. When clonidine was administered 90 minutes before induction at dose of 4.5 to 5 μg per kg, the MAC and MAC awake of sevoflurane decreases by as much as 35% compared with patients who receive no premedication. Studies show a similar reduction of MAC in animals and humans for halothane (up to 45% MAC reduction) and isoflurane (up to 40% MAC reduction). Clonidine premedication also decreases thiopentone requirements for induction of anesthesia. In addition, clonidine premedication reduces vital capacity rapid inhalation anesthetic induction time with sevoflurane. Patients who are administered clonidine chronically experience a decrease in their anesthetic requirements by as much as 10% to 20%.

Studies have demonstrated that clonidine premedication results in a decreased opioid requirement during general anesthesia. Via a reduction in sympathetic nervous system outflow, it is also effective in attenuating the hemodynamic response to a surgical stimulus. This is of particular importance in patients who require large doses of opioids to achieve hemodynamic stability, which may prolong recovery time. Owing to the sedating effects of α-2 adrenergic agonists, however, some studies have demonstrated postoperative sedation and delayed emergence in patients premedicated with clonidine.

SUGGESTED READINGS

Howie MB, Hiestand DC, Jopling MW, et al. Effect of oral clonidine premedication on anesthetic requirement, hormonal response, hemodynamics, and recovery in coronary artery bypass graft surgery patients. *J Clin Anesth.* 1996;8(4):263–272.

Inomata S, Yaguchi Y, Toyooka H. The effects of clonidine premedication on sevoflurane requirements and anesthetic induction time. *Anesth Analg.* 1999;89(1):204–208.

Katoh T, Ikeda K. The effect of clonidine on sevoflurane requirements for anaesthesia and hypnosis. *Anaesthesia.* 1997;52(4):377–381.

Miller RD, Eriksson LI, Fleisher LA, et al, eds. *Miller's Anesthesia.* 7th ed. Philadelphia, PA: Churchill Livingstone; 2009:284–285, 508, 1135.

Organ Donor: Bradycardia Rx

Generic, Clinical Sciences: Anesthesia Procedures, Methods, and Techniques

Jinlei Li

Edited by Benjamin Sherman

KEY POINTS

1. Postoperative bradycardia in cardiac transplant recipients may be sinus, junctional, or due to an atrioventricular block.
2. The loss of cardiac reflexes and a limited ability to compensate to changing physiologic conditions require an urgency of intervention.
3. Atropine is ineffective in a denervated heart because of its reliance on intact cardiac vagal innervation.
4. Treatment of bradycardia in transplanted hearts relies mostly on direct-acting beta adrenergic medications for rate and contractility augmentation, particularly isoproterenol and epinephrine.
5. Temporary or permanent pacing may be required.

DISCUSSION

Bradycardia with stable hemodynamics may not need treatment under anesthesia. However, patients who cannot increase stroke volume readily (i.e., those with aortic stenosis, hypertrophic cardiomyopathy, or ongoing ischemia) do not tolerate bradycardia well. Untreated bradycardia in these patients may quickly lead to hemodynamic instability. **Under normal conditions**, pharmacologic treatment of bradycardia generally includes atropine, glycopyrrolate, isoproterenol, epinephrine, and ephedrine. Antiarrhythmics such as amiodarone, lidocaine, procainamide, and bretylium should be avoided, as they may worsen bradycardia by slowing ventricular response rate.

During cardiac organ harvest, the neural plexus innervating the donor heart is transected, resulting in a denervated heart for implantation. Postoperative bradycardia in cardiac transplant recipients may be sinus or due to a junctional bradycardia or an atrioventricular block. The differential diagnosis includes inadequate preservation leading to ischemia, surgical injury or harvest injury to sinoatrial node, electrolyte imbalance, preoperative administration of amiodarone, or allograft rejection.

It is imperative to quickly establish and treat the underlying cause, as it may significantly affect mortality (Table 1). The loss of cardiac reflexes and a limited ability to compensate further support the urgency of intervention. Atropine is ineffective in a denervated heart because of its reliance on intact cardiac vagal innervation, although it may reverse

Table 1. Rx for Bradycardia in Donor Heart

Cause	Onset	Treatment
Sinus node preservation injury	Early	Resolve with time/temporary pacer
Conduction system injury at harvest	Early	Resolve with time/temporary or permanent pacer
Amiodarone	Early	Resolve with time/temporary pacer
Electrolyte derangement	Early or late	Electrolyte normalization
Allograft rejection	Early or late	To increase immunosuppression

From Wachter RM, Goldman L, Hollander H, eds. *Hospital Medicine*. 2nd ed. Philadelphia, PA: Lippincott Williams & Wilkins; 2005:373–379, with permission.

parasympathetically mediated peripheral vasodilation. Pharmacologic interventions for bradycardia in posttransplant patients include beta adrenergic medications such as isoproterenol or epinephrine. Pacing either by epicardial leads placed intraoperatively or by intravascular leads or transcutaneous pacing may be required if pharmacologic treatment is inadequate. Although postoperative bradycardia generally resolves within several days, between 3% and 15% of patients require a permanent pacemaker for definitive management.

SUGGESTED READING

Wachter RM, Goldman L, Hollander H, eds. *Hospital Medicine*. 2nd ed. Philadelphia, PA: Lippincott Williams & Wilkins; 2005:373–379.

Organophosphate Poisoning Rx

Generic Clinical Sciences: Anesthesia Procedures, Methods, Techniques

Ashley Kelley

Edited by Ala Haddadin

KEY POINTS

1. Symptoms of organophosphate (OP) poisoning result from stimulation of muscarinic and nicotinic acetylcholine (ACh) receptors and affect a wide range of organ systems.
2. Treatment of OP poisoning centers around oxime therapy, treatment with atropine, and prevention of seizure activity with the use of benzodiazepines.
3. Patients may require mechanical ventilation if symptoms progress to respiratory failure.
4. Experimental treatments that have shown great promise include magnesium, bioscavenger therapy with cholinesterase enzymes, and hemoperfusion.

DISCUSSION

OP poisoning results from exposure to pesticides and agents of chemical warfare. All agents work by inhibiting acetylcholinesterase (AChE), thus propagating the effects of ACh at the muscarinic and nicotinic ACh receptors. Symptoms resulting from muscarinic receptor stimulation include salivation, tearing, papillary constriction, and diarrhea. Symptoms resulting from nicotinic receptor stimulation include muscle weakness and may progress to fasciculation or paralysis. CNS effects include seizures with possible progression to coma. Effects on the cardiovascular system are wide ranging and may result in hypo- or hypertension and tachycardia or bradycardia.

The treatment of OP poisoning is a three-pronged approach: neutralize the toxin, counteract the effects of the OP with anticholinergics, and administer seizure prophylaxis. Oxime drugs (such as pralidoxime) cleave the bond between the OP and AChE, thereby allowing the OP to be metabolized. Atropine is administered to counteract the hemodynamic effects of OP poisoning, at a dose of 2 to 5 mg every 5 to 10 minutes. Even at therapeutic doses, however, atropine may cause adverse reactions that can limit its use. Glycopyrrolate, although more expensive (the relative cost of 0.2 mg of glycopyrrolate to 0.6 mg of atropine is approximately 2:1), has significantly fewer central side effects and may be used with similar efficacy. Overstimulation of central receptors is an important cause of early death in OP poisoning. Pretreatment with benzodiazepines has been shown to increase survival; thus, diazepam administration is considered standard therapy. If symptoms have progressed to respiratory failure, patients may require intubation and ventilatory support.

Some medications have shown great promise in the treatment of OP poisoning, but are not yet used routinely because of insufficient evidence regarding their efficacy. Magnesium may be helpful in reducing the stimulatory effect of ACh on muscle and may prevent drug-induced torsades de pointes. Bioscavenger therapy with cholinesterase enzymes has shown great promise as a future potential treatment to neutralize the unbound OP before reaching its target site. Hemoperfusion, although expensive, may be a useful adjunct in enhancing OP elimination in people who present early after exposure.

SUGGESTED READINGS

Barash PG, Cullen BF, Stoelting RK, et al, eds. *Clinical Anesthesia.* 6th ed. Philadelphia, PA: Lippincott Williams & Wilkins; 2009:1573–1574.

Hines RL, Marschall KE, eds. *Stoelting's Anesthesia and Co-existing Disease.* 5th ed. Philadelphia, PA: Churchill Livingstone; 2008:551–552.

Peter JV, Moran JL, Pichamuthu K, et al. Adjuncts and alternatives to oxime therapy in organophosphate poisoning—is there evidence of benefit in human poisoning? A review. *Anaesth Intensive Care.* 2008;36:339–350.

Oxygen Delivery Index Determinants

Physiology

Archer Martin

Edited by Ala Haddadin

1. Oxygen delivery index, or DO2I, is an equation that calculates the amount of oxygen being delivered into the tissue of the body.
2. DO2I can be calculated by the following equation: $DO2I$ $(mL/min/m^2)$ = $CI \times CCaO_2$, where CI = cardiac index, $CCaO_2$ = oxygen-carrying capacity of arterialized blood.

Oxygen delivery index is an equation that calculates the amount of oxygen being delivered to the body. Cardiac index is calculated by multiplying the heart rate times the stroke volume, and dividing by the body surface area.

The oxygen-carrying capacity of arterialized blood equals the components of bound oxygen and dissolved oxygen. The determinants of the equation include hemoglobin concentration, arterial oxygen saturation, and dissolved oxygen concentration. Hemoglobin concentration and arterial oxygen saturation can be measured by direct blood gas measurements and pulse oximetry, respectively.

As the bound component of oxygen-carrying capacity is significantly greater than the dissolved component, most clinicians ignore the dissolved component when calculating DO2I. The importance of supplemental oxygen is best demonstrated during conditions of anemia where the relative percentage of contribution of the dissolved component of oxygen is less than trivial.

Miller RD, Eriksson LI, Fleisher LA, et al, eds. Postoperative intravascular fluid therapy. In: *Miller's Anesthesia.* 7th ed. Philadelphia, PA: Churchill Livingstone; 2009:2796.

Oxygen Delivery to Fetus during Labor

Subspecialties: Obstetric Anesthesia and Pediatrics

Meredith Brown and Margaret Rose

Edited by Lars Helgeson

KEY POINTS

1. During labor, blood flow to the placenta becomes restricted during contractions.
2. Fetal pathology may limit its ability to tolerate normal transient reductions in placental blood flow. Examples include fetal anemia, congenital anomalies, or other factors causing chronic fetal stress.
3. Continuous monitoring of fetal heart rate (FHR), variability, and uterine contractions can help practitioners to identify fetal stress, which is most often due to hypoxemia.

DISCUSSION

While in utero, fetal respiration is dependent on the placenta for the exchange of oxygen and carbon dioxide. Placental compromise will affect fetal well-being and may lead to in utero growth restriction, hypoxemia, or fetal demise. During labor, blood flow to the placenta becomes restricted during contractions. A placenta able to maintain a healthy fetus may not be able to provide adequate oxygenation during the stress of contractions and delivery. Of all perinatal deaths, 3% are due to intrauterine hypoxia or birth asphyxia. Umbilical or placental complications account for 2%. Maternal pathology, such as pregnancy-induced hypertension, pulmonary or cardiac disease, diabetes, and nutrition derangements can also impair placental respiration, thereby contributing to fetal mortality. Fetal pathology such as fetal anemia, cardiac and congenital anomalies, and other factors causing chronic fetal stress may limit its ability to tolerate normal transient reductions in placental blood flow.

During periods of inadequate fetal respiration, as fetal PaO_2 decreases, CO_2 and lactate accumulate. This potentially results in respiratory and metabolic acidosis. Fetal hypoxemia can cause physiologic responses such as bradycardia, gasping movements, an overall decrease in fetal movements, and a redistribution of blood flow to vital organs. These stressors can result in increased fetal catecholamines, resulting in tachycardia and systemic hypertension.

1. ***Continuous monitoring of the pattern of FHR variability can help practitioners to identify fetal stress.***
   - The *baseline FHR* should be between 110 and 160 beats per minute (bpm).
   - *Variability*: Long-term variability is evaluated over 3 to 6 minutes and should demonstrate variation of 6 to 10 bpm of FHR. Fetal ECG can demonstrate short-term variability (beat-to-beat variability—see below).

2. ***The pattern of FHR during contractions can identify a fetus in distress or susceptible to hypoxemia. Continuous monitoring of FHR coupled to uterine contractions is necessary to identify these patterns.***
   - An *acceleration* occurring with contractions (of 15 bpm lasting 15 seconds) demonstrates well-balanced autonomic tone and is associated with good fetal outcome.
   - *Early decelerations* are a decrease in FHR less than 20 bpm, occurring only during contractions (tracings may appear as "mirror images"). This pattern denotes fetal head compression, causing brief hypoxia and vagal stimulation, with good fetal recovery.

- *Variable decelerations* are irregular decelerations in FHR often resulting from umbilical cord compression and vagal bradycardia. Their variability in onset, duration, and amplitude reflects inconsistent degrees of cord compression and resultant fetal hypoxia. Although no intervention is required when the fetus exhibits a good recovery, increasing severity (amplitude and duration) may denote increasing hypoxia or fetal compromise.
- *Late decelerations* are a decrease in FHR, beginning 10 to 20 seconds after the contraction begins and enduring after the contraction subsides. This FHR pattern signifies uteroplacental insufficiency and is associated with fetal intolerance of prolonged periods of hypoxia.
- FHR below 60 bpm is unable to sustain fetal life. When prolonged, it signifies hypoxic insult. Emergent delivery may be warranted to prevent permanent fetal damage or demise.

3. ***Antenatal and perinatal testing helps to identify susceptible or stressed fetuses, which can improve overall outcomes.***

- The *nonstress test* simply monitors the FHR, which should demonstrate variability (an increase by 15 bpm over normal baseline, lasting at least 5 seconds) with fetal movements, occurring at least twice in 20 minutes.
- During a *contraction stress test*, FHR patterns are monitored during natural or induced contractions. This test is performed when uteroplacental insufficiency is suspected.
- The *biophysical profile* measures by ultrasound fetal tone, breathing, and movements as well as amniotic fluid volume and takes into account the results of a nonstress test.

4. ***After rupture of the amniotic sac, further testing can be performed to further evaluate fetal well-being.***

- *Fetal scalp sampling* can provide blood gas measurements. Interpretation of values must include consideration of the stage of labor, presence of maternal acidosis, and whether the sample was drawn during a contraction.
- Normal: pH $\geq$ 7.25; $PO_2 \geq$ 20; $PCO_2 \leq$ 50; $HCO_3 \leq$ 20; base excess less than–6.
- *Fetal pulse oximetry* can also be performed. Normal fetal O_2 saturation is between 30% and 70%. Prolonged periods (more than 10 minutes) of saturations less than 30% suggest fetal acidosis. However, studies have failed to demonstrate improved outcomes and suggest that normal values may falsely reassure clinicians.
- *Continuous fetal ECG* using an internal scalp electrode is under investigation in Europe. During fetal hypoxemia, ST segment changes and PR:RR interval changes may be seen. When used in conjunction with other monitoring techniques, this technique may reduce intrauterine hypoxia and unnecessary cesarean deliveries, while decreasing incidence of fetal acidosis at birth.

Braveman FR. *Obstetric and Gynecologic Anesthesia: The Requisites in Anesthesiology.* Edinburgh, UK: Elsevier Mosby; 2006:39–50.

SUGGESTED READING

Oxytocin: Electrolyte Effects

Subspecialties: Obstetric Anesthesia

Dallen Mill

Edited by Lars Helgeson

KEY POINTS

1. Oxytocin, a hormone structurally similar to vasopressin, is released by the posterior pituitary.
2. At high doses, oxytocin can induce hyponatremia because of antidiuretic effects similar to that of vasopressin.
3. Rapid metabolism of dextrose in dextrose-containing carrier solutions can lead to dilutional hyponatremia, thereby exacerbating oxytocin-induced hyponatremia.
4. The risk of hyponatremia can be minimized by administering oxytocin using low-rate protocols, and with isotonic carrier solutions.

DISCUSSION

Oxytocin is one of two hormones synthesized in the hypothalamus, and released from the posterior pituitary gland. Oxytocin is a cyclic nonapeptide differing from vasopressin (antidiuretic hormone), the other hormone released by the posterior pituitary, by two amino acids. It is postulated that this structural similarity contributes to oxytocin's most clinically significant electrolyte effect of hyponatremia. Oxytocin binds to vasopressin receptors in the kidney, causing an antidiuretic effect, particularly at iatrogenic supraphysiologic levels encountered in the peripartum period. Data from both animal and human studies suggest that V_2 receptors and renal aquaporin-2 (AQP2) may mediate the antidiuretic action of oxytocin.

The risk of oxytocin-induced hyponatremia is especially high when infused rapidly (20 mU per minute) with dextrose-containing solutions. D5W is a problematic carrier solution because of the dilutional hyponatremia resulting from the rapid metabolism of dextrose. The hyponatremia induced by this combination can be profound. When infused at high rates, oxytocin in D5W has been implicated in the development of acute hyponatremia, seizure, and coma in the setting of postpartum hemorrhage. Thus, the administration of low-rate oxytocin protocols using isotonic carrier solutions, such as normal saline, has been advocated for nearly two decades. Studies have demonstrated that when infused with isotonic solutions, the risk of hyponatremia is extremely small (even when administered at high rates of up to 300 mU per minute).

Asymptomatic hyponatremia can often be treated with water restriction or administration of isotonic saline. If patients show signs of hyponatremia such as confusion, coma, and convulsions, oxytocin must be discontinued, and the hyponatremia should be corrected. Care should be taken to correct the hypernatremia slowly; if corrected too quickly, osmotic demyelination syndrome (central pontine myelinolysis) can occur.

SUGGESTED READINGS

Bergum D, Lonnée H, Hakli TF. Oxytocin infusion: acute hyponatraemia, seizures and coma. *Acta Anaesthesiol Scand.* 2009;53:826–827.

Joo KW, Jeon US, Kim GH, et al. Antidiuretic action of oxytocin is associated with increased urinary excretion of aquaporin-2. *Nephrol Dial Transplant.* 2004;19:2480–2486.

Ophir E, Solt I, Odeh M, et al. Water intoxication—a dangerous condition in labor and delivery rooms. *Obstet Gynecol Surv.* 2007;62:731–738.

Smith JG, Merrill DC. Oxytocin for induction of labor. *Clin Obstet Gynecol.* 2006;49:594–608.

Pacemaker Designation
Organ-based Clinical: Cardiovascular

Roberto Rappa

Edited by Qingbing Zhu

Roberto Rappa

Edited by Qingbing Zhu

KEY POINTS

1. Pacemakers are categorized by a five-letter code (the NBG pacemaker identification code).
2. The five-letter code describes the cardiac chamber(s) paced, sensed, their response to sensing, their programmability, and their arrhythmia functions.
3. Pacemakers can pace the atrium, the ventricle, or both (dual-chamber pacemakers).
4. Pacemakers can be programmed in one of three pacing modes: asynchronous pacing, single-chamber demand pacing, or dual-chamber atrioventricular (AV) sequential demand pacing.

DISCUSSION

Pacemakers are categorized by a five-letter code that is set forth by the North American Society of Pacing and Electrophysiology (NASPE) [aka the Heart Rhythm Society] and the British Pacing and Electrophysiology Group (BPEG). This five-letter designation is also called the NBG pacemaker identification code. It describes the chamber(s) paced, sensed, their response to sensing, their programmability, and their arrhythmia functions. For simplicity, we will not discuss the last two letters of the code.

A general understanding of pacemaker modes and their associated identification codes is essential in the perioperative management of patients with artificial cardiac devices. The following will provide a brief overview of pacemakers functionality and their pacing options.

Modern day pacemakers have a variety of complex pacing algorithms. They additionally vary according to their placement, location, and functionality of their pacing leads. Fortunately, understanding several simple concepts can make one's life a lot easier. The first step is to identify the chamber(s) that is/are paced. Pacemakers (and their associated leads) can pace the atrium, the ventricle, or both (dual-chamber pacemakers). This distinction is in fact the first letter of the NBG code. There are only four first-letter options: 0 (none/no pacing), A (atrial-paced pacemaker), V (ventricular-paced pacemaker), or D (dual-chamber pacemaker).

The next two letters of the NBG code are designed to describe how the pacemaker senses and responds to the different cardiac chamber(s) that is/are paced. In general, pacemakers can only be programmed in one of three pacing modes: asynchronous pacing, single-chamber demand pacing, or dual-chamber AV sequential demand pacing.

In asynchronous pacing mode feature, the pacemaker paces the atrium, ventricle, or both chambers at a preset-fixed rate. If the patient can produce an intrinsic heartbeat, the pacemaker will still deliver at a preset rate. The danger of this mode is apparent when a pacing "spike" is delivered during a patient's normal spontaneous ventricular repolarization period. If this occurs, a possible "R-on-T" phenomenon could induce a ventricular fibrillation rhythm.

The single-chamber demand pacing feature on pacemakers is analogous to a backup mode. In this type of pacing, the pacemaker is designed to pace either the atrium or the ventricle according to a preset-fixed rate. If the patient's spontaneous electrical activity and heart rate (HR) is above the preset level, the pacemaker could sense this intrinsic activity (second NBG identifier letter) and choose to inhibit further pacing (third NBG identifier letter). If the patient's spontaneous rhythm is "sensed" to be below the preset level, the pacemaker will then generate a pacing spike to pace the designated cardiac chamber at its programmed rate. As a result, you have a programmable fail-safe mechanism where the patient can automatically be paced in the setting of an inadequate spontaneous HR.

Dual-chamber sequential AV pacemaker devices enable the pacemaker to sense and inhibit both cardiac chambers according to a minimum preset pacing period. This mode of pacing additionally has an obligatory PR interval delay that is preprogrammed. This feature will sense for intrinsic ventricular activity only after an obligatory delay period. If it does not sense spontaneous ventricular electrical activity after the designated PR delay, it will pace the ventricle. For example, let us consider a programmed dual-chamber pacemaker with a rate of 60 beats per minute (bpm) and a PR delay interval of 150 milliseconds. If the patient's intrinsic sinus rate falls below the obligatory 60 bpm, the pacemaker will then be triggered to pace the atrium. The device will then wait 150 milliseconds to sense for intrinsic ventricular activity. If it does not sense such activity, it will similarly be triggered to pace the ventricle.

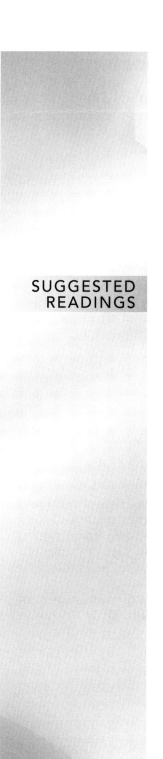

SUGGESTED READINGS

Barash PG, Cullen BF, Stoelting RK, et al., eds. *Clinical Anesthesia.* 6th ed. Philadelphia, PA: Lippincott Williams & Wilkins; 2009:1586–1587.

Cheng A, Yao F. Pacemakers and implantable cardioverter-defibrillators. In: Yao FF, Fontes ML, Malhotra V, eds. *Yao and Artusio's Anesthesiology: Problem Oriented Patient Management.* 6th ed. Philadelphia, PA: Lippincott Williams & Wilkins; 2008:229–251.

Morgan GE, Mikhail MS, Murray MJ, eds. *Clinical Anesthesiology.* 4th ed. New York, NY: Lange Medical Books/McGraw-Hill; 2005:487–488.

Pacer Lead Placement: ECG Morph
Organ-based Clinical: Cardiovascular

Kellie Park

Edited by Benjamin Sherman

1. The morphology of the ECG in a person with a pacemaker is dependent on the location of the pacer wire(s) in the heart.
2. In a single-chamber atrial pacemaker, the electrical signals travel through the atrioventricular (AV) node and the morphology of the QRS complex appears normal.
3. In a single-chamber ventricular pacemaker, the impulse from the pacemaker appears before the QRS complex, creating a characteristically wide QRS waveform.
4. In a dual-chamber pacemaker, a combination of both atrial and ventricular pacing may be observed on ECG.

P

Cardiac pacemakers are indicated for patients in whom symptomatic bradycardia is either present or highly probable. The pacemaker generally consists of two parts: the pulse generator, which has a battery and electronic circuitry, and the leads, which are threaded through the central venous system into the heart and implanted into the heart muscle. In a single-chamber pacemaker, the lead is implanted in the right atrium or right ventricle; in a dual-chamber pacemaker, the leads are implanted into the right atrium and ventricle; and in a biventricular pacemaker, the leads are placed in both the right atrium, right ventricle, and deep in the coronary sinus toward the left ventricle. The morphology of the ECG in a person with a pacemaker is dependent on the location of the pacer wire(s) in the heart.

In a single-chamber atrial pacemaker (indicated in a person with symptomatic sinus bradycardia or junctional rhythms), the electrical signals travel through the AV node and the morphology of the QRS complex appears normal (Fig. 1).

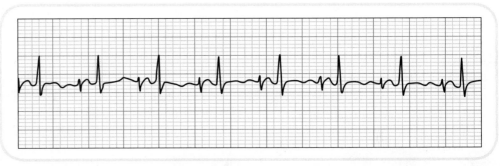

Figure 1. ECG tracing in a person with atrial pacemaker wire. (Adapted from Barash PG, Cullen BF, Stoelting RK, et al., eds. *Clinical Anesthesia*. 5th ed. Philadelphia, PA: Lippincott Williams & Wilkins; 2009:1588, with permission.)

In a single-chamber ventricular pacemaker (indicated in AV block and certain cases of atrial fibrillation), there is typically no P wave present. Instead the impulse from the pacemaker appears before the QRS complex creating a characteristically wide QRS waveform (Fig. 2).

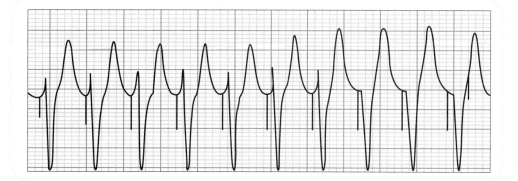

Figure 2. ECG tracing in a person with ventricular pacemaker wire. (Adapted from Barash PG, Cullen BF, Stoelting RK, et al., eds. *Clinical Anesthesia*. 5th ed. Philadelphia, PA: Lippincott Williams & Wilkins; 2009:1588, with permission.)

In a dual-chamber pacemaker, the most commonly used pacemaker, a combination of both atrial and ventricular pacing may been observed on ECG (Fig. 3). If the electrical signals conduct appropriately through the atrium and subsequently through the AV node, the ventricular signal is inhibited. Typically, a P wave will be present immediately preceding its QRS complex. However, if the atrial impulse is not conducted after a set amount of time, the pacer will generate a ventricular impulse and a ventricular pacing pattern will be observed.

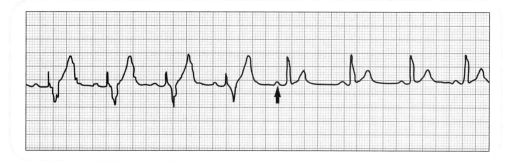

Figure 3. ECG in a person with dual-chamber pacemaker wires; the *arrow* indicates the point after which subsequent atrial activity is conducted through the AV node, thereby inhibiting ventricular pacing. (Adapted from Barash PG, Cullen BF, Stoelting RK, et al, eds. *Clinical Anesthesia*. 5th ed. Philadelphia, PA: Lippincott Williams & Wilkins; 2009:1588, with permission.)

In a biventricular pacemaker, one may see a wide QRS complex or a narrow QRS complex depending on the timing of the pacemaker. If both the left and right ventricles are stimulated simultaneously, the QRS will be narrow. If there is a delay between the two ventricular stimulations, the QRS will appear wide.

SUGGESTED READINGS

Barash PG, Cullen BF, Stoelting RK, et al, eds. *Clinical Anesthesia*. 5th ed. Philadelphia, PA: Lippincott Williams & Wilkins; 2009:1588.

Stone KR, McPherson CA. Assessment and management of patients with pacemakers and implantable cardioverter defibrillators. *Crit Care Med*. 2004;32:S155–S165.

PACU Bypass: Rationale

Generic Clinical Sciences: Anesthesia Procedures, Methods, Techniques

Bijal Patel

Edited by Hossam Tantawy

P

KEY POINTS

1. Phase I recovery area refers to the unit in which patients recover immediately after the completion of a surgical procedure, where the patient is expected to regain core physiologic functions including the stability of hemodynamics, pulmonary function, and the airway.
2. Phase II recovery area is considered a short-stay unit that patients go to after being discharged from the Phase I area, where the patient gains increased cognitive functions to the point where he or she would be able to effectively participate in activities of daily living at home.
3. Fast-tracking is the process of going directly from the operating room (OR) to Phase II recovery, bypassing Phase I.
4. Possible advantages of fast-tracking include cost-savings, faster discharge times, and the patient may be more comfortable, faster than in a Phase I setting, as it requires less invasive and less frequent monitoring and care.

DISCUSSION

The recovery process after ambulatory anesthesia can be broken down into three phases. Phase I refers to the primary postanesthesia care unit (PACU) in which patients recover immediately after the completion of a surgical procedure. During this phase, the patient is expected to regain core physiologic functions including the stability of hemodynamics, pulmonary function, and the airway. Phase I requires a high level of care, usually with a 2:1 patient to nursing ratio.

The Phase II recovery area is considered a short-stay unit that patients go to after being discharged from the Phase I area. During Phase II recovery, the patient gains increased cognitive functioning to the point where he or she would be able to effectively participate in activities of daily living at home. The level of care is less than what is required in the Phase I area, and less frequent monitoring is needed. Generally, an assessment called the modified Aldrete score is used to move patients from Phase I to Phase II of the recovery process. The scoring system assesses activity, respiration, circulation, consciousness, and oxygen saturation, with each category worth two points. An acceptable score for transferring patients from Phase I to Phase II recovery is 8 to 10, with at least 1 point in each of the five categories.

At times, patients can also be sent directly from the OR to the Phase II area, also called fast-tracking. Similar to the modified Aldrete score, White and Song scoring system is often used as a criterion for acceptable fast-tracking. Level of consciousness, physical activity, hemodynamic stability, respiratory stability, oxygen saturation, postoperative pain status, and postoperative emetic symptoms are assessed under this system. Again, each category is worth two points, with a minimum of 12 points needed, and at least 1 point in each category.

Some of the possible advantages with fast-tracking include cost-savings and faster discharge times, with a lower rate of unplanned hospital admissions. In addition, the patient may be more comfortable, faster than in a Phase I setting, as it requires less invasive and less frequent monitoring and care. Generally, a limited number of family and friends are allowed in the Phase II area. Oral intake is usually introduced at this point, and the patient is placed in a sitting position as tolerated. With the advent of minimally invasive surgical techniques, short-acting anesthetic agents, and multimodal techniques for pain (including the use of regional blocks and limiting central acting opioids) and emesis control, fast-tracking may be an option to a greater number of patients.

Possible disadvantages related to fast-tracking include increased staffing requirements and cross-training of staff, and revenue loss associated with Phase I recovery. In addition, there is some evidence that patients who bypass the PACU may experience a higher rate of nursing interventions for symptoms such as nausea or pain.

Phase III of the recovery process usually occurs at home. Here, the patient returns to his or her baseline activity level that was present before the procedure.

SUGGESTED READINGS

Springman SR, ed. *Ambulatory Anesthesia: The Requisites in Anesthesiology*. Philadelphia, PA: Mosby Elsevier; 2006:109–116.

Twersky RS, Philip BK, eds. *Handbook of Ambulatory Anesthesia*. 2nd ed. New York, NY: Springer Science and Business Media; 2008:326.

Williams BA, Kentor ML, Williams JP, et al. PACU bypass after outpatient knee surgery is associated with fewer unplanned hospital admissions but more Phase II nursing interventions. *Anesthesiology*. 2002;97:981–988.

PACU Stage I Bypass Criteria

Generic Clinical Sciences: Anesthesia Procedures, Methods, Techniques

Kristin Richards

Edited by Ala Haddadin

KEY POINTS

1. The Aldrete score, the criteria typically used to determine whether a patient may be discharged from a Phase I postanesthesia care unit (PACU), requires that patients must first achieve a score of 8 to 10, with no score of 0 in any category.
2. In fast-tracking, which involves bypassing the Phase 1 PACU, patients are brought directly from the operating room to a less-extensively monitored Phase II step-down unit.
3. In the White and Song scoring method, which is commonly used for fast-tracking, a minimal score of 12, with no score of 0 in any category, is required for a patient to be fast-tracked after general anesthesia.

DISCUSSION

After emergence from anesthesia, patients are transported to a Phase I PACU. This area typically has a nurse to patient ratio of 1:2, and the capability for monitoring is similar to that of the operating room. On arrival to a Phase I PACU, patients' pulse oximetry, blood pressure, and ECG, and temperature are monitored. In addition, the level of consciousness is determined, as are the pain score and extent or recovery of a regional nerve block (if one was done).

Before discharge from a Phase I recovery unit, supplemental oxygen is weaned to maintain an oxygen saturation of greater than 92%, or to preoperative levels, if the baseline oxygen saturation was lower than 92%. Although in Phase 1 recovery, patients' pulse oximetry is continuously monitored. Pain and nausea are treated if necessary, and postoperative regional blocks are performed if indicated.

It is necessary for patients to meet certain criteria in order to be discharged from a Phase I PACU. These discharge criteria were initially established in 1970 with a scoring system commonly referred to as the *Aldrete scale* (Table 1). A score of 8 to 10, with no score of 0 in any category, is considered safe to discharge a patient from a Phase I PACU. This scoring system (or a similar, modified scoring system) is the most common criteria used for discharging patients from a Phase I PACU.

Table 1. The Aldrete Scale

Activity	Score
Able to move four extremities voluntarily or on command	2
Able to move two extremities voluntarily or on command	1
Unable to move extremities voluntarily or on command	0
Respiration	
Able to breathe deeply and cough freely	2
Dyspnea or limited breathing	1
Apnea	0
Circulation	
Blood pressure ±20% of preanesthetic level	2
Blood pressure ±20% to 49% of preanesthetic level	1
Blood pressure ±50% of preanesthetic level	0

(continued)

Table 1. The Aldrete Scale *(continued)*

Activity	Score
Consciousness	
Fully awake	2
Arousable on calling	1
Not responding	0
O_2 Saturation	
Able to maintain O_2 saturation >92% on room air	2
Needs O_2 inhalation to maintain O_2 saturation >90%	1
O_2 saturation <90% even with O_2 supplement	0

Adapted from Springman SR, ed. *Ambulatory Anesthesia: The Requisites in Anesthesiology.* Philadelphia, PA: Mosby Elsevier; 2006:110–111, with permission.

Fast-tracking is the process of bypassing a Phase I PACU. There is some evidence that bypassing Phase 1 recovery can shorten the time to discharge. Fast-tracking involves transferring a patient from the operating room directly to a Phase II step-down unit, which is less-extensively monitored. A Phase II unit may not be appropriate for patients who have had a general anesthetic because side effects that are generally treated in a Phase I PACU (including nausea, vomiting, and pain) are not taken into consideration. Thus, in the scoring system commonly used for fast-tracking, the White and Song scale, scoring is similar to a modified Aldrete PACU discharge approach except that the criteria of pain and nausea/vomiting are added (Table 2). Using these criteria, a minimal score of 12, with no score of 0 in any category, is required for a patient to be fast-tracked after general anesthesia.

Table 2. The White and Song Scale

Level of Consciousness	Score
Awake and oriented	2
Arousable with minimal stimulation	1
Responsive only to tactile stimulation	0
Physical Activity	
Able to move all extremities on command	2
Some weakness in movement of extremities	1
Unable to voluntarily move extremities	0
Hemodynamic Stability	
Blood pressure <15% of baseline MAP value	2
Blood pressure 15% to 30% of baseline MAP value	1
Blood pressure >30% below baseline MAP value	0
Respiratory Stability	
Able to breathe deeply	2
Tachypnea with good cough	1
Dyspnea with weak cough	0
Oxygen Saturation Status	
Maintains value <90% on room air	2
Requires supplements oxygen (nasal prongs)	1
Saturation <90% with supplemental oxygen	0
Postoperative Pain Assessment	
No or mild discomfort	2
Moderate to severe pain controlled with intravenous analgesics	1
Persistent severe pain	0

Table 2. The White and Song Scale *(continued)*

Level of Consciousness	Score
Postoperative Emetic Symptoms	
No or mild nausea with no active vomiting	2
Transient vomiting or retching	1
Persistent moderate to severe nausea and vomiting	0

Adapted from Springman SR, ed. *Ambulatory Anesthesia: The Requisites in Anesthesiology.* Philadelphia, PA: Mosby Elsevier; 2006:110–111, with permission.

SUGGESTED READINGS

Aldrete JA. The post-anesthesia recovery score revisited. *J Clin Anesth.* 1995;7:89–91.

Springman SR, ed. *Ambulatory Anesthesia: The Requisites in Anesthesiology.* Philadelphia, PA: Mosby Elsevier; 2006:110–111.

White PF. Criteria for fast-tracking outpatients after ambulatory surgery. *J Clin Anesth.* 1999;11:78–79.

Pain Management: Rib Fracture

Subspecialties: Pain

Jodi Sherman

Edited by Jodi Sherman

1. Multiple rib fractures (MRFs) cause severe pain that can seriously compromise respiratory mechanics and exacerbate underlying lung injury, predisposing to respiratory failure.
2. There are many approaches to pain control for MRF, including systemic opioids, regional techniques, and nonsteroidal anti-inflammatory drug (NSAID) adjuvants.
3. The most beneficial regional approaches include paravertebral and epidural catheters, but intercostal, interpleural, or intrathecal techniques may also play a helpful role.
4. Local anesthetic toxicity is highest with techniques near the intercostal vessels, where absorption is highest and made worse by rib fractures.
5. No single method can be safely and effectively used in all MRF cases, and a multimodal approach is best applied after weighing risks and benefits of each technique.

MRFs cause severe pain that can seriously compromise respiratory mechanics and exacerbate underlying lung injury, predisposing to respiratory failure. Early institution of effective pain control is therefore essential. There are many approaches to pain control for MRF, including systemic opioids, regional techniques, and NSAID adjuvants. The most beneficial regional approaches include paravertebral and epidural catheters, but intercostal, interpleural, or intrathecal techniques may also play a helpful role. No single method can be safely and effectively used in all MRF cases, and a multimodal approach is best applied after weighing risks and benefits of each technique.

Chest wall trauma accounts for 8% of all trauma admissions, and rib fractures are the most common. They contribute significantly to morbidity and mortality, particularly in the elderly and in those with reduced respiratory reserve. Rib fractures often coincide with pulmonary contusions and flail chest that further compromise respiratory function. Pain from MRF is often more harmful than the injury itself, as the pain limits deep breathing and coughing. Poor pulmonary effort leads to atelectasis, ventilation-perfusion mismatch, hypoxemia, respiratory distress, and even respiratory failure. Early and effective MRF pain control maximizes pulmonary function, permits aggressive pulmonary toilet, aids early mobilization, and is therefore essential to minimize pulmonary complications.

Systemic opioids are often the first approach to relieving MRF pain. They may be administered IV by clinicians or by patient-controlled analgesia (PCA). IV opioids improve visual analog pain scores and vital capacity, but also cause sedation, respiratory depression, and cough suppression. Systemic opioids better serve as an adjuvant to regional techniques in supplementing incomplete blocks or covering pain from concomitant traumatic injuries.

An *intercostal nerve block* (ICNB) entails placement of local anesthetic at the intercostal nerve proximal to the injury site of a single rib. Because sensory innervation involves contributions from segments above and below each affected level, multiple level blocks are typically required to adequately treat even single rib fracture pain. These can be time-consuming and painful to perform, and also predispose patients to local anesthetic toxicity because of multiple injections and the high rate of absorption from the intercostal vessels. Multiple injections further increase the risk of iatrogenic pneumothorax. Successful ICNBs can result in improved pulmonary function; however, the effect wears off with the

429

local anesthetic dose. A single ICN continuous catheter can be placed, but is not prudent, given overlapping sensory contributions.

An *intrapleural catheter* can be placed percutaneously. It has the advantage over ICNBs in that it covers multiple sensory levels. However, they are technically challenging to perform with a high failure rate, have increased risk of pulmonary injury, and are of poor and variable efficacy, as local anesthetic spread is gravity dependent and therefore difficult to predict. Furthermore, there is a risk of phrenic nerve anesthetization.

Thoracic epidural catheter (TEC) in MRF patients who are older than 60 years is an independent predictor of both decreased mortality and decreased incidence of pulmonary complications. An epidural catheter for MRF pain control is superior to systemic opioids. TEC patients are alert and able to breathe, cough deeply, and tolerate chest physiotherapy (PT). The results are increased functional residual capacity and vital capacity, significantly increased PaO_2, shorter intensive care unit, and hospital stays with reduced costs. TECs can be technically challenging to place and typically result in significant hypotension. With any needle technique, there is risk of infection, bleeding, and failed or incomplete block, and with TECs, there is a further serious risk of spinal cord injury. Local anesthetic is typically used, although opioids can also serve as a neuraxial adjuvant. Opioids can also be used as the primary agent to eliminate secondary hypotension but with inferior effect when compared with local anesthetic. Any opioids increase the risk of sedation, respiratory depression, as well as nausea and vomiting, urinary retention, and pruritus.

Paravertebral catheter. A recent meta-analysis demonstrated that paravertebral and thoracic epidural blocks provided comparable pain relief and were superior to PCA alone. Furthermore, paravertebral blocks had a better side-effect profile (no urinary retention and much reduced incidence of hypotension) as well as reduced pulmonary complications. Both paravertebral and epidural catheters demonstrate superior pulmonary function tests (PFTs) over PCA, intercostal, and intrapleural techniques. Paravertebral blocks had the greatest PFTs overall, even over epidurals, presumably because of unilateral as opposed to bilateral anesthetization of accessory intercostal muscles. For bilateral rib fractures, either bilateral paravertebral or epidural catheters could be used; however, hypotension could be seen with either, and bilateral paravertebral catheters carry the risk of bilateral pneumothoraces.

NSAIDs, administered either orally or through IV, serve as helpful adjuvants in a multimodal approach to MRF pain management. Advantages include pain control from an alternative pathway than regional or opioid mechanisms, and importantly without respiratory depression or sedation. Disadvantages include increased platelet dysfunction, renal injury, and gastrointestinal upset (e.g., from ketorolac), or hepatic injury (e.g., from acetaminophen).

Early and effective MRF pain control maximizes pulmonary function, permits aggressive pulmonary toilet, aids early mobilization, and is therefore essential to minimize pulmonary complications. The ideal approach to MRF pain management is safe, easy to perform, and of adequate duration; permits deep breathing and clearance of secretions; and facilitates chest PT and early mobilization, with minimal sedation. No single method can be safely and effectively used in all MRF cases, and a multimodal approach is best applied after weighing risks and benefits of each technique.

SUGGESTED READINGS

Carrier FM, Turgeon AF, Nicole PC, et al. Effect of epidural analgesia in patients with traumatic rib fractures: a systematic review and meta-analysis of randomized controlled trials. *Can J Anaesth.* 2009;56(3):230–242.

Davies RG, Myles PS, Graham JM. A comparison of the analgesic efficacy and side-effects of paravertebral vs epidural blockade for thoracotomy—a systemic review and meta-analysis of randomized trials. *Br J Anaesth.* 2006;96(4):418–426.

Karmakar MK, Ho AM. Acute pain management of patients with multiple fractured ribs. *J Trauma.* 2003;54: 615–625.

Paired vs. Unpaired *t*-test

Mathematics, Statistics, Computers

Svetlana Sapozhnikova

Edited by Raj K. Modak

KEY POINTS

1. Paired *t*-test requires the same sample size in both study groups. Sample groups analyzed by an unpaired *t*-test can have different sample sizes.
2. The number of degrees of freedom is *n*–1 for the paired *t*-test and *n*–2 for the unpaired *t*-test.
3. *p*-Value can be obtained using *t*-distribution table after calculating *t*-test statistic and the degrees of freedom.
4. *t*-Test allows comparison of the **mean values of two populations** even when population variances are not known.

DISCUSSION

t-Test allows comparison of the mean values of two populations even when population variances are not known. It is performed via calculation of a *t*-statistic, where sample variances are used instead of unknown population variances. Once the *t*-statistic is determined, it can be used to obtain a *p*-value from a *t*-distribution table. If a *p*-value is less than a threshold value alpha chosen for statistical significance (alpha is frequently 0.05 for a one-tailed *t*-test), then the null hypothesis of no difference between the population means is rejected. When population variance is known, *z*-statistic is used.

t-Tests can be paired or unpaired. Paired *t*-tests require either two groups of the same sizes and with the same variances matched exactly except for the characteristics studied or, most commonly, same study subjects, who had two measurements taken on them (x_i and y_i). The first measurement (x_i) on each subject is used for the first study group and the second measurement (y_i) for the second group. For example, patients' heart rates during preoperative evaluation and intraoperatively can be compared using paired *t*-test.

t-Statistic for paired *t*-test can be calculated as follows:

$$t = \frac{\bar{d}}{SE\,\bar{d}},$$

where $\bar{d} = \Sigma_{i=1}^{n}(x_i - y_i)/n$ is an average of differences between both measurements in a pair and *n* is the number of study subjects. $SE\,\bar{d}$, a standard error for both of the means, is calculated as $SE\,\bar{d} = SD/\sqrt{n}$, where *SD* is a standard deviation. In order to obtain *p*-value from the *t*-distribution table, one needs to know degrees of freedom. For paired *t*-test, degrees of freedom are calculated as sample size *n*–1.

When measurements are taken on two independent groups of subjects, they cannot be analyzed using paired *t*-test. Instead, unpaired *t*-test is used. Unpaired *t*-test does not require two sample groups of equal sizes. To calculate *t*-statistic, one has to calculate each sample mean $\bar{x}$ and $\bar{y}$.

The denominator is a weighted average of the *SD*s of each sample. Degrees of freedom

$$t = \frac{\bar{x} - \bar{y}}{\sqrt{\left(\sqrt{\frac{1}{n_x} + \frac{1}{n_y}}\right)\left(\frac{(n_x - 1)s_x^2 + (n_y - 1)s_y^2}{n_x + n_y - 2}\right)}}$$

432

used for the unpaired *t*-test equal to the total number of subjects in both groups minus two (*n*–2).

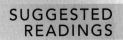

Barash PG, Cullen BF, Stoelting RK, et al, eds. *Clinical Anesthesia*. 6th ed. Philadelphia, PA: Lippincott Williams & Wilkins; 2009:195–200.

Hemmings HC, Hopkins PM, eds. *Foundations of Anesthesia*. 2nd ed. Mosby, an Imprint of Elsevier; 2005:chap 18. http://www.mdconsult.com.

P

Parental Presence: Indications
Subspecialties: Pediatric Anesthesia

Kevan Stanton

Edited by Mamatha Punjala

1. Current studies are inconclusive as to the effect parental presence has on the child's emotional outcome.
2. The decision to allow a parent to be present during induction must be made in the child's best interest, not the parents'.
3. Parental presence should not be used in place of premedication in a child requiring premedication.
4. The child's level of development should be considered when deciding whether to allow the presence of a parent.

Parents often request to be present for the induction of their child's anesthesia. Current studies have been inconclusive as to the degree of effect this has on the child's anxiety level or emotional outcome, but in practice, does appear to be helpful in certain situations. It also helps the parents to feel more involved, although the decision of whether to allow a parent to be present should always be based on the child's best interest, not the parents.

In most cases, parental presence is limited to one parent. In some instances, the presence of a parent can reduce the amount of, or eliminate entirely, the need for premedication. However, the presence of a parent should not be used in place of premedication in a child that truly needs to be premedicated.

The most common situation in which parental presence is indicated is when the child is highly anxious of parental separation (children undergoing surgery are often more anxious of parental separation than of the surgery itself). Another situation in which parental presence is indicated and can be very helpful is in the case of a handicapped child. Parents of handicapped children are likely to know how to better interact with their child and help them remain calm and cooperative. Parental presence in the recovery room can also be helpful in calming a child and can help determine whether a child is crying because of pain or because of anxiety and parental separation.

When deciding whether to allow a parent to be present for induction, the level of the child's development must be taken into consideration. If the child has not yet developed anxiety toward strangers, it serves no benefit to the child to have a parent present during induction. Also, if the child is heavily premedicated, there will likely be no benefit to the child in allowing a parent to be present. Anxious parents may only worsen the situation and most often should not be allowed to be present for induction. The final decision of whether to allow a parent to be present for induction is at the anesthesiologist's discretion, and must be based on his or her best clinical judgment.

Barash PG, Cullen BF, Stoelting RK, et al, eds. *Clinical Anesthesia*. 6th ed. Philadelphia, PA: Lippincott Williams & Wilkins; 2009:1207.

Lerman J, Steward D, Cote CJ. *Manual of Pediatric Anesthesia*. 6th ed. Philadelphia, PA: Churchill Livingstone; 2010:6.

Miller RD, Eriksson LI, Fleisher LA, et al., eds. *Miller's Anesthesia*. 7th ed. Philadelphia, PA: Churchill Livingstone; 2010:2576–2577.

Patent Ductus Arteriosus: Dx
Subspecialties: Pediatric Anesthesia

Alexander Timchenko

Edited by Mamatha Punjala

KEY POINTS

1. The incidence of isolated patent ductus arteriosus (PDA) is 1 in 2,500 live births, and is associated with prematurity and prenatal exposure to rubella.
2. The physical examination findings that can help identify PDA in children include the classic "continuous machine" murmur, pulsus bisferiens, bounding pulses, and a wide pulse pressure.
3. Signs and symptoms that can help support a diagnosis of PDA include signs of heart failure, recurrent respiratory infections, lobar emphysema and collapse, pulmonary hemorrhage, renal insufficiency, and bacterial endocarditis.
4. Echocardiography is the gold standard in confirming the diagnosis of PDA; ECG and chest X-ray findings are nonspecific and are usually normal.
5. Brain natriuretic peptide (BNP) levels can be used to screen for PDA and help guide its treatment; in addition, low levels of cortisol in the first week of life are associated with PDA.
6. During the first 2 weeks of life for the term infant (or the first several weeks of extrauterine life for the preterm infant), the neonate may revert back to fetal circulation during periods of hypoxia, acidosis, or decreases in temperature.

P

DISCUSSION

The ductus arteriosus is an important component of fetal circulation that normally closes in the first few hours after birth. In full-term infants, the incidence of an isolated PDA is 1 in 2,500 live births, accounting for 10% of congenital heart defects. A PDA is associated with prematurity and prenatal exposure to rubella, especially in the first trimester. The ratio of female neonates to male neonates affected is almost 2:1.

When PDA presents asymptomatically, it is usually identified by its classic murmur on routine physical examination. The murmur heard in PDA, which is heard best at the first or second intercostal space at the left sternal border, has been described as a "continuous machine" sound and is loudest during systole. Other prominent physical examination findings include pulsus bisferiens (two different peaks separated by a deep cleft on the arterial waveform), which is both a sensitive and specific finding, as well as bounding pulses and a wide pulse pressure.

If untreated, a PDA with significant left-to-right shunting can lead to heart failure. When PDA is suspected in a child, the signs and symptoms can help support the diagnosis. Signs of heart failure and respiratory distress, including tachypnea, diaphoresis, pulmonary edema, failure to thrive, and decreased exercise tolerance can be present. In addition, children may present with recurrent respiratory infections, lobar emphysema and collapse, pulmonary hemorrhage, renal insufficiency, and bacterial endocarditis.

Echocardiography is the gold standard for confirming the diagnosis of PDA. Continuous-wave Doppler can detect abnormal flow, and color-flow Doppler can give important information regarding the size and shape of the ductus. ECG and chest X-ray findings are nonspecific and are usually normal. With severe left-to-right flow, evidence of left ventricular hypertrophy or left atrial enlargement can be present.

Laboratory studies can also have some diagnostic value. BNP is a biomarker that has been used to identify heart failure in children caused by PDA and can help guide its treatment. BNP levels more than 1,110 pg per mL have been associated with a sensitivity of 100% and a specificity of 95% for symptomatic PDA. Low levels of cortisol in the first week of life are also associated with PDA.

SUGGESTED READINGS

Hamrick SE, Hansmann G. Patent ductus arteriosus of the preterm infant. *Pediatrics*. 2010;125:1020–1030.

Holzman RS, Mancuso TJ, Polaner DM, eds. *A Practical Approach to Pediatric Anesthesia*. Philadelphia, PA: Lippincott Williams & Wilkins; 2008:603–604.

Lake CI, Booker PD, eds. *Pediatric Cardiac Anesthesia*. 4th ed. Philadelphia, PA: Lippincott Williams & Wilkins; 2005:413–414.

P

PDP Headache: Risk Factors

Regional Anesthesia

Ira Whitten

Edited by Jodi Sherman

KEY POINTS

1. Several characteristics of the spinal needle determine the risk of postdural puncture headache (PDPH), including the type and gauge of the spinal needle and orientation of the bevel (relative to the dural fibers).
2. Other major factors that determine the risk of developing a PDPH include the age of the patient, anatomy, skill of the person performing the procedure, and a history of PDPH.
3. Factors that do not seem to influence the risk of PDPH include the duration of bed rest after spinal anesthesia, hydration prior to spinal needle placement (intravenous or oral), and patient positioning during the procedure.

DISCUSSION

PDPH is one of the most common complications of spinal anesthesia, yet it can also occur after accidental dural puncture during epidural anesthesia. The incidence of PDPH following spinal anesthesia has decreased dramatically with the advent of smaller gauge needles and newer tip designs.

Several characteristics of the spinal needle determine the risk of developing a PDPH, the most important of which are the type and gauge of the needle. The risk of developing a PDPH directly correlates with the diameter of the needle. The incidence is approximately 40% with a 22G needle, 25% with a 25G needle, 2% to 12% with a 26G needle, and 2% with a 29G needle. The type of needle tip is also important, as cutting needle tips result in larger holes in the dura. The modern "pencil-point" needle tips are thought to spread the fibers of the dura, leaving a smaller hole. In addition, the risk of PDPH is thought to be higher if the bevel of the spinal needle is inserted perpendicular, instead of parallel, to the dural fibers. A "wet-tap" during attempted epidural catheter placement is more likely to cause a PDPH compared to modern spinal needles because of the large diameter of the needle and the trauma caused by the sharp needle point.

PDPH is rare in children, is more common following puberty, and less common with increasing age. The number of attempts at spinal anesthesia is thought to directly correlate with the risk of PDPH. Therefore, the anesthesiologist's skill is an important factor in determining the risk of developing a PDPH. A history of PDPH is also a risk factor for the development of a subsequent PDPH, though the underlying reason is unknown.

Factors that do not seem to influence the risk of PDPH after spinal anesthesia include the duration of bed rest after spinal anesthesia, hydration prior to spinal needle placement (intravenous or oral), and patient positioning during the procedure.

SUGGESTED READINGS

Ahmed SV, Jayawarna C, Jude E. Post-lumbar puncture headache: diagnosis and management. *Postgrad Med J.* 2006;82:713–716.

Barash PG, Cullen BF, Stoelting RK, eds. *Clinical Anesthesia.* 5th ed. Philadelphia, PA: Lippincott Williams & Wilkins; 2009:947–948.

Miller RD, Stoelting RK, eds. *Basics of Anesthesia.* 5th ed. Philadelphia, PA: Churchill Livingstone; 2007:260–261.

Turnbull DK, Shepherd DB. Post-dural puncture headache: pathogenesis, prevention, and treatment. *Br J Anesth.* 2003;91:718–729.

Peak vs. Plateau Airway Pressure

Subspecialties: Critical Care

Neil Sinha

Edited by Shamsuddin Akhtar

1. Lung expansion requires overcoming the elastic and structural tissues in the major airways and surface tension in the alveoli as well as the pressure exerted by chest wall recoil.
2. Peak airway pressure is the maximum amount of pressure in a patient's airway.
3. Plateau airway pressure reflects the pressure in the airway once the target tidal volume has been achieved and airway flow is static.
4. Increases in the peak airway pressure in the absence of change to the plateau airway pressure can typically be attributive to airway obstruction from asthma, foreign masses, excess secretions, or kinking of the ventilator tubing.

Airway pressures in mechanical ventilation are functions of pulmonary compliance and resistance. In order for the lungs to expand during positive pressure ventilation, elastic and structural tissues in the major airways and surface tension in the alveoli must be overcome. In addition, near total lung capacity, the pressure exerted by chest wall recoil also contributes to resistance to lung expansion. In volume-control ventilation (in the absence of spontaneous effort), the pressure required to overcome these two opposing forces and deliver the pre-set tidal volume can be broken down into peak and plateau pressure (see Fig. 1).

P

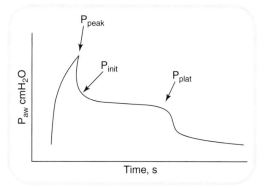

Figure 1. Peak and plateau pressures in a mechanically ventilated patient. (From Jain M, Sznajder JI. Bench-to-bedside review: distal airways in adult respiratory distress syndrome. *Crit Care.* 2007;11:206, with permission.)

Peak airway pressure is the maximum amount of pressure in a patient's airway and is most often recorded at the end of inspiration. Peak airway pressure is the sum of PEEP, elastic, and resistive pressures. Excess airway pressure (>35 cm H_2O) may lead to overdistention of alveoli and barotrauma. Plateau airway pressure reflects the pressure in the airway once the target tidal volume has been achieved and airway flow is static. It is a marker of the small airways and alveoli and is the sum of the elastic pressure and PEEP within the system.

There are many disease processes that cause an increase in both the peak and plateau airway pressures. Intrinsic lung disease such as pneumonia, atelectasis, and pulmonary edema as well as thoracic cage deformities cause an increase in both peak and plateau pressures. Airway obstruction from asthma, foreign masses, excess secretions, or kinking of the ventilator tubing may cause an increase in peak airway pressure without changing the plateau airway pressure.

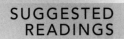

Hall JB, Schmidt GA, Wood LDH, eds. *Principles of Critical Care*. 3rd ed. New York, NY: McGraw-Hill; 2005:427–430.

Jain M, Sznajder JI. Bench-to-bedside review: distal airways in adult respiratory distress syndrome. *Crit Care*. 2007;11:206.

Marino, PL. *The ICU Book*. 3rd ed. Philadelphia, PA: Lippincott William & Wilkins; 2007:462–468.

P

PEEP: Effect on PAOP
Organ-based Clinical: Respiratory

Brooke Albright

Edited by Shamsuddin Akhtar

Brooke Albright

KEY POINTS

1. Positive end-expiratory pressure (PEEP) stents alveoli open at end expiration, thereby increasing lung volumes (especially the functional residual capacity [FRC]), decreasing the shear stress associated with opening and closing of alveoli, improving V/Q mismatching, and decreasing the magnitude of right-to-left intrapulmonary shunting.
2. The optimal level of PEEP correlates with the highest total respiratory compliance, the highest mixed venous oxygen tension, and the lowest V_D/V_T.
3. PEEP can cause an erroneous effect on pulmonary artery occlusion pressure (PAOP) due to the transmission of increased intra-alveolar pressure to the pulmonary capillaries.
4. The adverse cardiovascular effects of PEEP depend on the severity of respiratory failure, the level of PEEP, the contractility of the heart, and the pulmonary vasculature.

DISCUSSION

PEEP stents alveoli open at end expiration, thereby increasing lung volumes (especially the FRC), decreasing the shear stress associated with opening and closing of alveoli, improving V/Q mismatching, and decreasing the magnitude of right-to-left intrapulmonary shunting. PEEP is indicated when high concentrations of inspired oxygen ($FiO_2 > 0.5$) are needed for prolonged periods of time to maintain adequate PaO_2. PEEP is usually added in 2.5 to 5.0 cm H_2O increments until the PaO_2 is at least 60 mm Hg with an FiO_2 greater than 0.5. Most patients show maximal improvement in oxygen transport and pulmonary compliance with levels of PEEP greater than 15 cm H_2O. The optimal level of PEEP correlates with the highest total respiratory compliance, the highest mixed venous oxygen tension, and the lowest V_D/V_T.

An important adverse effect of PEEP is decreased cardiac output due to increased intrathoracic pressure interfering with venous return (decreased preload). Excessive levels of PEEP can decrease the PaO_2 by overdistending alveoli and compressing pulmonary capillaries. Therefore, PEEP can cause an erroneous effect on PAOP. High levels of PEEP also can increase pulmonary pressure and resistance to the point of right ventricular dilation, resulting in leftward displacement of the interventricular septum, causing restriction of left ventricular filling. In addition, unilateral pulmonary hyperinflation can cause decreased heart rate and cardiac output from neural reflex. Finally, high levels of PEEP may increase the incidence of barotrauma. The adverse cardiovascular effects of PEEP depend on the level of PEEP, severity of respiratory failure, the contractility of the heart, and the pulmonary vasculature. They are exaggerated in the presence of hypovolemia.

SUGGESTED READINGS

Hines RL, Marschall K. *Stoelting's Anesthesia and Co-existing Disease*. 5th ed. Philadelphia, PA: Saunders Elsevier; 2002:127–128.

Yao F, Fontes M, Malhotra V. *Anesthesiology Problem Oriented Patient Management*. 6th ed. Philadelphia, PA: Lippincott Williams & Wilkins; 2008:69.

PEEP: Lung Volume Effect
Organ-based Clinical: Respiratory

Emilio Andrade

Edited by Veronica Matei

Emilio Andrade

Edited by Veronica Matei

KEY POINTS

1. Positive end-expiratory pressure (PEEP) is positive pressure applied during the expiratory phase of the respiratory cycle.
2. Functional residual capacity (FRC) is the volume of air at the end of a normal expiration.
3. Patients on ventilators have collapse of distal airspaces at the end of expiration, resulting in reduced FRC, atelectasis, and impairment of gas exchange.
4. PEEP is added to counterbalance this alveolar collapse and improve gas exchange by increasing aerated lung.

DISCUSSION

FRC is the volume of air at the end of a normal expiration. Closing capacity is the volume at which airways begin to close in the dependent part of the lungs. FRC is normally more than the closing capacity, but with aging and anesthesia, the closing capacity can be more than the FRC. This causes ventilation/perfusion abnormalities.

PEEP is applied at the end of expiration to prevent the collapse of distal airways, which is a common occurrence with ventilator-dependent patients. PEEP stents the airway open by opposing the elastic recoil of the lungs. PEEP can open collapsed alveoli and reverse atelectasis (lung recruitment). Areas of collapsed parenchyma are seen in as much as 90% of intubated anesthetized patients.

During mechanical ventilation, the use of PEEP increases FRC above the closing capacity, improving arterial oxygenation. Effect of PEEP applied to airways can be followed by the PaO_2/FiO_2 ratio. If PEEP is effective, this ratio will increase. If it is harmful, the ratio will decrease. PEEP can increase deadspace by overdistention of normal alveoli. PEEP can also compress surrounding capillaries and increase intrapleural pressure, thereby decreasing cardiac output. Barotrauma can be seen with levels of PEEP greater than 20 cm H_2O.

SUGGESTED READINGS

Chomka C. Cardiopulmonary effects of positive end expiratory pressure. In: *Anesthesiology Clinics of North America*. Vol 5(4). Philadelphia, PA: WB Saunders Company; 1987:778–780.

Marino PL. Modes of assisted ventilation. *The ICU Book*. 3rd ed. Philadelphia, PA: Lippincott Williams & Wilkins; 2007: 481–485.

Morgan G, Mikhail M, Murray M. *Clinical Anesthesiology*. 4th ed. New York, NY: Lange Medical Books/ McGraw-Hill; 2006:1038–1039, 544–546.

P

PEEP: LV Effects
Organ-based Clinical: Respiratory

Trevor Banack

Edited by Shamsuddin Akhtar

KEY POINTS

1. Positive end-expiratory pressure (PEEP) refers to the use of positive pressure during the respiratory cycle. The pressure at the end of the expiratory phase is higher than ambient pressure which increases the functional residual capacity (FRC).
2. In general, PEEP raises intrathoracic pressures and impairs venous return.
3. The most likely cause of decreased cardiac output with PEEP is lower venous return or preload to the left ventricle.
4. Another physiological explanation for decreased left ventricular function is the increased right ventricular volume load.

DISCUSSION

PEEP refers to the use of positive pressure during the respiratory cycle. The pressure at the end of the expiratory phase is higher than ambient pressure which increases FRC. This increase in FRC leads to the recruitment of alveoli during inspiration and prevents alveoli collapse during expiration. Overall, the goal is to improve V/Q matching with use of PEEP, because it decreases intrapulmonary shunting of blood.

However, application of PEEP also has cardiopulmonary side effects. In general, PEEP raises intrathoracic pressures and impairs venous return. Specifically, with respect to the heart, as PEEP is increased, there is a simultaneous decrease in cardiac output. The most likely cause of decreased cardiac output is lower venous return or preload to the left ventricle. As pressure increases on pulmonary parenchyma, small capillary beds within that tissue are squeezed. This increases pulmonary vascular resistance, and subsequently there is less blood volume delivered to the left atrium.

Another physiological explanation for decreased left ventricular function is the increased right ventricular volume load. As capillary beds are compressed from PEEP, less blood volume is allowed to leave the right ventricle. The overdistended right ventricle distorts the intraventricular septum and impairs diastolic filling of the left heart. Subsequently, the cardiac output is impaired.

SUGGESTED READINGS

Barbas CS, de Matos GF, Pincelli MP, et al. Mechanical ventilation in acute respiratory failure: recruitment and high positive end-expiratory pressure are necessary. *Curr Opin Crit Care.* 2005;11:18–28.

Marini JJ, Wheeler AP. *Critical Care Medicine: The Essentials.* 3rd ed. Lippincot Williams & Wilkins; 2006:167–169.

Morgan GE, Mikhail MS, Murray MJ, eds. *Clinical Anesthesiology.* 4th ed. New York, NY: Lange/McGraw-Hill; 2006:1039.

P

PEEP to Treat Hypoxia

Subspecialties: Critical Care

Garth Skoropowski

Edited by Veronica Matei

1. Positive end-expiratory pressure (PEEP) increases functional residual capacity (FRC) and prevents alveolar collapse.
2. PEEP decreases intrapulmonary shunting and improves arterial oxygenation. The effectiveness of PEEP can be assessed by increased PaO_2/FiO_2 ratio.
3. By increasing intrathoracic pressure, PEEP can decrease the cardiac output and can increase the intracranial pressure (ICP).

PEEP can be an effective method for improving oxygenation and treating hypoxia in mechanically ventilated patients. Decreased lung compliance contributes to atelectasis in patients receiving mechanical ventilation, and PEEP serves to counteract collapsing forces by stabilizing and expanding alveoli. PEEP can also reverse atelectasis in collapsed alveoli in an effect known as recruitment. PEEP thus increases the surface area of the lung that is available for gas exchange. This improves ventilation/perfusion mismatch and can decrease intrapulmonary shunting, resulting in improved arterial oxygenation. PEEP also increases FRC.

By exerting positive pressure, PEEP increases intrathoracic pressure, which results in decreased venous return or a reduction in preload causing a drop in cardiac output. By decreasing venous return and essentially raising central venous pressure, compliance of the intracranial ventricles is diminished, causing an increase in ICP. Therefore, PEEP is contraindicated in patients with pulmonary embolism, pneumothorax, bronchopleural fistulas, recent pulmonary surgery, and patients with intracranial abnormalities. Excessive PEEP can also cause overdistention of alveoli and barotrauma, which is typically seen at PEEP levels greater than 20 cm H_2O. If there are no atelectatic areas within the lungs, PEEP can cause overdistension and lung damage.

The effectiveness of PEEP can be evaluated by examining the PaO_2/FiO_2 ratio. If the addition of PEEP increases the ratio, this indicates that atelectatic areas of the lungs have been recruited and are now being aerated and contributing to gas exchange. However, if the ratio worsens, PEEP causes lung overdistension and possible lung injury. In this case, there may be no atelectatic areas in the lungs available for recruitment.

SUGGESTED READINGS

Acosta P, Santisbon E, Varon J. The use of positive end-expiratory pressure in mechanical ventilation. *Crit Care Clin.* 2007;23:251–261.

Marino PL. *The ICU Book.* 3rd ed. Philadelphia, PA: Lippincott Williams & Wilkins; 2007:481–486.

Morgan GE, Mikhail MS, Murray MJ. *Clinical Anesthesiology.* 4th ed. New York, NY: Lange Medical Books/ McGraw-Hill; 2005:1037–1039.

Roberts JR, Hedges JR, Custalow C, eds. Mechanical ventilation. In: *Clinical Procedures in Emergency Medicine.* 4th ed. Philadelphia, PA: Saunders; 2004:139–141.

Peripheral Nerves: Sensory versus Motor
Subspecialties: Pain

Anjali Vira

Edited by Thomas Halaszynski

KEY POINTS

1. Peripheral nerves can be categorized in several ways, including by function, speed of conduction, nerve size, sensory versus motor, nerve fiber type (A, B, and C), etc.
2. Large myelinated A-fibers conduct both sensory and motor transmission very rapidly.
3. Large myelinated A-fibers are typically one of the last nerve fibers to be blocked by local anesthetic administration.
4. Small, nonmyelinated C-fibers slowly transmit an array of sensory information such as pain and temperature.
5. Small, nonmyelinated C-fibers are one of the first nerve fiber types to be blocked by local anesthetics.

DISCUSSION

Nerve fiber type A has functions of proprioception and large motor function. In addition, type A nerves also function in small motor function, touch, pressure, and are responsible for muscle tone, temperature, and sharp pain. Type B nerve fibers function in a preganglionic autonomic capacity. Type C nerve fibers are unmyelinated and function in dull pain, temperature, and touch sensations. Peripheral nerves are often categorized by their physical properties, including nerve fiber diameter, and whether the nerves are myelinated. This differentiation is important because these two properties affect speed of conduction and function of each nerve type. Myelination and large diameter nerve fibers favor fast conduction velocity. Large diameter nerves are better conductors intrinsically, and myelination increases conduction velocity by salutatory conduction as well as by providing electrical insulation.

Sensory motor nerve differentiation is based on the different sizes of nerves and evidence of myelination of nerve fibers involved in pain conduction (Aα- and C-fibers) as compared with those involved in motor function (Aα-fibers). Large diameter myelinated A-fibers are located in muscles and joints and are able to transmit motor and proprioceptive signals at a high velocity (5 to 100 m per second). Conversely, small unmyelinated C-fibers located in afferent sensory nerves and in the sympathetic plexus conduct autonomic, pain, and temperature signals more slowly (1.2 m per second). Intermediate in conduction velocity are the preganglionic autonomic B nerve fibers (3 to 14 m per second).

Effect of local anesthetics is another way to help understand the differentiation between sensory and motor peripheral nerves. Each local anesthetic has a minimal concentration necessary to completely block a nerve fiber depending upon whether the nerve is sensory or motor. The concentration of local anesthetic depends not only on the potency but also on the intrinsic physical properties of the nerve fibers it is acting upon. In general, larger diameter nerve fibers are more resistant to blockade than smaller diameter nerve fibers. However, the intrinsic conductibility of individual fibers also affects susceptibility to blockade so that not all small diameter fibers are blocked before all large diameter fibers. This leads to a differential blockade of temperature sensation and proprioception prior to motor blockade, followed by loss of sensation of sharp pain and light touch.

SUGGESTED READINGS

Barash PG, Cullen BF, Stoelting RK, et al., eds. *Clinical Anesthesia*. 6th ed. Philadelphia, PA: Lippincott Williams & Wilkins; 2009:532–535.

Morgan GE, Mikhael MS, Murray MJ, eds. *Clinical Anesthesiology*. 4th ed. New York, NY: Lange McGraw-Hill; 2006:266.

Peripheral TPN: Complications

Subspecialties: Critical Care

Chi Wong

Edited by Ala Haddadin

1. The osmolarity of the peripheral parenteral nutrition (PPN) solution is limited to 900 mOsm per L to avoid phlebitis.
2. The most common complication of PPN is thrombophlebitis.
3. The metabolic complications are similar compared with those of total parenteral nutrition (TPN) and include hypokalemia, hypocalcemia, hypophosphatemia, and hypomagnesemia.
4. Regardless of continuing or discontinuing PPN in the operating room, the most important intraoperative management is frequent blood glucose monitoring to guide subsequent therapy.
5. Lipid infusions containing oxidizable lipids increase the risk of oxidation-induced cell injury and may promote organ injury.

PPN is indicated in patients who are unable to tolerate enteral feeding. Patients requiring less than 2,000 calories per day with a brief period of nutritional support (< 14 days) may have parenteral nutrition delivered through a peripheral vein, to avoid the many complications associated with central-line access. The osmolarity of the PPN solution is limited to 900 mOsm per L with short catheters to avoid phlebitis. Due to the osmolarity limits of these low-flow blood vessels, large fluid volumes are required to approach protein and energy requirements for hypermetabolic patients, which may not be practical in an ICU setting. If large fluid volumes are required, a potential complication in patients with compromised cardiac function is fluid overload and congestive heart failure.

Technical complications of PPN are minimal compared to TPN. The most common complication is thrombophlebitis that necessitates frequent peripheral catheter replacement. Another common complication is intravenous catheter infiltration and extravasation. Catheter site inspection must be performed regularly. Most peripheral vein catheters will last between 48 and 72 hours and will require systematic site rotation. Heparin and corticosteroids can be added to the infusion, and local glyceryl nitrate patch can be applied locally to reduce the occurrence of thrombophlebitis, thus prolonging catheter life. Infectious complications include catheter site skin infections and septic phlebitis.

Although less common than with TPN, PPN may lead to increased production of carbon dioxide (CO_2) secondary to metabolism of a large glucose load. Increased ventilatory work is required to eliminate the CO_2 produced. Elevated CO_2 production may require initiating mechanical ventilation, or it may make it more difficult to wean patients from long-term ventilatory support. Reducing total calories (glucose and fat) may benefit patients with pulmonary disease fed parenterally who develop worsening hypercapnia.

The metabolic complications are similar compared with those of TPN. Acute metabolic events most commonly involve glucose and electrolytes. Hyperchloremic metabolic acidosis is a complication secondary to amino acid metabolism that liberates hydrochloric acid. Other electrolyte abnormalities include hypokalemia, hypocalcemia, hypophosphatemia, and hypomagnesemia. Deficiencies in potassium, magnesium, and calcium can lead to cardiac arrhythmias. Hypophosphatemia can precipitate rhabdomyolysis, severe muscle weakness, and respiratory failure. Hypomagnesemia can cause muscle weakness and seizures.

PPN complications in the operating room include rebound hypoglycemia if it is abruptly stopped. Anesthetic management includes either continuing the PPN infusion or stopping it and providing a substitute such as a 10% dextrose solution. However, the stress response of surgery may cause glucose intolerance, and the concomitant PPN infusion may result in excessive hyperglycemia leading to hyperosmolar nonketotic coma or keto-acidosis. Regardless of continuing or discontinuing PPN, the most important intraoperative management is frequent blood glucose monitoring to guide subsequent therapy and maintain glucose levels between 100 and 150 mg per dL. Last, a dedicated IV catheter for PPN should not be violated by infusing anesthetic agents, blood products, or IV fluids.

Hepatobiliary dysfunction is a common manifestation of long-term parenteral nutrition and is less likely to occur with PPN. Bypassing the portal circulation may lead to biliary stasis and lack of gallbladder contraction. This can result in acalculous cholecystitis. If possible, stimulating gallbladder contractility with enteral feeding will reverse this process. Excess glucose calories and lipids in parenteral nutrition may result in hepatic steatosis and abnormal liver function tests, with an eventual progression to liver cirrhosis.

Lipid infusions used in PPN increase the risk of oxidation-induced cell injury. PPN wvcontaining oxidizable lipids promotes organ injury and is associated with impaired oxygenation and prolonged respiratory failure.

Complications can be minimized by regularly monitoring plasma electrolytes, blood glucose, and serum triglycerides. Regular insulin should be added to PPN to maintain blood glucose in the normal range.

SUGGESTED READINGS

Marino PL. *The ICU Book.* 3rd ed. Philadelphia, PA: Lippincott Williams & Wilkins; 2007:859–869.

Miller RD, Eriksson LI, Fleisher LA, et al., eds. *Miller's Anesthesia.* 7th ed. Philadelphia, PA: Churchill Livingstone; 2009:2944–2950.

Morgan GE, Mikhail MS, Murray MJ, eds. *Clinical Anesthesiology.* 4th ed. New York, NY: McGraw-Hill; 2006:1060–1062.

P

pH Buffering: Bicarbonate
Subspecialties: Critical Care

Holly Barth

Edited by Hossam Tantawy

1. Acid–base disorders refer to imbalances of hydrogen and bicarbonate ions in the blood. Normal pH of plasma is important for regulating enzyme activity, myocardial activity, hemoglobin saturation, and chemical reactions.
2. Buffering systems of the human body include bicarbonate, proteins including hemoglobin, ammonia, and phosphates.
3. The most critical buffer for maintaining pH is bicarbonate.

Acid–base disorders refer to imbalances of hydrogen and bicarbonate ions in the blood. Normal pH of plasma is important for regulating enzyme activity, myocardial activity, hemoglobin saturation, and chemical reactions. The body maintains the pH of blood 7.35 to 7.45.

The mechanisms to prevent changes in pH are buffer systems, pulmonary response, and renal response. The buffer system adds either an acid or a base to correct the pH and can work instantly. After buffer systems are exhausted, pulmonary mechanisms respond to correct pH in minutes, whereas renal compensation requires hours to days to restore pH to appropriate physiologic values.

Buffering systems of the human body include bicarbonate, proteins including hemoglobin, ammonia, and phosphates. The most critical buffer for maintaining pH is bicarbonate. The bicarbonate buffer system can be described by the following chemical equation:

$$CO_2 + H_2O \leftrightarrow H_2CO_3 \leftrightarrow H^+ + HCO_3^-$$

In this readily reversible reaction, carbon dioxide reacts with water to form carbonic acid through the enzyme carbonic anhydrase. Carbonic acid spontaneously forms hydrogen and bicarbonate.

An ideal physiologic buffer should have a pKa of 7.40, but the bicarbonate system has a pKa of 6.1. However, the bicarbonate system is effective because the concentration of bicarbonate in the blood is high and can readily be adjusted by the elimination or retention of CO_2 by the lungs. CO_2 is highly diffusible in tissues and blood, and carbonic anhydrase will quickly and effectively convert all available CO_2 into bicarbonate to defend against decreases in pH. Although bicarbonate is very effective for metabolic acid–base derangements, it should be noted that it is not effective for respiratory acid–base derangements together with resultant increase in CO_2.

Morgan GE, Mikhail MS, Murray MJ, eds. *Clinical Anesthesiology.* 4th ed. New York, NY: Lange/McGraw-Hill; 2006:711–712, 719.

Stoelting RK, Miller RD, eds. *Basics of Anesthesia.* 5th ed. Philadelphia, PA: Elsevier; 2007:311–318.

Pheochromocytoma: Dx Markers

Organ-based Clinical: Endocrine/Metabolic

Laurie Yonemoto

Edited by Mamatha Punjala

Laurie Yonemoto

Edited by Mamatha Punjala

KEY POINTS

1. Pheochromocytomas produce and secrete excess catecholamines independent of neurogenic control.
2. Diagnosis of pheochromocytoma is made by free catecholamine concentration and catecholamine metabolites in urine.
3. The blood level of catecholamine metabolites is a function of creatinine clearance.
4. Urine metabolite concentration is not always elevated, and diagnosis may depend on clinical suspicion and additional nonspecific findings such as elevated hematocrit, left ventricular hypertrophy (LVH), cardiomegaly, and nonspecific T-wave changes on an ECG.
5. Chromogranin A (CgA) is gaining acceptance as a serum marker of neuroendocrine tumors.

P

DISCUSSION

Pheochromocytomas are tumors of the adrenal medulla that produce, store, and secrete excess amounts of catecholamines (epinephrine and norepinephrine) independent of neurogenic control. Approximately 80% to 90% of tumors are solitary, confined to a single adrenal gland, and 5% of cases are inherited as a familial autosomal dominant trait.

Pheochromocytomas are also associated with other syndromes and diseases such as MEN IIA/IIB, Von Recklinghausen neurofibromatosis, and Von Hippel–Lindau disease, and usually present in young to mid-adult life. Symptoms can include paroxysmal or sustained HTN, palpitations, headache, flushing, and even myocardial infarction.

The diagnosis of pheochromocytoma is crucial, as greater than 90% of cases are curative with surgical removal. The diagnosis is based on identification of free catecholamine concentration and identification of catecholamine metabolites in urine. A 24-hour urine collection is performed on a patient suspected of having a pheochromocytoma to evaluate for elevated levels of urinary vanillylmandelic acid (VMA), unconjugated norepinephrine, and epinephrine (Fig. 1). VMA is an end product of catecholamine metabolism. These levels are expressed as a function of the creatinine clearance.

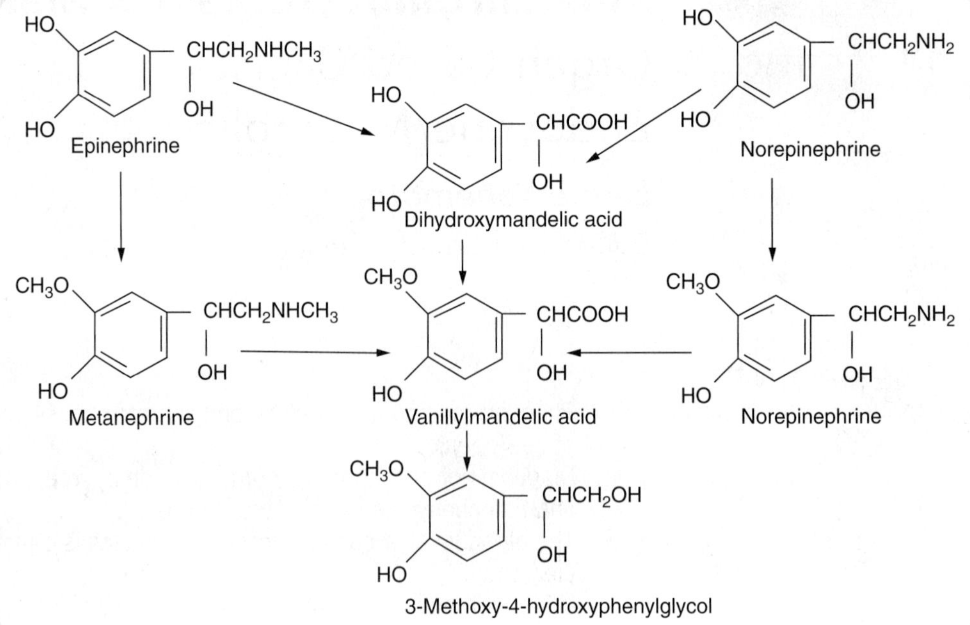

Figure 1. Catecholamine Metabolites. (Redrawn from Berne RM, Levy MN, eds. *Physiology*. New York, NY: CV Mosby Co.; 1983:1062, with permission.)

Although the measurement of catecholamine metabolites is the most common diagnostic assay, it is not always reliable. Urinary levels are not always elevated to a significant degree, and some patients with paroxysmal HTN have normal values in between attacks. Other helpful diagnostic markers include ECG changes such as LVH or nonspecific T wave changes, cardiomegaly on CXR, or elevated HCT secondary to intravascular volume depletion. CT and MRI are the standardized imaging methods used to localize pheochromocytomas.

Chromogranin A (CgA) is gaining acceptance as a serum marker of neuroendocrine tumors. Its specificity in differentiating between neuroendocrine and nonneuroendocrine tumors, its sensitivity to detect small tumors, and its clinical value, compared with other neuroendocrine markers, have not clearly been defined, however. Serum CgA was most frequently increased in subjects with gastrinomas (100%), pheochromocytomas (89%), carcinoid tumors (80%), nonfunctioning tumors of the endocrine pancreas (69%), and medullary thyroid carcinomas (50%). The highest levels were observed in subjects with carcinoid tumors.

SUGGESTED READINGS

Barash PG, Cullen BF, Stoelting RK, et al., eds. *Clinical Anesthesia*. 6th ed. Philadelphia, PA: Lippincott Williams & Wilkins; 2009:1292–1295.
Morgan GE, Mikhail MS, Murray MJ, eds. *Clinical Anesthesiology*. 4th ed. New York, NY: McGraw Hill; 2006: 253–254, 812–813.

Pheochromocytoma: Hypertension Rx

Organ-based Clinical: Endocrine/Metabolic

Meredith Brown

Edited by Mamatha Punjala

KEYWORD

SECTION

KEY POINTS

1. The first-line treatment for hypertension associated with pheochromocytoma is phenoxybenzamine, a noncompetitive presynaptic (alpha-2) and postsynaptic (alpha-1) blocker. The starting dose is 10 mg every 8 hours with incremental increases up to 80 to 200 mg per day.
2. The other possible first-line treatment is the use of a selective alpha-1 blockers such as prazosin.
3. If the patient is experiencing tachycardia or cardiac dysrhythmias, beta-adrenergic blockade may be added to alpha blockade.
4. Treatment of hypertension should be initiated 10 to 14 days prior to surgery.

DISCUSSION

The traditional medication used to treat hypertension associated with pheochromocytoma is phenoxybenzamine. This medication is a long-acting (24 to 48 hours), noncompetitive presynaptic (alpha-2) and postsynaptic (alpha-1) blocker with a starting dose of 10 mg every 8 hours, with incremental increases up to 80 to 200 mg per day. Side effects of phenoxybenzamine include blunting of cardiovascular reflexes and postural hypotension. Other medications that have been used effectively include selective alpha-1 blockers including doxazosin, prazosin, and terazosin, all of which induce postural hypotension. Once alpha-blockade has been instituted, beta-adrenergic blockade may be added to the alpha-blockade if patients are experiencing tachycardia or cardiac dysrhythmias. Beta-blockade should not be instituted until adequate alpha-blockade has been established due to the risk of unopposed alpha-mediated vasoconstriction. If the pheochromocytoma has metastasized or surgery cannot be performed, initiation of therapy with alpha-methyl tyrosine, a tyrosine hydroxylase inhibitor, may occur. By inhibiting tyrosine hydroxylase, catecholamine biosynthesis is limited.

Intraoperatively, treatment of hypertension associated with pheochromocytoma can be accomplished with phentolamine, nitroprusside, or nicardipine. Recommendations for treatment of the hypertension associated with pheochromocytoma include initiation of treatment 10 to 14 days prior to surgery, during which hypovolemia and anemia return to normal and hypertension is controlled.

SUGGESTED READINGS

Barash PG, Cullen BF, Stoelting RK, et al, eds. *Clinical Anesthesia.* 6th ed. Philadelphia, PA: Lippincott Williams & Wilkins; 2009:1293–1295.

Morgan GE, Mikhail MS, Murray MJ, eds. *Clinical Anesthesiology.* 4th ed. New York, NY: Lange/McGraw-Hill; 2006:813.

P

Pheochromocytoma: Pre-op Preparation

Organ-based Clinical: Endocrine/Metabolic

Martha Zegarra

Edited by Mamatha Punjala

KEY POINTS

1. Preoperative preparation for a patient with pheochromocytoma focuses on adrenergic blockage and volume replacement as well as a thorough preoperative evaluation of symptoms.
2. Alpha-blockade should be performed prior to beta-blockade; otherwise, unopposed vasoconstriction will lead to increased peripheral vascular resistance and hypertension.

DISCUSSION

Pheochromocytomas are catecholamine-secreting tumors of embryonic neural crest origin, whose presenting signs and symptoms include intermittent hypertension, headache, diaphoresis, and tachycardia. Pheochromocytomas release both epinephrine and norepinephrine, which leads to increased peripheral vascular resistance and arterial blood pressure. Hypertension can lead to intravascular volume depletion, renal failure, and cerebral hemorrhage. Increased peripheral vascular resistance increases myocardial work, leading to myocardial ischemia, ventricular hypertrophy, and congestive heart failure. Prolonged exposure to epinephrine and norepinephrine may lead to catecholamine-induced cardiomyopathy.

Preoperative preparation focuses on adrenergic blockage and volume replacement as well as a thorough preoperative evaluation. Specifically, resting arterial blood pressure, orthostatic blood pressure, heart rate, presence of ventricular ectopy, and ECG evidence of ischemia should be evaluated.

Preoperative treatment with phenoxybenzamine produces alpha-blockade and helps correct volume deficit in addition to correcting hypertension and hyperglycemia. Administration of phenoxybenzamine, an alpha-1 antagonist, results in effective vasodilation, leading to a drop in arterial blood pressure and an increase in intravascular volume. A decrease in red cell mass and plasma volume contributes to severe chronic hypovolemia in patients with pheochromocytoma. Hematocrit can be normal or elevated and does not reliably reflect volume status. Phenoxybenzamine can be administered orally and is longer acting than phentolamine, another alpha-1 antagonist. IV phentolamine can be used intraoperatively to control hypertensive episodes; however, it has a long onset time and duration of action, and tachyphylaxis often develops.

Beta-blockade is recommended in patients with tachycardia or ventricular arrhythmias. Alpha-blockade should be performed before beta-blockade; otherwise, unopposed alpha-stimulation causing vasoconstriction will lead to an increase in peripheral vascular resistance and myocardial work. In addition, without the inotropic effect of beta-1 stimulation, the increase in workload may not be tolerated by the heart, leading to ischemia, hypertrophy, and heart failure.

There are many intraoperative considerations when caring for a patient presenting for pheochromocytoma resection. Potentially life-threatening variations in blood pressure, particularly during induction of anesthesia and manipulation of the tumor, indicate the need for direct arterial pressure monitoring. Large intraoperative fluid shifts underscore the importance for large bore intravenous access and urinary output monitoring. Patients with evidence of catecholamine cardiomyopathy may benefit from placement of a pulmonary arterial catheter.

SUGGESTED READINGS

Barash PG, Cullen BF, Stoelting RK, et al, eds. *Clinical Anesthesia*. 6th ed. Philadelphia, PA: Lippincott Williams & Wilkins; 2009:1292–1294.

Morgan GE, Mikhail MS, Murray MJ, eds. *Clinical Anesthesiology*. 4th ed. New York, NY: Lange Medical Books/McGraw Hill; 2006:253–254, 812–813.

P

Physician Impairment: Referral

Generic Clinical Sciences: Anesthesia Procedures, Methods, Techniques

Anna Clebone

Edited by Raj K. Modak

KEY POINTS

1. A national system of Physician Health Programs (PHPs) exists for physicians with addiction problems.
2. The PHPs have a good 5-year success rate at returning physicians (all specialties) to practice.
3. The rate of substance abuse disorders is higher for anesthesiologists than for other medical specialties.
4. Anesthesiology presents unique concerns for drug addiction.

DISCUSSION

Physicians with addiction problems are often referred to a national system of PHPs. Substance abuse should not be tolerated in any physician. However, a system that is only punitive (e.g., permanently revoking licensure) could lead to hesitancy in seeking help or delays in reporting colleagues. The Physician Health Program seeks to address these concerns by advocating early detection and then providing comprehensive, long-term treatment. The program involves a residential facility for greater than 1 month. Physicians in this program receive follow-up care for greater than 5 years, including random urine drug tests. Seventy-eight percent remain drug free for the first 5 years of the program, as measured by random urine testing. Seventy-one percent keep their license and remain in practice at the 5-year point. These statistics, however, include all specialties.

Anesthesiology presents several unique concerns for both patient and practitioner. First, access to potentially addictive substances is part of the day-to-day practice of anesthesiology, leading to many potential situations for relapse. Second, anesthesiology requires constant alertness while on duty and quick action when problems arise. The margin for error is much less due to the immediacy of the specialty. The anesthesiologist is often the only one making decisions critical to the patient's well-being. Contrast this with a practitioner working in a clinic. The practitioner decides to give a prescription that is often written down by a nurse, always filled by a pharmacist, and frequently checked for interactions by the pharmacy's computer. An impaired practitioner could be more easily detected before a fatal error occurs.

The rate of substance abuse disorders is higher for anesthesiologists than for other medical specialties. Due to the unique nature of anesthesiology, some advocate a zero tolerance policy for addicted anesthesiologists. Although time-consuming, retraining in a different specialty may be the best option for formerly drug-addicted anesthesiologists.

SUGGESTED READINGS

DuPont RL, McLellan AT, Carr G, et al. How are addicted physicians treated? A national survey of Physician Health Programs. *J Subst Abuse Treat.* 2009;37(1):1–7.

Skipper GE, Campbell MD, Dupont RL. Anesthesiologists with substance use disorders: a 5-year outcome study from 16 state physician health programs. *Anesth Analg.* 2009;109(3):891–896.

Placenta Accreta: Risk Factors
Subspecialties: Obstetric Anesthesia

Frederick Conlin
Edited by Lars Helgeson

KEY POINTS

1. A placenta that has attached itself to myometrium is known as a placenta accreta.
2. Placenta increta is a variant of a placenta accreta, where the placenta has grown into the myometrium. Placenta percreta refers to one that has penetrated the uterine serosa.
3. Risk factors include previous uterine surgery, placenta previa, advanced maternal age, and a thin decidual layer.
4. Profound hemorrhage is a likely complication often requiring cesarean hysterectomy to control the bleeding.

DISCUSSION

Normal placentae attach to the decidual layer of the uterus, which allows for easy separation from the uterus after delivery of the fetus. Placenta accreta is a condition where the placenta has attached onto the myometrium, resulting in excessive bleeding after its removal. Placenta increta is a variant of a placenta accreta, where the placenta has penetrated into the myometrium. Placenta percreta refers to one that has penetrated the uterine serosa. Placenta percreta is the most severe and may adhere on or into neighboring organs or blood vessels, leading to more extensive bleeding and injury to the involved organs.

Placenta accreta occurs in about 1 in 2,500 pregnancies. Risk factors include previous uterine surgery (such as cesarean section, fibroid excision, or dilation and curettage), placenta previa, a thin decidual layer, and advanced maternal age. The most significant risk factors are uterine scar and placenta previa. The risk of accreta with placenta previa increases significantly with the number of cesarean sections. The risk of accrete is 1% with no uterine scar and no previa. That risk increases to 4% with previa, 10% to 25% with previa plus one previous section, and 67% with placenta previa and multiple previous sections.

Elective cesarean section with hysterectomy is the standard management of known placenta percreta, increta, and many accretas. In addition, elective embolization of the uterine vessels supplying the area may be of benefit in reducing blood loss in some patients. Large-bore intravenous access and readily accessible blood products are required. Unfortunately, the presence of a placenta accreta is often not known before delivery.

SUGGESTED READINGS

Datta S, ed. *Anesthetic and Obstetric Management of High-Risk Pregnancy.* 3rd ed. New York, NY: Springer; 2004:121.
Hines RL, Marschall KE, eds. *Anesthesia and Coexisting Disease.* 5th ed. Philadelphia, PA: Churchill Livingstone; 2008:567.
Morgan GE, Mikhail MS, Murray MJ, eds. *Clinical Anesthesiology.* 4th ed. New York, NY: McGraw-Hill; 2005:908.

P

Placental Transfer: Anticholinergic

Subspecialties: Obstetric

Gregory Albert

Edited by Lars Helgeson

Gregory Albert

Edited by Lars Helgeson

KEY POINTS

1. The transfer of any medication across the placenta depends on a number of factors including its lipid solubility, ionization, and degree of protein binding.
2. Atropine and scopolamine easily cross the placenta.
3. Glycopyrrolate does not significantly cross the placenta.

DISCUSSION

When caring for a pregnant patient, the anesthesiologist must have an understanding of the effects of medications administered to both parturient and fetus. A number of medications prescribed have profound effects on the fetus. The degree of the effect depends on its lipid solubility, ionization, and protein-binding capability.

Measurable umbilical drug levels of atropine and scopolamine occur within 1 minute of administration. Atropine requires about 5 minutes to reach equilibrium between fetal and maternal blood with a ratio of nearly one. Scopolamine has similar pharmacokinetics. Glycopyrrolate, however, does not cross the placenta easily. The fetal to maternal ratio of glycopyrrolate is roughly 0.2. As a result, glycopyrrolate lacks any apparent physiologic effects on the fetus.

P

SUGGESTED READING

Chestnut D, ed. *Obstetric Anesthesia: Principals and Practice*. Philadelphia, PA: Mosby Inc.; 2004:60.

Placental Transfer: Local Anesthetics
Subspecialties: Obstetrics

Ashley Kelley

Edited by Lars Helgeson

1. Small, nonionized, lipophilic molecules including amide local anesthetics cross the placenta easily.
2. Once transferred, local anesthetics can become "trapped" in the fetus by ionization in the more acidemic environment.
3. Accumulated local anesthetic agents in the fetus can cause cardiovascular depression and arrhythmias as well as decreased muscular tone.

When administering drugs to parturients, anesthesiologists must remember factors affecting placental transfer of drugs to the fetus and potential effects on the fetus from these medications. Factors affecting placental transfer include ionization, lipid solubility, and molecular weight. Small, nonionized, lipophilic molecules cross the placenta most easily. Most local anesthetics possess these characteristics and are thus easily transferred to the fetus via the placenta.

The ionization of a molecule depends on the local pH as well as the pKa, the pKa being the pH at which the concentration of ionized and nonionized forms of a molecule is equal. This is expressed in the Henderson–Hasselbalch equation:

$$pH = pKa + \log (base)/(cation).$$

Amide local anesthetics are weak bases at physiologic pH, and this leaves a significant portion of nonionized molecule available for placental transfer. Ester local anesthetics are metabolized by maternal plasma cholinesterase, and this decreases the amount available for placental transfer.

When local anesthetics cross the placenta into the fetus, they become "ion trapped." The pH in the fetal blood is generally lower than that of maternal blood by approximately 0.1 point. The lower pH means that a greater proportion of the local anesthetic will become ionized and thus will be unable to diffuse back to the maternal circulation. The result is decreased concentration of the nonionized portion while maintaining the concentration gradient between the maternal blood and the fetal blood, and this allows for continued diffusion to the fetus across the placenta. If the fetus is acidemic from fetal distress, the proportion of ion-trapped molecules becomes even higher.

The fetus possesses enzymes for degradation of local anesthetics, but the elimination half-life is longer than that of the mother because of an increased volume of distribution. Accumulated local anesthetic in the fetus can cause decreased neuromuscular tone, and inadvertent intravascular injection may cause depression of fetal cardiac function and generate cardiac arrhythmias.

Barash PG, Cullen BF, Stoelting RK, et al, eds. *Clinical Anesthesia*. 6th ed. Philadelphia, PA: Lippincott Williams & Wilkins; 2009:1140–1148.
Stoelting RK, Miller RD, eds. *Basics of Anesthesia*. 5th ed. Philadelphia, PA: Churchill Livingstone; 2007:298, 481–488.

P

PONV after Pediatric Surgery

Subspecialties: Pediatrics

Terrence Coffey

Edited by Mamatha Punjala

KEY POINTS

1. Postoperative nausea and vomiting (PONV) occurs in as many as 30% of patients who are not treated with antiemetics.
2. Children and women are most susceptible to PONV; however, children younger than 2 years have a decreased risk of PONV.
3. Risk factors for PONV include type of surgery, duration of surgery, type of anesthesia, and prior history of PONV.
4. The use of two or more antiemetics is more effective than a single prophylactic agent.

DISCUSSION

PONV is the most common cause of postanesthetic complication (20% to 30% of pediatric cases). Children (older than 2 years) and women are most susceptible. Other risk factors include prior history of PONV, motion sickness, surgical procedure longer than 1 hour, and intraabdominal, intracranial, middle ear, ophthalmologic, laparoscopic, and genital operations. There is increased risk of nausea after intraoperative opioid administration. Finally, postoperative pain can cause PONV in children.

Propofol anesthetic decreases risk of PONV. Other antiemetics include ondansetron, metoclopramide, transdermal scopolamine, dexamethasone, and droperidol. The use of two or more antiemetic agents is more effective than a single agent prophylactically. The use of nitrous oxide or induction with etomidate increases the incidence of PONV.

PONV poses medical risks such as increased risk of aspiration, increased risk of jeopardizing suture lines, and increased central venous pressure, which increases morbidity after tympanic, ocular, or intracranial procedures. Before treating PONV, serious causes for nausea and vomiting should be ruled out such as hypotension, hypoxemia, hypoglycemia, and increased intracranial pressure.

SUGGESTED READINGS

Barash PG, Cullen BF, Stoelting RK, et al, eds. *Clinical Anesthesia*. 6th ed. Philadelphia, PA: Lippincott Williams & Wilkins; 2009:1131–1133.

Bready LL, Noorily SH, Dillman D. *Decision Making in Anesthesiology*. 4th ed. Philadelphia, PA: Mosby; 2007.

P

PONV Prophylaxis

Pharmacology

Nicholas Dalesio

Edited by Lars Helgeson

1. Postoperative nausea and vomiting (PONV) risks are increased on the basis of patient profile as well as the type of surgery.
2. Multiple receptors are believed to be involved in PONV. This allows for multiple drug classes to be effective in treating PONV.
3. A multimodal approach to treat PONV is the best one.

PONV is the most common adverse event in patients in the postanesthesia care unit. Risk factors that increase the incidence of PONV include female gender, pregnancy, nonsmokers, history of PONV and motion sickness, surgery within 1 to 7 days of menstruation, perioperative narcotic use, and the type of surgery. PONV is increased after lithotripsy, laparoscopy, major breast, ENT, and gynecologic surgeries. In pediatrics, PONV is increased with orchidopexy, tonsillectomy, and strabismus surgeries. PONV is twice as likely in children as in adults. Prophylaxis is similar to that of adults.

The vomiting pathway propagates via the vagus nerve to the area postrema in the brainstem, also known as the *vomiting center*. Serotonin receptors have been shown to be involved in nausea and vomiting, and antagonist drugs such as ondansetron can alleviate these symptoms with minimal side effects. Other effective drugs include dopamine receptor antagonists, anticholinergics, and antihistamines; however, these medications sometimes have serious side effects. Other treatments shown to decrease PONV include clonidine, dexamethasone, and anesthetic choice for intraoperative anesthesia. Propofol has PONV-decreasing properties. Nitrous oxide increases the incidence of PONV.

Multimodal therapy is likely the most effective way to treat PONV. Supplemental fluid therapy and O_2 therapy decrease the incidence of PONV. In children, acupuncture at the P6 acupuncture point located on the wrist can be as effective as droperidol to treat PONV. Use of alternative pain control modalities can also decrease PONV. Cost-effectiveness, efficacy, and side-effect profiles must be considered when deciding PONV prophylaxis. Despite multiple studies, a universal treatment plan for all patients has not been established.

Barash PG, Cullen BF, Stoelting RK, et al, eds. *Clinical Anesthesia*. 6th ed. Philadelphia, PA: Lippincott Williams & Wilkins; 2009:841–842, 1214.

Post-CPB Creatinine Increase: DDx

Organ-based Clinical: Renal: Urinary/Electrolytes

Nehal Gatha

Edited by Benjamin Sherman

KEY POINTS

1. According to various studies, the incidence of acute kidney injury (AKI) after cardiopulmonary bypass (CPB) varies from 4% to 7%.
2. The most common predictor of increased creatinine post-CPB is preoperative increased creatinine.
3. AKI after CPB can be secondary to a low cardiac output state during CPB or immediately after separation of CPB in the perioperative period.
4. The differential diagnosis of an increase in creatinine post-CPB is wide and includes previous renal impairment, inadequate flow rates during CPB, persistent hypotension post-CPB, tamponade, arrhythmia, hemodilution, bleeding, elevated circulating free hemoglobin, and embolic events.

DISCUSSION

According to various studies, the incidence of AKI after CPB varies from 4% to 7%. AKI can be a very serious complication, leading to increased morbidity and mortality in post-CPB patients. During CPB, there are multiple etiologies of AKI, and it is important to differentiate the possible causes of rising creatinine in this patient population.

The most common predictor of increased creatinine post-CPB is preoperative increased creatinine. Baseline renal dysfunction will be exacerbated in the post-CPB period; therefore, it is important to note preoperative glomerular filtration rate and creatinine and to optimize them before surgery when possible. Commonly, patients with advanced heart failure and long-standing diabetes will have compromised renal function before CPB.

A second cause of increased creatinine after CPB is low cardiac output state during CPB or immediately after separation of CPB in the intraoperative period. The causes of a low cardiac output state are numerous. Common causes are decreased CPB flows intraoperatively or postoperative hypotension due to low systemic vascular resistance, hypovolemia, or heart failure. Heart failure is attributed to stunned myocardium, myocardial ischemia, cardiac tamponade, and/or arrhythmias. To avoid low cardiac output states during CPB, it is critical to work closely with the perfusion team to maintain an appropriate mixed venous oxygen saturation, blood gas values, and chemistries through adequate flow rates and medications. It is important to adequately treat hypotension while attempting to separate from CPB with volume, vasopressors, or inotropes to ensure adequate end-organ perfusion. Transesophageal echocardiography will help guide the anesthesiologist and surgeon in the assessment of left heart function and/or the presence of tamponade. Finally, arrhythmias must be identified and treated quickly to avoid a low cardiac output.

Hematocrit and volume status must be continuously reassessed to determine whether the kidneys are adequately perfused. CPB leads to profound hemodilution, which causes a relative anemia. Similarly, if there is persistent bleeding causing inadequate intravascular volume, perfusion of the kidneys will be insufficient. If hypotension is persistent, chest tube output is high, and creatinine continues to rise post-CPB, reexploration should be considered by the surgical team.

CPB that utilizes nonpulsatile flow and increased nephrotoxic substances such as free hemoglobin and serum ferritin can further injure the kidneys. Both mechanisms can lead to AKI and increased creatinine in the post-CPB period.

P

Finally, there is a risk with CPB of embolic or thrombotic events. Whether it is an air embolus from cannulation or emboli showers from clamping and unclamping of vessels, these cause AKI because they block blood flow through renal vasculature.

SUGGESTED READINGS

Davis CL, Kausz AT, Zager RA, et al. Acute renal failure after cardiopulmonary bypass is related to decreased serum ferritin levels. *J Am Soc Nephrol.* 1999;10:2396–2402.

Hensley F, Martin D, Gravlee G. *A Practical Approach to Cardiac Anesthesia.* 3rd ed. Philadelphia, PA: Lippincott Williams & Wilkins; 2003:135, 254–260.

Morgan GE, Mikhail MS, Murray MJ. *Clinical Anesthesiology.* 4th ed. New York, NY: Lange Medical Books/McGraw-Hill; 2006:chap 17:743–744.

P

Post-op Jaundice: DDx
Generic Clinical Sciences: Anesthesia Procedures, Methods, Techniques

Jinlei Li

Edited by Hossam Tantawy

1. Jaundice is caused by hyperbilirubinemia and can appear in up to 20% of patients after major surgery.
2. The most common cause of postoperative jaundice is prehepatic in nature and includes resorption of a large hematoma or a transfusion reaction resulting in red blood cell breakdown.
3. Hepatocellular dysfunction may also result in postoperative jaundice and may be triggered by underlying liver disease (hepatitis, congenital disease, hepatocellular carcinoma [HCC], fatty liver), intraoperative hypotension/hypoxia, surgical sympathetic stimulation, and drug toxicity.
4. Posthepatic causes of postoperative jaundice include cholestasis, which can be observed in chronically and severely ill patients and pregnant patients. Postoperative cholecystitis and pancreatitis, bile duct injury, and extrahepatic obstruction from calculi, stricture, or neoplasm must also be considered in the differential diagnosis.

P

Jaundice is caused by hyperbilirubinemia and can appear in up to 20% of patients after major surgery. The causes of postoperative jaundice generally fall under one of three categories: prehepatic (increased bilirubin production), hepatic (hepatocellular dysfunction), or posthepatic (biliary obstruction). The most common cause of postoperative jaundice is prehepatic in nature and includes resorption of a large hematoma or a transfusion reaction resulting in red blood cell breakdown. Other prehepatic causes include senescent (old) red cell breakdown and other types of hemolytic reactions (drug induced, disease related, etc.). Disease-related hemolytic reactions include sickle cell disease and G6PD deficiency.

Hepatocellular dysfunction may also result in postoperative jaundice. It is possible for signs of postoperative liver dysfunction to occur hours after surgery or even days or weeks later, depending on the cause. For example, hypoxic liver injury can generally become apparent within hours, whereas anesthesia-induced hepatitis may take weeks to present. Postoperative jaundice can also be the result of underlying liver disease, at times unknown to both the patient and the clinician. Preexisting diseases include viral hepatitis, alcoholic hepatitis, fatty liver, cirrhosis, congenital disease, and HCC. The congenital disease, Gilbert syndrome, presents as unconjugated hyperbilirubinemia and is a benign disorder. In this case, postoperative jaundice can be triggered by the stress of surgery, fever, infection, or being NPO. Other congenital disorders resulting in hyperbilirubinemia include Crigler–Najjar, Dubin–Johnson, and Rotor syndromes.

Anesthesia and surgical stress can induce further hepatic malfunction. Intraoperative hypotension may result in decreased hepatic blood flow and cellular injury. Isoflurane is the inhalational agent that causes the least decrease in hepatic blood flow. Intraoperatively, hepatic surgical injury, as well as systematic disease such as sepsis and shock, can contribute to hepatic injury through hypotension. Surgical activation of the sympathetic system results in vasoconstriction of the splanchnic vasculature and hepatic artery and results in decreased portal flow, which can lead to possible injury.

Drug toxicity is a possible cause of hepatic injury and postoperative jaundice. Halothane-induced hepatitis has been well established. Antibiotics and ketamine are also among the drugs reported to cause hepatic toxicity. Nitrous oxide inhibits methionine synthase and, therefore, in theory, may affect liver function adversely, although no clinical evidence supports this in acute nitrous use.

Posthepatic causes of postoperative jaundice include cholestasis, which can be observed in chronically and severely ill patients and pregnant patients. Postoperative cholecystitis and pancreatitis, bile duct injury, and extrahepatic obstruction from calculi, stricture, or neoplasm must also be considered in the differential diagnosis.

Workup for postoperative jaundice includes a detailed history and physical examination; laboratory studies; imaging such as ultrasound, CT, and endoscopic retrograde cholangiopancreatography; and interventions such as liver biopsy. Laboratory studies include, but are not limited to, complete blood counts, liver function tests, complete metabolic profile, haptoglobin, lactate dehydrogenase, prothrombin time, partial prothrombin time, and international normalized ratio. In terms of management, the key is prevention with careful anesthetic planning preoperatively. Postoperatively, the mainstay is to treat underlying disease and reversible cause of injury and supportive care. Fulminant hepatic failure is treated by supportive therapy, and if it does not improve, would proceed to liver transplant.

SUGGESTED READINGS

Barash PG, Cullen BF, Stoelting RK, et al, eds. *Clinical Anesthesia.* 6th ed. Philadelphia, PA: Lippincott Williams & Wilkins; 2009:1247–1276.
Morgan GE, Mikhail MS, Murray MJ. *Clinical Anesthesiology.* 4th ed. New York, NY: McGraw Hill; 2006:773–780.

Postop. Vomiting: Peds vs. Adults
Subspecialties: Pediatric Anesthesia

Thomas Gallen

Edited by Mamatha Punjala

KEY POINTS

1. It is difficult to readily identify nausea in children, and as a result, a pediatric postoperative vomiting (POV) is commonly used as the measurement of postoperative nausea and vomiting (PONV) in children.
2. PONV/POV is a common complaint among both children and adults with peak incidences (of high-risk populations) of up to 50% to 70%.
3. Surgical duration of greater than 30 minutes increases pediatric POV risk.
4. Strabismus surgery, ENT surgery, dental procedures, orchidopexy, and craniofacial procedures are commonly known to increase pediatric POV risk.
5. POV peaks in school-aged children and is greater in children than in adults.
6. Anesthesia-related risk factors for PONV include use of volatile anesthetics, nitrous oxide, intravenous opioids, ketamine, and etomidate.

DISCUSSION

It is difficult to readily identify nausea in children, and as a result, POV is commonly used as the measurement of PONV in children. PONV/POV is a common complaint among both children and adults with peak incidences (of high-risk populations) of up to 50% to 70%. The following are the risk factors with a focus comparing adult and pediatric patients:

1. Peak incidence is school-aged children.
2. Children have no difference in gender rates until postpubescence, when female rates of PONV predominate as they do with adults.
3. Children with parents or siblings that have PONV/POV are at increased risk.
4. There is a weak correlation with increased rates of PONV/POV.
5. In both children and adults, opioids increase risk of POV/PONV, whereas midazolam probably reduces risk.
6. Smoking reduces the risk of PONV in adults, whereas neither first-hand nor second-hand smoke has been studied in children.
7. There is an increased incidence in children with strabismus surgery, ENT surgeries, dental procedures, orchidopexy, and craniofacial procedures.
8. Surgical duration of greater than 30 minutes increases pediatric POV risk.
9. In children and adults, volatile anesthetics (including nitrous oxide), narcotics, ketamine, and etomidate increase risk, whereas propofol decreases risk.
10. Increased volume replacement decreases risk.
11. In both adults and children, pain is an independent risk factor, and nonnarcotic/peripheral nerve blockade may decrease PONV incidence, whereas opioids increase it.

Once a patient has been appropriately risk stratified, prophylaxis and treatment should be considered. In addition, medications should be considered in relation to their side-effect profiles (see Table 1). Ondansetron and dexamethasone generally have the highest benefit to side-effect profile in pediatrics. Use of multiregimen treatments are more efficacious, and in a large clinical trial, increasing number of antiemetics reduced PONV from 52% without any antiemetic to 37%, 28%, and 22% when one, two, or three agents were used. The antiemetic agents commonly used fall into one (or more) of six categories provided in Table 1.

P

Table 1. Drugs used in PONV

Class	Receptor Site of Action	Drugs	Side Effects
Anticholinergics	Muscarinic, histaminergic (H_1)	Atropine, scopolamine	Dry mouth, visual disturbances, confusion, hallucination, sedation
Antihistamines	Histaminergic (H_1)	Cyclizine, dimenhydrinate, diphenhydramine	Sedation
Butyrophenones	D_2	Droperidol	Sedation, agitation, *extrapyramidal effects, QT prolongation*
Phenothiazines	D_2	Promethazine, prochlorperazine, perphenazine	Sedation, agitation, extrapyramidal effects
Benzamides	D_2, 5-HT_3	Metoclopramide	*Dystonia, extrapyramidal effects*
Serotonin antagonists	5-HT_3	Ondansetron, dolasetron, granisetron	Headache, dizziness, *QT prolongation*

D_2, dopamine type 2; 5-HT_3, 5-hydroxytryptamine type 3.

SUGGESTED READINGS

Blum RH. Postanesthetic recovery. In: Holzman RS, Mancuso TJ, Polaner DM, eds. *A Practical Approach to Pediatric Anesthesia.* Philadelphia, PA: Lippincott Williams & Wilkins; 2008:146–148.

Ho K-Y, Gan TJ. Postoperative nausea and vomiting. In: Lobato EB, Gravenstein N, Kirby RR, eds. *Complications in Anesthesiology.* Philadelphia, PA: Lippincott Williams & Wilkins; 2008:571–579.

Lichtor LJ. Ambulatory anesthesia. In: Barash PG, Cullen BF, Stoelting RK, et al, eds. *Clinical Anesthesia.* 6th ed. Philadelphia, PA: Lippincott Williams & Wilkins; 2009:839–843.

Postoperative ATN: DDx

Organ-based Clinical: Renal: Urinary/ Electrolytes

Archer Martin

Edited by Hossam Tantawy

1. Acute tubular necrosis (ATN) is an intrinsic renal cause of acute renal failure and is the most common reason for renal failure in the perioperative period, accounting for up to 75% of cases of failure.
2. The two major causes of ATN include ischemia and nephrotoxins.
3. Renal ischemia may be caused by perioperative hypotension, sepsis, volume depletion, procedures directly involving the renal circulation (including cardiac surgery and abdominal aortic aneurysm repair), and inhibition of prostaglandin synthesis.
4. The list of nephrotoxic agents possible for causing ATN includes antibiotics (aminoglycosides, cephalosporins, penicillins, vancomycin, sulfonamides, and amphotericin B), intravenous radiologic contrast, anesthetic agents (methoxyflurane and enflurane), nonsteroidal anti-inflammatory drugs (NSAIDs), myoglobin and chemotherapeutic agents.

P

The causes of acute renal failure are generally categorized into prerenal, renal, and postrenal. Prerenal causes of renal failure are a result of decreased renovascular flow, and include cardiomyopathy, hypovolemia, aortic stenosis, mechanical ventilation, and dissecting aneurysms. Intrinsic renal failure generally falls under ATN or acute interstitial nephritis. Finally, causes of postrenal failure include papillary bilateral ureter obstruction, retroperitoneal masses, prostatic hypertrophy, and urethral strictures.

ATN is an intrinsic renal cause of acute renal failure and is the most common reason for renal failure in the perioperative period, accounting for up to 75% of cases of failure. ATN occurs when there is insult to the renal tubular epithelial cells. The two major causes of ATN include ischemia and nephrotoxins. Ischemia may be caused by perioperative shock, sepsis, volume depletion, procedures directly involving the renal circulation (including cardiac surgery and abdominal aortic aneurysm repair), and inhibition of prostaglandin synthesis.

The list of nephrotoxic agents possible for causing ATN is wide and varied. They inflict renal damage by either disrupting oxygen delivery or oxygen utilization. These agents include antibiotics, intravenous radiologic contrast, anesthetic agents (methoxyflurane and enflurane), NSAIDs, and chemotherapy. The most common antibiotics associated with postoperative ATN are aminoglycosides, but the disorder can also occur with cephalosporins, penicillins, vancomycin, sulfonamides, and amphotericin B. Chemotherapy agents including cisplatin and methotrexate have also been associated with ATN and should be included in the differential of postoperative ATN if given in the immediate perioperative period. Immunosuppressive agents, such as cyclosporin A and tacrolimus, have also been associated with acute kidney injury.

Rhabdomyolysis, stemming from crush injuries, burn injuries, and extensive muscle injuries, may cause ATN through the effect of myoglobin on the kidneys. Myoglobin can collect in the renal tubules, leading to failure. Hemoglobin may also cause acute kidney injury, but less so compared with myoglobin. In the setting of acidosis and hypovolemia, the toxicity of both hemoglobin and myoglobin may increase.

There is controversy regarding the nephrotoxicity of volatile agents such as sevoflurane. Toxicity is thought to occur secondary to fluoride ion and compound A formation; however, this association has not been proven in the human population.

SUGGESTED READINGS

Barash PG, Cullen BF, Stoelting RK, et al, eds. *Clinical Anesthesia*. 6th ed. Philadelphia, PA: Lippincott Williams & Wilkins; 2009:1354–1355.

Marino PL. *The ICU Book*. 3rd ed. New York, NY: Lippincott Williams & Wilkins; 2007:581–582.

P

Preeclampsia: Lab Abnormalities

Subspecialties: Obstetric Anesthesia

Marianne Saleeb

Edited by Lars Helgeson

1. Preeclampsia is a pregnancy-induced syndrome that usually occurs after 20 weeks of gestation. It is characterized by new-onset hypertension (>140/90), proteinuria (>2 g per day), and often generalized edema. It can be either mild or severe, potentially resulting in liver and renal failure, disseminated intravascular coagulopathy, eclampsia, and central nervous system (CNS) abnormalities such as headache, visual changes, confusion, and unconsciousness.
2. Preeclamptic patients tend to be hypovolemic and hypoproteinemic secondary to fluid shifts into the extravascular space, which may be worsened by proteinuria.
3. Preeclampsia may result in decreased renal blood flow and glomerular filtration rate (GFR), leading to elevated serum creatinine and urea.
4. HELLP syndrome is a variant of severe preeclampsia. Additional findings include *h*emolysis, *e*levated *l*iver enzymes, and thrombocytopenia (*l*ow *p*latelets). It is possible to see elevated liver enzymes and thrombocytopenia (seen in 15% of preeclamptic patients) without the presence of HELLP syndrome.

P

Preeclampsia is a pregnancy-induced syndrome that usually occurs after 20 weeks of gestation. It is characterized by new-onset hypertension (>140/90), proteinuria (>2 g per day), and often generalized edema (not necessary for diagnosis). It can be either mild or severe, leading to liver and renal insufficiency, disseminated intravascular coagulopathy, and CNS abnormalities including headache, visual changes, confusion, and loss of consciousness. If seizures occur, the diagnosis becomes eclampsia. Severe preeclampsia is classified as blood pressure greater than 160/110, proteinuria greater than 5 g per day, or evidence of severe end-organ damage. The signs and symptoms of preeclampsia are a result of endothelial cell injury causing microangiopathy of target organs such as brain, liver, kidney, and placenta. Treatment for preeclampsia is delivery, and generally, there is significant improvement of signs and symptoms within 48 hours after delivery.

Preeclamptic patients are at risk for hypovolemia and hypoproteinemia secondary to fluid shifting into the extravascular space, which may be further compounded by proteinuria. As a result, there may be an elevated hematocrit despite an underlying anemia. Women with preeclampsia have a mean plasma volume 9% less than that found in normal pregnancy and up to 30% to 40% less if severe disease is present. Preeclampsia may result in decreased renal blood flow and GFR, which may lead to elevated serum creatinine and urea.

Thrombocytopenia is seen in approximately 15% of women with preeclampsia. The decrease in platelets is generally mild, and counts range from 100,000 to 150,000. This decrease results from platelet aggregation at sites of endothelial damage. Abnormal liver enzyme concentrations may also be seen in preeclampsia. It is possible to have elevated aspartate aminotransferase, lactate dehydrogenase, and alkaline phosphatase. HELLP syndrome is a form of severe preeclampsia. Characteristics of this syndrome include hemolysis, elevated liver enzymes, and thrombocytopenia.

Barash PG, Cullen BF, Stoelting RK, et al, eds. *Clinical Anesthesia.* 6th ed. Philadelphia, PA: Lippincott Williams & Wilkins; 2009:1149–1152.

Block DR, Saenger AK. Preeclampsia: prediction, diagnosis, and management beyond proteinuria and hypertension. *Clinical Laboratory News.* 36(2):8–10.

Hines RL, Marschall KE. *Stoelting's Anesthesia and Co-existing Disease.* 5th ed. Philadelphia, PA: Churchill Livingstone; 2008:562–565.

Pregnancy: Hematologic Changes
Subspecialties: Obstetric Anesthesia

Garth Skoropowski

Edited by Lars Helgeson

KEY POINTS

1. Plasma volume increases between 45% and 50% by the 34th week of pregnancy and remains at that level until term.
2. RBC volume only increases by 30% over prepregnancy levels, resulting in a dilutional anemia of pregnancy.
3. Pregnancy is a hypercoagulable state with an increase in fibrinogen (doubles in mass) and coagulation factors VII, VIII, IX, X, and XII. Only factor XI and XIII levels are decreased.
4. Thrombocytopenia with platelet counts below 150,000 can be seen in the third trimester in about 8% of pregnant women.

DISCUSSION

Pregnancy has multiple effects on the hematologic system. The plasma volume increases between 45% and 50% by the 34th week of pregnancy and remains at that level until term. Elevated estrogen and progesterone levels during pregnancy increase both plasma renin and aldosterone, resulting in increased sodium and water retention, thereby contributing to the increase in plasma volume. The red cell mass initially decreases and then starts increasing after the 8th week of pregnancy and continues to increase until term when it is 30% above prepregnancy values. Total blood volume at term is about 90 cc per kg compared with 65 cc per kg in the average adult female. However, since the plasma volume increases more than the red blood cell mass, there is a relative anemia of pregnancy. To maintain oxygen delivery during pregnancy, cardiac output is increased, the arterial partial pressure of oxygen is increased, and there is a right shift of the oxyhemoglobin dissociation curve.

Despite the overall increase in the absolute amount of plasma proteins during pregnancy, the plasma protein concentration actually decreases to values less than 6 g per dL. This is also due to the dilutional effect of increased plasma volume. This decrease in protein concentration results in the increase of the active form of protein-bound drugs. In addition, there is a 25% reduction in plasma cholinesterase level.

Pregnancy is a hypercoagulable state. Both the prothrombin time and the partial thromboplastin time are reduced. Fibrinogen (doubles in mass) and most factors including VII, VIII, IX, X, and XII are increased. Only factor XI and XIII levels are decreased. Meanwhile, there is a decrease in protein S concentrations and resistance to activated protein C, resulting in a decrease in anticoagulant activity.

Thrombocytopenia with platelet counts below 150,000 can be seen in the third trimester in about 8% of pregnant women. White blood cell counts are generally between 8,000 and 10,000 throughout pregnancy.

SUGGESTED READINGS

Barash PG, Cullen BF, Stoelting RK, et al, eds. *Clinical Anesthesia.* 6th ed. Philadelphia, PA: Lippincott Williams & Wilkins; 2009:1138.

Chestnut DH, Polley LS, Tsen LC, et al. *Chestnut's Obstetric Anesthesia Principles and Practice.* 4th ed. Philadelphia, PA: Mosby Elsevier; 2009:21–23.

Miller RD. *Miller's Anesthesia.* 6th ed. Philadelphia, PA: Elsevier Churchill Livingstone; 2005:2309–2310.

Morgan GE, Mikhail MS, Murray MJ. *Clinical Anesthesiology.* 4th ed. New York, NY: McGraw-Hill; 2006:696, 876–877.

Pregnancy: Non-OB Surg Risks

Subspecialties: Obstetric

Glenn Dizon

Edited by Lars Helgeson

1. Elective operations should be postponed until approximately 6 weeks or later after delivery. The most common emergencies requiring immediate surgery include trauma, ovarian torsion or ruptured cyst, acute cholecystitis, and acute appendicitis.
2. Anesthetic considerations are related to the physiologic changes associated with pregnancy, the possible teratogenicity of anesthetic drugs, the potential for abortion or premature delivery, and the indirect effects of anesthesia on uteroplacental circulation.

About 1% to 2% of pregnant women require surgery during their pregnancy. All elective operations should be postponed until 6 weeks or longer after delivery. Only situations requiring immediate surgery should be performed. The most common indications include trauma, acute cholecystitis, ovarian torsion or ovarian cyst rupture, and acute appendicitis.

When surgical intervention is required, anesthetic considerations are primarily related to the physiologic changes associated with pregnancy. Additional considerations include potential pharmacologic teratogenicity, the potential for abortion or premature delivery, and the indirect effects of anesthesia on uteroplacental circulation.

1. Physiologically, there is a reduction in gastric motility, decreased lower esophageal sphincter tone, and gastric acid hypersecretion. All these changes increase the risk of pulmonary aspiration and lung injury. Other physiologic changes include decreased FRC and increased oxygen consumption, both promoting rapid oxygen desaturation during apnea. Combining this with capillary engorgement of the respiratory mucosa (predisposing the upper airways to trauma, bleeding, and obstruction), there is a significantly increased risk for failed intubation.
2. Teratogenic influences on the fetus are another consideration. In the first 2 weeks, teratogens have an all-or-nothing effect, either being lethal or nonlethal to the fetus. In 3 to 8 weeks, organogenesis occurs, and anesthetic exposure can cause major developmental abnormalities. After the 8th week, drug exposure has less effect on morphology and more effect on growth and physiology of the fetus. Therefore, the fewest number of drugs should be used, with some avoided completely (benzodiazepines). The potential for spontaneous abortion is increased in women who had received general anesthesia during the first or second trimesters. It is unclear how much anesthesia versus the stress of the procedure and the underlying disease process may precipitate abortion or preterm labor (especially after intraabdominal surgery near the uterus).
3. The adequacy of uteroplacental circulation is easily affected by anesthesia. Hypoxemia, hypotension, hypovolemia, severe anemia, and increased sympathetic tone can cause fetal stress and hypoxia by inhibiting the transfer of oxygen and nutrients across the placenta. Severe hyperventilation of the mother and increased uterine activity may also reduce uterine blood flow.

Barash PG, Cullen BF, Stoelting RK. *Clinical Anesthesia.* 5th ed. Philadelphia, PA: Lippincott Williams & Wilkins; 2006:1175–1178.

Morgan GE, Mikhail MS, Murray MJ. *Clinical Anesthesiology.* 4th ed. New York, NY: McGraw-Hill; 2005:876–877, 919–920.

P

Pregnancy: SVT Rx
Pharmacology

Dan Froicu

Edited by Lars Helgeson

1. Pregnancy is a risk factor for supraventricular tachycardia (SVT).
2. Adenosine is the drug of choice for termination of SVT.
3. Avoid hypotension during regional anesthesia in pregnancy.
4. Treatment should take into account the severity of the condition, the moment in pregnancy, and possible harmful effects of pharmacotherapy on the fetus.

SVT is any arrhythmia with a heart rate above 120 beats per minute, with an atrial or atrioventricular (AV) junctional origin. It is the most frequent arrhythmia in women of reproductive age. Reported incidence varies from 1 in 1,000 to 1 in 8,000 pregnant women, with half being symptomatic.

Pregnancy is associated with an increase in premature atrial complexes and premature ventricular complexes, which is considered to be a risk factor for SVT. The increase in circulating volume, heart rate, and sympathetic tone and the increase in estrogen levels are a few of the factors that favor the development of SVT. Some of the drugs used in pregnancy, such as tocolytics, may also predispose to SVT. Vasodilatation caused by regional anesthesia decreases atrial filling, which is arrhythmogenic in itself. Furthermore, ephedrine used to correct the subsequent hypotension may lead to tachyarrhythmia.

Safety of the fetus must be considered when choosing treatment options. Adenosine temporarily depresses sinoatrial nodal activity and decreases AV conduction. It has an elimination half-life of 8 to 10 seconds and has excellent results in termination of SVT (dosage is 6 to 12 mg IV). Beta-blockers are agents of choice in Wolff–Parkinson–White syndrome, but their use may be limited to the third trimester (atenolol should not be used; it is a class "D" drug). Calcium channel blockers such as verapamil are effective in terminating SVT, but their negative inotropic effect needs to be taken into consideration. Synchronized cardioversion is a safe way to treat symptomatic SVT, which is refractory to drugs. Fetal heart rate should be monitored at all times during pharmacologic and electrical treatment of SVT. Persistent SVT can also be treated surgically with ablation of the accessory pathway. Rarely, ablation of the AV node itself is possible, which would require the insertion of a permanent pacemaker. Ablation therapy can be performed during the second trimester.

Barash PG, Cullen BF, Stoelting RK et al. *Clinical Anesthesia*. 6th ed. Philadelphia: Lippincott Williams & Wilkins, 2009.

P

Pregnancy GE Reflux Mechanism

Subspecialties: Obstetric Anesthesia

Neil Sinha

Edited by Lars Helgeson

KEY POINTS

1. The prevalence of gastroesophageal reflux disease (GERD) in the pregnant population is estimated to be 22%, 39%, and 72% in the first, second, and third trimesters, respectively. The severity of symptoms parallels the progression of pregnancy.
2. Clinical manifestations of GERD in pregnancy are similar to those in the general population.
3. The cause of the increased incidence of GERD in pregnancy is multifactorial—a decrease in the lower esophageal sphincter (LES) tone, delayed gastric emptying, and increased intragastric pressure (as a consequence of the gravid uterus), all contribute.

DISCUSSION

GERD is one of the most common clinical conditions found in pregnancy. The prevalence of GERD in the pregnant population is estimated to be 22%, 39%, and 72% in the first, second, and third trimesters, respectively. The severity of symptoms parallels the progression of pregnancy. Most women have a significant reduction or complete resolution of symptoms shortly after delivery. The clinical manifestations of GERD in pregnancy are similar to those in the general population, with heartburn being the most common complaint. The heartburn is typically exacerbated by the supine position, large fatty meals, and citrus beverages. Extraintestinal characteristics of GERD, such as asthma, hoarseness, and cough, are also common in the pregnant population.

The cause of the increased incidence of GERD in pregnancy is multifactorial.

1. Manometric evaluation reveals that pregnancy results in a steady decline in LES tone, which rapidly returns to normal levels after delivery. LES pressure in pregnancy shows a blunted response to pentagastrin, metacholine, edrophonium, and a protein meal. In the general population, these agents significantly increase the LES pressure. Estrogen and progesterone individually decrease the LES pressure. The pronounced decline during pregnancy is attributed to the combination of both. Women on estrogen alone, or sequential estrogen and progesterone oral contraceptives do not have a change in LES pressure at baseline. They do show a marked reduction in LES pressure while the two sex hormones are taken together. This is likely to be the primary cause of GERD during pregnancy.
2. Gastric emptying time (mouth-to-cecum transit time) is significantly reduced in the third trimester of pregnancy (when compared to controls 4 weeks postpartum). The impact of the delayed gastric emptying times on GERD is uncertain.
3. As a consequence of the gravid uterus, intragastric pressure in the full-term pregnancy is almost twice that of controls. After delivery, the intragastric pressure returns to baseline levels. Surprisingly, there is no direct correlation between the size of the gravid uterus and severity of symptoms. Consequently, the increase of intragastric pressures has slight impact in the development of GERD during pregnancy. Alternatively, the mechanical change of the angle at the gastroesophageal junction plays a significant role.

SUGGESTED READINGS

Charan M, Katz P. Gastroesophageal reflux disease in pregnancy. *Curr Treat Options Gastroenterol*. 2001;3(1):73–81.

Katz PO, Castell DO. Gastroesophageal reflux disease during pregnancy. *Gastroenterol Clin North Am*. 1998;27(1):153–167.

Preop Renal Failure Predictors

Organ-based Clinical: Renal: Urinary/ Electrolytes

Anjali Vira

Edited by Ala Haddadin

KEY POINTS

1. Preexisting renal disease, advanced age, major trauma, certain types of surgical procedures (cardiopulmonary bypass [CPB] and aortic surgery), congestive heart failure (CHF), and exposure to nephrotoxic drugs are some of the predictors for the development of acute renal failure.
2. Patients who are already intravascularly depleted or receive inadequate intraoperative fluid resuscitation have also shown to be at high risk for development of renal failure.
3. A urine output of greater or equal to 0.5 cc/kg/h, maintenance of cardiac output, and avoidance of large swings in systemic arterial blood pressure may help maintain adequate renal perfusion and function.

DISCUSSION

There are many predictors and contributing factors that can be linked with the development of acute peri-operative renal failure. Preexisting renal disease, advanced age, certain types of surgical procedures, and exposure to certain nephrotoxic drugs are only some of these predictors. Also, patients with specific medical conditions such as CHF or other cardiovascular disease that can be linked to renovascular disease are at increased risk for renal failure.

Patients who have undergone massive trauma such as crush injuries, major hemolytic reactions, and rhabdomyolysis are considered to be at high risk for the development of acute renal failure. Trauma leading to multiorgan system dysfunction places a patient at greater risk for failure as well. Patients who are already intravascularly depleted or receive inadequate intraoperative fluid resuscitation have also shown to be at high risk. Sepsis and the delayed treatment of sepsis may lead to acute renal failure. In addition to these, recent exposure to nephrotoxic agents such as intravenous contrast dye, aminoglycoside antibiotics, nonsteroidal anti-inflammatory medications, and angiotensin-converting enzyme inhibitors is also an important risk factor.

Patients with preexisting renal insult and those who are at risk for development of peri-operative acute renal failure require close monitoring for signs of deteriorating renal function and careful management of intravascular volume status. Monitoring hourly intraoperative urine output and intravascular volume is important in all surgical procedures, especially in patients who are at high risk for development of peri-operative acute renal failure. A urine output of greater or equal to 0.5 cc/kg/h, maintenance of cardiac output, and avoidance of large swings in systemic arterial blood pressure may help maintain adequate renal perfusion and function.

Certain surgical procedures such as cardiac surgery and major aortic surgery are associated with a high-enough incidence of peri-operative acute renal failure that prophylaxis with generous hydration with intravenous crystalloid and diuresis may be indicated. Mannitol 0.5 g per kg may be started during or even before induction and is thought to function by the maintenance of adequate renal blood flow by preventing obstruction of tubules and also by preserving the cellular architecture within the renal tubules.

SUGGESTED READINGS

Hines RL, Marschall KE. *Stoelting's Anesthesia and Co-existing Disease.* 5th ed. Philadelphia, PA: Churchill Livingstone; 2008:327.

Morgan GE, Mikhail MS, Murray MJ. *Clinical Anesthesiology.* 4th ed. New York, NY: McGraw Hill; 2006:736, 751, 754.

P

Preop Testing: Bayes' Theorem

Generic Clinical Sciences: Anesthesia Procedures, Methods, Techniques

Chi Wong

Edited by Raj K. Modak

KEY POINTS

1. Bayes' theorem relates the chance of the patient having the disease before the test is performed (pretest probability) with sensitivity and specificity.
2. Bayes' theorem is a conditional probability and can be expressed as P (D+|T+), which is the probability of having the disease (D+) given a positive test (T+) and follows the product rule.
3. The utility of a given preoperative test is reliable when applied to a population of patients with high pretest probability. It is unwise to perform tests in populations with either a very low prevalence of disease (high false positives) or very high prevalence of disease (high false negatives).

DISCUSSION

In preoperative testing, the appropriate use of diagnostic tests is vital in making therapeutic and prognostic decisions. For example, a false positive test may result in unnecessary delay or cancellation of surgery. Only after a thorough history and physical exam should diagnostic tests be considered that would help rule in or rule out a specific diagnosis. When a test result is positive, the decision to accept the result as being true depends on knowledge of the test characteristics and its performance pitfalls. Furthermore, test results cannot be adequately interpreted without knowing the prevalence of the disease in the population under study. Because test results inherently carry a degree of uncertainty, they should be scrutinized to determine if they are consistent with the overall clinical picture of the patient.

In preoperative testing, clinical decision making is based on Bayes' theorem, which predicts that the posttest probability of disease is dependent on the test's sensitivity, specificity, and the pretest probability of disease. This theorem provides a method to evaluate the predictive ability of diagnostic tests and improve uncertainty about a diagnosis. The pretest probability of disease is dependent on the patient's history and physical examination and denotes the probability of disease being present prior to testing. It includes prior probability or disease prevalence.

Bayes' theorem is a conditional probability and can be expressed as P (D+|T+), which is the probability of having the disease (D+) given a positive test (T+) and follows the product rule. Mathematically, Bayes' theorem is as follows:

$$P(D+ \mid T+) = \frac{P(D+ \text{ and } T+)}{P(T+)} = \frac{\text{prevalence} \times \text{sensitivity}}{(\text{prevalence} \times \text{sensitivity}) + [(1 - \text{prevalence})(1 - \text{specificity})]}$$

Hence, Bayes' theorem can be used to calculate the posttest probability of disease if the diagnostic test's sensitivity, specificity, and pretest probability or disease prevalence are known.

Clinically, diagnostic tests should be performed on patients suspected of a disease who are likely to test positive. For example, if patients have a high pretest probability of disease, a positive test is confirmatory and a negative test may more likely be a false negative rather than a true negative. Conversely, if patients have a low pretest probability of disease, a negative result is confirmatory and a positive test is likely to be a false positive rather than a true positive.

SUGGESTED READINGS

Miller RD, Eriksson LI, Fleisher LA, et al, eds. *Miller's Anesthesia*. 7th ed. Philadelphia, PA: Churchill Livingstone; 2010:3082–3083.

Sackett DL. The rational clinical examination. A primer on the precision and accuracy of the clinical examination. *JAMA*. 1992;267(19):2638–2644.

Preoperative Anxiolysis in Children
Subspecialties: Pediatrics

Samantha Franco

Edited by Mamatha Punjala

1. Preoperative anxiolysis in children involves communication between the child, the parents, and all involved health care providers.
2. Pharmacologic and behavioral methods, such as operating room tours, acupuncture, music, and coloring books, can help address preoperative anxiety and stress in children.
3. Midazolam via the oral route is the most commonly used premedication in the United States, as it has a rapid onset and predictable effect without causing cardiorespiratory depression.
4. Various sedatives other than midazolam, such as ketamine, clonidine, dexmedetomidine, and so forth, as well as different routes of administration (oral, rectal, intranasal, intramuscular), can prove efficacious to alleviate preoperative anxiety depending on the clinical situation.

P

Anesthesia and surgery cause a substantial amount of stress and hardship on both the child and parents. Anxiety in children undergoing surgery is characterized by subjective feelings of tension, apprehension, nervousness, and worry, and may be expressed in many forms. Some children verbalize their fears explicitly, whereas for others anxiety is expressed only behaviorally. Many children may become agitated, look scared, breathe deeply, tremble, stop talking or playing, and start to cry. These behaviors, which may prolong the induction of anesthesia, could give children some sense of control in the situation, and thereby diminish a damaging sense of helplessness. To cope with the preoperative stress, there needs to be consistent communication between the child, the parents, and all involved health care providers during the preoperative period. Therefore, the sphere of communication encompasses not only the child's immediate needs but also those of the family and providers.

Although discussion and communication are key factors toward a successful and smooth transition from preoperative to intraoperative care for the child, various pharmacologic and behavioral methods can be used to address the issue of perioperative anxiety in children and their parents. Behavioral interventions include tours of the operating room, written and audiovisual materials, coloring books, handling and familiarity with the anesthesia mask, and patient care representatives skilled in the preoperative preparation of children. To date, most studies suggest that preoperative preparation programs reduce anxiety and enhance coping in children. Some hospitals and programs allow parents to be present for the induction of anesthesia, but the efficacy of this intervention is uncertain and the availability of such programs is not universal. There are also other nonpharmacologic interventions, such as acupuncture, music, and hypnosis, that have been shown to reduce the anxiety in perioperative environments. Pharmacologic methods such as midazolam are very effective treatment for preoperative anxiety. Sedation before surgery is an effective method that is widely used for young children for decreasing anxiety. Other effects that may be achieved by pharmacologic preparation of the patient include amnesia, anxiolysis, prevention of physiologic stress, and analgesia. In addition, children who are sedated before coming to the operating room may have fewer stress-related behavioral changes in the immediate postoperative time compared with groups of patients who receive no sedation.

Recent research has documented that a child's fear on the day of surgery might extend beyond the immediate postoperative period. About 50% of all children undergoing routine outpatient surgery present at 2 weeks postoperatively with new-onset anxiety, nighttime crying, enuresis, separation anxiety, temper tantrums, and sleep or eating disturbances. Usually, the majority of these behaviors disappear within 3 to 4 weeks postoperatively. Primary health care providers should be aware of these behaviors and assure parents that these behavioral changes are self-limited. Children with postoperative behavioral changes that persist beyond 3 to 4 weeks after surgery should be referred to a trained mental health provider.

Upon establishing that preoperative anxiolysis is paramount for the successful preoperative anesthetic care of the child, various preparations and routes of administration should be considered and discussed in relation to their efficacy (Table 1). Oral premedications, such as midazolam, are commonly used in the United States. More than 85% of all preoperative sedation in the United States is performed using midazolam. Midazolam has a rapid onset and predictable effect without causing cardiorespiratory depression. Midazolam, in doses of 0.5 to 0.75 mg per kg PO (per os), can have a peak effect in about 30 minutes, and studies have shown that in surgeries lasting an hour or more, oral midazolam in doses of 0.25 to 0.5 mg per kg does not appear to lengthen recovery time. Although very effective in most children, about 14% of children may not respond to a midazolam dose of 0.5 mg per kg. This group of children is reported to be younger (4.2 ± 2.3 vs. 5.9 ± 2.0 years) and to have high levels of preoperative emotionality. Therefore, using higher doses of midazolam (0.75 mg per kg) may be more appropriate in these nonresponders. Strict adult supervision is required in children who receive this drug, even though serious side effects after oral midazolam are uncommon. Midazolam has been shown to be superior to parental presence in decreasing perioperative stress for patients and families; however, parental presence does result in increased parental satisfaction from the overall perioperative experience. If the effects of midazolam need to be reversed, then flumazenil, a competitive benzodiazepine antagonist, can be given to children at 0.05 mg per kg intravenously titrated to 1.0 mg total dose.

Other oral agents have also been employed with variable success for preoperative sedation in children. Oral ketamine, for instance, has been used in doses of 5 to 6 mg per kg for children 1 to 6 years of age, with maximal sedation occurring in 20 minutes. The combination of ketamine and midazolam has also been used as an oral sedative premedication mixture though nausea and vomiting rates were slightly increased in children who received oral ketamine. Oral transmucosal fentanyl has also been used to sedate children prior to induction of anesthesia; however, due to side effects such as facial pruritus, high incidence of postoperative nausea and vomiting, and arterial oxygen desaturation, this drug is not currently used routinely in the perioperative setting. Clonidine and most recently dexmedetomidine have been used as preoperative sedatives. Clonidine, an alpha-2 agonist, given in combination with atropine, does produce satisfactory preoperative sedation, easy separation from parents, and mask acceptance within 45 minutes, even though it has a slower onset time than midazolam. Orally administered clonidine in a dose of about 4 μg per kg can reliably cause sedation, decrease anesthetic requirements, decrease requirement for postoperative analgesics, and attenuate the response to tracheal intubation. Dexmedetomidine, a more selective alpha-2 agonist than clonidine, at 1 μg per kg transmucosally or 3 to 4 μg per kg orally, has similar sedative and axiolytic effect to clonidine or midazolam.

Other routes of administration of these medications have varying efficacy for preoperative anxiolysis in children. The intranasal route can provide rapid absorption and avoidance of first-pass hepatic metabolism; however, most children cry on administration because it transiently irritates the nasal passages. Midazolam can be administered intranasally in a dose of 0.2 mg per kg. Other agents, such as sufentanil, used intranasally have been abandoned because of side effects like chest wall rigidity and hypoxia. Rectal administration of midazolam (0.5 to 1.0 mg per kg) can reduce anxiety of children prior to induction, but the provider must ensure that the drug is not expelled immediately. Barbiturates, such as methohexital and thiopental, can also be administered rectally at 25 mg per kg, but they have an onset time of about 10 minutes and may lead to respiratory depression and oxygen desaturation due to the variable reabsorption in the rectum. Intramuscular administration is another and perhaps better alternative to the intravenous route than the rectal or intranasal paths. Intramuscular midazolam in a dose of 0.3 mg per kg provides anxiolysis in 5 to 10 minutes, and ketamine at a dose of 3 to 4 mg per kg IM can produce a quiet, breathing, yet minimally responsive patient in about 5 minutes. Overall, the oral route is the most commonly used and preferred method of preoperative sedative administration in children; however, nasal, rectal, and intramuscular routes can also be efficacious in specific cases, such as in cognitively challenged patients, for perioperative anxiolysis.

Table 1. Premedication: Drug Options and Doses

Medication	Route	Dose (mg/kg)	Time to Onset (min)	Elimination Half-Life $T_{1/2}$ (h)
Midazolam	Oral	0.25–1.0	10	2
	Intranasal	0.2–0.3	<10	2–3
	Rectal	0.3–1.0	10	2–3
Ketamine	Oral	3.0–6.0	10	2–3
	Intranasal	3.0–5.0	<10	3
	Rectal	5.0–6.0	20–30	3
Clonidine	Oral	0.002–0.004	45	8–12

From Barash PG, Cullen BF, Stoelting RK, et al, eds. *Clinical Anesthesia.* 6th ed. Philadelphia, PA: Lippincott Williams & Wilkins; 2009:1211.

SUGGESTED READINGS

Barash PG, Cullen BF, Stoelting RK, et al, eds. *Clinical Anesthesia.* 6th ed. Philadelphia, PA: Lippincott Williams & Wilkins; 2009:chap 45: Pediatric anesthesia:1206–1220.

Cote CJ, Cohen IT, Suresh S, et al. A comparison of three doses of commercially prepared oral midazolam syrup in children. *Anesth Analg.* 2002;94:37.

Kain ZN, Caldwell-Andrews AA, Maranets I, et al. Preoperative anxiety and emergence delirium and postoperative maladaptive behaviors. *Anesth Analg.* 2004;99:1648.

Kain ZN, MacLaren J, McClain BC, et al. Effects of age and emotionality on the effectiveness of midazolam administered preoperatively to children. *Anesthesiology.* 2007;107:545.

McCann ME, Kain ZN. The management of perioperative anxiety in children: an update. *Anesth Analg.* 2001;93:98.

Shannon M, Albers G, Burkhart K, et al. Safety and efficacy of flumazenil in the reversal of benzodiazepine-induced conscious sedation. *J Pediatr.* 1997;131:582.

Wang SM, Hofstadter MB, Kain ZN. An alternative method to alleviate postoperative nausea and vomiting in children. *J Clin Anesth.* 1999;11:231.

Pre-renal Oliguria: Dx

Organ-based Clinical: Renal/Urinary/ Electrolytes

Xing Fu

Edited by Hossam Tantawy

KEY POINTS

1. Oliguria is defined as inadequate urinary output, often considered to be less than 400 cc per day or anything less than 0.5 mL/kg/h.
2. Pre-renal causes of oliguria include hypovolemia, mechanical ventilation, cardiomyopathy, aortic stenosis, and medications that impair renal autoregulation (i.e., nonsteroidal anti-inflammatory drugs [NSAIDs], angiotensin-converting-enzyme [ACE] inhibitors, angiotensin receptor blockers [ARBs]).
3. Prerenal oliguria results in renal hypoperfusion, which causes the activation of compensatory systemic and renal responses that increase tubular reabsorption of sodium and water, resulting in low urine output.
4. The urinary indices for prerenal oliguria are specific gravity greater than 1.018, osmolality greater than 500 mmol per kg, urine/plasma urea nitrogen ratio greater than 8, urine/plasma creatinine ratio greater than 40, urine sodium less than 10 mEq per L, fractional excretion of sodium (FENa) less than 1%, and renal failure index less than 1.

P

DISCUSSION

Oliguria is defined as inadequate urinary output, often considered to be less than 400 cc per day or anything less than 0.5 mL/kg/h. The causes of oliguria are generally classified as prerenal, renal, or postrenal in nature. Prerenal causes include hypovolemia, mechanical ventilation, cardiomyopathy, aortic stenosis, and medications that impair renal autoregulation (i.e., NSAIDs, ACE inhibitors, ARBs). Renal causes for oliguria generally fall under acute tubular necrosis or acute interstitial nephritis. Some of the potential causes of postrenal oliguria are a retroperitoneal mass, prostatic hypertrophy, papillary necrosis, and urethral stricture.

Prerenal oliguria results in renal hypoperfusion, which causes the activation of compensatory systemic and renal responses that increase tubular reabsorption of sodium and water that results in low urine output. The diagnosis of prerenal oliguria can be made using various history and physical and laboratory findings. Orthostatic hypotension, low central venous pressure (CVP), skin tenting, and dry mucous membranes may point to hypovolemia as a cause. In addition, a decrease in blood pressure after lung inflation in a mechanically ventilated patient may suggest inadequate preload and hypovolemia.

The urinary indices for prerenal oliguria are specific gravity greater than 1.018, osmolality greater than 500 mmol per kg, urine/plasma urea nitrogen ratio greater than 8, urine/ plasma creatinine ratio greater than 40, urine sodium less than 10 mEq per L, FE_{Na} less than 1%, and renal failure index less than 1. Of the various urinary indices, FE_{Na} is considered one of the most reliable at differentiating prerenal from renal oliguria.

SUGGESTED READINGS

Marino PL. *The ICU Book*. 3rd ed. Philadelphia, PA: Lippincott Williams & Wilkins; 2007:579–584.
Morgan GE, Mikhail MS, Murray MJ. *Clinical Anesthesiology*. 4th ed. New York, NY: McGraw-Hill; 2005:151, 1046–1047.

Pressure vs. Volume Vent: ICU

Generic Clinical Sciences: Anesthesia Procedures, Methods,Techniques

Laurie Yonemoto

Edited by Raj K. Modak

1. Pressure-cycled modes of ventilation deliver fixed pressures.
2. Volume-cycled modes of ventilation deliver fixed volumes.
3. Changes in lung compliance affect the performance of both pressure and volume modes of ventilation.
4. The key advantage of pressure-controlled ventilation (PCV) is lower risk of barotrauma, which comes with the disadvantage of greater potential for hypoxemia and hypercarbia.
5. The key disadvantage of volume-controlled ventilation (VCV) is higher risk of barotrauma, which comes with the advantage of less potential for hypoxemia and hypercarbia.

Many patients in the intensive care unit (ICU) develop respiratory failure and require mechanical ventilation. Mechanical ventilation is typically achieved by the generation of positive pressure, forcing a volume of gas into the lungs. Although the terminology used to describe ventilators is varied, a facile way to examine differences between the use of pressure and volume can be seen with controlled mechanical ventilation (CMV). In this mode of ventalation, it will be assumed that the patient being ventilated cannot make any respiratory effort, as seen with patients receiving muscle relaxation. In this mode, patients could be ventilated under VCV or PCV. Advantages and disadvantages of the use of pressure or volume are best seen by understanding fundemental concepts in lung compliance.

Lung compliance (*C*) is defined as the change in lung volume (*V*) divided by the change in lung pressure (*P*) (Fig. 1). As such, $C = V/P$. Many clinical circumstances alter lung compliance. The usual senario is a reduction in lung compliance. In such a situation, at a given reduced compliance, a higher pressure is required to achieve fixed lung volume, or a smaller lung volume is seen at a fixed change in pressure.

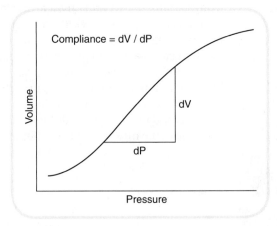

Figure 1. Static compliance curve. Compliance equals the change in volume divided by the change in pressure.

In VCV, the tidal volume is set or "fixed." The peak airway pressure is inversely related to the compliance ($P = V/C$). If a patient's condition changes, reducing the pulmonary compliance, the result is an increase in the mean and peak airway pressures. The risk of elevated airway pressures is barotrauma to the lung and alterations in hemodynamics (elevated central venous pressure [CVP], low cardiac output, low systemic blood pressure) related to increased intrathoracic pressure. However, VCV allows a consistent alveolar and minute ventilation affording less risk of hypoxemia and hypercarbia.

In PCV, the airway pressure is limited or "fixed." Airway pressures will not exceed the set pressure limit. The tidal volume is directly related to the compliance of the lung ($V = P \times C$). If a patient's condition changes, reducing the pulmonary compliance, the result is decrease in the tidal volume. As can be deduced, the fixed pressure setting decreases the risks of barotrauma. However, alterations in tidal volume can result in impaired alveolar ventilation causing hypoxemia; reductions in minute ventilation can increase blood concentrations of carbon dioxide, resulting in acute respiratory acidosis.

As the technology used in ventilators is improving, intermittant and assisted/supported modes of ventilation are now commonly mixing and matching methods of volume and pressure. However, the basic concepts surrounding lung compliance remains the same.

SUGGESTED READINGS

Barash PG, Cullen BF, Stoelting RK, et al, eds. *Clinical Anesthesia*. 6th ed. Philadelphia, PA: Lippincott Williams & Wilkins; 2009:1457–1358.

Morgan GE, Mikhail MS, Murray MJ. *Clinical Anesthesiology*. 4th ed. New York, NY: McGraw Hill; 2006:1031–1033.

Preterm Labor: Treatment
Subspecialties: Obstetrics

Jorge Galvez

Edited by Lars Helgeson

1. Preterm labor is defined as labor occurring before 37 weeks of gestation.
2. Women in preterm labor who receive tocolytic therapy often deliver approximately 48 hours after presentation despite therapy.
3. Tocolytic therapy is administered in combination with antenatal steroids to promote fetal lung maturity and improve neonatal outcomes.
4. If successful in arresting preterm labor, the patient remains at risk for preterm labor. Maintaining therapy/bed rest may be warranted.
5. Tocolytic agents used in the treatment of preterm labor include beta agonists, magnesium sulfate, calcium channel blockers, and prostaglandin synthetase inhibitors.

Preterm labor is defined as labor that occurs before the 37th week of gestation. Women in preterm labor may be difficult to distinguish from women with premature uterine contractions, who are not in active labor. Criteria developed by Creasy help in the identification of preterm labor. The most accepted criterion is cervical change, which is subject to examiner bias. Others include the following:

- More than four uterine contractions every 20 minutes
- Cervical dilation (>2 cm in nulliparous women, >3 cm in multiparous women)
- Cervical effacement greater than 80%
- Uterine contractions combined with cervical change (requires serial examinations)

The therapeutic goal for preterm labor is to suppress uterine activity, thus prolonging the pregnancy. This allows for further fetal development with improved neonatal outcomes. Women in preterm labor who receive tocolytic therapy go on to deliver an average of 48 hours after presentation despite the therapeutic regimen administered. Therefore, it is important to combine tocolytic therapy with antenatal corticosteroids to promote fetal lung maturity, should the fetus be delivered prematurely.

Absolute contraindications to tocolytic therapy include the following:

- Severe preeclampsia
- Severe bleeding
- Severe placental abruption
- Chorioamnionitis
- Severe fetal growth restriction
- Severe fetal distress
- Fetal death or anomaly incompatible with life
- Mature lung studies via amniocentesis
- Certain maternal cardiac arrhythmias

Relative contraindications to tocolytic therapy include the following:

- Chronic hypertension
- Mild placental abruption
- Stable placenta previa

P

- Maternal cardiac disease
- Hyperthyroidism or uncontrolled diabetes mellitus
- Mild fetal distress
- Fetal anomaly
- Cervical dilation greater than 4 cm.

Pharmacologic Therapy

Beta-agonists, ritodrine (intravenous [IV]), and terbutaline (IV or subcutaneous) may be administered in incremental doses until successful or maternal or fetal side effects prevent further therapy. Side effects of beta-agonists include maternal tachycardia, hypotension, hyperkalemia, pulmonary edema, decreased urine output, hypertension, palpitations, agitation, arrhythmias, myocardial infarction, decreased gastric emptying, postpartum cardiomyopathy, and death. Fetal side effects include tachycardia, redistribution of blood flow, increased thickness of the interventricular septum, supraventricular tachycardia, myocardial ischemia and necrosis, hydrops fetalis, and hypoglycemia.

Although magnesium sulfate ($MgSO_4$) is the most widely used tocolytic agent today, its efficacy is falling under scrutiny. Widespread use was adopted without well-designed placebo controlled trials. Several randomized trials have shown $MgSO_4$ to be no more effective than placebo as a tocolytic. Meta-analysis has concluded that $MgSO_4$ is not effective at delaying or preventing preterm birth and that its use is associated with increased neonatal mortality. It is typically administered with an IV loading dose of 4 to 8 g over 20 minutes followed by an infusion of 2 to 4 g per hour. Adjustments are based on uterine contraction activity, serum magnesium levels, and maternal side effects. Therapy can be stopped when contractions stop for 12 to 24 hours. Maternal side effects include flushing, headache, nystagmus, nausea, dizziness, and lethargy. Serious side effects include pulmonary edema, neuromuscular blockade, osteopenia, and respiratory depression. Fetal side effects include decreased fetal heart rate variability, central nervous system depression, decreased muscle tone, poor respiratory effort, and low Apgar scores.

Calcium channel blockers work as nonspecific relaxants of smooth muscle, which can result in cessation of contractions. Side effects include maternal hypotension, potentiation of neuromuscular blockade from magnesium sulfate, fetal heart block, neonatal acidosis, and stillbirth.

Prostaglandins are intimately involved in the process of cervical ripening and labor, and thus inhibition of prostaglandins via cyclooxygenase (COX) inhibition can prevent preterm labor. Nonsteroidal anti-inflammatory drug agents (such as indomethacin) can be useful as a tocolytic agent. Fetal contraindications to indomethacin are growth restriction, renal anomalies, chorioamnionitis, oligohydramnios, ductal dependent cardiac lesions, and twin-twin transfusion syndrome. Maternal side effects with long-term therapy include gastrointestinal bleeding, coagulopathies, exacerbation of asthma, and renal injury.

Other agents include oxytocin analogs, nitroglycerine, COX-2 inhibitors, ketorolac, progestins, and nitric oxide inhibitors, although most of these have not been widely tested or have not received approval by the U.S. Food and Drug Administration for tocolysis.

Ancillary Therapy for Women in Preterm Labor

Antenatal corticosteroids (betamethasone 12 mg intramuscularly [IM] every 24 hours × 2 doses or dexamethasone 6 mg IM every 12 hours × 4 doses) significantly improve neonatal outcomes, including lower incidence of respiratory distress syndrome, intraventricular hemorrhage, and death. ACOG and NIH recommend that all women at risk for preterm labor before 34 weeks of gestation receive a course of preterm corticosteroids.

SUGGESTED READING

Gibbs RS, Karlan BY, Haney AF, et al. *Danforth's Obstetrics and Gynecology*. 9th ed. Philadelphia, PA: Lippincott Williams & Wilkins; 2008:165–185.

Propofol Infusion Syndrome: Dx

Pharmacology

Amit Mirchandani

Edited by Hossam Tantawy

1. Propofol infusion syndrome is a rare and sometimes fatal condition described in critically ill patients undergoing long-term propofol infusion at high doses.
2. The main features of the syndrome consist of cardiac failure, rhabdomyolysis, severe metabolic acidosis, and renal failure.
3. The syndrome can be lethal, and literature suggests caution when using prolonged (>48 hours) propofol sedation at doses higher than 5 mg/kg/h, especially in patients with acute neurologic or inflammatory illnesses.

Propofol infusion syndrome is a process that can be fatal to patients on long-term propofol infusion at high doses. Most of these patients have been described as critically ill patients, with acute neurologic illnesses or acute inflammatory diseases, complicated by severe infections and even sepsis. These patients may have also been receiving catecholamines and/or steroids in addition to propofol during intubation.

Central nervous system activation produces catecholamines and glucocorticoids, while systemic inflammation produces cytokine factors. These factors in combination are priming factors for cardiac and peripheral muscle necrosis and dysfunction. To add potential insult in these critically ill patients, high-dose propofol for sedation in those already on catecholamine support may also act as triggering factors.

At cellular level, propofol interferes with free fatty acid utilization and mitochondrial activity. Imbalance between energy demand and utilization is a key pathologic process that leads to peripheral and cardiac muscle necrosis.

In the end, propofol infusion syndrome is multifactorial. Propofol, particularly when combined with catecholamines and/or steroids, acts as a triggering factor. The syndrome can be lethal, and literature suggests caution when using prolonged (>48 hours) propofol sedation at doses higher than 5 mg/kg/h, particularly in patients with acute neurologic or inflammatory illnesses. In these cases, alternative sedative agents, such as narcotics and benzodiazepines, should be considered. If these agents are unsuitable for sedation, the care provider should pursue strict monitoring of signs of myocytolysis.

VasileB, Rasulo F, Candiani A, et al. The pathophysiology of propofol infusion syndrome: a simple name for a complex syndrome. *Intensive Care Med.* 2003;29(9):1417–1425.

Prostaglandin for Congenital Heart: Cx
Subspecialties: Pediatrics

Samantha Franco

Edited by Mamatha Punjala

KEY POINTS

1. E-type prostaglandins dilate and maintain patency of the ductus arteriosus in order to improve pulmonary blood flow, reduce hypoxemia, and acidosis in patient with ductal-dependent pulmonary blood flow lesions and also maintain systemic blood flow and prevent congestive heart failure in patients with ductal-dependent aortic or systemic blood flow conditions.
2. Prostaglandins provide medical management as a bridge to surgery in patients with congenital heart disease, especially preterm infants, where surgical delay may be advantageous for further growth.
3. Side effects with Prostaglandin infusions vary, but are mainly characterized by cardiovascular and respiratory changes, thereby requiring close monitoring of hemodynamic parameters, pulse oximetry, heart rate, and arterial blood pressure.

DISCUSSION

The E-type prostaglandins have been in use for various types of congenital heart defects, such as pulmonary atresia, critical pulmonary stenosis, or severely hypoplastic right ventricle, which depend almost entirely on a patent ductus arteriosus for the maintenance of pulmonary blood flow. Likewise, interruption of the aortic arch requires ductal patency for blood flow to the lower half of the body. Patients can become extremely sick once the ductus constricts, and therefore, without intervention can die in the first month of life. The original demonstration by Oceani and Olley that E-prostaglandins are potent relaxants of the ductus arteriosus, confirmed by further animal studies in vivo and in vitro, suggested their use in these patients.

Administration of prostaglandin to reverse ductus constriction and increase pulmonary blood flow should improve tissue oxygenation, correct metabolic acidosis, and improve the chances of successful surgery. Several lines of investigation support that endogenous prostaglandins help to control muscle tone in the fetal ductus arteriosus. Therefore, comprehension of the uses and side effects of prostaglandins is needed in congenital heart disease.

Broadly, there are two subgroups of congenital heart disease, namely, ductus-dependent pulmonary blood flow lesions and ductus-dependent aortic or systemic blood flow conditions. The former group includes pulmonary atresia with ventricular septal defect or pulmonary stenosis, in which patency of the ductus arteriosus is vital in maintaining pulmonary blood flow and to relieve hypoxemia and acidosis. Prostaglandin E_1 (PGE_1) infusions, by relaxing the smooth muscle of the ductus arteriosus, will dilate and open the ductus arteriosus and lead to subsequent improvement in pulmonary blood flow via left-to-right shunting.

The latter, ductal-dependent aortic or systemic blood flow lesions, such as hypoplastic left heart syndrome, aortic atresia, interruption of the aortic arch, and coarctation of the aorta, require patency of the ductus arteriosus to maintain systemic blood flow and vital organ perfusion and to prevent congestive heart failure. Therefore, closure of the ductus will result in severe reduction in systemic blood flow, hypotension, shock, and congestive heart failure. PGE_1 infusion will maintain ductus patency and dilatation and maintain systemic blood flow by way of right-to-left shunting. It also helps to maintain perfusion to vital organs and prevent congestive heart failure and shock. In coarctation of the aorta, PGE_1 infusion reduces the pressure difference between the ascending and descending aorta and is attributed to the relaxation/dilatation of the aortic end of the ductus arteriosus. The only admixture lesion in which PGE$_1$ infusion was found to be useful was in transposition of the great arteries. Opening of the ductus arteriosus and facilitating large left-to-right shunting through it helps to improve pulmonary blood flow and hence improved oxygenation by improved atrial mixing. As prostaglandin infusion helps to maintain hemodynamic stability through ductal patency and dilatation, it serves as a bridge to surgery, especially in preterm infants, where surgical delay via medical management allows for further growth and development.

The preferred route of administration is intravenous, and the infusion usually starts at 0.05 ug/kg/min and can even be reduced to 0.01 ug/kg/min or titrated to higher doses of 0.2 to 0.4 ug/kg/min to achieve the desired effect. Patients should be continuously monitored for blood pressure, heart rate, and pulse oximetry.

Various studies have also reviewed the side effects of prostaglandin infusions in patients with congenital heart disease. Cardiovascular events like hypotension, edema, and rhythm disturbances were more common (18%), followed by central nervous system effects like seizures and hyperthermia (16%). Respiratory depression leading to apnea or hypoventilation was noted in 12% of patients receiving PGE$_1$ infusion. Other side effects relating to metabolic, infectious, gastrointestinal, hematologic, and renal systems together contributed to less than 10% of side effects related to PGE$_1$ infusion. As there is a dominance of cardiovascular and respiratory side effects, arterial blood pressure and respiratory activity should be monitored carefully to initiate timely measures and careful titration of the infusion.

SUGGESTED READINGS

Barash PG, Cullen BF, Stoelting RK, et al, eds. *Clinical Anesthesia*. 6th ed. Philadelphia, PA: Lippincott Williams & Wilkins; 2009.

Reddy SC, Saxena A. Prostaglandin E1: first stage palliation in neonates with congenital cardiac defects. *Indian J Pediatr*. 1998;65(2):211-216.

Taylor WJ, Alpert BS. Prostaglandins and the management of congenital heart disease. *Am Fam Physician*. 1982;26(6):127-132.

Pyloric Stenosis: Metab Abnormality
Subspecialties: Pediatric Anesthesia

Martha Zegarra

Edited by Mamatha Punjala

KEY POINTS

1. Pyloric stenosis is not a surgical emergency; rather, it is a medical emergency requiring normalization of fluid, electrolyte, and acid–base derangements before surgical intervention.
2. Progressive emesis causes a hypochloremic, hypokalemic metabolic alkalosis with a compensatory respiratory acidosis.
3. Correction of fluid and electrolyte derangements requires hydration with a sodium chloride containing solution supplemented with potassium.
4. Postoperatively, there is an increased risk of delayed awakening, respiratory depression, and hypoventilation or periodic apnea because of persistent metabolic or cerebrospinal fluid (CSF) alkalosis.

DISCUSSION

Pyloric stenosis is a common cause of gastric outlet obstruction in children, which occurs when a hypertrophic pylorus obstructs the passage of food from the stomach into the small intestine. Pyloric stenosis is not a surgical emergency; rather, it is a medical emergency requiring normalization of fluid, electrolyte, and acid–base derangements before surgical correction.

Projectile vomiting is pathognomonic for this disease process, but a more common clinical manifestation is chronic nonbilious vomiting after feeds. Progressive emesis results in a loss of sodium, potassium, chloride, and hydrogen ions from the extracellular space. Initially, as chloride and hydrogen ions are lost through vomiting, the kidney attempts to maintain a normal serum pH by excreting potassium and sodium bicarbonate. With persistent vomiting, volume contraction occurs and the kidneys respond by conserving sodium and excreting hydrogen, thereby defending extracellular volume in preference to serum pH. The initially alkaline urine becomes acidic, and this paradoxical aciduria worsens the existing metabolic alkalosis. Thus, the most frequent hallmark presentation is a hypokalemic, hypochloremic metabolic alkalosis with a compensatory respiratory acidosis. However, severe dehydration and hypovolemic shock may present as metabolic acidosis with hyperventilation and a respiratory alkalosis. Hyponatremia, though present, may not be appreciated because of hypovolemia, and an associated hypocalcemia may also be present.

Correction of fluid and electrolyte derangements requires hydration with a sodium chloride containing solution. Potassium supplementation should be commenced once urine output is adequate. Lactated Ringer's solutions should be avoided, as lactate is metabolized to bicarbonate and can worsen the alkalosis.

Definitive treatment of pyloric stenosis requires pyloromyotomy, which can be undertaken after the volume deficit and electrolyte abnormalities have been corrected. General anesthesia is induced in the usual manner, with prior thorough emptying of the stomach with a large nasogastric (NG) or orogastric (OG) tube. These children are at increased risk for delayed awakening, respiratory depression, and hypoventilation or periodic apnea in the recovery room because of persistent metabolic or CSF alkalosis.

SUGGESTED READINGS

Hines RL, Marschall KE. *Stoelting's Anesthesia and Coexisting Disease.* 5th ed. Philadelphia, PA: Churchill Livingstone/Elsevier; 2010:599–600.

Litman RS. *Pediatric Anesthesia: The Requisites in Anesthesiology.* Philadelphia, PA: Elsevier/Mosby; 2004:233.

Morgan GE, Mikhail MS, Murray MJ. *Clinical Anesthesiology.* 4th ed. New York, NY: Lange Medical Books/McGraw Hill; 2006:942–943.

Renal Failure: CPB Surgery
Organ-based Clinical: Cardiovascular

Veronica Matei

Edited by Qingbing Zhu

1. Renal dysfunction is a frequent complication of cardiac operations using cardiopulmonary bypass (CPB).
2. The etiology of CPB-induced renal injury is multifactorial, and includes systemic inflammatory response and renal hypoperfusion.
3. The treatment of CPB-induced renal dysfunction is largely supportive, although early recognition is important.

Renal dysfunction is a frequent complication of cardiac operations using CPB. The extent of CPB-induced renal dysfunction ranges from subclinical injury to established renal failure requiring dialysis. The incidence of renal dysfunction varies considerably, depending on the definition and criteria used in the various studies. Acute renal insufficiency occurs in 8% to 20% of these patients depending on the diagnostic criteria used, and 1% to 5% of patients who require postoperative dialysis. Comorbidities, including diabetes mellitus, impaired left ventricular function, and advanced age, are recognized predisposing factors.

The pathophysiology is multifactorial and is thought to be related to the systemic inflammatory response and renal hypoperfusion secondary to extracorporeal circulation.

Nonpulsatile flow during CPB is thought to be an important etiological factor, resulting in renal vasoconstriction and ischemic renal injury. However, studies examining pulsatile blood flow and renal outcomes have not shown definitive results.

Strategies for prevention of CPB-induced renal injury have included manipulation of perfusion pressure, off-pump procedures to preserve the pulsatile flow, and promotion of renal vasodilatation by pharmacologic agents. The treatment of acute renal insufficiency is largely supportive. Early recognition is important because timing of treatment may be crucial to assure the best possible outcome.

Barash PG, Cullen BF, Stoelting RK, et al, eds. *Clinical Anesthesia*. 6th ed. Philadelphia, PA: Lippincott Williams & Wilkins; 2009.

Renal Failure: Electrolytes

Generic, Clinical Sciences: Anesthesia Procedures, Methods, Techniques, and Organ-based Clinical: Renal/ Urinary/Electrolytes

Tori Myslajek

Edited by Ala Haddadin

KEY POINTS

1. Renal failure may lead to electrolyte abnormalities such as hyponatremia, hyperkalemia, hyperphosphatemia, hypermagnesemia, and hypocalcemia.
2. Hyponatremia results when the increase in water exceeds the increase in sodium, as can occur with renal failure.
3. Hypocalcemia is thought to occur as a result of calcium deposition into bone, secondary to hyperphosphatemia, parathyroid hormone (PTH) resistance, and low intestinal absorption secondary to decreased synthesis of 1,25-dihydroxycholecalciferol by the kidneys.

DISCUSSION

Chronic renal failure is a progressive disease that results in irreversible decline in renal function. The full manifestation, known as uremia, is seen when the glomerular filtration rate decreases below 25 mL per minute. Many patients with decompensated renal failure manifest metabolic disease in the form of metabolic acidosis, hyperkalemia, hyponatremia, hypermagnesemia, hyperphosphatemia, hypocalcemia, and hyperuricemia. The anesthetic management of patients with renal failure can be complex and must take several factors into consideration.

Hyperkalemia usually occurs when the creatinine clearance is less than 5 mL per minute, but can occur in other renal failure patients when large potassium loads are encountered. The most significant effect of hyperkalemia is on the heart and its conduction system. Elevated potassium levels may result in peaked T-waves, P-R interval prolongation, ST segment elevation, and arrhythmias.

Conditions contributing to acidosis, such as hypoventilation, will contribute to hyperkalemia through shift in compartments from intracellular to extracellular. Administration of succinylcholine will also contribute to hyperkalemia in amounts up to 0.5 mEq per L in patients, regardless of renal failure. Patients who may have an exaggerated release of potassium include those with burns, upper and lower motor neuron diseases, closed-head injuries, and prolonged immobilization. Generally, elective surgeries are postponed until dialytic patients have been dialyzed and lab values are relatively normalized, such as potassium less than 5.5 mEq per L. If a surgery is truly emergent and hyperkalemia is of concern, one can treat a patient intravenously with glucose and insulin as well as by hyperventilation to drive potassium into the cell. Furthermore, calcium may be used to stabilize the myocardium in the setting of hyperkalemia.

There are several disorders that cause edema and are characterized by an increase in both total body sodium and water content. Hyponatremia results when the increase in water exceeds the increase in sodium, as can occur with renal failure, congestive heart failure, cirrhosis, and nephritic syndrome. In renal failure, water and sodium retention result in hyponatremia in the setting of extracellular fluid overload. Hyponatremia may cause mental status changes, lethargy, seizures, and changes in deep tendon reflexes. Correcting sodium intraoperatively is rarely an issue. However, in the setting of severe hyponatremia, values less than 120 mEq per L, rapid correction may result in central pontine myelinolysis.

Hyperphosphatemia has virtually no symptoms, and hypermagnesemia is usually mild, with symptoms mostly neurologic and cardiovascular in nature. Dietary restrictions should be in place, and if severe, dialysis may be indicated for elimination.

Hypocalcemia is thought to occur as a result of calcium deposition into bone, secondary to hyperphosphatemia, PTH resistance, and low intestinal absorption secondary to decreased synthesis of 1,25-dihydroxycholecalciferol by the kidneys. It is usually asymptomatic, but if severe, may have cardiovascular and neurologic effects. The goal of treatment in the acute setting is to eliminate symptoms and not necessarily to return values to normal.

SUGGESTED READINGS

Morgan GE, Mikhail MS, Murray MJ. *Clinical Anesthesiology*. 4th ed. Philadelphia, PA: McGraw-Hill Professional; 2005:597–623, 669–673.
Rose BD, Rennke HG. *Renal Pathophysiology*. Baltimore, MD: Lippincott Williams & Wilkins; 1994:176–184, 280, 288–290.
Stoelting RK, Miller RD. *Basics of Anesthesia*. 5th ed. Philadelphia, PA: Churchill Livingstone; 2007:429–430.

R

Renal Failure: Platelet Function

Organ-based Clinical: Renal/Urinary/ Electrolytes

Donald Neirink

Edited by Hossam Tantawy

KEY POINTS

1. Renal failure results in a decline in urine production and glomerular filtration, causing accumulation of nitrogenous wastes, leading to uremia.
2. Uremia predisposes patients to bleeding by inhibiting ADP, interfering with the production of von Willebrand factor (vWF), and interfering with platelet binding at the GPIIb-IIIa receptor.
3. Decreased fibrinolysis and increased coagulability are other resulting effects from uremia, leading to thrombogenesis.

DISCUSSION

Renal failure results in a decline in urine production and glomerular filtration. Patients can accumulate nitrogenous wastes such as urea in the blood, leading to uremia. Uremia has a deleterious effect on platelet function. Uremia can predispose patients in renal failure to bleeding through a variety of mechanisms. ADP is necessary for platelet aggregation. However, uremic patients accumulate guanidinosuccinic acid, which is a direct inhibitor of ADP, thereby resulting in decreased platelet aggregation. Accumulated metabolites may also interfere with the production of vWF. Decreased levels of vWF lead to decreased platelet adhesiveness. These metabolites may also interfere with platelet binding at the GPIIb-IIIa receptor, again leading to decreased platelet aggregation.

DDAVP can be used in uremic patients to increase platelet aggregation and adhesiveness. Administration of DDAVP causes release of vWF from endothelial cells, which can quickly improve platelet function.

Patients in renal failure have also been shown to be in a prothrombotic state. This is due to decreased fibrinolysis and increased coagulability in uremic patients. Activated platelets also release small vesicles with procoagulant activity, which contributes to this overall state and may be involved in clinical thrombogenesis.

SUGGESTED READINGS

Barash PG, Cullen BF, Stoelting RK, et al, eds. *Clinical Anesthesia*. 6th ed. Philadelphia, PA: Lippincott Williams & Wilkins; 2009:401–402.

Miller RD. *Miller's Anesthesia*. 6th ed. Philadelphia, PA: Elsevier, Churchill, and Livingstone; 2006:2238–2239.

Renal Failure: Relaxants

Organ-based Clinical: Renal/Urinary/Electrolytes

Adrianna Oprea

Edited by Ala Haddadin

KEY POINTS

1. Succinylcholine is safely used in patients with renal failure as long as the potassium is less than 5 at the moment of the induction.
2. The nondepolarizing muscle relaxants that can be used safely in renal failure are atracurium, cisatracurium, mivacurium, and rocuronium.
3. Atracurium and cisatracurium undergo Hofmann degradation, a process of spontaneous breakdown at body temperature and pH, as well as metabolism by nonspecific esterases in the plasma.

DISCUSSION

In renal disease, there are a number of factors that alter the pharmacokinetics and pharmacodynamics of the neuromuscular blocking drugs. These factors include reduced elimination of the drug, accumulation of active metabolites, altered fluid compartment size, and acid–base/electrolyte disturbances.

Depolarizing Neuromuscular Blockade

In renal failure, there is reduced plasma cholinesterase activity, and prolonged neuromuscular block following succinylcholine is possible. Succinylcholine administration results in a mild and transient increase in serum potassium concentration. In persons with normal renal function, the serum potassium increases by 0.5 to 1 mmol per L within 3 to 5 minutes of a dose and returns to normal after 10 to 15 minutes. Patients with chronic kidney disease do not demonstrate an exaggerated hyperkalemic response, and succinylcholine (1.5 mg per kg) can be used safely if the serum potassium concentration is less than 5 mEq per L at the time of induction.

Nondepolarizing Neuromuscular Blockade

In patients with chronic kidney disease, the initial dose of a nondepolarizing neuromuscular blocking drug is larger than in normal persons.

Benzylisoquinoliniums

The long-acting benzylisoquinoliniums, D-tubocurarine, metocurine, and doxacurium, are dependent on renal excretion for elimination. When given to patients with renal failure, they have a duration of action that is not only prolonged, but also considerably less predictable than in healthy patients. Atracurium, cisatracurium, and mivacurium all undergo breakdown in the plasma and can be safely used in renal failure.

The pharmacokinetics and pharmacodynamics of atracurium are not altered by chronic kidney disease. Atracurium undergoes Hofmann degradation, a process of spontaneous breakdown at body temperature and pH (45%), as well as metabolism by nonspecific esterases in the plasma (45%). Only about 10% of a bolus dose is excreted in the urine over 24 hours in healthy patients.

Owing to its stereochemistry, cisatracurium is metabolized mostly by Hofmann degradation (80%) and less by ester hydrolysis. About 15% of a bolus dose is excreted in the urine over 24 hours in healthy patients. In patients with renal failure, cisatracurium clearance is reduced by 13% and the terminal elimination half-life is prolonged by 4.2 minutes.

Mivacurium is metabolized by plasma cholinesterase and may accumulate in renal failure, but it is generally considered safe.

Aminosteroids

Pancuronium is excreted mainly in the urine (70%), although 35% undergoes hepatic metabolism with biliary excretion of the metabolites. The clearance of pancuronium is reduced and the half-life prolonged in patients with chronic kidney disease.

Vecuronium predominantly undergoes biliary excretion, although up to 30% may be excreted in the urine. Only a small fraction of the drug undergoes hepatic metabolism to 3-hydroxyvecuronium, which is active at the neuromuscular junction. In patients with renal failure, the elimination half-life is increased and the duration of action is prolonged.

The elimination of rocuronium depends mostly on biliary excretion of the unchanged drug, but up to 33% is excreted in the urine within 24 hours. A small fraction is metabolized in the liver, producing a metabolite with insignificant neuromuscular blocking activity. Although the clearance of rocuronium is reduced by 39% in renal failure, it is a suitable agent to use, especially in the setting of rapid sequence intubation in patients with hyperkalemia.

SUGGESTED READINGS

Barash PG, Cullen BF, Stoelting RK. *Clinical Anesthesia*. 5th ed. Philadelphia, PA: Lippincott Williams & Wilkins; 2006:426–436.

Morgan GE, Mikhail MS, Murray MJ. *Clinical Anesthesiology*. 4th ed. New York, NY: McGraw-Hill; 2005:205–226.

R

Renal Function: Periop Preservation

Organ-based Clinical: Renal/Urinary/ Electrolytes

Gabriel Pitta

Edited by Hossam Tantawy

1. Prevention of perioperative renal failure relies on a high-risk patient identification, optimization of overall renal function, and avoidance of nephrotoxins.
2. Preventative strategies as well as active interventions by the anesthesiologist are key in preserving perioperative renal function.

Renal failure is a source of grave morbidity and mortality in the perioperative period. Anesthesiologists should recognize patients at high risk for such failure, optimize overall renal function, and avoid nephrotoxins if possible to promote perioperative preservation of renal function.

Preventative strategies as well as active interventions by the anesthesiologist are key in preserving perioperative renal function. Preventative strategies include the optimization of intravascular volume, appropriate control of the blood pressure to avoid hypotension and hypertension, and assessment for optimization of any preexisting prerenal, renal, or postrenal conditions, which may antagonize perioperative renal preservation.

Interventions should be aimed at maintaining oxygen delivery and tubular blood flow. Intraoperatively, urine flow should be maintained greater than or equal to 0.5 mL/kg/h. Avoidance of hypoxemia, hypercarbia, and inappropriate cardiac output will aid in the maintaining of oxygen delivery to the kidneys. It should be noted that chronically hypertensive patients may require higher perfusion pressures than those with normal blood pressure, and this fact should be taken into consideration when planning to optimize renal perfusion perioperatively.

Procedures at higher risk for renal dysfunction include the following: procedures where intraabdominal pressure rises above 18 mm Hg, the use of cardiopulmonary bypass, and aortic cross clamping.

The use of loop diuretics, mannitol, calcium channel blockers, dopamine, fenoldopam, *N*-acetylcysteine, and atrial natriuretic peptide (ANP) has been studied in the preservation of renal function perioperatively. Although some studies have shown promise, none of the above drugs have been proven to prevent the development of renal failure. The preservation of renal function perioperatively can be best accomplished through preventative strategies and interventions designed to optimize volume, cardiac output, and renal perfusion.

Agarwal RC, Jain RK, Yadava A. Prevention of perioperative renal failure. *Indian J Anaesth*. 2008;52(1):38–43.

R

Renal Insufficiency: Dx

Organ-based Clinical: Renal/Urinary/Electrolytes

Margaret Rose

Edited by Ala Haddadin

KEY POINTS

1. Acute kidney injury (AKI) and chronic kidney disease (CKD) have been associated with increasing morbidity and mortality.
2. AKI is characterized by abrupt increase of serum creatinine greater than or equal to 1.5 to 2 times baseline, with a decrease in urine output to less than 0.5 mL/kg/h for over 6 hours.
3. CKD is diagnosed by decreased glomerular filtration rate (GFR) that persists for over 3 months.
4. Other markers of kidney damage are important, may occur within the setting of a normal GFR or creatinine, and include abnormal urine chemistries or sediment and abnormalities found on imaging. These must be further investigated, so that permanent kidney damage can be minimized.

DISCUSSION

Renal insufficiency or renal failure can be separated into *acute* or *chronic*.

Acute Kidney Injury

AKI occurs in patients both acutely and chronically ill, in a variety of settings, resulting from a wide variety of etiologies. Even small, short-term changes in serum creatinine have been associated with increasing morbidity and mortality.

The Acute Kidney Injury Network (AKIN) defines AKI as:

> An abrupt (within 48 hours) reduction in kidney function currently defined as an absolute increase in serum creatinine of >0.3 mg/dl (>25 micromole/L), a percentage increase of 50% or a reduction in urine output (documented oliguria of <0.5 ml/kg/hr for >6 hours).

The AKIN has further classified AKI into stages as explained in Table 1. AKI frequently occurs in the setting of CKD, necessitating the clinician to consider baseline serum creatinine percentage of increase, rather than absolute values.

Table 1. Staging system for AKI

Stage	Creatinine Criteria	Urine Output Criteria
1	Increase in serum creatinine of ≥0.3 mg/dL (≥26.4 μmol/L) or increase of ≥150%–200% (1.5 to 2-fold) above baseline	<0.5 mL/kg/h for >6 h
2	Increase in serum creatinine of >200%–300% (>2 to 3-fold) above baseline	<0.5 mL/kg/h for > 12 h
3	Increase in serum creatinine of >300% (>3–fold) above baseline, or serum creatinine ≥4.0 mg/dL (≥354 μmol/L) with an acute rise of ≥0.5 mg/dL (≥44 μmol/L)	<0.3 mL/kg/h × 24 h or anuria × 12 h

From Levin A, Warnock DG, Mehta RL, et al. Improving outcomes from acute kidney injury: report of an initiative. *Am J Kidney Dis.* 2007;50(1):1–4.

Chronic Kidney Disease

CKD is more loosely defined as "either kidney damage or decreased kidney function (decreased GFR) for 3 or more months."

The National Kidney Foundation recommends that the use of serum creatinine not be used solely to estimate renal function, because in the setting of decreased muscle mass (elderly, chronically ill), it cannot accurately represent renal function.

More specifically, GFR is considered to be the best measure of kidney function, despite disease state. GFR, however, varies according to age, sex, race, and body size, and must be calculated using these patient variables and measured serum creatinine. The Cockcroft-Gault* formula for creatinine clearance is generally used:

$$\text{Cr Cl} = \frac{(140 - \text{age}) \times \text{weight} \times (0.85 \text{ if female})}{72 \times P_{\text{Cr}}}$$

Age in years; weight in kg; P_{Cr} in mg per dL; Cr Cl in mL per minute.

Normal GFR for a young adult is 120 to 130 mL/min/1.73 m². This "normal" declines with age. Although this decline with age normally occurs, a decreased GFR in the elderly should not merely be attributed to age. A decrease of GFR is an independent predictor of adverse outcomes.

A GFR less than 60 mL/min/1.73 m² represents a loss of half of the normal kidney function. Below this, complications of kidney disease increase. Kidney failure occurs when the GFR declines below 15 mL/min/1.73 m² with signs of uremia, when dialysis is required.

Other markers of kidney damage are important, and may occur within the setting of a normal GFR. These include abnormal urine chemistries or sediment and abnormalities found on imaging. These findings are associated with adverse outcomes and progression of kidney disease, despite a normal GFR. Therefore, further evaluation is a requisite, since the finding may represent a progressive condition causing kidney damage.

SUGGESTED READINGS

Levey AS, Coresh J, Balk E, et al. National Kidney Foundation practice guidelines for chronic kidney disease: evaluation, classification, and stratification. *Ann Intern Med.* 2003;139(2):137–149.

Levin A, Warnock DG, Mehta RL, et al. Improving outcomes from acute kidney injury: report of an initiative. *Am J Kidney Dis.* 2007;50(1):1–4.

R

---

*Another formula the MDRD (Modification of Diet in Renal Disease) adds an adjustment of 1.2 for African Americans.

Renal Insufficiency: Hyperkalemia
Organ-based Clinical: Renal/Urinary/Electrolytes

Christian Scheps

Edited by Hossam Tantawy

1. Hyperkalemia is a common complication in patients with impaired renal function, which can lead to morbidity and even mortality in extreme cases.
2. Hyperkalemia has many etiologies and may result in patients with renal insufficiency secondary to alterations of potassium intake, intracellular release, and excretion.

DISCUSSION

Hyperkalemia is a common and serious cause of morbidity in patients with chronic renal insufficiency secondary to an inability to clear potassium from the circulation at a normal rate. Dangerous and even fatal levels of potassium can thus accumulate, leading to many untoward effects such as cardiac arrhythmia and arrest. The anesthesiologist must be acutely aware of this possible complication when caring for this growing population, as some commonly used anesthetic adjuncts derange the body's normal potassium levels.

For example, one must be extremely careful when administering succinylcholine to patients with renal insufficiency, as this can lead to increased serum potassium levels from intracellular release.

Many other factors can contribute to an increase in serum potassium, and it is best to organize them as aspects of potassium *intake*, *release*, and *excretion*.

- *Intake*. Patients with chronic renal insufficiency must be very careful regarding potassium intake. Certain foods, such as banana, spinach, and salt substitutes, contain high levels of potassium, and excessive intake of these foods can lead to increased potassium levels. In the hospitalized patient, care must again be taken by the patient and staff, as exogenous intake of potassium in the form of intravenous solution, potassium salts, and blood transfusion can have deleterious effects.
- *Intracellular release*. Many factors can contribute to increased intracellular potassium release. Metabolic derangements such as sepsis and metabolic acidosis can lead to severe augmentations in serum potassium. Medications such as beta-blockers, digoxin, and succinylcholine can all encourage release.
- *Excretion*. Patients with chronic renal insufficiency excrete potassium at a reduced rate, and outside factors can contribute to this and make the condition fatal. For example, a rapid drop in glomerular filtration rate in a patient with an already reduced rate can cause potassium levels to rise. Therefore, it is important to maintain baseline renal function in a patient whose filtration is already impaired. Medications can also lead to an increase in potassium excretion impairment. For example, angiotensin-converting enzyme inhibitors, potassium-sparing diuretics, and heparin can all lead to hyperkalemia when administered to a patient with chronic renal insufficiency.

SUGGESTED READING

Barash PG, Cullen BF, Stoelting RK, et al, eds. *Clinical Anesthesia*. 6th ed. Philadelphia, PA: Lippincott Williams & Wilkins; 2009:1019–1020.

R

Renal Replacement Rx Selection

Organ-based Clinical: Renal/ Urinary/ Electrolytes

Milaurise Cortes

Edited by Ala Haddadin

KEY POINTS

1. Renal replacement therapy (RRT) is used to treat patients with renal failure. The options available for RRT include hemodialysis (HD), peritoneal dialysis (PD), and renal transplant.
2. Dialysis can be used to treat fluid overload, clear toxins, and correct electrolyte abnormalities.
3. RRT can be intermittent, where 1 to 4 L are removed at one session, or continuous, in which fluids are removed slowly.
4. In general, continuous RRT is better tolerated in critically ill patients who cannot tolerate wide fluid shifts.
5. Patients on dialysis suffer from anemia, hypoalbuminemia, secondary hyperparathyroidism, and infection.

DISCUSSION

RRT is a supportive measure used to treat patients with renal failure. There are concerns for a patient's volume status, ability to clear toxins, and maintain electrolyte levels once a patient is diagnosed with renal failure. RRT may include HD, PD, and renal transplant.

The indications for the initiation of RRT include metabolic acidosis, electrolyte disturbances, intoxications, fluid overload, and uremia. However, the time course to initiate RRT is not clearly defined; RRT may be initiated before the blood urea nitrogen (BUN) levels reach levels consistent with acidemia. If the indications mentioned previously are not present, one can start RRT when BUN levels are 100 mg per dL and/or certain signs and symptoms manifest (depending on age), even if the above criteria are not met.

RRT can be further broken down into intermittent dialysis and continuous dialysis. Intermittent dialysis is the first treatment option available for patients with acute renal failure. However, in instances of hemodynamic instability, continuous dialysis is theoretically the best therapy because it is better tolerated by critically ill patients (especially those who are hypotensive). In addition, continuous regulation of fluid can help hyper- and hypovolemia, as continuous HD removes fluids slowly. On the other hand, intermittent HD removes 1 to 4 L of fluids typically within a few hours.

PD, such as continuous HD, is slow and continuous. The advantages of PD include a decrease in the risk of bleeding because anticoagulation is not used, providing the patient with the freedom to do dialysis at home, and its effectiveness with kids since needles are not used.

Long-term complications of patients with renal failure on RRT include anemia, hypoalbuminemia, secondary hyperparathyroidism, and infection.

SUGGESTED READINGS

Bajaj P. Renal replacement therapy [editorial]. *Indian J Anaesth.* 2008;52(6):753.

Barash PG, Cullen BF, Stoelting RK, et al, eds. *Clinical Anesthesia.* 6th ed. Philadelphia, PA: Lippincott Williams & Wilkins; 2009:1460.

Goldman L, Ausiello DA. *Cecil Medicine.* 23rd ed. Philadelphia, PA: Saunders; 2007:940–941.

Kellum JA, Angus DC, Johnson JP, et al. Continuous versus intermittent renal replacement therapy: a meta-analysis. *Intensive Care Med.* 2002;28(1):29–37.

Murray P, Hall J. Renal replacement therapy for acute renal failure. *Am J Respir Crit Care Med.* 2000;162(3): 777–781.

R

Renin–Angiotensin CV Physiology
Physiology

Laurie Yonemoto

Edited by Hossam Tantawy

KEY POINTS

1. The renin–angiotensin–aldosterone system (RAAS) regulates systemic vascular resistance and intravascular volume.
2. Renin release is stimulated by three factors: beta-1 receptor activation, a decrease in afferent arteriole pressure in the kidneys, and decreased sodium delivery to the distal tubules.
3. Angiotensin II causes direct vasoconstriction by stimulating angiotensin II receptors on blood vessels. It also stimulates the release of vasopressin and aldosterone.
4. Aldosterone increases intravascular volume by increasing sodium reabsorption and water retention.

DISCUSSION

The RAAS plays an integral part in regulating systemic vascular resistance and intravascular volume in the body, thus influencing arterial blood pressure and cardiac output. The first hormone of this system, renin, is a proteolytic enzyme stored primarily in the juxtaglomerular cells of the kidney. Release of renin is stimulated by three main influences: decreases in afferent arteriole pressure, sympathetic stimulation via beta-1 receptor activation, and decreases in sodium delivery to the distal tubules of the kidney (sensed by macula densa cells located adjacent to the juxtaglomerular cells). Renin then acts on the circulating plasma substrate, angiotensinogen, to form angiotensin I.

The next hormone in this system, angiotensin I, undergoes further transformation by angiotensin-converting enzyme (ACE) located in the vascular endothelium, especially the one located in the lungs, to the active hormone, angiotensin II. Angiotensin II has many functions, all of which serve to increase systemic vascular resistance and intravascular volume. Angiotensin II causes direct vasoconstriction by stimulating angiotensin II receptors on blood vessels, facilitates norepinephrine release from sympathetic nerve endings, and causes cardiac and vascular hypertrophy. Furthermore, angiotensin II stimulates the release of vasopressin from the posterior pituitary, thereby increasing fluid retention by the kidneys, and it also stimulates the release of aldosterone from the adrenal cortex. The final hormone of this system, aldosterone, serves to increase sodium reabsorption and water retention by the kidneys, resulting in increased intravascular volume.

ACE inhibitors, angiotensin II receptor blockers, and aldosterone receptor blockers are all used to treat hypertension and heart failure by blocking the key components in this pathway (Fig. 1).

R

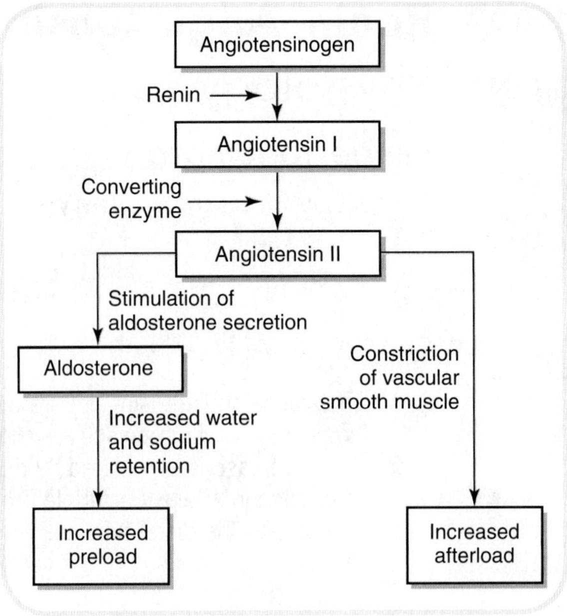

Figure 1. Renin Angiotensin Pathway (Images: http://www.gcrweb.com/HeartDSS/epicomp.htm.)

SUGGESTED READINGS

Barash PG, Cullen BF, Stoelting RK, et al, eds. *Clinical Anesthesia*. 6th ed. Philadelphia, PA: Lippincott Williams & Wilkins; 2009:343, 1348–1349.

Morgan GE, Mikhail MS, Murray MJ. *Clinical Anesthesiology*. 4th ed. New York, NY: McGraw Hill; 2006:675.

R

Rheumatoid Arthritis Complications

Generic, Clinical Sciences: Anesthesia Procedures, Methods, Techniques

Robert Schonberger

Edited by Jodi Sherman

KEY POINTS

1. Rheumatoid arthritis is a systemic disease, which affects nearly every organ system of the body.
2. A thorough airway examination with particular attention to neck mobility is crucial in patients with rheumatoid arthritis.
3. Coronary artery disease is more prevalent in patients with rheumatoid arthritis than in age-matched controls.
4. Interstitial lung disease is a common manifestation of rheumatoid arthritis.
5. Renal dysfunction may occur as a result of vasculitis as well as toxicity from therapeutic drugs for rheumatoid arthritis.

DISCUSSION

The most pressing problems for the anesthesiologist caring for a patient with rheumatoid arthritis generally occur during attempts to control the airway. Neck immobility may complicate attempts at intubation, and a careful assessment of airway flexibility as well as associated neurologic impairment is a critical element of the preoperative history and physical examination. Atlantooccipital subluxation is another common finding in rheumatoid arthritis and is assessed by radiologic examinations, particularly the lateral X-ray of the neck during neck flexion. If atlantooccipital subluxation or instability is present, neck movement should be minimized during airway management. Rheumatoid arthritis can also affect the cricoarytenoids, and their dislocation is possible during endotracheal intubation. This may present as hoarseness, pain on swallowing, laryngeal tenderness, and stridor.

Rheumatoid arthritis is a systemic disease, which causes potential functional impairment of organs, including the heart, lungs, and kidneys. For example, coronary artery disease is twice as common in patients with rheumatoid arthritis than in controls. The heart may also have valvular abnormalities as well as conduction abnormalities. A variety of lung pathologies may arise in patients with rheumatoid arthritis, but the most common is pleural effusion followed by interstitial lung disease. Renal disease may also develop in these patients, particularly as a result of nephrotoxic drug use such as gold or penicillamine. Systemic sequelae from rheumatoid arthritis should be familiar to anesthesiologists.

SUGGESTED READING

Hines R, Marschall KE, eds. *Stoelting's Anesthesia and Co-existing Disease.* 5th ed. Philadephia, PA: Elsevier; 2008:455–457.

R

Robotic Prostatectomy: Contraindications

Generic, Clinical Sciences: Anesthesia
Procedures, Methods, Techniques

James Shull
Edited by Ala Haddadin

KEY POINTS

1. Robotic prostatectomy is an increasingly popular method of prostate resection that may have unique advantages.
2. Most contraindications to robotic prostatectomy can be readily deduced through a general familiarity with the procedure.
3. Relative/absolute contraindications stem from the ability to tolerate positioning and abdominal insufflation.

DISCUSSION

Robotic-assisted prostatectomy is an increasingly popular technique for patients in need of a radical prostatectomy. In skilled hands, a robotic prostatectomy may result in less blood loss, postoperative pain, and improved return of urinary continence and sexual function.

Although there may be benefits to the robotic technique, it is of the utmost importance to carefully select suitable candidates to optimize patient outcome. Many of these contraindications can be easily deduced by considering the aspects of the surgery unique to this approach.

The first consideration is the steep Trendelenburg positioning in conjunction with insufflation of the abdomen with carbon dioxide. These conditions can cause undesirably elevated airway pressures in obese patients and in those with severe pulmonary disease. This positioning may also shift the blood volume so as to overload a failing heart, which would make this technique a poor choice for patients with significant congestive heart failure. Another subset of patients that may not tolerate Trendelenburg positioning are those with cerebral aneurysms or other intracranial pathology that cannot tolerate increased intracranial pressure.

Another consideration is the surgical technique itself. It is best suited for a contained surgical field in a precise area. For this reason, the technique is relatively contraindicated for patients with extensive previous abdominal surgeries, those with very large prostates, and those with widespread cancer.

SUGGESTED READING

Shah N, Kaul S, Menon M. Surgical robotics in urology: robotic assisted radical prostatectomy. *Oper Tech Gen Surg.* 2005;7(4):201–208.

Root Cause Anal: Essential Elements

Generic Clinical Sciences: Anesthesia Procedures, Methods, Techniques

Tomalika Ahsan-Paik

Edited by Raj K. Modak

KEY POINTS

1. Root cause analysis (RCA) is a retrospective analysis of a problem that attempts to identify the root cause of a problem with the goal that correcting the root cause of the problem is the optimal approach of solving the problem itself.
2. The approach to root cause involves identifying the defects in the system that result in errors as opposed to the people involved in the system.
3. The most critical flaw should be corrected to prevent recurrences (also known as the 100-year fix).
4. The solutions should be subsequently implemented, and further data collection should occur to ensure effectiveness.

DISCUSSION

RCA is a retrospective analysis of a problem that attempts to identify the root cause of a problem with the goal that correcting the root cause of the problem is the optimal approach of solving the problem itself. RCA is the preferred approach, since identifying and subsequently correcting the root cause should decrease the recurrence of the original problem as opposed to correcting the consequential symptom, which does not address the original problem. RCA is a tool for continuous improvement. The traditional applications of RCA are resolution of customers and complaints, disposition of nonconforming material, and corrective action plans resulting from internal audits.

The approach to root cause involves identifying the defects in the system that result in errors as opposed to the people involved in the system. The root cause can be identified by "asking why a problem occurred" repeatedly until the fundamental flaw in the process is determined. Subsequently, the most critical flaw should be corrected to prevent recurrences (also known as the 100-year fix). RCA involves a systemic investigation into the sequence of events to determine the causal relationship between individual events.

The five basic classes of RCA are safety based, originating from accident analysis, occupational safety, and health; production based, originating from quality control; process based, mostly used for business process; failure based, which focuses on failure analysis used in the field of engineering; and system based, which originated from ideas combined from fields of risk management, change management, and system analysis.

To perform an RCA, one must first define the problem and gather data and evidence. Subsequently, the "why?" should be repeatedly asked until the corrective action(s) that will prevent recurrence of the problem is ascertained (the "100-year fix"). Ultimately, these solutions should be implemented and further data collection should occur to ensure effectiveness (see Fig. 1).

R

500

Problem: the washing machine does not work—Machine makes loud noise while washing the fourth load

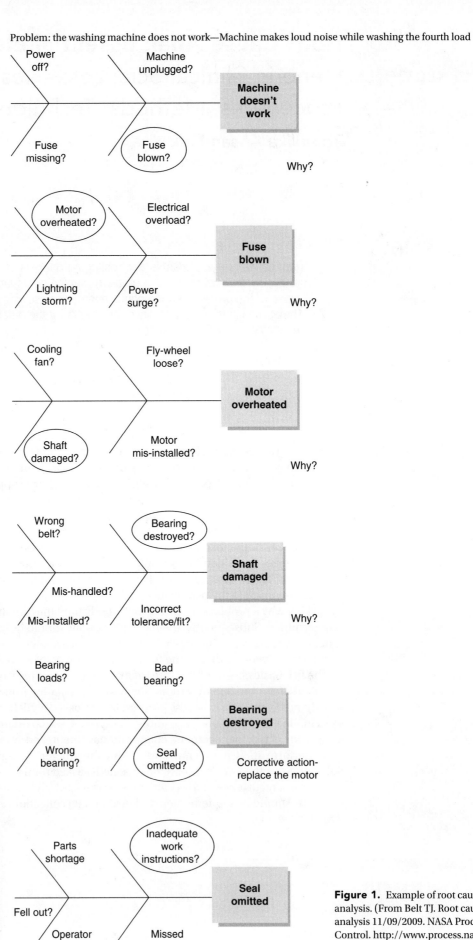

Figure 1. Example of root cause analysis. (From Belt TJ. Root cause analysis 11/09/2009. NASA Process Control. http://www.process.nasa.gov/documents/RootCauseAnalysis, with permission.)

So, the root cause was concluded to be inappropriate instructions.

501

The tools used in RCA include brainstorming, Pareto chart, fishbone diagram, run and flow chart, histogram, control chart, scatter diagram, and tree diagram (see Fig. 2).

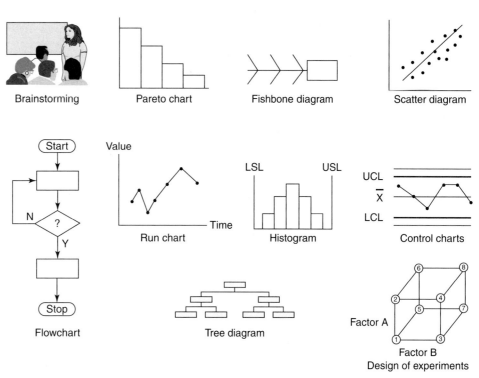

Figure 2. Techniques used in RCA. (From http://aacesubajou.wordpress.com/2011/04/03/w2_swastioko-budhi_-conducting-a-root-cause-analysis-in-project-management-division/, with permission.)

Belt TJ. Root cause analysis 11/09/2009. NASA Process Control. http://www.process.nasa.gov/documents/RootCauseAnalysis.

http://aacesubajou.wordpress.com/2011/04/03/w2_swastioko-budhi_-conducting-a-root-cause-analysis-in-project-management-division/

Rx: Antithrombin III Deficiency
Organ-based Clinical: Hematologic

Dmitri Souzdalnitski

Edited by Benjamin Sherman

1. Antithrombin III is an important hematologic factor involved in prevention of clot formation both in healthy vessels and in impaired vessels undergoing active bleeding.
2. Thrombophilia due to decreased antithrombin III is congenital, being an autosomal dominant trait.
3. Pregnant women with antithrombin III deficiency should be anticoagulated during pregnancy.
4. Heparin resistance can be a manifestation of reduced blood concentrations of antithrombin III.
5. Delivery of fresh-frozen plasma can restore antithrombin III concentrations, reducing heparin resistance.

Antithrombin III is an important hematologic factor in the coagulation cascade, responsible for preventing clot formation within the blood stream of both healthy vessels and pathologic vessels undergoing active bleeding.

Deficiency of antithrombin III is an autosomal dominant trait with a frequency reported to be between 1 in 1,000 and 1 in 5,000 patients. Although those with the deficiency are up to 20 times more likely to have a venous thromboembolism than someone without it, the deficiency is often clinically silent until a venous thromboembolism occurs, usually in conjunction with another risk factor of hypercoagulability.

Anesthetic considerations include standard thrombosis prophylaxis perioperatively (compression boots intraoperatively). Discussion should be had with the surgeons regarding the patient's perioperative pharmacologic interventions, whether at baseline or given by the primary team at the time of surgery. It should be noted that pregnant women should be anticoagulated throughout the duration of their pregnancy, and this should be considered before the use of neuraxial analgesia in the labor setting.

In cardiac and vascular procedures where heparin is used for anticoagulation, antithrombin III deficiency is manifested by low concentrations of the substance, which, in turn, can cause heparin resistance. This is commonly associated with patients with nephrotic syndrome, where the antithrombin III is lost via the kidneys through proteinuria. Careful checking of the Activated Clotting Time (ACT) before initiation of cardiopulmonary bypass should be kept in mind. In these patients, the heparin sensitivity can be reestablished by the delivery of fresh-frozen plasma, which has antithrombin III molecules.

Hines RL, Marschall KE, eds. *Stoelting's Anesthesia and Co-existing Disease.* 5th ed. Philadelphia, PA: Churchill Livingstone; 2002:430–433.

Saline: Hyperchloremic Acidosis

Physiology

Stephanie Cheng

Edited by Ala Haddadin

KEY POINTS

1. Metabolic acidosis can be categorized as being either an anion gap or a nonanion gap metabolic acidosis.
2. Administration of normal saline in excess of 30 mL per kg is one of the most common causes of hyperchloremic metabolic acidosis.
3. Treatment of hyperchloremic metabolic acidosis includes mechanical ventilation and sodium bicarbonate administration in certain situations.

DISCUSSION

Metabolic acidosis occurs when the body's pH falls below 7.35 as a result of accumulating acids other than CO_2. There are two types of metabolic acidosis, which is determined on the basis of the anion gap. The anion gap is calculated by taking the sum of chloride and HCO_3 anions and subtracting the total from sodium cations. This results in the concentration of other anions in the serum, primarily albumin anions, usually falling between 3 and 11 mEq per L. The presence of a high anion gap indicates acidosis secondary to increased unmeasured anions such as lactic acidosis or ketoacidosis. A nonanion gap metabolic acidosis indicates bicarbonate wasting from either the kidneys (renal tubular acidosis) or the gastrointestinal (GI) tract (diarrhea).

One such mechanism for nonanion gap metabolic acidosis is the infusion of normal saline in excess of 30 mL/kg/h. As a result of the law of mass action, excessive chloride in the body impairs reabsorption of bicarbonate by the kidneys.

Similar to other types of metabolic acidosis, hyperchloremic acidosis causes the body to compensate by hyperventilation in an attempt to increase CO_2 elimination. In healthy patients, hyperchloremic acidosis secondary to saline infusion usually requires no treatment. If, however, the patient does not have the capability of physically compensating for the acidosis (the equivalent of respiratory acidosis), there are a number of treatment strategies. If the patient is truly unable to ventilate appropriately by himself or herself, it may be necessary to provide extracorporeal support. The patient may need to be intubated and minute ventilation increased until underlying causes can be fixed. Bicarbonate administration is recommended in settings of metabolic acidosis causing pH <7.1. This treatment should only be given to patients who are able to ventilate adequately, because bicarbonate administration generates increased CO_2 in the body and will worsen the acidosis if patient is unable to eliminate it. Dosing of HCO_3 is as follows:

$$\text{Weight (kg)} \times (24 - \text{plasma } HCO_3) \times (0.3) = NaHCO_3 \text{ dose}$$

Only half of the calculated dose is administered initially, followed by measurement of pH to evaluate effect. Administration of $NaHCO_3$ remains controversial, as there is limited evidence of clinical improvement.

SUGGESTED READINGS

Barash PG, Cullen BF, Stoelting RK, et al, eds. *Clinical Anesthesia*. 6th ed. Philadelphia, PA: Lippincott Williams & Wilkins; 2009:290–296.

Miller RD, Stoelting RK. *Basics of Anesthesia*. 5th ed. Philadelphia, PA: Churchill Livingstone; 2007:317–323.

Scheingraber S, Rehm M, Sehmisch C, et al. Rapid saline infusion produces hyperchloremic acidosis in patients undergoing gynecologic surgery. *Anesthesiology*. 1999;90:1265–1270.

SBE Prophylaxis

Pharmacology

Michael Tom

Edited by Benjamin Sherman

1. The indications for antibiotic prophylaxis to prevent infective endocarditis have dramatically decreased from previous recommendations.
2. Prophylaxis is reserved for only high-risk patients undergoing dental or invasive respiratory tract procedures that require incision or biopsy.
3. High-risk patients are defined as those with:
   a. prosthetic heart valves including bioprosthetic and homograft valves;
   b. prosthetic material used for cardiac valve repair;
   c. a prior history of infective endocarditis;
   d. unrepaired cyanotic congenital heart disease including palliative shunts and conduits;
   e. completely repaired congenital heart defects, within 6 months, that utilize prosthetic materials or a device, either through surgery or through a catheter intervention;
   f. incomplete congenital repairs with residual defects close to prosthetic materials;
   g. cardiac transplant with a valvulopathy.
4. Prophylaxis is not recommended for gastrointestinal (GI) or genitourinary (GU) tract procedures unless active infection is suspected.
5. The choice of antibiotic for prophylaxis has not changed from previous recommendations.

In 2007, a significant change in the Guidelines for the Prevention of Infective Endocarditis occurred. The new recommendations reduced the indications for antibiotic prophylaxis for endocarditis. These recommendations are based on data that suggest infective endo-carditis is more likely to result from exposure to bacteremia associated with daily activities, rather than with dental, GI, or GU procedures.

Endocarditis prophylaxis may prevent an extremely small number of cases of endocarditis in high-risk patients. The benefits of routine use of endocarditis prophylaxis do not exceed the risks of antibiotic-associated adverse events and the promotion of antibiotic-resistant organisms. The American Heart Association narrowed down the patients at high risk for developing severe forms and complications of endocarditis, and has recommended that only these patients should receive endocarditis prophylaxis (Table 1). In addition to dental procedures, prophylaxis is recommended for invasive procedures of the respiratory tract and infected skin, skin structures, or musculoskeletal tissue. Antibiotic prophylaxis is not recommended for GI or GU tract procedures unless active infection is suspected. For patients who meet those criteria, the antibiotics to use are not different from previous recommendations, and are listed in Table 2.

S

Table 1. Cardiac Conditions Associated with the Highest Risk of Adverse Outcomes from Endocarditis for Which Prophylaxis for Dental Procedures is Reasonable

1. Prosthetic cardiac valve or prosthetic material used for cardiac valve repair
2. Previous infective endocarditis
3. Congenital heart disease:
   Unrepaired cyanotic congenital heart disease, including palliative shunts and conduits
   Completely repaired congenial heart defect with prosthetic material or device, whether placed by surgery or by catheter intervention, during the first 6 mo after the procedure[a]
   Repaired congenital heart disease with residual defects at the site or adjacent to the site of a prosthetic patch or prosthetic device (which inhibit endothelialization)
4. Cardiac transplantation recipients who develop cardiac valvulopathy

Except for the conditions listed above antibiotic prophylaxis is no longer recommened for any other of congenital heart disease.
[a]Prophylaxis is reasonable because endothelialization of prosthetic material occurs within 6 months after the procedure.
From Wilson W, Taubert KA, Gewitz M, et al. Prevention of infective endocarditis. Guideliness from the American Heart Association. *Circulation.* 2007;116:1736–1754, with permission.

Table 2. Antibiotic Prophylaxis Regiments for a Dental Procedure

Situation	Agent	Regimen: Single Dose 30 to 60 min before Procedure	
		Adults	**Children**
Oral	Amoxicillin	2 g	50 mg/kg
Unable to take oral medition	Ampicillin OR cefazion or ceftriaxone	2 g	50 mg/kg
Allergic to penicillins or ampicillin—oral	Cephatexin[-1]	2 g	50 mg/kg
	OR Clindamycin[-1]	600 mg	20 mg/kg
	OR Azithromycin or cianthromycin	500 mg	15 mg/kg
Allergic to penicillins or ampicillin and unable to take oral medication	Cefazolin or ceftriaxone*	1 g IM or IV	50 mg/kg IM or IV
	OR Clindamycin	600 mg IM or IV	20 mg/kg Im or IV

[a]Or other first or second generation oral cephalosporin in equivalent adult or a pediatric dosage.
[b]Cephalosporins should not be used in an individual with a history of anaphylaxis, or urticaria with penicillins or ampicillins.
From Wilson W, Taubert KA, Gewitz M, et al. Prevention of infective endocarditis. Guideliness from the American Heart Association. *Circulation.* 2007;116:1736–1754, with permission.

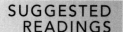

SUGGESTED READINGS

Hines RL, Marschall KE, eds. *Stoelting's Anesthesia and Co-existing Disease.* 5th ed. Philadelphia, PA: Churchill Livingstone; 2002:30–31.

Wilson W, Taubert KA, Gewitz M, et al. Prevention of infective endocarditis. Guideliness from the American Heart Association. *Circulation.* 2002;116:1726–1754.

S

SE vs. SD calculation
Mathematics, Statistics, Computers

Milaurise Cortes
Edited by Raj K. Modak

KEY POINTS

1. Standard deviation is the variation of data from the mean or average.
2. The standard error measures the ambiguity in a sample statistic. It indicates the uncertainty in a mean value from a sample as an estimate of the mean value of a population.
3. Standard error is calculated by dividing standard deviation by the square root of the sample size. Therefore, the larger the sample size, the smaller the standard error.

DISCUSSION

Standard deviation is the variation of data from the mean or average. A low standard deviation would indicate that the various data values are close to the value of the mean, while a high standard deviation would indicate that the data values range far from the value of the mean. In other words, standard deviation measures the spread of distribution. Standard deviations are often used when studying normal distributions.

The standard error measures the ambiguity in a sample statistic. Essentially, it indicates the uncertainty in a mean value from a sample as an estimate of the mean value of a population. Standard error is calculated by dividing standard deviation by the square root of the sample size. Therefore, the larger the sample size, the smaller the standard error.

Standard deviation is useful when one is studying the variation between individuals, and standard error is useful when one is studying summary statistics, that is, means and differences. Standard error is also useful when used to help produce confidence intervals.

$$\sigma = \sqrt{\frac{\sum\left(\bar{x} - x\right)^2}{n-1}}$$

where σ = standard deviation, $\sum$ = sum, $\bar{x}$ = average of the data, x = individual data point, n = sample size.

$$S = \frac{\sigma}{\sqrt{n}}$$

where S = standard error, σ = standard deviation, n = sample size.

SUGGESTED READINGS

Altman DA, et al. *Statistics with Confidence: Confidence Intervals and Statistical Guidelines*. 2nd ed. BMJ Books; 2000:25.
Barash PG, et al. *Clinical Anesthesia*. 6th ed. Philadelphia, PA: Lippincott Williams & Wilkins; 2009:196,199.
Coggon D. *Statistics in Clinical Practice*. 2nd ed. BMJ Books; 2003:16.

Septic Shock: Vasopressin Rx

General Clinical Sciences: Anesthesia Procedures, Methods, Techniques

Mary DiMiceli

Edited by Hossam Tantawy

KEY POINTS

1. In septic shock, early goal-directed therapy has been shown to reduce morbidity and mortality. Important end points include central venous pressure (CVP) 8 to 12 mm Hg, mean arterial pressure (MAP) $\geq$65 mmHS, and mixed venous oxygen saturation (SvO$_2$) $\geq$70%.
2. If hypotension is refractory to fluid resuscitation, inotropic/vasopressor medications must be initiated.
3. Recent arguments propose use of vasopressin given its deficient state in patients in septic shock.
4. Vasopressin works on V1 receptors on vascular smooth muscle to cause not only vasoconstriction, and therefore resulting in increased MAP, but also decreased cardiac output.

DISCUSSION

The systemic inflammatory response syndrome (SIRS) is the body's response to systemic inflammation, including a febrile response and leukocytosis. The criteria involved in diagnosing SIRS require at least two of the following: (1) fever greater than 38.0° C or less than 36.0° C, (2) heart rate greater than 90 beats per minute, (3) respiratory rate greater than 20 breaths per minute or PaCO$_2$ less than 32 mm Hg, and (4) WBC greater than 12,000 per mm^3, less than 4,000 per mm^3, or greater than 10% immature (band) forms. Sepsis is the condition characterized by SIRS, which is secondary to an infection. A patient is said to have severe sepsis when there is organ dysfunction of one or more vital organs, which can progress to septic shock that requires vasopressors to maintain arterial blood pressure (BP).

Early goal-directed therapy is geared toward making adjustments in resuscitation end points, that is, afterload, preload, and contractility (CVP 8 to 12 mm Hg, MAP $\geq$65 mmHS, but $\leq$90 mm Hg, and SvO$_2$ $\geq$70%) to affect oxygen delivery and demand. Treatment includes control of infection with early initiation of antibiotic therapy and source control, fluid resuscitation to achieve aforementioned end points to indicate adequate perfusion or early initiation of vasopressor support if persistent hypotension, and finally supportive treatment of any complications secondary to organ failure.

It is important to stress that one of the main components to treating septic shock is early management of hypotension by initially treating with fluid replacement to achieve MAP greater than 65 mm Hg to improve tissue and end-organ perfusion. If hypotension is recalcitrant to fluid resuscitation (if not corrected after approximately 3 L of fluids), an inotrope/vasopressor, such as norepinephrine, dopamine, epinephrine, or vasopressin, should be used. Choice of the infusion should be individualized depending on the hemodynamic parameters.

Vasopressin is a peptide hormone, related to oxytocin, which is synthesized in the hypothalamus and stored and released by the pituitary gland. It has both vasopressor and antidiuretic effects by binding to V1 receptors on vascular smooth muscle and V2 receptors in the kidney, respectively. In many recent studies, the role of vasopressin in septic shock has been discussed, but typically has been used in cases of hypotension refractory to dopamine or norepinephrine. Endogenous levels are decreased in shock state. Therefore, the theory behind using vasopressin as the initial vasopressor of choice is that it serves as a replacement for the endogenously deficient levels in patients with septic shock.

508

In addition, because levels are deficient, V1 receptors exhibit increased sensitivity to vasopressor effect when exposed to exogenous vasopressin. Vasopressin mainly acts as a vasoconstrictor at the V1 receptors, ultimately resulting in increased BP, MAP, organ perfusion, and neurologic function, with the undesired effect of decreasing cardiac output. As a result, it must be used in caution with heart failure patients. It is given at a rate of 0.01 to 0.04 units per minute intravenously. Adding vasopressin to norepinephrine infusion could result in decreasing the level of norepinephrine infusion.

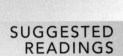

Howland RD, Mycek MJ. *Pharmacology*. 3rd ed. Philadelphia, PA: Lippincott Williams & Wilkins; 2006:276–277.

Marino PL. Infection, inflammation and multiorgan injury.In:*The ICU book*. 3rd ed. Philadelphia, PA: Lippincott Williams & Wilkins; 1998:737–743.

Morgan GE Jr, Mikhail MS, Murray MJ. *Clinical Anesthesiology*. 4th ed. New York, NY: Lange Medical books/ McGraw Hill; 2006:1051–1057.

Rivers E, Nguyen B, Havstad S, et al. Early goal-directed therapy in the treatment of severe sepsis and septic shock. *N Engl J Med*. 2001;345:1368–1377.

Russell JA, Walley KR, Singer J, et al. Vasopressin versus norepinephrine infusion in patients with septic shock. *N Engl J Med*. 2008;358:877–887.

Stoelting RK, Miller RD, eds. *Basics of Anesthesia*. 5th ed. Philadelphia, PA: Churchill Livingstone; 2007:605.

S

Shunt: Effect of Increased FiO$_2$
Organ-based Clinical: Respiratory

Francis vanWisse

Edited by Veronica Matei

Francis vanWisse

Edited by Veronica Matei

KEY POINTS

1. The normal ventilation to perfusion ratio (V/Q) is 0.8.
2. The shunt effect occurs when V/Q is less than 1, but greater than 0.
3. True shunts (V/Q = 0) represent perfused but not ventilated alveolar capillary segments.
4. There are three types of shunts: physiologic, postpulmonary, and pathoanatomic.
5. The oxygen challenge test can be used to differentiate refractory shunts from those responding to oxygen.

DISCUSSION

The normal V/Q ratio is 0.8. The shunt effect occurs when V/Q is less than 1, but greater than 0. True shunts (V/Q = 0) represent perfusion without ventilation. There are three types of shunts: physiologic (atelectasis/consolidation of alveoli), postpulmonary (secondary to bronchial, mediastinal, pleural, and thebesian veins), and pathoanatomic (congenital or traumatic anomalies and intrapulmonary tumors). Significant shunts are between 20% and 30% of cardiac output with fatal shunts being greater than 30%.

Denitrogenation associated with Fraction of inspired oxygen (FIO$_2$) of 1.0 increases Partial Pressure of Alveolar Oxygen (PAO$_2$) in the underventilated alveolus to ensure saturated Hgb, thus correcting hypoxemia. The lower the V/Q ratio, the higher the required FIO$_2$ to correct the associated hypoxemia. Hypoxemia from shunt effect responds to O$_2$ therapy as long as blood is exposed to alveolar gas.

A true shunt (V/Q = 0) does not have blood exposed to alveolar gas, and thus will not respond to increases in FIO$_2$. One can consider a shunt refractory to oxygen with an arterial blood gas (ABG) showing PaO$_2$ less than 55 mm Hg and FIO$_2$ greater than 0.35. A simple test to differentiate refractory shunts from those responding to oxygen is to follow the oxygen challenge test. This consists of obtaining a baseline ABG, increasing the FIO$_2$ by 0.2, repeating the ABG in 30 minutes, and comparing the PaO$_2$. If the PaO$_2$ has increased by greater than 10 mm Hg from baseline, the hypoxemia is responsive to oxygen.

SUGGESTED READING

Morgan GE, Mikhail MS, Murray MJ. Respiratory physiology: the effects of anesthesia. In: *Clinical Anesthesiology*. 4th ed. New York, NY: McGraw-Hill; 2005:555.

S

SIADH: Lab Values

Organ-based Clinical: Endocrine/Metabolic

Alexey Dyachkov

Edited by Mamatha Punjala

1. Diagnostic criteria of syndrome of inappropriate antidiuretic hormone secretion (SIADH) include plasma hypoosmolality (<270 mOsm per L), inappropriately elevated urine osmolality relative to plasma and urinary sodium excretion (>20 mEq per L), and clinical euvolemia with hyponatremia (serum sodium <130 mEq per L).
2. Supportive criteria for diagnosis of SIADH include inappropriately low uric acid and plasma vasopressin levels.

In SIADH, the main laboratory value is an inappropriate value of antidiuretic hormone (ADH) compared with plasma osmolality. In order to be diagnostic, the ADH level must be assessed in conjunction with plasma hypoosmolality. It is interesting to note that 10% to 20% of patients fulfilling other criteria of SIADH, in fact, have an appropriate level of ADH.

The first of the diagnostic criteria for SIADH is the presence of true plasma hypoosmolality less than 275 mmol/L. Normal values are 280 to 295 mmol/L, calculated either directly or indirectly using the following formula:

$$\text{Plasma osmolality (mmol/L)} = 2 \times [Na^+] \text{ (mEq per L)} + \text{glucose (mg per dL)}/18 + \text{BUN (mg per dL)}/2.8$$

Causes of "false" hypoosmolality, such as pseudohyponatremia (produced by marked elevations of either lipids or proteins, occupying larger proportion of plasma volume, leading to artifactual decrease in $[Na^+]$, measured by flame photometry) or hyperglycemia (an osmotic shift of water from intracellular fluid to extracellular fluid, which in turn produces a dilutional decrease in serum $[Na^+]$), must be excluded. When the plasma contains significant amounts of unmeasured solutes, such as osmotic diuretics, radiographic contrast agents, and some toxins (ethanol, methanol, and ethylene glycol), plasma osmolality cannot be calculated accurately. In these situations, osmolality must be obtained by direct measurement.

Another criterion for SIADH is urine osmolality inappropriate for plasma osmolality. This means that urine osmolality must be greater than *maximally* dilute (maximal dilution in normal adults is > 100 mOsm per kg H_2O). Also, urine osmolality need not be elevated inappropriately at all levels of plasma osmolality, because in the reset osmostat variant form of SIADH, vasopressin secretion can be suppressed with resultant maximal urinary dilution if plasma osmolality is decreased to sufficiently low levels.

Other diagnostic criteria include clinical euvolemia and elevated urinary sodium excretion while on a normal salt and water intake. Patients with SIADH can have low urine Na^+ excretion if they subsequently become hypovolemic or solute depleted, conditions that sometimes follow severe salt and water restriction. It is also important to note an absence of other potential causes of euvolemic hypoosmolality: hypothyroidism, hypocortisolism (Addison's disease or pituitary adrenocorticotropic hormone insufficiency), and diuretic use.

Some supportive criteria include low uric acid and plasma vasopressin levels. Volume expansion and vasopressin acting on V1 receptors in the kidney increase the clearance of uric acid, so hypouricemia is found with SIADH. When patients are hyponatremic, values of uric acid are reported to be less than 4 mg per dL (< 0.24 mmol per L).

Patients with SIADH generally require only fluid restriction. Very rarely is hypertonic saline needed for the treatment of SIADH.

SUGGESTED READINGS

Becker KL, Kahn CR, Rebar RW, eds. *Principles and Practice of Endocrinology and Metabolism*. Philadelphia, PA: Lippincott Williams & Wilkins; 2002:297–306.

Kronenberg HM, Melmed S, Polonsky KS, et al, eds. *Williams Textbook of Endocrinology*. 11th ed. Philadelphia, PA: Saunders Elsevier; 2008:275–285.

S

Side Effects of Tocolytics
Subspecialties: Obstetric Anesthesia

Jeffrey Widelitz

Edited by Lars Helgeson

1. Commonly used tocolytic medications include terbutaline and ritodrine (β^2 agonists), magnesium sulfate, calcium channel blockers, and indomethacin.
2. The side-effect profiles of tocolytics are attributed to their pharmacologic class and their effects on maternal and fetal physiology.

Terbutaline

- *Maternal side effects*: Cardiac arrhythmias, pulmonary edema, myocardial ischemia, hypotension, tachycardia, anxiety.
- *Fetal and neonatal side effects*: Fetal tachycardia, hyperinsulinemia, hypoglycemia, myocardial and septal hypertrophy, myocardial ischemia.

Ritodrine

- *Maternal side effects*: Metabolic hyperglycemia, hyperinsulinemia, hypokalemia, antidiuresis, altered thyroid function, physiologic tremor, palpitations, nervousness, nausea or vomiting, fever, hallucinations.
- *Fetal and neonatal side effects*: Tachycardia, hypoglycemia, hypocalcemia, hyperbilirubinemia, hypotension, intraventricular hemorrhage.

Magnesium Sulfate

- *Maternal side effects*: Flushing, lethargy, headache, muscle weakness, diplopia, dry mouth, pulmonary edema, cardiac arrest. Increased sensitivity to neuromuscular blocking agents and decreased MAC.
- *Fetal and neonatal side effects*: Lethargy, hypotonia, respiratory depression, bone demineralization with prolonged use.

Calcium Channel Blockers

- *Maternal side effects*: Flushing, headache, dizziness, nausea, transient hypotension. Caution should be exercised in patients with renal disease and hypotension. In addition, concomitant use with magnesium sulfate can result in cardiovascular collapse. Cardiovascular depression is enhanced with volatile anesthetics, but can lead to postpartum uterine atony, which is unresponsive to prostaglandins and oxytocin.
- *Fetal and neonatal side effects*: Heart block, acidosis.

Indomethacin

- *Maternal side effects*: Nausea, heartburn, upper gastrointestinal bleeding, renal injury.
- *Fetal and neonatal side effects*: Constriction of the ductus arteriosus, pulmonary hypertension, reversible decrease in renal function in presence of oligohydramnios, intraventricular hemorrhage, hyperbilirubinemia, necrotizing enterocolitis.

Note: Combining tocolytic drugs potentially increases maternal morbidity and should be used with caution.

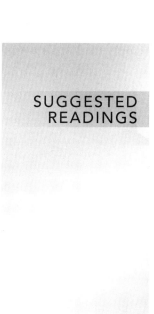

SUGGESTED READINGS

American College of Obstetricians and Gynecologists (ACOG). *Management of Preterm Labor*. Washington, DC; 2003:9 (ACOG Practice Bulletin; No. 43).

Datta S. *Obstetric Anesthesia Handbook*. 4th ed. New York, NY: Springer Science+Business Media, Inc; 2006: 270–273.

S

Sitting Position: BP Measurement
Organ-based Clinical: Neurologic and Neuromuscular

Johnny Garriga
Edited by Ramachandran Ramani

1. There are significant changes in hemodynamics in the sitting compared with the supine position.
2. Accurate and reliable measurements of blood pressure (BP) are imperative, and therefore, intraarterial invasive BP monitoring is usually employed, with the transducer flushed free of air and zeroed at the level of the mastoid process.

Positioning in surgery is critical depending on the procedure. From performing operations in the supine position to having patients in the prone position, positioning is often decided on the basis of the anatomical exposure of the operation. An unusual position that is used often in neurosurgical procedures involving posterior fossa is the sitting position. There are several explanations for the rationale of this particular position. Not only does it give the surgeon optimal access to the surgical site, but the operative surgical site is also elevated above the level of the heart, thus decreasing cerebral blood flow and the venous pressure, thereby decreasing the bleeding during surgery. The sitting position also affords advantages to the anesthesiologist. Diaphragmatic excursion is unhindered, making ventilation easier. The position also affords easier access to the endotracheal tube and airway, access to the chest wall if resuscitative measures are necessary, and the ability to monitor cranial nerves considering the unobstructed view of the face as shown in Figure 1.

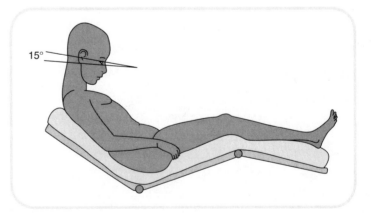

Figure 1. Sitting position

However, there are inherent disadvantages to the sitting position. The changes in position cause many hemodynamic changes. More specifically, gravity and anesthetic agents affect the cardiovascular function. In healthy adult patients, stroke volume and cardiac output are decreased by approximately 12% to 20% and cerebral perfusion pressure reduces by 15%, with minimal change in heart rate in the sitting position. Because of the hemodynamic instability, it is important to accurately measure the BP. When measuring BP, there tends to be differences in the values between the sitting versus the supine position. It is widely known that diastolic pressure measured while sitting is higher than when measured supine (by approximately 5 mm Hg). However, there is less agreement about the changes found in systolic pressures (some say it is 8 mm Hg higher in the supine than in the sitting position).

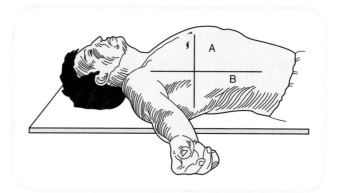

Figure 2. Phlebostatic Axis

By convention, BP measurement is carried out, so that the cuff or the arterial line transducer is at the level of the right atrium in both positions. This is where blood measurements are to be leveled and zeroed, in the case of the arterial line. This is accomplished by aligning the stopcock on top of the transducer (the air–fluid interface of the monitoring system) with the phlebostatic axis, essentially the anatomical reference on the chest that reflects the right atrium of the heart. This is usually found by drawing vertical line out from the fourth intercostal space at the sternum and a horizontal line drawn through the midpoint of the intercostal space and the midaxillary line as shown in Figure 2.

Accurate and reliable BP is absolutely critical in the sitting position. In the sitting position, because of the effect of gravity, the perfusion pressure in the brain is lower than the pressure measured at the level of the heart. For every 2.5 cm increase in height, there is a 2 mm per Hg drop in arterial pressure. If the head is 20 cm above the heart, the arterial perfusion pressure in the brain would be 16 mm Hg lower than what is recorded at the level of the heart (fourth intercostal space). Hence, it is recommended that the arterial pressure transducer should be positioned at the level of the mastoid process (level of the circle of Willis) during sitting position surgery. Similarly in beach chair position surgery for shoulder, arterial pressure should be measured at the level of the mastoid process (cerebral perfusion pressure).

SUGGESTED READINGS

Gottlieb JD, Ericsson JA, Sweet RB. Venous air embolism: a review. *Anesth Analg.* 1965;44:773–779.

Marshall WK, Bedford RF, Miller ED. Cardiovascular responses in the seated position—impact of four anesthetic techniques. *Anesth Analg.* 1983;62:648–653.

Matjasko J, Petrozza P, Cohen M, et al. Anesthesia and surgery in the seated position: analysis of 554 cases. *Neurosurgery.* 1985;17:695–702.

Winsor T, Burch GE. Phlebostatic axis and phlebostatic level: reference levels for venous pressure measurement in man. *Proc Soc Exp Biol Med.* 1945;58:165–169.

Smoking Cessation: Resp Physiol
Organ-based Clinical: Respiratory

Caroline Al Haddadin and Zhaodi Gong

Edited by Veronica Matei

KEY POINTS

1. Smoking has several effects on the respiratory system, including decreased ciliary motility, increased sputum production, and increased airway reactivity.
2. Smoking is one of the most prevalent risk factors for postoperative mortality.
3. Anesthesiologists and physicians should advise patients to stop smoking at least 2 months prior to elective surgery.

DISCUSSION

Approximately 40% of cigarette smokers will die prematurely unless they quit. Smoking increases the likelihood of developing atherosclerotic disease, peripheral vascular disease, chronic obstructive pulmonary disease, and cancers.

The effects of tobacco burning can be divided into two phases: the aerosol phase and the vapor phase. The aerosol phase settles in the alveoli and has many carcinogenic compounds. The vapor phase contains carbon monoxide (CO) and toxins that affect the cilia motility and irritate the respiratory tract.

Smoking is one of the most prevalent risk factors for postoperative mortality. Smokers have a 2- to 6-fold increase risk of postoperative pneumonia. All patients are advised to stop smoking before surgery.

It is has been shown that there is a definite benefit to smoking cessation greater than 8 weeks prior to surgery. However, it is controversial whether cessation less than 8 weeks is beneficial or harmful. The elevated carboxyhemoglobin levels seen in smokers compared with nonsmokers can decrease to near normal levels with smoking cessation of only 12 to 24 hours. Normalization of the mucociliary dysfunction seen in smokers takes at least 3 weeks, and during that time, there is actually an increase in sputum production. It is for this reason that some studies have shown an increase in postoperative pulmonary complications such as pneumonia in patients who stop smoking less than 8 weeks preoperatively compared with those who continue to smoke.

Nicotine is the principal constituent of tobacco responsible for the addiction of smokers. When tobacco is burned, the resultant smoke contains nicotine, carbon monoxide, and thousands of compounds that result from pyrosynthesis, volatilization, and pyrolysis of tobacco.

Several genes have been associated with nicotine addiction. Some will reduce the clearance of nicotine and others with increased likelihood of dependence. Genetic alterations that involve the neurotransmitter dopamine and possibly the serotonergic and cholinergic regulatory pathways are being investigated. The acidic pH of cigarettes limits absorption of the nicotine in the mouth (as opposed to cigars and pipes, which have an alkaline pH) and requires the inhalation of smoke into the larger surface of the lungs for adequate absorption to satisfy the addiction.

There are five adjunct drugs recommended by the Public Health Service to help with smoking cessation, including bupropion SR, nicotine gum, nicotine inhaler, nicotine nasal spray, and nicotine patch. In a study of bupropion-assisted smoking cessation, it was demonstrated that there was a decreased risk of postoperative complications after 4 weeks of smoking cessation. Consequently, anesthesiologists and physicians should advise patients to stop smoking at least 2 months prior to elective surgery.

S

SUGGESTED READINGS

Barash PG, Cullen BF, Stoelting RK, et al, eds. *Clinical Anesthesia.* 6th ed. Philadelphia, PA: Lippincott Williams & Wilkins; 2009:252.

Braunwald E, Fauci AS, Kasper DL, et al. *Harrison's Principles of Internal Medicine.* 15th ed. New York, NY: McGraw Hill Professional; 2001.

Scanlon PD, Connett JE, Waller LA, et al. Smoking cessation and lung function in mild-to-moderate chronic obstructive pulmonary disease. The Lung Health Study. *Am J Respir Crit Care Med.* 2000;161:381–390.

Verbanck S, Schuermans D, Paiva M, et al. Small airway function improvement after smoking cessation in smokers without airway obstruction. *Am J Respir Crit Care Med.* 2006;174(8):853–857.

S

Spinal Anes Complic: MRI Indications
Subspecialties: Regional Anesthesia

Shaun Gruenbaum
Edited by Thomas Halaszynski

KEY POINTS

1. When motor and sensory functions do not adequately recover after spinal anesthesia, or other neurologic symptoms persist, an MRI study should be performed immediately to determine whether the underlying pathology is surgically treatable or reversible.
2. A neuraxial (spinal–epidural) abscess will often present with back pain, fever, and variable neurologic symptoms, and when suspected, it should be investigated without delay by MRI.
3. Persistent lower extremity numbness or weakness after spinal anesthesia should raise the suspicion of spinal hematoma and should also be evaluated immediately by MRI because a delayed diagnosis often results in less favorable outcomes.
4. Spinal anesthesia should not be performed in a patient with a spinal tumor or when signs of spinal cord or spinal nerve root compression are present; such underlying pathology should be investigated with MRI imaging.
5. If new neuraxial or progressive neurologic symptoms develop (whether neuraxial procedures were performed or not performed), an immediate neurosurgical consult and MRI of the spine should be obtained.

DISCUSSION

Spinal anesthesia is generally considered safe and neurologic complications rare. However, patients should always be carefully monitored postoperatively after spinal anesthesia administration. When motor and sensory function do not adequately recover after spinal anesthesia, or when other neurologic symptoms persist, an MRI study and neurosurgical consultation should be performed immediately to determine whether the underlying pathology is treatable or reversible. Other imaging modalities, including computerized axial topographical scan (CT scan) and myelography, are less sensitive and may fail to demonstrate a developing neurologic lesion. Thus, an MRI should be done without delay if suspicions exist.

Neurologic complications after spinal anesthesia are often nonspecific, the most serious being paraplegia, cauda equina syndrome, and paresthesias. The differential diagnosis can be large and includes direct trauma by the spinal needle, extrinsic compression from an abscess, hematoma formation, neuraxial tumor, toxicity from local anesthetics, and spinal cord ischemia.

Spinal–epidural abscess is a rare complication from spinal or epidural anesthesia. A neuraxial abscess classically presents with a triad of back pain, fever, and variable neurologic symptoms. Neurologic symptoms typically occur late, and diagnostic studies can often be delayed. Therefore, a timely diagnosis is imperative for prompt treatment of a neuraxial abscess with neurosurgical decompression and antibiotics, as this is associated with a favorable outcome. The presence of any symptoms (particularly fever, which is often the first symptom) should warrant diagnostic imaging. MRI is the recommended imaging modality and offers the most accurate definitive diagnosis. MRI produces high-resolution images with a sensitivity exceeding 90%, and can detect the degree of spinal cord compression. MRI is especially useful in distinguishing spinal–epidural abscess from other causes of infection including discitis, osteomyelitis, spondylitis and meningitis, as well as noninfectious etiologies.

Spinal hematoma that often presents with persistent lower extremity numbness or weakness is a rare, but potentially devastating complication of spinal anesthesia. When the

S

519

diagnosis of spinal hematoma is delayed more than 8 hours, the damage caused by spinal cord compression has a much less favorable outcome. MRI is very sensitive in diagnosing spinal hematoma, and is indicated in patients with a high index of suspicion (especially patients with coagulation defects in whom the risk is higher).

MRI is indicated before spinal anesthesia when preoperative neurologic examination reveals signs of spinal root or cord compression, especially in patients with a malignancy or history of malignancy. Performing a spinal anesthesia in a patient with a metastatic spinal tumor can result in serious neurologic complications, including paraplegia.

SUGGESTED READINGS

Barash PG, Cullen BF, Stoelting R, et al, eds. *Clinical Anesthesia*. 5th ed. Philadelphia, PA: Lippincott Williams & Wilkins; 2009:947–950.
Cherng YG, Chen IY, Liu FL, et al. Paraplegia following spinal anesthesia in a patient with an undiagnosed metastatic spinal tumor. *Acta Anaesthesiol Taiwan*. 2008;46:86–90.
Grewal S, Hocking G, Wildsmith JA. Epidural abscesses. *Br J Anaesth*. 2006;96:292–302.

Spinal Anesthesia Spread: Factors

Regional Anesthesia

Christina Mack

Edited by Jodi Sherman

1. Baricity and patient position are the two most important factors affecting spread of local anesthetic in spinal anesthesia.
2. Gravity causes hyperbaric solutions to move downward in the cerebrospinal fluid (CSF).
3. Hypobaric solutions move in the opposite direction of gravity in the CSF.
4. Other factors that affect the spread of anesthetic solutions in the subarachnoid space include the speed of injection, direction of the needle aperture, hydrophilic/lipophilic nature of anesthetic, and the local anesthetic dose.

In spinal blocks, local anesthetic can be injected directly into the subarachnoid space to provide a dense motor and sensory block. Opioids can also be administered in this fashion, either as an adjuvant to local anesthetic or as a sole agent. Several factors that affect the spread of spinal anesthesia are discussed below.

Characteristics of the injectate solution can influence the cephalad spread of local anesthetics within the CSF. The principle factor with the most influence is the baricity. The baricity of the CSF is 1.0003 ± 0.0003 g per mL at 37° C. Solutions whose baricity is less than 0.9990 are hypobaric and will flow upward in the CSF; those whose baricity is greater than 1.0015 are hyperbaric and will flow downward in the CSF because of the influence of gravity. Solutions whose baricity falls in between these two values are isobaric and gravity will not have an influence on their flow in the CSF. Mixing local anesthetics with dextrose, typically from 5% to 8%, can create hyperbaric solutions. Mixing local anesthetics in distilled water creates hypobaric solutions. Isobaric solutions are prepared in normal saline or with aspirated CSF. Other factors that can affect spread of spinal drugs include volume, concentration, temperature, lipophilicity, and viscosity.

The other major factor that influences spinal anesthesia spread is patient positioning. For instance, a saddle block, which is restricted to the lower lumbar and sacral regions, can be accomplished by either injecting a hyperbaric solution while the patient is in the sitting position or by injecting a hypobaric solution with the patient in the prone jackknife position. Manipulating patient position is especially helpful in situations where surgery is performed on one side of the body. To provide anesthesia for a right knee surgery, for example, a hyperbaric solution can be injected while the patient is in the right lateral decubitus position or a hypobaric solution can be injected while the patient is in the left lateral decubitus position.

Patient characteristics such as age, height, weight, gender, spinal anatomy, and increased intraabdominal pressure have some effects on spread of local anesthetic. Pregnant patients, obese patients, and patients with ascites can have altered levels of spinal spread, as increased abdominal pressure may engorge epidural veins and thereby compress the CSF space. The net effect can result in increased cephalad spread at standard doses and volumes.

Opioids can also be administered in spinal anesthesia, either as an adjuvant to local anesthetic or as a sole agent. Hydrophilic opioids such as morphine take longer to penetrate tissues and therefore have a slower onset and longer duration of action than lipophilic agents such as fentanyl and sufentanil. Slow penetration into tissues also allows more time for cephalad spread of the agent, thereby increasing chances for respiratory depression. In contrast, lipophilic opioids such as fentanyl and sufentanil have faster tissue penetration, allowing faster onset and shorter duration of action.

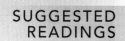

Bernards C. Epidural and spinal anesthesia. In: Barash PG, Cullen BF, Stoelting RK, et al, eds. *Clinical Anesthesia.* 6th ed. Philadelphia, PA: Lippincott Williams & Wilkins; 2009:932–940.

Hocking G, Wildsmith JA. Intrathecal drug spread. *Br J Anaesth.* 2004;93(4):568–578.

S

Spinal Cord Stimulation: Reprogramming

Subspecialties: Pain

Adnan Malik

Edited by Jodi Sherman

KEY POINTS

1. Spinal cord stimulation (SCS) can be used as an effective means of chronic pain management.
2. Reprogramming involves adjustments of electrode configurations and changes to the amplitude, width, and frequency of electrical impulses.
3. Cathodes are 30 times more effective than anode electrodes at stimulating dorsal column fibers.
4. Amplitudes between 2 and 4 V typically result in paresthesias for most patients.
5. The greater the pulse width, the broader the paresthesia effect.
6. Frequency has no significant clinical effect, and personal preference often determines settings utilized.

DISCUSSION

SCS has been utilized to manage patients with failed back surgery syndrome (FBBS) and those in whom conservative medical therapy has failed. Although many mechanisms are proposed, it is felt that inhibition of sympathetic outflow and activation of the descending modulating systems play key roles in pain relief.

Programming a spinal cord stimulator involves manipulation of electrode configurations, amplitude, width, and frequency of electrical impulses. The cathode is approximately 30 times more effective at stimulating the dorsal column fibers as the anode is. The ideal placement of the electrodes is best achieved by stimulating the cathodes. Newer stimulator systems allow "current steering," whereby multiple configurations can be achieved by allowing for partial cathode and anode arrangements at different electrode pairs.

The amplitude is measured in volts and is typically set for a range between 0 and 10 V depending on the type of electrode and the types of nerves being stimulated. This allows for adjustment of the intensity of stimulation. Although most patients sense paresthesias between 2 and 4 V, the threshold can depend on prior epidural scarring, changes to dorsal column fibers, and the posterior CSF space.

The width of electrical impulses ranges from 100 to 400 μs. Widening of the pulse width results in a greater area of paresthesias invoked. The frequency can range from 20 to 120 Hz and is determined by patient preference, with some choosing a lower-frequency beating sensation compared with others who prefer higher-frequency buzzing. It must be kept in mind, however, that there is no correlation with frequency and clinical response.

Selecting the lowest settings that are clinically effective allows for extended battery life in those spinal cord stimulators that are nonrechargeable. In addition, cycling of stimulation can also be utilized to extend battery life.

SUGGESTED READINGS

Barash PG, Cullen BF, Stoelting RK, et al, eds. *Clinical Anesthesia*. 6th ed. Philadelphia, PA: Lippincott Williams & Wilkins; 2009:1525–1526.

Kunnumpurath S, Srinivasagopalan R, Vadivelu N. Spinal cord stimulation: principles of past, present and future practice: a review. *J Clin Monit Comput*. 2009;23:333–339.

Morgan GE, Mikhail MS, Murray MJ, eds. *Clinical Anesthesiology*. 4th ed. New York, NY: Lange McGraw-Hill; 2006:393.

S

Spinal Hypotension Rx
Subspecialties: Regional Anesthesia

Jordan Martin

Edited by Thomas Halaszynski

KEY POINTS

1. Hypotension is often common after spinal anesthesia, and treatment should routinely be initiated when blood pressure is 25% to 30% below baseline or systolic blood pressure is less than 90 mm Hg.
2. Pretreatment with a crystalloid bolus may decrease the severity, but does not prevent hypotension after a spinal anesthetic.
3. In theory, ephedrine (both an alpha-agonist and a beta-agonist) is preferable to phenylephrine (alpha-agonist alone) in the management of spinal hypotension because ephedrine is more effective at increasing venous tone (thus increasing preload), which is the major cause of spinal hypotension, and it can also increase the heart rate.
4. Placing the patient in the head down position is also effective as part of the treatment strategy for spinal hypotension after spinal anesthesia.

DISCUSSION

Neuraxial anesthesia can be a useful technique for many surgeries, as well as in the labor and delivery area for pregnant patients. As with all types of anesthesia, neuraxial anesthesia is not without its own complications. Hypotension is the most common side effect after spinal anesthesia, with an incidence that ranges from 0% to 50% in nonpregnant patients and can be as high as 50% to 90% in pregnant patients. Risk factors for developing hypotension include aspects such as hypovolemia, age older than 40 years, obesity, concurrent use of general anesthesia, and an anesthetic level reaching as high as the thoracic-5 (T5) vertebra or above. The risk of developing hypotension increases with a rising height of the spinal block; however, the severity of cardiovascular effects has not always been shown to correlate with spinal block level. There are no set guidelines as to when to initiate treatment for hypotension, but the commonly accepted parameters include a blood pressure 25% to 30% below baseline or a systolic blood pressure less than 90 mm Hg in previously normotensive patients.

Hypotension that can result when performing spinal anesthesia is created by blockade of sympathetic efferents (sympathectomy) that often leads to both venous and arterial vasodilation. The venodilation decreases preload that leads to decreased cardiac output, and arterial dilation causes a decrease in systemic vascular resistance. The goal of treating hypotension due to a sympathectomy created during spinal anesthesia is to counteract these physiologic effects. First-line therapy to treat hypotension after spinal anesthesia often includes administration of crystalloid solutions; however, this may be ineffective in normovolemic patients. Pretreatment with crystalloids before performing spinal anesthesia may also decrease the incidence of hypotension, but does not completely prevent hypotension from occurring.

A more reliable solution to treating hypotension that often results from a spinal anesthetic is with administration of vasopressors. The hypotension caused by spinal anesthesia is due to a decrease in preload more extensively and to a greater degree than by a decrease in afterload. Therefore, a joint alpha- and beta-agonist (ephedrine) that increases venous and arterial tone is preferable and usually more effective than a pure alpha agonist, such as phenylephrine, which proves less effective at increasing venous tone. However, low-to-moderate doses of dopamine may also be used to avoid tachyphylaxis sometimes associated with prolonged use of ephedrine. If these measures fail to adequately treat hypotension created during spinal anesthesia, epinephrine could be another medication

S

of choice. In conjunction with medications and fluids, positioning the patient in a head down position may allow gravity to relieve some of the hypotension created during spinal anesthesia.

In pregnant patients, the addition of inferior venocaval compression secondary to the gravid uterus can increase and worsen the hypotension effects from neuraxial anesthesia. Because of this potential deleterious effect, preventative measures such as leg wrapping, left uterine displacement, and/or pre-spinal block crystalloid administration are used more frequently. Once again, ephedrine is most commonly used, as it helps to maintain uterine blood flow. However, phenylephrine can also be safely used, especially when an increase in maternal heart rate would not be tolerated or fetal acidosis is of concern.

SUGGESTED READINGS

Barash PG, Cullen BF, Stoelting RK, et al, eds. *Clinical Anesthesia.* 6th ed. Philadelphia, PA: Lippincott Williams & Wilkins; 2009:945–947.

Finucane BT. *Complications of Regional Anesthesia.* 2nd ed. New York, NY: Springer; 2007:149–151.

Lobato EB, Gravenstein N, Kirby RR, eds. *Complications of Anesthesia.* 3rd ed. Philadelphia, PA: Lippincott Williams & Wilkins; 2008:675–676.

Morgan GE, Mikhail MS, Murray MJ, eds. *Clinical Anesthesiology.* 4th ed. New York, NY: Lange McGraw-Hill; 2006:316–318.

S

Spinal Stenosis: Dx

Subspecialties: Pain

Harika Nagavelli

Edited by Thomas Halaszynski

KEY POINTS

1. Spinal stenosis is a narrowing of the spinal cord caused by a wide range of etiologies.
2. Diagnosis of spinal stenosis relies heavily on clinical severity and is secondarily validated through radiologic evidence.
3. Patients often present with leg pain and/or lower back pain associated with activity such as walking, standing, sitting, and going up and down stairs or hills. The pain is usually immediately alleviated with the cessation of such activity.
4. Conservative pain management with lifestyle modifications, nonsteroidal anti-inflammatory drugs (NSAIDs), and epidural steroid injections has proven to alleviate many of the symptoms very well.
5. MRI is the gold standard for radiologic diagnosis of spinal stenosis.

DISCUSSION

Spinal stenosis is a narrowing of the spinal canal. The narrowing that occurs in the canal can involve the central canal, the lateral recess, or can involve narrowing of the foramina. Spinal stenosis is also classified according to whether it is a congenital or acquired stenosis. The direct etiology is predominately due to broad disk bulges, osteophytes, or hypertrophy of the ligamentum flavum. However, eventually all adults acquire, to some extent, spinal stenosis because of the natural process of aging, leading to a degenerative stenosis with the loss of disk height.

The presentation of spinal stenosis often correlates to the type of spinal canal narrowing that may be involved. For example, stenosis caused by narrowing of the foramina tends to produce symptoms along a certain dermatome of the exiting nerve root that is being compressed.

A typical patient with spinal stenosis usually presents as an elderly person with low back pain and progressive leg pain (often bilateral) that is typically triggered by going down stairs or walking, with immediate relief on cessation of that activity. Patients often experience pain associated with neurogenic claudication such as numbness, tingling, loss of sensation, and pain of both legs while active. This is in contrast to pain associated with claudication of the vascular system that often takes a longer time for relief after cessation of the inciting activity and involves diminished peripheral pulses. Furthermore, leaning forward or positions that increase lumbar flexion alleviate pain for patients with spinal stenosis because it reduces the narrowing of the spine created by extension.

Diagnosis and treatment of spinal stenosis have become increasingly important in anesthesia, with surgical treatment increasing by at least 8-fold in a 20-year period. In addition, with the rising availability for diagnosis of spinal stenosis by MRI or CT scan along with the association of lower back pain in the aging population to degenerative stenosis, conservative treatments for any associated radicular pain has also been emphasized. Epidural corticosteroid treatments have been used to treat acute exacerbation, and have proven to deliver degrees of pain relief.

Conservative management of spinal stenosis involves a wide range of treatment modalities starting from lifestyle changes to narcotics. The majority of patients afflicted with spinal stenosis have moderate limitations with daily tasks. Exercise programs have proven to have better results than bed rest for long-term reductions of radicular pain. Acute exacerbations can be treated at a pain clinic with periodic and incremental epidural steroid injections. In particular, with those patients afflicted with narrowing of the foramina, a

S

pain specialist may inject corticosteroids transforaminally and target the exact area that triggers patient discomfort.

Anti-inflammatory medications such as NSAIDs and corticosteroids are often the best approach when stenosis of the spinal canal is due to soft-tissue hypertrophy and inflammation. In contrast, bony narrowing of the canal secondary to osteophytes or broad-based disk bulges is best treated surgically.

Low back pain and radiculopathy do not have a direct correlation to radiologic evidence to the extent of stenotic pathology for any given patient. Surgical treatment is initiated and dependent on clinical presentation, severity of symptoms, and response to conservative treatments. Although MRI is the gold standard in visualizing soft-tissue and stenotic narrowing of the spinal canal, radiologic gradation of the stenosis is secondary to clinical presentation and severity in diagnosing spinal stenosis toward determining a treatment plan.

Somatosensory evoked potentials (SSEPs) may also be helpful in identifying the nerve root level generating the symptoms; however, it has a high false-positive rate, and is often used in conjunction with imaging. SSEPs are helpful in the sense that they test dorsal spinal columns involved in the sensory uptake of pain, temperature, and pressure information. Likewise, CT enhanced with intrathecal contrast myelography can aid in delineating the source of a patient's radiculopathy when MRI is contraindicated in such patients (those with implantable cardiac devices and other metal containing implants). Ultimately, however, clinical presentation triumphs all in the diagnosis of spinal stenosis and hence patient management.

SUGGESTED READINGS

Aebi M, Gunzburg R, Szpalski M, eds. *The Aging Spine.* Berlin, Germany: Springer; 2005:94–98.
Cohen SP, Rowlingson J, Abdi S. Low back pain. In: Warfield CA, Bajwa ZA, eds. *Principles and Practice of Pain Medicine.* 2nd ed. New York, NY: McGraw-Hill; 2004: chap 28: 273–284. http://www.accessanesthesiology.com/content/3412674.
Hurley C. *Spine.* 7th ed. Philadelphia, PA: Lippincott Williams & Wilkins; 2004:105–111.

S

Statistical analysis: Power and Study Design
Mathematics, Statistics, Computers

Roberto Rappa and Jennifer Dominguez
Edited by Raj K. Modak

KEY POINTS

1. Statistical power calculations are often done during the planning stages of a study to help estimate an adequate sample size that will prevent alpha and beta type errors.
2. The power of a statistical test is the probability of the test in rejecting a false null hypothesis (type II error).
3. Statistical power = 1 – beta error, where beta error = false negative error.
4. The statistical power of a test depends on four factors: the statistical significance criterion used in the study, the magnitude of the experimental effect in the population, the sample size used to measure the effect, and the study design.
5. One can achieve greater statistical power by increasing the alpha value, decreasing population variability, increasing sample size, or by making the magnitude of the experimental effect higher.

DISCUSSION

To accurately describe power analysis in the context of study design, a few statistical terms must be reviewed:

- **Null hypothesis:** A general position in statistical hypothesis testing that stipulates that there is no relationship between two measured outcomes or that the proposed treatment has no effect.
- **Type I error:** A type I error is made when one *incorrectly rejects* the null hypothesis. This is also known as a false positive or alpha error. This occurs when the investigators observe a difference when, in truth, there is none. This indicates that the test has poor specificity (see below).
- **Type II error:** A type II error is made when one *incorrectly accepts* the null hypothesis. This is also known as a false negative or beta error. This occurs when the investigators fail to observe a difference when, in truth, there is one. This indicates that the test has poor sensitivity (see below).
- α **(alpha error):** The probability of making a type I error.
- β **(beta error):** The probability of making a type II error.
- **Specificity:** The proportion of correctly identified negatives (the percentage of healthy people who are correctly identified as not having the condition).
- **Sensitivity:** The proportion of correctly identified positives (the percentage of sick people who are correctly identified as having the condition).

A statistical hypothesis states the relationship between study variables anticipated by the researchers. A null hypothesis is also formulated that assumes the hypothesis is false. Two types of errors (alpha and beta) can arise from this approach. They are described in the table below (see Fig. 1).

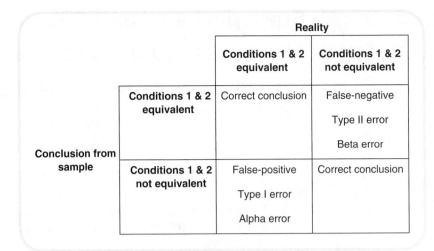

		Reality	
		Conditions 1 & 2 equivalent	**Conditions 1 & 2 not equivalent**
Conclusion from sample	**Conditions 1 & 2 equivalent**	Correct conclusion	False-negative Type II error Beta error
	Conditions 1 & 2 not equivalent	False-positive Type I error Alpha error	Correct conclusion

Figure 1. Errors in hypothesis testing: Two-way truth table. (From Barash PG, et al. *Clinical Anesthesia*. 6th ed. Philadelphia, PA: Lippincott Williams & Wilkins; 2009:197.)

The alpha or type 1 error refers to finding a difference between conditions when one does not exist. The value of alpha is generally set at 0.05. If a data set fails to achieve significance, where $p > 0.05$, there may truly be no difference between the variables, or the study may have had too few data points to find a statistical difference.

The latter explanation illustrates the type II or beta error that estimates the probability of missing a true finding. Beta errors occur when the null hypothesis is not rejected, although it is false. Therefore, the hypothesized difference exists, but the study is not large enough to detect it.

Statistical power calculations are often done during the planning stages of a study to help estimate an adequate sample size that will prevent these errors. The statistical power of a study refers to its ability to detect a difference between conditions if one is truly there. Mathematically, power is calculated as 1 – beta error, and it is generally set at 80% or greater.

$$\text{Statistical power} = 1 - \text{beta error}$$

Power is influenced by a number of factors including effect size (magnitude of expected differences between conditions), sample size, response variability (standard deviation), and significance level (alpha level). A small effect size is associated with a greater chance of making a type II error. Larger sample size yields greater power, where achieving adequate power must be balanced with feasibility and expenditure of resources. Increased variability between conditions reduces power, as does selecting a smaller alpha value.

Barash PG, Cullen BF, Stoelting RK, et al. *Clinical Anesthesia*. 6th ed. Philadelphia, PA: Lippincott Williams & Wilkins; 2009:192–204.

Boslaugh S, Watters PA. *Statistics in a Nutshell*. Sebastopol, CA: O'Reilly Media Inc.; 2008:358.

Cleophas TJ, Zwinderman AH, Cleophas TF, et al. *Statistics Applied to Clinical Trials*. New York: Springer; 2008:81.

Feinstein AR. *Principles of Medical Statistics*. Boca Raton, FL: Chapman & Hall; 2002:489

Jekel JF, Katz DL, Elmore JG, et al. *Epidemiology, Biostatistics and Preventive Medicine*. 3rd ed. Philadelphia, PA: Saunders Elsevier; 2007:198.

SUGGESTED READINGS

Statistics: Median
Mathematics, Statistics, Computers

Juan Egas

Edited by Raj K. Modak

1. The three statistical methods of measuring the central tendency of a distribution are the mean, the median, and the mode.
2. The median can be found by arranging the list of values in a distribution from low to high and finding the number that lies exactly in the middle.

There are three ways to measure central tendency of a distribution in inferential statistics: the mean, the median, and the mode. The median is the middle position of a distribution, and it is not affected by extreme or large deviations from the mean score. The median can be found by arranging the list of values in a distribution from the lowest value to the highest and selecting the middle number. If the number of items in a given set is an odd number, then the median would be the number in the middle of the distribution. For example, the median of the distribution shown below is 4:

$$1, 2, 3, \mathbf{4}, 5, 6, 7$$

When the total amount of observed individuals is an even number, then the median can be calculated by averaging the two middle scores of the distribution. For example, the median of the distribution shown below would be 4.5:

$$1, 2, 3, 4, 5, 6, 7, 8$$

The mode is the most frequent number or most common value in a frequency distribution. The mean is also called the arithmetic average, and it is the most commonly used measure of central tendency. To calculate the mean, one must add all of the values within the distribution and then divide the total by the number of items in the distribution. Between all the measures of central tendency, the mean may be the most effective measure in calculating the central tendency in a group because it accounts for all of the observed values in a distribution and also accounts for their distance from the central tendency. The mean is the most affected measure by few extreme values in a distribution.

Barash P, Cullen BF, Stoelting RK, et al. *Clinical Anesthesia*. 6th ed. Philadelphia, PA: Lippincott Williams & Wilkins; 2009:196.

S

Stats: ANOVA indications
Mathematics, Statistics, Computers

Soumya Nyshadham

Edited by Raj K. Modak

KEY POINTS

1. Analysis of variance (often called ANOVA) is a method by which **means** can be statistically compared when **more than two groups** are involved.
2. The following assumptions are required for ANOVA:
   a. Each of the *z* populations should be randomly sampled.
   b. The *z* populations have means that are compared with variances of normal distributions.
3. The test statistics for ANOVA are *F* ratios and follow *F* distributions when the null hypothesis is true. These statistical tests are used to determine whether the null hypothesis is upheld or rejected.
4. Three classes of ANOVA models primarily exist: fixed-effects models, random-effects models, and mixed-effects models.

DISCUSSION

Paired *t*-tests are often used when comparing two populations. This method most commonly involves the difference between means and comparing these values with the variability. If *t*-tests were used (as they can be for two populations), it would result in an increased chance of type I error (error of rejecting the null hypothesis when it is true—a false positive). If paired *t*-tests were used to compare more than two populations, numerous combinations would need to be performed resulting in a higher type I error rate than the standard 0.05, thus creating results that are falsely statistically significant.

ANOVA is a method by which **means** can be statistically compared when **more than two groups** are involved. ANOVA is based on the following hypotheses: $H_0 = x_1 = x_2 = x_3 \cdots = x_z$; $H_1 = $ Not all x ($y = 1, 2, ..., z$). Statistical tests are used to determine whether the null hypothesis is upheld or rejected. The following assumptions are required for ANOVA: Each of the *z* populations should be randomly sampled, the *z* populations have means (x) that are equal or not with variances of normal distributions. The test statistics for ANOVA are *F* ratios and follow *F* distributions when the null hypothesis (H_1) is true.

Three classes of ANOVA models primarily exist: fixed-effects models, random-effects models, and mixed-effects models. Fixed-effects models are those in which the levels of the treatments under analysis are fixed such that the conclusion is valid only for the treatments involved. Random-effects models are those in which the levels of the treatments under analysis are chosen randomly from a population such that the conclusion is valid for the entire population from which the treatments are chosen. Mixed-effects models are those that involve both fixed and random factors.

SUGGESTED READINGS

Aczel AD, Souderpandian J. *Complete business statistics.* 7th ed. Columbus, OH: McGraw-Hill/Irwin; 2009:349–355, 379.

Barash PG, Cullen BF, Stoelting RK, et al. *Clinical Anesthesia.* 6th ed. Philadelphia, PA: Lippincott Williams & Wilkins; 2009:200–201.

S

Stellate Ganglion Block: Effects
Subspecialties: Pain

Jammie Ferrara

Edited by Jodi Sherman

KEY POINTS

1. Indications for a stellate ganglion block include complex regional pain syndromes, phantom limb pain, herpetic zoster pain, and circulatory compromise from vasospastic or thromboembolic events.
2. The stellate ganglion is also known as the cervicothoracic ganglion, as it lies between C7 and T1.
3. The C6 transverse process is also known as *Chassaignac tubercle* and is a palpable landmark for the anterior paratracheal (most common) approach to this block.
4. Horner syndrome is indicative of a sympathectomy of the head and face.
5. A 1.0° to 1.5° C increase in temperature of the block side versus core temperature or contralateral side is indicative of a successful sympathetic block of the arm.

DISCUSSION

Indication. The stellate ganglion block is one of the most commonly used regional blocks of the face and upper extremity. Stellate ganglion blocks are indicated for sympathetically driven pain syndromes such as complex regional pain syndrome, phantom limb pain, herpes zoster pain, frostbite, or tumor invasion of neurovascular structures. Other indications include thromboembolic or vasospastic events that cause circulatory insufficiency in the upper extremities.

Anatomy. The inferior cervical ganglion is fused with the first thoracic ganglion, giving it a stellate appearance. It receives preganglionic sympathetic fibers from the intermediolateral cell column in the spinal cord of T1 – T6. The stellate ganglion is anterior to the first rib, extending along the C7 – T1 interspace, and may lie over the anterior tubercle of C7. It is bordered inferiorly by pleura, medially by longus colli muscle, and laterally by the scalene muscles. It is bordered anteriorly by the subclavian vertebral artery and posteriorly by the C7 transverse process and T1. Along the superior border of the stellate ganglion is the transverse process of the sixth cervical vertebrae, the palpable edge of which is also known as *Chassaignac tubercle*. This palpable landmark is a prominence along the paratracheal region of the neck and is the hallmark for the anterior paratracheal approach to a block. It serves as bony protection for the vertebral artery, thereby also protecting the artery from accidental local anesthetic injection during a block. Chassaignac tubercle lies within the same plane as the prevertebral fascia, thus permitting mediastinal and contralateral spread of the local anesthetic injectate (Fig. 1).

S

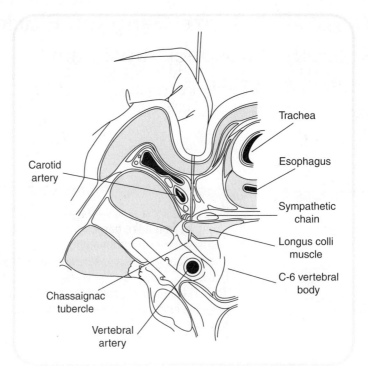

Figure 1. Transverse section at the C6 level. (From Warfield CA, Bajwa ZH, eds. *Principles and Practice of Pain Medicine*. 2nd ed. New York, NY: McGraw-Hill; 2004:696–698, with permission. Courtesy of http://www.accessanesthesiology.com.)

Technique. The anterior paratracheal approach is the most popular approach, as it is the easiest and the least painful for the patient and has the least amount of risk when performed correctly. With the patient in the supine position, the neck in slight extension, and the mouth slightly opened, the injection site is over the C6 transverse process (Chassaignac tubercle), lateral to cricoid cartilage and medial to the carotid artery. Ultrasound, fluoroscopy, or CT can be used to guide accurate needle placement. If the sympathetic block is not achieved at the level of Chassaignac tubercle, a repeat block at C7 or T1 can be done. However, a block at this level increases the risk of a brachial plexus block, as well as potential pneumothorax. Large volumes (20 mL) can produce a more complete sympathectomy of the arm and hand (C5–T1 dermatomes), but are associated with hoarseness (80%), dysphagia (60%), and brachial plexus block (10%) secondary to the spread of local anesthetic onto nearby laryngeal nerves and cervical nerve roots. Horner sign (ipsilateral ptosis, miosis, anhydrosis, and conjunctival engorgement) indicates a sympathetic block of the head and face. However, it does not suggest a sympathectomy of the upper extremity. A 1.0° to 1.5° C increase in temperature of the block side versus core temperature or contralateral side is indicative of a successful sympathetic block of the arm.

Complications. Dysphagia and hoarseness are common complications with the anterior paratracheal approach because of the proximity of the laryngeal nerves to the stellate ganglion. If the patient is unable to say "ee" or has difficulty swallowing water, there is likely incidental recurrent laryngeal blockade. The patient should also be assessed for motor block of the upper extremity, as the brachial plexus is also adjacent. Other major, yet rare, complications include intravascular injection, chylothorax, pneumothorax, diaphragm hemiparesis, and esophageal perforation.

Warfield CA, Bajwa ZH, eds. *Principles and Practice of Pain Medicine*. 2nd ed. New York, NY: McGraw-Hill; 2004:696–698.

SUGGESTED READING

Steroid Prophylaxis Indications
Organ-based Clinical: Endocrine/Metabolic

Gabriel Jacobs

Edited by Mamatha Punjala

KEY POINTS

1. Chronic steroid usage can cause pituitary–adrenal axis suppression, and the patient may be unable to respond to perioperative stress.
2. Patients with adrenal insufficiency and pituitary–adrenal axis suppression should receive steroid prophylaxis.
3. There are several possible risks associated with steroid prophylaxis, but the data are very limited.
4. Intravenous (IV) hydrocortisone 100 to 200 mg can be given as prophylaxis depending on the nature of the surgery and patient.

DISCUSSION

Patients with adrenal insufficiency and hypothalamic–pituitary–adrenal (HPA) axis suppression will require additional steroid coverage to mitigate the normal stress response of surgery. Exogenous steroid administration may cause pituitary–adrenal axis suppression, and it is often impossible to predict the degree of suppression without costly provocative testing with adrenocorticotropic hormone stimulation.

Because of the low risk of deleterious effects, generally patients who have received steroid therapy within the last 9 to 12 months before surgery may receive prophylactic supplemental steroids. Patients who are on chronic steroids should receive supplementation because of the increased stress of surgery and anesthesia. Perioperative stress includes the depth of anesthesia along with the degree of trauma. Also, deep general anesthesia and regional anesthesia can delay the usual release of endogenous glucocorticoids. Cases of perioperative cardiovascular derangements have been reported in patients with chronic adrenal suppression. Patients with known acute adrenal insufficiency should receive steroid prophylaxis. Also, a single dose of corticosteroids in patients with chronic obstructive pulmonary disease or asthma may help ameliorate increases in airway resistance postoperatively.

For patients who are on chronic steroid therapy, one can administer hydrocortisone IV. The dose administered is dependent on the nature of the surgery. For minor surgical procedures, 100 mg of IV hydrocortisone is an appropriate dose. Major surgical procedures may warrant 200 mg of IV hydrocortisone for a 70-kg man. The IV dose can then be decreased 25% each day until the patient can resume oral steroid intake as long as there is no contraindication to continue IV steroids (e.g., post-op infection).

Possible risks of steroid therapy include abnormal wound healing, infection, exacerbation of preexisting hypertension, formation of stress ulcers, psychosis, and fluid retention.

Abnormal wound healing and postoperative infection are the two complications that have been studied heavily with no definitive evidence either way.

SUGGESTED READINGS

Barash PG, Cullen BF, Stoelting RK, et al., eds. *Clinical Anesthesia*. 6th ed. Philadelphia, PA: Lippincott Williams & Wilkins; 2009:251.

Miller RD, Eriksson LI, Fleisher LA, eds. *Miller's Anesthesia*. 7th ed. Philadelphia, PA: Churchill Livingstone; 2009:1082–1083.

Stroke Volume: A. Fib Effects
Physics, Monitoring, and Anesthesia Delivery

Tara Paulose

Edited by Benjamin Sherman

1. Atrial fibrillation is a common cardiac arrhythmia.
2. Atrial fibrillation is a disorganized pattern of atrial contraction associated with decreased ventricular filling.
3. Ventricular volumes are frequently irregular, leading to overall decreased stroke volume, cardiac output, and blood pressure.
4. Because synchronized atrial contractions normally contribute 15% to 30% of the ventricular end-diastolic volume, patients with atrial fibrillation have a decreased ability to increase cardiac output in response to stress or increased physical activity.

Atrial fibrillation has emerged as one of the most common cardiac arrhythmias, with an incidence strongly increasing with age. It is characterized by disorganized waves of excitation through the atria, causing contractions of the atria upwards of 300 beats per minute, leading to haphazard triggering of ventricular contractions through the AV node. This ineffectual triggering of atrial contraction has complex physiologic effects.

As the atria contract in a disordered fashion, the volume of blood transmitted to the left ventricle is lessened, thereby resulting in decreased left ventricular volumes and essentially a decreased stroke volume, which in turn leads to decreased cardiac output and lower blood pressure. If atrial fibrillation is accompanied by a rapid ventricular response, cardiac output can be substantially lowered because of minimal myocardial filling time. Synchronized atrial contractions normally contribute 15% to 30% of the volume entering the ventricle during diastole, yet in patients with diastolic dysfunction, this percentage can be substantially greater. Therefore, the development of atrial fibrillation in these patients with increased myocardial stiffness and resistance to filling may have severe alterations in hemodynamics acutely. In conditions of increased physical activity or stress, it is not surprising that patients experience symptoms of increased fatigue, dyspnea, and palpitations because of their limited ability to increase cardiac output.

Treatment of patients with atrial fibrillation can be complex. Therapy is centered on restoration of sinus rhythm; if that is not possible, rate control therapies are used to optimize filling time. Lastly, anticoagulation therapy is frequently utilized to decrease the incidence of stroke that occurs from stasis and thrombosis of blood in the atrium.

Barash PG, Cullen BF, Stoelting RK, et al., eds. *Clinical Anesthesia*. 6th ed. Philadelphia, PA: Lippincott Williams & Wilkins; 2009:123–124, 211.

Garratt C. *Mechanisms and Management of Cardiac Arrhythmias*. London, UK: BMJ Books; 2009:43–49.

Nguyen T, Hu D, Kim M. *Management of Complex Cardiovascular Problems: The Evidence-Based Medicine Approach*. John Wiley & Sons Ltd; 2008:288.

S

Subarachnoid Bleed: ECG Effects

Organ-based Clinical: Cardiovascular

Hyacinth Ruiter

Edited by Ramachandran Ramani

KEY POINTS

1. ECG effects in patients with subarachnoid bleed may resemble changes associated with coronary ischemia, myocardial infarction, or arrhythmias.
2. Patients experience significant ECG changes during the first 48 to 72 hours after subarachnoid bleed.
3. ECG changes associated with subarachnoid bleed suggest repolarization abnormalities involving the QT interval, ST segment, T wave, and U wave.
4. ECG changes and arrhythmias resolve within 12 days.

DISCUSSION

Subarachnoid bleed is most frequently caused by a rupture of a saccular aneurysm at the base of the brain. The classic signs and symptoms of a subarachnoid bleed include sudden severe headache, nausea, vomiting, and transient loss of consciousness. The presence of ECG abnormalities unexplained by preexisting cardiac risk factors is often not recognized, potentially placing patients at risk for inappropriate care.

ECG effects in patients with subarachnoid bleed may resemble changes associated with coronary ischemia, myocardial infarction, or arrhythmias. A plausible explanation has been the reversible myocardial injury caused by severe hypertension and autonomic discharge with catecholamine release. Studies have shown that patients with subarachnoid bleed are at increased risk for ventricular arrhythmias, including ventricular tachycardia, torsades de pointes, and ventricular fibrillation. Patients experience significant ECG changes during the first 48 to 72 hours after subarachnoid bleed, suggesting the importance of early monitoring.

ECG changes associated with subarachnoid bleed suggest repolarization abnormalities involving the QT interval, ST segment, T wave, and U wave. Abnormal canon T waves and changes in ST segment elevation or depression in patients with subarachnoid bleed often increase suspicions of myocardial ischemia or infarction. Repeat ECGs reflect resolution of all ECG changes and arrhythmias within 12 days. ST elevation normalizes within 1 week, but T-wave changes may persist for months. Morbidity and mortality associated with subarachnoid bleed do not appear to be contributed by cardiac abnormalities.

SUGGESTED READINGS

Miller RD, ed. *Miller's Anesthesia.* 6th ed. Philadelphia, PA: Churchill Livingstone; 2005:2148–2149.

Sommargren CE. Electrocardiographic abnormalities in patients with subarachnoid hemorrhage. *Am J Crit Care.* 2002;11:48–56.

S

Subarachnoid Hemorrhage: Nimodipine

Organ-based Clinical: Neurologic and Neuromuscular and Subspecialties: Critical Care

Ervin Jakab

Edited by Ramachandran Ramani

KEY POINTS

1. Nimodipine is FDA (U.S. Food and Drug Administration) approved for improvement of neurologic outcome in patients with subarachnoid hemorrhage (SAH) from ruptured intracranial aneurysms.
2. It is given orally, 60 mg every 4 hours for 21 days. This dose should be adjusted on the basis of the interaction with the inducers/inhibitors of CYP 3A4.
3. It has the typical side effects of the dihydropyridines, requiring blood pressure monitoring. It is a class C drug for pregnancy.

DISCUSSION

Nimodipine is a dihydropyridine that blocks voltage-gated "L-type" calcium channels, thus decreasing intracellular calcium in the cardiac and smooth muscle. It is currently approved for the management of vasospasm following SAH secondary to intracranial aneurysm bleeding. Vasospasm is the leading cause of mortality and morbidity in aneurysmal SAH. Nimodipine was initially marketed for this mechanism.

Subsequent studies have shown that although nimodipine does not significantly decrease vasospasm, it improves the odds of a good outcome, especially in patients with a good or fairly good clinical condition. The precise mechanism of action is unknown; arteriographic studies failed to demonstrate prevention or relief of vasospasm by nimodipine. The other possible mechanism is reversal of the ischemic cascade induced by vasospasm.

Nimodipine is typically administered in doses of 60 mg every 4 hours for 21 days after a SAH. It should be always given by an enteral route (orally or through a feeding tube). Intravenous or other parenteral administration has been associated with life-threatening side effects and deaths. If oral administration is not possible, it should be replaced with an intravenous dihydropyridine, such as nicardipine.

Nimodipine is metabolized in the liver by the cytochrome P450 system, and hence the dose should be decreased in patients with advanced liver disease. The inhibitors of CYP 3A4 (e.g., ketoconazole, erythromycin, valproic acid, cimetidine, ritonavir, and grapefruit juice) increase the plasma concentration of nimodipine, whereas the inducers (e.g., phenytoin, carbamazepine, and phenobarbital) decrease it. Also, rifampin accelerates the metabolism of nimodipine through a different mechanism.

The most frequent side effects are hypotension (13%), reversible liver/biliary system (12%), and gastrointestinal (11%) abnormalities.

Nimodipine is a category C drug for pregnancy (i.e., animal studies have shown an adverse effect on the fetus, although there are no adequate and well-controlled studies in humans, and potential benefits outweigh the risks in pregnant women).

SUGGESTED READINGS

Feigin VL, Rinkel GJ, Algra A, et al. Calcium antagonists in patients with aneurysmal subarachnoid hemorrhage: a systematic review. *Neurology.* 1998;50:876–883.

Nimotop Labeling Sheet, approved by FDA, retrieved on October 15, 2009 from http://www.accessdata.fda.gov/drugsatfda_docs/label/2006/018869s014lbl.pdf.

S

Succinylcholine: Normal K Increase
Organ-based Clinical: Renal/Urinary/ Electrolytes

Sharif Al-Ruzzeh

Edited by Hossam Tantawy

KEY POINTS

1. Succinylcholine administration may increase serum potassium by 0.5 mEq per L in normal patients.
2. This normal rise can be detrimental in patients with already elevated serum potassium levels because of acute or chronic reasons.
3. Cardiac arrest developing as a result of this rise in serum potassium levels can be difficult to manage.

DISCUSSION

Succinylcholine is a depolarizing neuromuscular blocker that imitates acetylcholine at the neuromuscular junction; this opening of the receptor causes the efflux of potassium. A typical increase of potassium serum concentration after administration of succinylcholine in normal patients is 0.5 mEq per L. This increase in potassium is transient in normal patients and generally does not result in adverse effects below a concentration of 6.5 to 7 mEq per L. Severe hyperkalemia causes changes in cardiac electrophysiology, which, if severe, can result in cardiac asystole. If the subsequent cardiac arrest proves to be refractory to routine cardiopulmonary resuscitation methods, rapid and aggressive management with calcium, insulin and glucose, bicarbonate, epinephrine, and even hemodialysis should be instituted to remove potassium from circulation promptly.

This expected normal increase in serum potassium could be detrimental in certain patients where serum potassium levels are elevated because of the certain pathologies such as burns, massive trauma, spinal cord transections or paralysis, and neurologic disorders. As there is no effective way to prevent the release of potassium after administration of succinylcholine, succinylcholine should be avoided in patients with preexisting elevated serum potassium. Pretreating the patients with magnesium sulfate (at a dose of 60 mg per kg intravenously) may limit an increase in serum potassium likely secondary to the prevention of potassium efflux from the myocardial cells. In addition, hyperventilation before the administration of succinylcholine may provide some degree of protection by reducing serum potassium (10- mm- Hg decrease in $PaCO_2$ reduces plasma $[K^+]$ by about 0.5 mmol per L).

SUGGESTED READINGS

Morgan G, Mikhail M, Murray M. *Clinical Anesthesiology*. 4th ed. New York, NY: McGraw-Hill Medical; 2005:214.
Reddy VG. Potassium and anaesthesia. *Singapore Med J*. 1998;39(11):511–516.
Stoelting R, Miller R. *Basics of Anesthesia*. 5th ed. Philadelphia, PA: Churchill Livingstone; 2007:141.

S

Succinylcholine and Bradycardia
Pharmacology

Rongjie Jiang

Edited by Mamatha Punjala

KEY POINTS

1. Succinylcholine can cause profound bradycardia. In adults, this commonly happens after the second bolus dosing of succinylcholine. However, in children, even teenagers, the first dose of succinylcholine may lead to cardiac arrest when given without atropine.
2. The mechanism of succinylcholine leading to sinus bradycardia is stimulation of muscarinic receptors in the sinus node.

DISCUSSION

Succinylcholine consists of two acetylcholine molecules linked through the acetate methyl groups (Fig. 1). It activates all cholinergic receptors just like acetylcholine because of its structural configuration. The receptors include nicotinic on both sympathetic and para-sympathetic ganglia and muscarinic in the sinus node of the heart. The end result is typically sinus bradycardia. Succinylcholine is metabolized by plasma cholinesterase to suc-cinylmonocholine and choline. These metabolites may sensitize the heart to a subsequent dose. It may explain why there is higher incidence of bradycardia after a second dose of succinylcholine in adults.

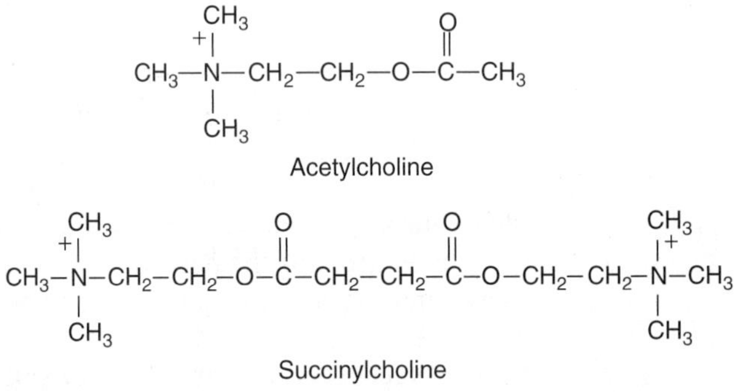

Figure 1. Acetylcholine and succinylcholine.

Succinylcholine is problematic in patients with predominantly vagal tone, such as children. The bradycardia, which sometimes progresses to asystole, may be prevented by the administration of thiopental, atropine, ganglion-blocking drugs, and nondepolarizing neuromuscular blockers. If a child needs a rapid-sequence induction, intravenous atropine at a dose of 0.02 mg per kg is recommended to prevent the bradycardia. It should be given before the induction agent and succinylcholine.

SUGGESTED READING

Miller RD, Eriksson LI, Fleisher LA, et al, eds. *Miller's Anesthesia.* 7th ed. Philadelphia, PA: Elsevier, Churchill, and Livingstone; 2009:863–865, 2572.

Superior Laryng N Anatomy

Anatomy

Jonathan Tidwell

Edited by Jodi Sherman

1. The superior laryngeal nerve arises from the vagus nerve and divides into an internal branch and an external branch.
2. The internal branch provides sensation to the laryngeal mucosa above the vocal cords, and the external branch provides motor innervation to the cricothyroid muscle.
3. The superior laryngeal nerve block is utilized to anesthetize the laryngeal mucosa above the vocal cords during awake intubation.

The superior laryngeal nerve is a branch of the vagus nerve arising from the inferior vagal ganglion at the superior end of the carotid triangle. Within the carotid sheath, the superior laryngeal nerve divides into an autonomic/sensory internal branch and a motor external branch (Fig. 1). The internal laryngeal nerve branches off the superior laryngeal nerve just lateral to the cornu of the hyoid bone before travelling through the thyrohyoid membrane into the piriform recess. The internal branch supplies sensory fibers to the laryngeal mucosa above the vocal cords (base of tongue, epiglottis, aryepiglottic folds, and arytenoids). The external laryngeal nerve provides motor innervation to the cricothyroid muscle and is responsible for contraction of the vocal cords during laryngospasm.

A superior laryngeal nerve block is achieved by blocking the internal laryngeal nerve to provide anesthesia of the laryngeal mucosa superior to the vocal folds and including their superior surface. This block is used during awake endotracheal intubation and is also used for perioral endoscopy, transesophageal echocardiography, and laryngeal and esophageal instrumentation.

S

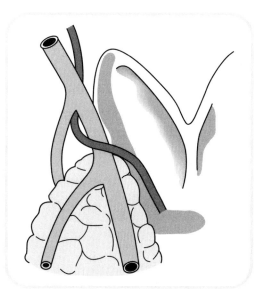

Figure 1 Relationship between superior laryngeal nerve and carotid artery. (From Duh QY. Surgical anatomy and embryology of the thyroid and parathyroid glands and recurrent and external laryngeal nerves. In: Clark OH, Duh QY, eds. *Textbook of Endocrine Surgery*. Philadelphia, PA: WB Saunders; 1997:11. http://www.elsevierimages.com/image/superior.htm.24487)

SUGGESTED READINGS

Barash PG, Cullen BF, Stoelting RK, et al, eds. *Clinical Anesthesia*. 6th ed. Philadelphia, PA: Lippincott Williams & Wilkins; 2009:775.

Finucane BT, Santora AH. *Principles of Airway Management*. 3rd ed. New York, NY: Springer-Verlag; 2003:5–7.

S

<table>
<tr><td>KEYWORD</td><td rowspan="2"># Surgical Stim: Effect on MAC
Physiology</td></tr>
<tr><td>SECTION</td></tr>
</table>

K. Karisa Walker

Edited by Raj K. Modak

KEY POINTS

1. Minimum alveolar concentration (MAC) is defined as the alveolar concentration of an anesthetic agent that prevents movement in response to a surgical stimulus in 50% of patients at 1 atm.
2. MAC can be defined based on other stimuli–response or concentration–response relationships.
3. MAC values are additive when multiple agents are used.
4. Surgical stimulation increases circulating catecholamine levels and therefore increases MAC-BAR.

DISCUSSION

MAC is defined as the alveolar concentration of an anesthetic agent that prevents movement in response to a surgical stimulus in 50% of patients at 1 atm. This is classically determined by skin incision at the abdomen. The concept of MAC allows for the comparison of potency between anesthetics and gives an impression of the partial pressure of inhaled anesthetic at its target site, the brain. Investigators have described concentrations of volatile anesthetic required to prevent movement in response to a variety of noxious stimuli, as depicted below.

MAC in a literal sense does not define adequate anesthesia for all patients. The dose of volatile anesthetic found to prevent movement in 95% of surgical patients is approximately 1.3 MAC. Other definitions for MAC exist depending on the criteria being used to define anesthesia. Self-awareness and recall are thought to be impaired at 0.4–0.5 MAC. MAC awake (the MAC associated with a patient opening his or her eyes on command) is 0.3 to

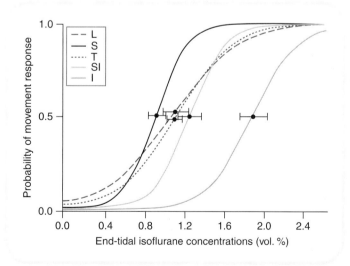

Figure 1. Logistic regression analysis of the end-tidal isoflurane concentration relative to the predicted probability of no movement response for different noxious stimuli. *Bars* indicate the 95% confidence intervals the end-tidal concentration with a 50% probability of response. I, laryngoscopy/intubation; L, laryngoscopy; S, trapezius muscle squeeze; SI, skin incision; T, tetanic nerve stimulation. (From Miller RD, Eriksson LI, Fleisher LA, et al. *Miller's Anesthesia.* 7th ed. Philadelphia, PA: Churchill Livingstone; 2009:1243 , with permission.)

0.4 MAC, with a range of 0.15 to 0.5 MAC, whereas the MAC required to lose consciousness is much less variable at 0.4 to 0.5 MAC. Whereas MAC is a measure of the amount of an anesthetic to prevent the somatic response to surgery, MAC-BAR is the concentration of volatile anesthetic, which 1 prevents sympathetic response to a noxious stimulus, and is approximately 1.5 MAC. Surgical stimulation increases circulating catecholamine levels and therefore increases MAC-BAR. Other factors that increase MAC include hyperthermia, chronic ethanol abuse, hypernatremia, and increased central neurotransmitter levels as can be seen in patients taking certain drugs such as cocaine, monoamine oxidase inhibitors (MAOIs), ephedrine, and levodopa.

MAC values are additive when more than one volatile anesthetic is in use. For example, 0.5 MAC of sevoflurane and 0.5 MAC of nitrous oxide would be roughly equivalent, in terms of the classical definition of MAC, to 1 MAC of a single agent.

SUGGESTED READINGS

Barash PG, Cullen BF, Stoelting RK, et al. *Clinical Anesthesia*. 6th ed. Philadelphia, PA: Lippincott Williams & Wilkins; 2009:424–425.

Miller RD, Eriksson LI, Fleisher LA, et al. *Miller's Anesthesia*. 7th ed. Philadelphia, PA: Churchill Livingstone; 2009:1242–1245.

Morgan GE, Mikhail MS, Murray MJ. *Clinical Anesthesiology*, 4th ed. New York, NY: McGraw-Hill; 2006:163–164.

S

SVO$_2$ Physiology

Physiology

Ashley Kelley

Edited by Veronica Matei

1. Mixed venous oxygen saturation (SVO$_2$) is the oxygen saturation of hemoglobin in pulmonary artery (PA) blood.
2. SVO$_2$ is used as a clinical surrogate for systemic blood flow.
3. Factors affecting the value of SVO$_2$ include cardiac output, hemoglobin concentration, arterial oxygen saturation, and whole-body oxygen consumption.

SVO$_2$ is the oxygen saturation of hemoglobin measured in a sample of blood originating from the PA. This sample can be obtained intermittently from a PA catheter, or SVO$_2$ can be monitored continuously from a specialized PA catheter using reflectance spectrophotometry.

SVO$_2$ is used as a clinical surrogate for systemic blood flow. The normal range of SVO$_2$ is 70% to 75%. Factors affecting the value of SVO$_2$ include cardiac output, hemoglobin concentration, arterial oxygen saturation, and whole-body oxygen consumption.

A decrease in SVO$_2$ indicates decreased systemic blood flow, increased oxygen extraction peripherally, or insufficient O$_2$ delivery to meet the consumption requirements. Decreased systemic blood flow is the result of various pathophysiologic events, for example, decreased cardiac output. Increased oxygen extraction may be caused by hypermetabolism. Decreased oxygen delivery results for such reasons as anemia and hypoxemia. The equation that demonstrates these relationships is $SVO_2 = DO_2/VO_2$, where DO_2 equals O$_2$ delivery and VO_2 equals O$_2$ consumption. In turn, these may be further broken down into their components. DO_2 equals cardiac output times the arterial O$_2$ content ($Q \times CaO_2$), and VO_2 equals cardiac output times the CaO$_2$ minus the venous O$_2$ content ($Q \times [CaO_2-CVO_2]$). Normal oxygen delivery is 900 to 1,100 mL per minute, and normal oxygen consumption is 200 to 270 mL per minute.

Common causes of an abnormally low SVO$_2$ are anemia or pathologic states leading to low CO, such as heart failure, myocardial infarction, or hypovolemia, whereas abnormally high SVO$_2$ values can be seen in sepsis, burns, certain toxicities such as cyanide or methemoglobinemia, or with a wedged PA catheter.

Marino PL. *The ICU Book*. 3rd ed. Philadelphia, PA: Lippincott Williams & Wilkins; 2007:21–24, 199–201, 390–392.
Morgan GE, Mikhail MS, Murray MJ. *Clinical Anesthesiology*. 4th ed. New York, NY: McGraw-Hill; 2006:141.
Stoelting RK, Miller RD, eds. *Basics of Anesthesia*. 5th ed. Philadelphia, PA: Churchill Livingstone; 2007:311.

Sympathetic Block Indications
Subspecialties: Pain

Dallen Mill

Edited by Thomas Halaszynski

1. Indications for sympathetic blockade include treatment of pain and some vascular disorders, reflex sympathetic dystrophy, herpetic neuralgia, peripheral vascular disease, and visceral pain.
2. Sympathetic blockade can be accomplished in several ways and is capable of treating numerous pain etiologies. These include general blocks of subarachnoid, epidural, or paravertebral blockade. More specific techniques include: stellate block, thoracic chain block, celiac plexus block, splanchnic nerve block, hypogastric plexus block, ganglion block, and intravenous regional sympathetic blockade, all of which have specific indications.

The primary indication for sympathetic blockade is the treatment of pain, but may also be indicated in the treatment of vascular disorders. Stellate ganglion block (also called *acervicothoracic sympathetic block*) is used primarily to treat complex regional pain syndrome (CRPS), but has also been used to treat refractory angina, phantom limb pain, vascular insufficiency (such as Raynaud disease or frostbite), hyperhidrosis, and other disorders. Lumbar sympathetic blocks (performed at second lumbar level) have been used for CRPS, as well as vascular insufficiency (e.g., in diabetic lower limb ischemia).

Pain:

- CRPS I and II (also called reflex sympathetic dystrophy)
- Acute herpetic and postherpetic neuralgia
- Visceral pain (typically associated with malignancy)
- Malignant and nonmalignant pelvic pain
- Phantom limb pain
- Frostbite
- Chronic donor site pain
- Postthoracotomy pain syndrome

Vascular pain:

- Peripheral vascular disease
- Raynaud disease

Spinal, epidural, peripheral nerve blocks, and paravertebral blocks can result in sympathetic blockade; however, they may also result in blockade of somatic fibers. In the specific diagnoses above, sympathetic blockade can be accomplished by a variety of techniques as indicated and discussed below:

- *Cervicothoracic (stellate) block.* This block usually blocks all the cervical and upper thoracic ganglia, and it is useful in patients with head, neck, arm, and upper chest pain, as well as vasospastic disorders of the upper extremity.
- *Thoracic sympathetic chain block.* Although this technique is very rarely used because of risk of pneumothorax, indications for this block are treatment of CRPS I or II, neuropathic pain in the thorax or chest wall, herpes zoster, postherpetic

neuralgia, and phantom pain after mastectomy. Vascular or vasospastic injury of the upper extremity can also respond to this block. Neoplastic or other painful pathology of the intrathoracic viscera, such as cancer of the esophagus, heart, trachea, or lung, can also respond well to this type of block.

- *Celiac plexus block.* The celiac block is indicated for pain in the abdominal visceral region, especially in patients with malignancy related to the abdominal wall or musculature.
- *Splanchnic nerve block.* Similar to the celiac plexus block, except without the additional blockade of the lumbar sympathetic chain, splanchnic nerve block results in postural hypotension.
- *Lumbar sympathetic block.* This block is indicated in patients with pain involving the pelvic region or lower extremities. Some patients with peripheral vascular disease involving the lower extremities leading to claudication pain may also benefit from this block.
- *Hypogastric plexus block.* With sensory fibers that bypass the lower spinal cord, this block is indicated in patients with cancer pain of the bladder, prostate, cervix, uterus, or rectum, mainly in those with pain in the pelvis in which epidural blocks have been unsuccessful.
- *Ganglion impar block.* A specific block for patients with pain in the perineal area, either sympathetic or visceral.
- *Intravenous regional sympathetic blockade.* A Bier block specifically using guanethidine can interrupt sympathetic innervations to an extremity for 3 to 7 days and is indicated in patients with pain in extremities with hemostatic compromise.

SUGGESTED READING

Morgan GE, Mikhail MS, Murray MJ. *Clinical Anesthesiology.* 4th ed. New York, NY: McGraw-Hill; 2006:383–387.

S

Synchronized Electrical Cardioversion

Generic, Clinical Sciences: Anesthesia Procedures, Methods, Techniques

Kellie Park

Edited by Qingbing Zhu

1. Synchronized cardioversion is the transient delivery of a current at a specific point in the ECG cycle, which causes depolarization of cardiac cells, allowing the sinus node to resume normal function and avoid ventricle arrhythmia.
2. It can be used for patients with reentrant tachycardia, stable ventricular tachycardia (VT), atrial fibrillation, atrial flutter, or other supraventricular tachycardia.
3. Synchronized cardioversion can be done externally or internally.
4. Sedation is usually needed, as cardioversion is uncomfortable in the awake patient.
5. Anesthesiologists must maintain safety practices in the same manner as with any other sedation they perform.

Electrical cardioversion is the use of direct current to treat reentrant-induced dysrhythmias, such as paroxysmal supraventricular tachycardia or VT, as well as atrial fibrillation, atrial flutter, or other supraventricular tachycardia. Pads or paddles are placed on the chest of the patient, and a shock is delivered specifically (synchronized) at the R wave of the QRS complex. This avoids shocking the patient during ventricular repolarization (T wave), which can lead to subsequent development of other arrhythmias, especially ventricular fibrillation. The delivery of current causes a brief depolarization of most cardiac cells, allowing the sinus node to "reset" and resume normal function.

When cardioverting a patient, it is critical to determine the type of device being used. The machines are either monophasic or biphasic. If a monophasic device is selected, after contacting the skin of the chest with the paddles, it can deliver 200 J to the patient's chest wall. If the rhythm does not convert, one can increase by 100 J with each shock for a maximum of 400 J. If using a biphasic device, starting dose is 100 J, as this device automatically adjusts to the patient's thoracic impedance. In patients with automatic implantable cardioverter defibrillators (AICDs) already in place, internal cardioversion is the method of choice to avoid using paddles on the skin, which can cause side effects such as skin discomfort and/or burns.

It is appropriate to use some sedation and analgesia in patients who are being electrically cardioverted because the procedure is often uncomfortable and distressing. Small amounts of barbiturates such as methohexital or propofol are often used, as well as benzodiazepines and narcotics, all being titrated to keeping the patient sedated, yet breathing spontaneously.

As with any other patient sedation, the anesthesiologist must make sure to have monitors including ECG, pulse oximetry, and blood pressure, as well as equipment readily available including suction, airway equipment, a working intravenous line, a bag mask valve device capable of delivering positive pressure ventilation, oxygen, and a crash cart with all drugs and equipment for cardiopulmonary resuscitation.

Marino PL. *The ICU Book*. 3rd ed. Philadelphia, PA: Lippincott Williams & Wilkins; 2007:346.
Morgan GE, Mikhail MS, Murray MJ. *Clinical Anesthesiology*. 4th ed. New York, NY: McGraw-Hill; 2006:533–535.

TEF: Other Abnormalities
Subspecialties: Pediatric Anesthesia

Margo Vallee

Edited by Mamatha Punjala

KEY POINTS

1. Tracheoesophageal fistula (TEF) is due to the failure of the endoderm of the trachea and esophagus to divide.
2. The most common TEF is type C, described by proximal esophageal atresia (EA) with a distal fistula between the trachea and the lower esophageal segment.
3. Congenital heart disease occurs in 25% to 30% of patients with TEF. Some of the anomalies that can be seen are ventricular septal defect, patent ductus arteriosus, tetralogy of Fallot, atrial septal defect, and coarctation of the aorta.
4. There are several musculoskeletal abnormalities that may be present including vertebral malformation, radial aplasia, polydactyly, and knee malformations.
5. Gastrointestinal abnormalities that may be encountered are midgut malrotations, pyloric stenosis, duodenal atresia, Meckel diverticulum, imperforate anus, and ectopic pancreas.
6. Associated genitourinary anomalies include renal malposition, renal agenesis, ureteral abnormalities, hydronephrosis, and hypospadias.

DISCUSSION

TEF has an incidence of approximately 1 in 3,000 to 3,500 live births. TEF is due to the failure of the endoderm of the trachea and esophagus to divide. Normally, by the 26th day of gestation, the trachea and esophagus separate. If the separation of the trachea from the esophagus occurs later than normal, the trachea, which grows faster than the esophagus, will separate the proximal and distal esophagus. The fistula tract is thought to be related to defective epithelial–mesenchymal interactions, which leads to EA and a TEF.

There are six types of TEF referred to by letters A through F. The most common TEF is type C, described by proximal EA with a distal fistula between the trachea and the lower esophageal segment. Type C accounts for nearly 90% of all TEF. Approximately 8% have EA without TEF. The other types are less common. Illustration of the types and relative frequencies can be found in Figure 1.

Overall, the incidence of TEF-associated anomalies is between 30% and 50%. Organ systems affected include cardiovascular, musculoskeletal, gastrointestinal, genitourinary, and craniofacial. Congenital heart disease occurs in 25% to 30% of patients with TEF. Some of the anomalies that can be seen are ventricular septal defect, patent ductus arteriosus, tetralogy of Fallot, atrial septal defect, and coarctation of the aorta. There are several musculoskeletal abnormalities that can be present, including vertebral malformation, radial aplasia, polydactyly, and knee malformations. Gastrointestinal abnormalities that may be encountered are midgut malrotations, pyloric stenosis, duodenal atresia, Meckel diverticulum, imperforate anus, and ectopic pancreas. Associated genitourinary anomalies include renal malposition, renal agenesis, ureteral abnormalities, hydronephrosis, and hypospadias. Lastly, cleft lip and cleft palate may be seen.

Some infants who have TEF have a well-recognized constellation of anomalies that fall into the category of VATER syndrome, which includes *V*ertebral anomalies, *A*nal malformations, *T*racheo*E*sophageal fistula, *R*adial limb dysplasia, and *R*enal deformities. Typically, the anomalies are responsible for the majority of the morbidity and mortality of these patients. Of particular importance is the recognition of coexisting cardiac defects. Notably, prematurity occurs in approximately 30% of these cases.

Before delivery, polyhydramnios is noted in about two-thirds of pregnancies involving an infant affected by EA/TEF. Despite this, many cases are not diagnosed prenatally. Signs

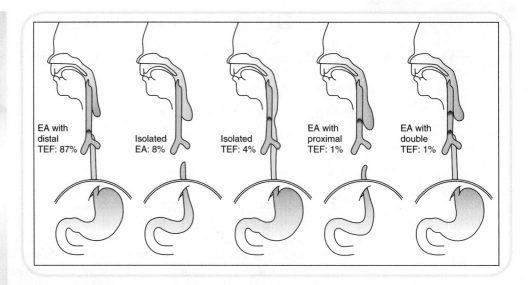

Figure 1. Classification from left to right: C, A, E, B, D. Not shown is type F, which is isolated esophageal stenosis. (From Clark DC. Esophageal atresia and tracheoesophageal fistula. *Am Fam Physician.* 1999;59:910–913, with permission.)

and symptoms of TEF include cyanotic episodes, coughing relieved by suctioning, excessive drooling, and inability to pass a soft catheter into the stomach. A catheter that stops at about 10 cm from the gum line is very suggestive of EA. Radiologic findings include a curled catheter located in the upper esophageal pouch and an air bubble in the stomach.

Preoperatively, the goal is to identify any associated congenital lesions and to assess the pulmonary system. Routine labs including complete blood count, electrolytes, glucose, calcium, and an arterial blood gas (ABG) should be obtained. Echocardiography should be done to rule out cardiac anomalies. Patients should remain NPO and be kept in the upright position with intermittent suctioning.

Pulmonary complications can be serious, as regurgitation and aspiration are common. Fluid in the pharynx cannot be swallowed because of the EA. In addition, the stomach can become significantly distended via the distal TEF. This can lead to impaired diaphragmatic function. Reflux is also common. Infants are frequently found to have pneumonitis and atelectasis. Hypoxemia and acidosis may ensue and should be monitored with serial ABGs.

Isolated TEF without EA is often not diagnosed immediately, and frequently presents in older infants and occasionally in adolescents or adults. Signs include coughing with feeding, choking, and pneumonitis. At times, a contrast esophageal study is sufficient to show the fistula, but if nonconfirmatory, a bronchoscopy should be done.

Often, the infants with TEF are intubated immediately in the delivery room. Positive pressure ventilation should not be used because it can significantly increase the air in the gut. The distal TEF is often just above the carina, making endotracheal tube placement difficult. A common approach is to push the endotracheal tube into the right main stem bronchus and pull back until bilateral breath sounds are heard. This typically places the tip just above the carina and usually distal to the fistula, so the stomach is not inflated.

A precordial stethoscope should be used to help in the detection of intraoperative obstruction in the event that the tube is dislodged by positioning or surgical manipulation. Standard monitors as well as arterial catheters are indicated. Nitrous oxide is contraindicated. If a sudden deterioration in heart rate, blood pressure, oxygen saturation, or lung compliance occurs, a contralateral pneumothorax should be considered in the differential diagnosis. In the case of pneumothorax, immediate treatment with chest tube insertion is of paramount importance. Pulmonary vascular resistance should be kept low, with the avoidance of hypoxia and hypercarbia. General recommendations are to keep the PaO_2 around 90 to 100 mm Hg and $PaCO_2$ in the 25 to 30 mm Hg range.

SUGGESTED READINGS

Gregory GA. *Pediatric Anesthesia.* 3rd ed. Philadelphia, PA: Churchill Livingstone; 1994:438–442.

Katz J, Steward DJ. *Anesthesia and Uncommon Pediatric Diseases.* 2nd ed. Philadelphia, PA: WB Saunders Company; 1993:109–112.

Motoyama EK, Davis PJ, eds. *Smith's Anesthesia for Infants and Children.* 7th ed. Philadelphia, PA: Mosby; 2006:550–552.

Tension Pneumocephalus: Dx
Anatomy

Caroline Al Haddadin

Edited by Ramachandran Ramani

1. Tension pneumocephalus is a rare complication of intracranial or craniofacial surgeries and could be rapidly life-threatening if not immediately diagnosed and treated.
2. Risk factors for the development of tension pneumocephalus include (a) type of surgery (posterior fossa interventions and burr hole, ventriculoperitoneal (VP) shunt, and lumbar drain placements conferring higher risk) and (b) position (sitting carries higher risk of air trapping).
3. Diagnosis of tension pneumocephalus relies on a high index of suspicion in patients who develop altered mental status or focal neurologic deficits after a high-risk surgery. CT scan of the head will reveal a dark, air-filled cavity compressing intracranial contents.

Pneumocephalus, defined as the presence of intracranial air (whether subdural, subarachnoid, epidural, or intraventricular), is common after neurosurgery. Virtually, all postcraniotomy patients have small amounts of free air secondary to surgical disruption of the bone or the dura. This is usually a benign condition that resolves spontaneously within a few days, as the body reabsorbs the small amount of air. In contrast, **tension** pneumocephalus, although rare occurring in approximately 0.1% to 3% of all craniotomies, carries a grave prognosis if not identified and corrected immediately.

Diagnosis of tension pneumocephalus begins with a high index of suspicion in patients at risk for the development of this complication. Risk factors include the following:

- *Type of surgery:* An increased risk is conferred by interventions such as posterior fossa operations, burr hole placement, craniofacial surgery, transsphenoidal hypophysectomy, VP shunt, or lumbar drain placement.
- *Position:* The sitting position during or after surgery carries the highest risk of air entrapment.
- *Facial fractures:* Fractures of the frontal and paranasal sinuses, orbital roof, cribriform plate, predispose to pneumocephalus during conditions of raised external pressure. Raised pressure can result from severe coughing, sneezing, vigorous nose-blowing or Valsalva maneuver, or with the use of continuous positive airway pressure (CPAP) or bilevel positive airway pressure (BiPAP) postoperatively in patients with facial fractures.
- Potentially, *intraoperative nitrous oxide use* may also worsen pneumocephalus, although published evidence for this is lacking. Nitrous oxide is known to diffuse from blood into air-filled cavities and may facilitate the development of tension pneumocephalus.

One of the proposed mechanisms for the development of pneumocephalus implicates the rapid removal of cerebrospinal fluid (CSF) to facilitate surgical exposure during neurosurgery. Known as the *inverted soda-pop bottle* hypothesis, it states that fluid leaving an inverted bottle creates a negative pressure or vacuum that sucks in and traps air at the top. Thus, during craniotomies, as the CSF is removed or drained to allow better visualization of the brain tissue, air can be trapped inside the calvarium. In addition, brain mass is decreased with Lasix, mannitol, and steroids during neurosurgery, and this creates additional space for air entrapment. For example, during the closing of a craniotomy for a posterior fossa tumor or C-spine surgery in a seated patient, the brain will be lying above the incision, which means that when CSF is drained downward, air can be trapped through the incision. In fact, air is retained in almost all craniotomies regardless of the position of the patient; however, the small amount of air is not usually of great concern because it is reabsorbed by the body within a few days.

As the brain reexpands during the postoperative period, any air that was not reabsorbed can begin to generate pressure on the intracranial contents (Fig. 1). Tension pneumocephalus can occur with as little as 25 cc of air. Air compressing the brain can lead to delayed awakening from anesthesia, changes in mental status post-op, focal neurologic deficits, or even sudden cardiovascular collapse. The diagnosis of tension pneumocephalus relies on a high index of suspicion in patients who have any one of the above risk factors, who become somnolent or develop focal deficits. The diagnosis can be confirmed with CT (gold standard), seen as a dark, air-filled cavity compressing the ventricles and cerebral tissue. Oftentimes, however, unstable patients with suspected tension pneumocephalus must be treated immediately with decompression (surgical evacuation or needle decompression of the air pocket through an existing burr hole), whereas closed water-seal systems are preferred in patients with drains.

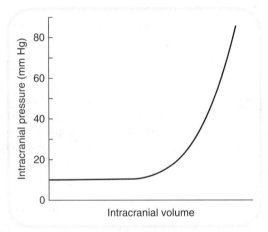

Figure 1. Tension pneumocephalus can occur when intracranial volume increases to the point that intracranial pressure is increased. (From Morgan GE, Mikhail MS, Murray MJ. Anesthesia for neurosurgery. In: *Clinical Anesthesiology*. 4th ed. McGraw-Hill Co; 2006:637–638. http://www.accessmedicine.com.)

SUGGESTED READINGS

Barash P, Cullen BF, Stoelting R, et al, eds. Patient positioning and related injuries. In: *Clinical Anesthesia*. 6th ed. Philadelphia, PA: Lippincott Williams & Wilkins; 2009:811.

Morgan GE, Mikhail MS, Murray MJ, eds. Anesthesia for neurosurgery. In: *Clinical Anesthesiology*. 4th ed. New York, NY: McGraw-Hill Co; 2006:637–638.

Newfield P, Cottrell JE, eds. *Handbook of Neuroanesthesia*. 4th ed. Philadelphia, PA: Lippincott Williams & Wilkins; 2007:141–142.

Webber-Jones JE. Tension pneumocephalus. *J Neurosci Nurs*. 2005;37(5):272–276.

Tension Pneumothorax: Dx and Rx
Organ-based Clinical: Respiratory

Bijal Patel

Edited by Shamsuddin Akhtar

KEY POINTS

1. Tension pneumothorax is a condition in which air or gas enters into the pleural cavity through a defect that acts as a one-way valve that may result in the compression of mediastinal structures and the contralateral lung.
2. Classic signs of tension pneumothorax are hypotension, neck vein distention, tracheal deviation, cyanosis, tachypnea, and absent/diminished breath sounds.
3. Definitive diagnosis is made via chest X-ray.
4. If tension pneumothorax is suspected in an unstable patient, one should not wait for radiographic confirmation and should proceed straight to treatment.
5. Treatment involves the insertion of a 14 G angiocatheter at the fourth intercostal space in the midaxillary line or at the second intercostal space at the midclavicular line.

DISCUSSION

Tension pneumothorax is a condition in which air or gas enters into the pleural cavity through a defect that acts as a one-way valve. This defect allows for air/gas to enter the cavity during inspiration, but does not allow it to exit during expiration. This creates increasing pressures within the cavity. Significant increase in intrapleural pressure results in the compression of mediastinal structures and the contralateral lung. The classic findings in a patient with tension pneumothorax are hypotension, neck vein distention, tracheal deviation, cyanosis, tachypnea, and absent/diminished breath sounds on the side of the pneumothorax side.

Tension pneumothorax can be confirmed on a chest X-ray. However, in a hemodynamically unstable/hypoxic patient, one should not wait for a radiograph to confirm the diagnosis. In this case, high clinical suspicion should allow one to proceed straight to treatment. Treatment involves the insertion of a 14 G angiocatheter at the fourth intercostal space in the midaxillary line. An alternate site for insertion is the second intercostal space at the midclavicular line. This maneuver allows the air to escape from the pleural cavity and decreases intrapleural pressure. Definitive treatment includes placement of a chest tube after the more immediate treatment of an angiocatheter placement.

SUGGESTED READINGS

Barash PG, Cullen BF, Stoelting RK, et al. *Clinical Anesthesia.* 6th ed. New York, NY: Lippincott, Williams & Wilkins; 2009:894.

Kumar V, Abbas AK, Fausto N. *Robbins and Cotran Pathologic Basis of Disease.* 7th ed. Philadelphia, PA: Elsevier Saunders; 2005:767–768.

T

Tetralogy of Fallot Rx
Subspecialties: Pediatrics

Samantha Franco

Edited by Mamatha Punjala

1. Tetralogy of Fallot (TOF) is a cyanotic congenital heart disease composed of a combination of ventricular septal defect (VSD), pulmonary valvular and/or right ventricular infundibular stenosis, right ventricular hypertrophy, and a large overriding aorta.
2. Hypercyanotic "tet" spells are caused by severe infundibular spasm, induced by changes in venous return and systemic vascular resistance (SVR), worsening a right-to-left shunt.
3. Prevention of hypercyanotic spells involves preanesthetic sedation, β-blockade, adequate anesthetic depth, and avoidance of hypovolemia and afterload reduction.
4. Patients with cyanotic TOF undergo either neonatal complete repair or neonatal palliation with an aortopulmonary shunt, followed by a complete repair at 4 to 6 months of age.
5. Complications following TOF repair can include atrial tachycardias, right bundle branch block (RBBB), ventricular ectopy, residual lesions or shunts, paradoxical emboli, and difficult vascular access.

TOF is the most common cause of cyanotic congenital cardiac disease in patients beyond the neonatal age, occurring in 3 of every 10,000 live births and accounting for up to one-tenth of all congenital cardiac lesions. TOF is composed of a combination of VSD, pulmonary valvular and/or right ventricular infundibular stenosis, right ventricular hypertrophy, and a large overriding aorta. The degree of right ventricular outflow and/or pulmonic obstruction determines the onset and severity of cyanosis.

Most patients will present with closure of the ductus arteriosus in the neonatal period with mild-to-moderate cyanosis, but typically without respiratory distress. Prostaglandin E_1 may be used to clinically stabilize the patient before surgical intervention. More uncommonly, patients with very mild right ventricular outflow tract obstruction at birth may be diagnosed at a couple months of age because the obstruction worsens, resulting in newly noticed cyanosis and a louder murmur. As patients with TOF have obstruction to pulmonary blood flow, they will not present with signs of heart failure such as failure to thrive. In TOF, both ventricles work at systemic pressure, but volume overload does not occur, and congestive heart failure is rare. Most patients will not exhibit lethargy or irritability unless in the setting of a "hypercyanotic (tet) spell" wherein cyanosis with hyperventilation and acidosis may occur. These "tet" spells are caused by severe infundibular spasm, probably induced by changes in venous return and SVR. When there is a reduction in SVR or decreased venous return, pulmonary blood flow decreases because blood tends to be shunted to the systemic circulation. In older children, the squatting posture may improve symptoms by increasing venous return from the lower extremities and by increasing SVR. The treatment of hypercyanotic spells is based on the goals of decreasing infundibular spasm by decreasing contractility and heart rate, and by increasing preload. Another goal (especially in fixed right ventricular outflow obstruction) is to increase SVR to decrease right-to-left shunting across the VSD. Some of the preventive measures and treatments for hypercyanotic spells are briefly outlined in Table 1.

Further examination in a patient suspected of TOF includes auscultation, ECG, and echocardiography. Upon auscultation, the second heart sound may be single and loud

Table 1. Prevention and Treatment Options for Hypercyanotic Tet Spells

Prevention	Treatment
Preanesthetic sedation	Prevent and relieve airway obstruction
Continued β-blockade	100% oxygen
Maintain adequate anesthetic depth	Deepen anesthesia or provide sedation
Avoid hypovolemia	Give fluid bolus
Avoid afterload reduction	Increase SVR—phenylephrine 1–2 µg/kg IV
	Esmolol 100–200 µg/kg/min
	Aortic compression

with a harsh systolic ejection murmur, emanating from the obstructed subpulmonary outflow tract; however, patients with severe obstruction may have very little antegrade flow across the subpulmonary outflow tract, be more significantly cyanotic, and have a less prominent murmur. Once the lesion is suspected, ECG and chest radiograph should be performed. The ECG will demonstrate right-axis deviation and prominent right ventricular forces, with large R waves in the anterior precordial leads and large S waves in the lateral precordial leads. Although the ECG is similar to that of a normal newborn, the right ventricular hypertrophy and right-axis deviation will not normalize in a patient with TOF. The classical chest radiograph will demonstrate a boot-shaped cardiac silhouette owing to displacement of the right ventricular apex from right ventricular hypertrophy. Diagnosis is confirmed with echocardiography.

Clinical management of a TOF patient is determined by the degree and type of subpulmonary obstruction, leading to the initiation of prostaglandin therapy to preserve ductal patency and provide a stable source of blood flow to the lungs with surgical intervention before hospital discharge, whereas others with adequate forward flow through the right ventricular outflow tract after ductal closure can be managed on an outpatient basis with close follow-up until a complete repair is performed. Patients with cyanotic TOF will either undergo neonatal complete repair or neonatal palliation with an aortopulmonary shunt, followed by a complete repair at 4 to 6 months of age. Complete neonatal repair provides prompt relief of the volume and pressure overload on the right ventricle, minimizes cyanosis, decreases parental anxiety, and eliminates the theoretical risk of stenosis occurring in a pulmonary artery resulting from a palliative procedure. Patients who undergo a successful complete repair during the neonatal period will be unlikely to require more than one intervention in the first year of life, but are not free from reintervention. Concerns regarding such neonatal complete repairs include exposure of the neonatal brain to cardiopulmonary bypass, and the increased need to place a patch across the ventriculopulmonary junction when compared with older age at repair. These so-called transannular patches create a state of chronic pulmonary regurgitation, which increases morbidity in young adults, producing exercise intolerance and ventricular arrhythmias. If left untreated, this increases the risk of sudden death. In summary, without randomized control trials, assessing the risk and benefits of the two surgical strategies has been notoriously difficult. Perioperative mortality rates for either surgical approach is less than 3%, and since neither strategy has shown superior results, surgical management remains dependent on the protocols preferred by the individual centers.

These patients should arrive in the operating room well sedated. Preoperative fluid restriction should be minimized to maintain adequate preload and/or maintenance fluid given intravenously (IV) to prevent hemoconcentration and hypovolemia. A smooth induction will help prevent increases in oxygen demand or hypercyanotic spells. The agents used should have minimal vasodilating properties, supporting halothane theoretically over isoflurane or sevoflurane, hence minimizing any increase in the right-to-left shunt. Mild myocardial depression is desirable, as it may relieve the infundibular obstruction. IV barbiturate dosages may be halved, and ketamine can be used, especially in very sick patients, because it maintains SVR and does not cause or worsen "tet" spells. With induction of anesthesia, arterial oxygen saturation generally increases in cyanotic patients, most likely because of the reduction in oxygen consumption during anesthesia and the increase in venous saturation. For major surgery, intra-arterial and/or central venous pressures should be measured directly, which aids in blood sampling and acid–base measurements, as well as central venous pressure estimation of stress on the right ventricle. Patients may still develop hypercyanotic spells perioperatively, because of the dynamic nature of the muscular infundibular obstruction present in TOF, and strategies listed in Table 1 may help alleviate the symptoms.

There are specific complications and sequelae following repair of TOF. Older repairs of TOF have resulted in right ventricular dysfunction due to pulmonary insufficiency, and a high incidence of dysrhythmias from right ventriculostomies. Incomplete relief of right ventricular outflow tract obstruction, demonstrated by RV:LV systolic pressure ratio of greater than 0.5, is an independent predictor of late mortality after repair. Repair at an older age is also associated with higher long-term mortality, as is the presence of a large outflow patch. The majority of patients are symptom free following repair. Some survivors of earlier repairs have a 6% incidence of sudden death, and at least a 10% incidence of inducible ventricular tachycardia, requiring AICD (an implantable cardioverter defibrillator) implantation. Patients should be consistently evaluated at follow-up visits for residual shunts and atrial and ventricular dysrhythmias.

SUGGESTED READINGS

Bailliard F, Anderson RH. Tetralogy of Fallot. *Orphanet J Rare Dis.* 2009;4:2.

Barash PG, Cullen BF, Stoelting RK, et al, eds. *Clinical Anesthesia.* 6th ed. Philadelphia, PA: Lippincott Williams & Wilkins; 2009:1155–1156.

Reed A, Yudkowitz F, eds. *Clinical Cases in Anesthesia.* 3rd ed. Philadelphia, PA: Elsevier, Churchill, Livingstone; 2005:409–418.

T

Thiopental: CMRO$_2$/CBF Relationship

Organ-based Clinical: Neurologic and Neuromuscular

Lisbeysi Calo

Edited by Ramachandran Ramani

KEY POINTS

1. Cerebral blood flow (CBF) is autoregulated over a wide range of mean arterial pressures (50 to 150 mm Hg) and averages 50 mL/100 g/min. Cerebral oxygen consumption is a major determinant of ischemic risk in the brain and is approximately 50 mL per minute.
2. Thiopental, like other intravenous (IV) anesthetics, decreases CBF and cerebral metabolic rate of oxygen consumption (CMRO$_2$) in parallel.
3. As a barbiturate, thiopental affords brain protection in cases of regional ischemia, but has not been shown to improve neurologic outcomes in cases of global brain ischemia.

DISCUSSION

CBF. The average CBF is approximately 50 to 55 mL/100 g/min, with gray matter having a higher flow than white matter. CBF is autoregulated, which means it is maintained constant over a wide range of mean arterial pressure (50 to 150 mm Hg), thus protecting the brain from ischemia.

CMRO$_2$. The CMRO$_2$ is an important determinant of the risk of ischemic insult. It averages 3 to 3.5 mL/100 g/min in adults (approximately 50 mL per minute for a 1,500 g brain). At high metabolic rates, a reduced CBF is more likely to produce neuronal damage. Decreased CMRO$_2$ makes ischemia less likely. IV anesthetics decrease CMRO$_2$ and CBF in parallel, with an associated reduction in cerebral blood volume and intracranial pressure. This is important with regard to the treatment of intracranial hypertension.

Thiopental is a barbiturate that depresses the reticular activating system; it suppresses transmission of excitatory neurotransmitters such as acetylcholine and enhances the transmission of inhibitory neurotransmitters (e.g., GABA). Thiopental decreases the CMRO$_2$ in a dose-dependent fashion, until a maximum effect is reached at a level of 50% to 55% reduction in oxygen consumption, at which point the electroencephalogram (EEG) becomes isoelectric. Secondarily, it also decreases the CBF, and therefore ICP, by causing cerebral vasoconstriction. With higher doses of thiopental, however, no further decrease in CMRO$_2$ are observed.

Thiopental can potentially provide cerebral protection during transient episodes of regional ischemia, particularly when given in anticipation of a potential ischemic event such as carotid artery cross-clamping during carotid endarterectomies. The dose of thiopental for the treatment of focal ischemia is titrated to EEG burst suppression. During global ischemia, however, thiopental does not seem to afford brain protection as measured by clinical neurologic outcomes.

Mechanisms proposed for the cerebral protection seen with thiopental include not only the decreases in CMRO$_2$ and CBF, but also the attenuation of neuronal injury, free radical scavenging, and alteration of fatty acid metabolism. As a barbiturate, thiopental has anticonvulsant properties. Thiopental may also help with membrane stabilization, calcium channel blockade, and maintenance of protein synthesis, all of which may contribute to improved neurologic outcome.

The Robin-Hood phenomenon, a reverse steal phenomenon, has been described with the use of thiopental, whereby vasoconstriction in normal brain tissue improves the perfusion of ischemic areas that are unable to vasoconstrict (ischemic vasomotor paralysis).

T

Extraperfusion of these at-risk areas helps reduce the risk of ischemia and may therefore afford neuronal protection in areas of injury and decreased blood flow.

SUGGESTED READINGS

Lobato EB, Gravenstein NK, Robert R, eds. *Complications in Anesthesiology*. Philadelphia, PA: Lippincott Williams & Wilkins; 2008:316.

Mantha S, Ochroch EA, Roizen MF, et al. Anesthesia for vascular surgery. In: Barash PG, Cullen BF, Stoelting RK, et al, eds. *Clinical Anesthesia*. 6th ed. Philadelphia, PA: Lippincott Williams & Wilkins; 2009:811.

Morgan GE, Mikhail MS, Murray MJ. Neurophysiology & anesthesia. In: *Clinical Anesthesiology*. 4th ed. New York, NY: McGraw-Hill Co; 2006:621.

Newfield P, Cottrell JE, eds. *Handbook of Neuroanesthesia*. 4th ed. Philadelphia, PA: Lippincott Williams & Wilkins; 2007:63.

Thoracoscopy: Hypoxemia Rx
Organ-based Clinical: Respiratory

Tiffany Denepitiya-Balicki

Edited by Veronica Matei

KEY POINTS

1. Lung separation for the purpose of controlling ventilation distribution is often needed to optimize surgical exposure in thoracoscopic cases and to prevent the spread of infected or bloody secretions.
2. Patients are often placed in the lateral decubitus position during thoracoscopic procedures. Positioning further increases the chances of hypoxemia by creating a potentially large shunt.

DISCUSSION

Thoracoscopy is a technique in which a fiberoptic scope is placed into the thorax, allowing inspection of thoracic contents as well as various diagnostic and surgical maneuvers. Although thoracoscopy may be carried out under local or regional anesthesia, it is most commonly performed under general anesthesia, often necessitating lung separation.

Multiple factors contribute to rendering the patients undergoing thoracoscopic procedures prone to developing hypoxemia. In the awake, upright patient, significant differences exist between the four lung zones in terms of ventilation and perfusion. The compliance of the alveoli differs between the apical portion (where alveoli are maximally inflated) and the basal portion. In addition, due to gravitational forces, the basal portion receives proportionally more blood flow than the apical portion. Taken together, these opposing forces create a V/Q mismatch that is accentuated when patients undergo general anesthesia (Fig. 1).

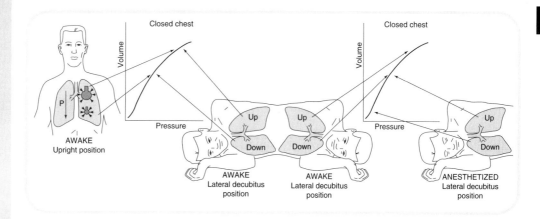

Figure 1. Effect of position on lung function (Reused from Morgan GE, Mikhail MS, Murray MJ. Anesthesia for thoracic surgery. In: *Clinical Anesthesiology.* 4th ed. New York, NY: McGraw-Hill Co; 2006:585–600. http://www .accessmedicine.com, with permission.)

Under anesthesia in the supine or lateral decubitus position, these physiologic changes become more pronounced. In the lateral decubitus position, the nondependent lung (the operative lung) is better ventilated than the dependent lung, which receives more blood flow. Once the nondependent lung is deflated for surgical purposes, that lung is no longer ventilated; however, it is still perfused, and thereby an inherent shunt is created.

Once hypoxemia has been identified in a thoracoscopic case using one-lung ventilation (OLV), initial steps that must be taken include the following:

1. Ensure the patient is breathing 100% oxygen during.
2. Inspect the endotracheal tube for positional movement.
3. Check for bilateral breath sounds, evaluating for the possibility of a pneumothorax in the dependent lung, secondary to barotrauma.
4. Inspect the breathing circuit to rule out disconnections or obstruction.
5. Suction the endotracheal tube for blood or secretions.
6. Severe hypoxemia mandates immediate conversion to double-lung ventilation.

If hypoxemia persists after these basic steps have been taken, alterations in ventilation may be appropriate. Maneuvers that mitigate the shunt created by one-lung ventilation may improve oxygenation; these include: (a) intermittent inflation on the nondependent lung and the application of a small amount of CPAP (5 to 10 cm H_2O) to the nondependent lung and (b) addition of PEEP to the dependent lung. Adding PEEP, however, may be a tenuous solution, as excessive PEEP may shunt blood away from the dependent lung, further worsening the shunt.

Finally, having the surgeon clamp the pulmonary artery that supplies blood to the nondependent lung may be necessary if all other maneuvers prove unsuccessful. This risky maneuver can eliminate the shunt created by the perfused but nonventilated operative lung, and is reserved for situations in which all other methods have failed to improve oxygenation.

SUGGESTED READINGS

Barash PG, Cullen BF, Stoelting RK, et al, eds. Patient anesthesia for surgical subspecialties. In: *Clinical Anesthesia*. 6th ed. Philadelphia, PA: Lippincott Williams & Wilkins; 2009:1040–1054.

Morgan GE, Mikhail MS, Murray MJ. Anesthesia for thoracic surgery. In: *Clinical Anesthesiology*. 4th ed. New York, NY: McGraw-Hill Co; 2006:585–600.

Reed A, Yudkowitz F. *Clinical Cases in Anesthesia*. 3rd ed. Philadelphia, PA: Elsevier Churchill Livingstone; 2005:73–84.

T

Thyroidectomy: Hypocalcemia
Organ-based Clinical: Endocrine/Metabolic

Jennifer Dominguez and Kristin Richards

Edited by Mamatha Punjala

KEY POINTS

1. Hypocalcemia can result from hypoparathyroidism after thyroid surgery.
2. Disruption of the blood supply to the parathyroid glands, rather than inadvertent removal, is the most common cause of hypoparathyroidism after thyroid surgery.
3. Symptoms of hypocalcemia usually manifest within 24 to 48 hours of surgery, and include anxiety, circumoral numbness, paresthesias, muscle cramps, stridor, laryngospasm, and positive Trousseau and Chvostek signs.
4. Immediate treatment with intravenous calcium is necessary, as well as long-term supplementation with calcium and vitamin D_3.

DISCUSSION

Thyroid surgery is commonly performed, with approximately 80,000 procedures done annually in the United States. Postoperative hypocalcemia resulting from acute hypoparathyroidism is a significant complication of total thyroidectomy, but it is unlikely to occur after unilateral thyroid lobectomy. In one recent series, it was found to occur in approximately 5% of patients undergoing total thyroidectomy. Although hypocalcemia can clearly result from inadvertent removal of all four parathyroid glands, it is much more likely to be caused by disruption of the blood supply to the parathyroid glands during thyroidectomy.

Symptoms of hypocalcemia usually occur between 24 and 48 hours postthyroid surgery and rarely occur in the postanesthesia care unit (PACU). Hypocalcemia produces neuronal irritability and tetany. The most common early symptoms are paresthesias of the fingers and toes, as well as circumoral numbess. Hypocalcemia may present to the anesthesiologist if these symptoms progress to tetany of the respiratory muscles that can cause stridor and laryngospasm. Hypocalcemia is associated with cardiovascular complications, as well as mental status changes. A detailed list of clinical manifestations is presented in Table 1. Hypocalcemia can also be sought with two clinical tests: tapping on the facial nerve to elicit *Chvostek* sign, and inflating a noninvasive blood pressure (NIBP) cuff 20 mm Hg above systolic blood pressure on the upper extremity to elicit carpal spasm or *Trousseau* sign. Both these tests elicit the resultant hyperexcitability of nerves secondary to hypocalcemia.

Table 1. Hypocalcemia: Clinical Manifestations

Cardiovascular	Respiratory
Dysrhythmias	Apnea
Digitalis insensitivity	Laryngeal spasm
ECG changes	Bronchospasm
Heart failure	
Hypotension	**Psychiatric**
	Anxiety
Neuromuscular	Depression
Tetany	Dementia
Muscle spasm	Psychosis
Papilledema	
Seizures	
Weakness	
Fatigue	

Treatment for severe hypocalcemia (ionized calcium less than 1.1 mmol per L or 4.4 mg per dL) or symptomatic hypocalcemia is intravenous calcium therapy with either calcium gluconate (1 g, 10 mL of 10% solution) or calcium chloride (1 g, 10 mL of 10% solution). Of note, the exact calcium salt selected (gluconate vs. chloride) may be important when only peripheral access is available in non-Operating Room (OR) locations, as calcium chloride is more irritating to peripheral veins and carries a higher risk of thrombophlebitis and venous infiltration, if not given centrally. When ordering calcium outside of the OR, it is also important to note that there is a 3-fold difference in the primary cation concentration between calcium gluconate, which contains 4.65 mEq Ca^{2+} per g, and calcium chloride, which contains 13.6 mEq Ca^{2+} per g. With severe hypocalcemia, an intravenous infusion for several days is usually necessary, and should be accompanied by ECG monitoring to detect adverse cardiac side effects, such as heart block or ventricular fibrillation. Electrolytes should be monitored regularly during repletion, until the ionized calcium stabilizes between 4 and 5 mg per dL. At that point, oral supplements can replace the IV infusion. If there is airway compromise, continuous positive airway pressure (CPAP) is usually effective. Plasma magnesium concentration should also be checked.

SUGGESTED READINGS

Barash PG, Cullen BF, Stoelting RK, et al, eds. *Clinical Anesthesia*. 6th ed. Philadelphia, PA: Lippincott Williams & Wilkins; 2009:1437.

Bhattacharyya N, Fried M. Assessment of the morbidity and complications of total thyroidectomy. *Arch Otolaryngol Head Neck Surg*. 2002;128(4):389–392.

Hines RL, Marshall KE, eds. *Stoelting's Anesthesia and Co-existing Disease*. 5th ed. Philadelphia, PA: Saunders Elsevier; 2008:388.

Time Constant Definition

Pharmacology

Kimberly Slininger

Edited by Raj K. Modak

1. Time constants are used to help characterize the exponential growth or decay of a system.
2. The time constant, or elimination rate constant (κ_e), is a first-order rate constant that helps describe elimination of a drug from the body. This is an overall constant describing elimination, which takes into account all factors, including excretion and metabolism.
3. Each compound has its own specific κ_e.
4. Systems are usually considered to be at steady state after 5 time constants have elapsed.

Time constants are composed of variables affecting the growth or decay of a system. Elimination rate constants, or time constants, are most commonly referenced in anesthesia in relation to pharmacokinetics and the achievement of steady state of a drug. This steady state can be either achieving a certain drug level in the body or the elimination of a drug. Under simple systems, steady state is considered to have occurred after 5 time constants.

In a first-order system, the time constant is the amount of time for the molecule to reach 63% of its goal concentration. To reach 95% of intended, 3 time constants are necessary, and to reach 100%, 5 time constants are necessary.

The time constant can be seen not only with drugs entering the body, but also for things such as gas flow of drugs through an anesthesia circuit reaching the patient. The time constant can be calculated by the following formula:

$$k \text{ (time constant)} = V/Cl$$

where Cl = clearance and V = volume of distribution.

Similarly, when discussing gas flows, k (time constant) can be calculated with the following formula:

$$\text{volume of the circuit in liters}/\text{amount of fresh gas flow in liters per minute.}$$

The mathematical relationship, which determines the change in concentration of a molecule with time, is represented by

$$y(t) = Ae^{(1-t/k)}$$

where k = time constant, $y(t)$ = change in concentration of the molecule, A = "initial" quantity, and e = mathematical constant.

This can then be extrapolated to certain substances/practices. For example, this equation governs the change in volatile agent when carried in gas fresh flow:

$$Fi = F_{set}e^{(1-t/k)}$$

where Fi = concentration inspired, F_{set} = concentration desired, k = timeconstant, and t = time.

Each substance has its own specific time constant in certain environments, which becomes important in determining the concentration of the molecule in a patient within a certain time frame.

SUGGESTED READINGS

Barash PG, Cullen BF, Stoelting RK, et al, eds. *Clinical Anesthesia*. 6th ed. Philadelphia, PA: Lippincott Williams & Wilkins; 2009:144–146.

Mapleson WW. The theoretical ideal fresh-gas flow sequence at the start of low-flow anesthesia. *Anaesthesia* 1998; 53:264–272.

Reese RL. *University Physics*. Pacific Grove, CA: Brooks/Cole; 2000:873.

Ritschel WA. *Handbook of Basic Pharmacokinetics*. 2nd ed. Washington, DC: Drug Intelligence Publications; 1980:413–426.

T

Total Knee Repl: Reg Anes Techniques

Anatomy

Juan Egas

Edited by Thomas Halaszynski

KEY POINTS

1. Dermatome distribution and nerve and nerve plexus involvement of knee innervation include both lumbar and lumbosacral nerves.
2. Regional anesthesia techniques used during knee surgery may include a lumbar plexus block, femoral and obturator block, and inguinal plexus block, combined with or without a sciatic nerve block.
3. Neuraxial anesthesia (usually spinal) or general anesthesia, together with the above-mentioned techniques for postoperative pain control, is an alternative option.
4. Epidural anesthesia/analgesia is another alternative during total knee replacement surgery.

DISCUSSION

There are two major nerve plexuses that innervate the knee of the lower extremity—lumbar and lumbosacral plexus. The *lumbar plexus* originates from the ventral rami of lumbar (L) 2 to 4 nerve rootlets and sometimes part of L1 and L5. This nerve plexus innervates the anterior aspect of the ipsilateral lower extremity. From cephalad to caudad, the major nerves of the lumbar plexus that innervate the knee of the lower extremity are (a) the lateral femoral cutaneous, (b) the obturator, and (c) the femoral.

A. The *lateral femoral cutaneous nerve* originates from the posterior divisions of L2 and L3 roots, and innervates the skin from the lateral portion of the buttock to the greater trochanter of the femur and the proximal two-thirds of the lateral aspect of the thigh.
B. The *obturator nerve* arises from the anterior divisions of L2–L4 and innervates the medial aspect of the thigh, including the skin, adductor muscle group, and hip, and medial aspect of the knee joint.
C. The *femoral nerve* forms from the posterior divisions of L2–L4, and provides innervation to the anterior muscles of the thigh, skin, anterior aspect of the knee, and hip joints. This nerve subsequently forms the saphenous nerve that innervates the medial aspect of the lower leg (below the knee).

The other major contributor to lower-leg innervation for knee surgery is *the lumbosacral plexus*, which arises from the ventral rami of L4 to sacral (S) 3 vertebra. The lumbosacral plexus innervates the posterior aspect of the lower extremity via the sciatic nerve. The *sciatic nerve* itself originates from L5 to S3 and innervates the posterior thigh and knee, before branching into the tibial and common peroneal nerves at the level of the popliteal fossa.

Combined blocks of the lumbar and lumbosacral plexus will often provide effective surgical anesthesia for the entire lower extremity, including the knee. Surgical anesthesia for knee surgery in which a tourniquet will be used may require blockade of the femoral, obturator, lateral femoral cutaneous, and sciatic nerves. Techniques that block all these nerves include the lumbar plexus block; femoral, lateral femoral cutaneous, and obturator blocks; or inguinal plexus block combined with a sciatic nerve block. Other modalities for knee surgery (including total knee replacement) may include an epidural anesthesia/analgesia or combining a spinal or general anesthetic with a lumbar plexus block for postoperative analgesia. Peripheral nerve blocks provide targeted anesthesia of the knee region, and can be very useful when neuraxial techniques might otherwise be contraindicated.

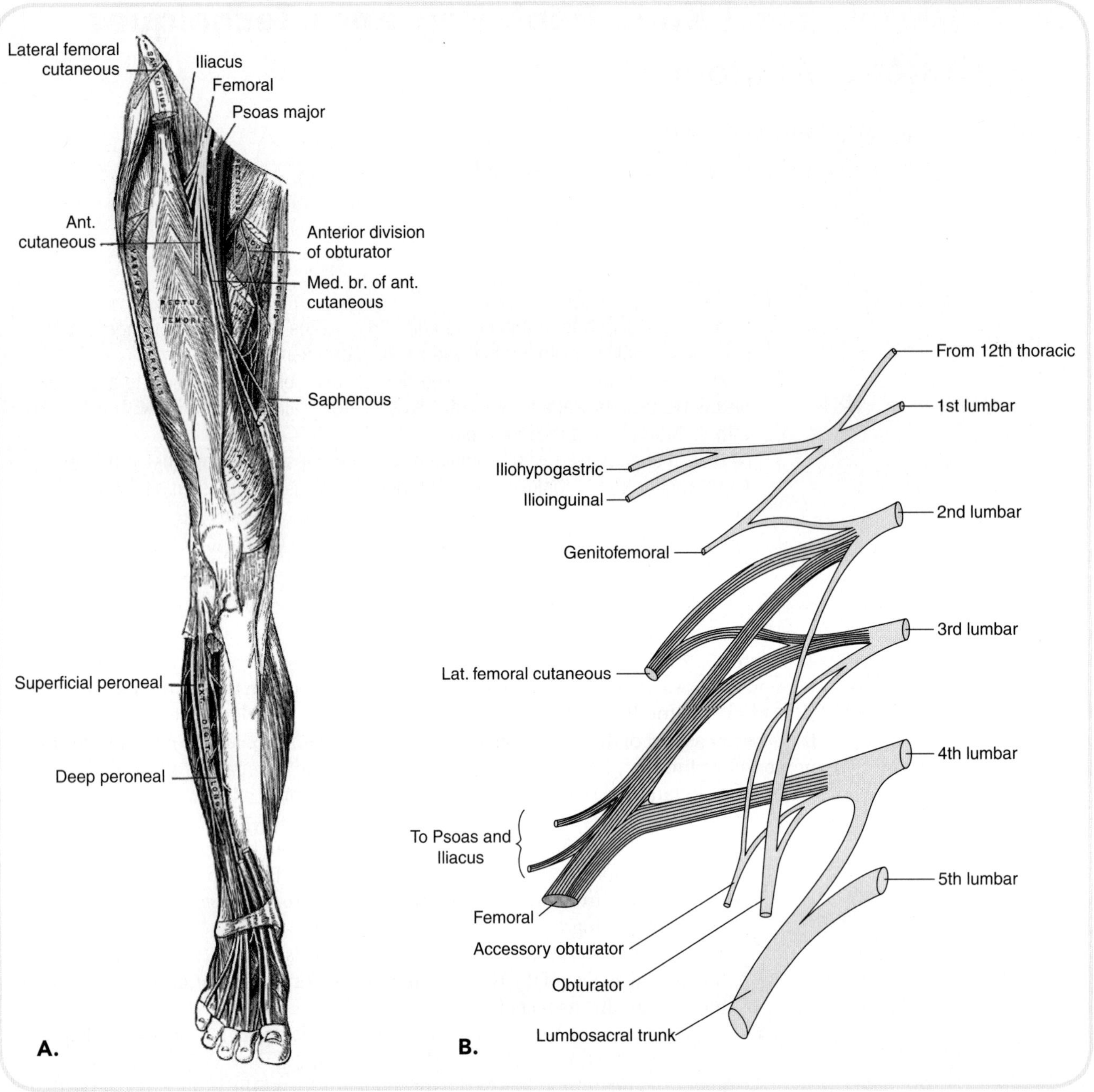

Figure 1. Images of the lumbosacral plexus. (A. From Gray H. *Anatomy of the Human Body*. 20th ed. Philadelphia, PA: Lea & Febiger; 1918. B. http://www.bartleby.com/107/ (images are in the public domain). Accessed January 12, 2009, with permission.)

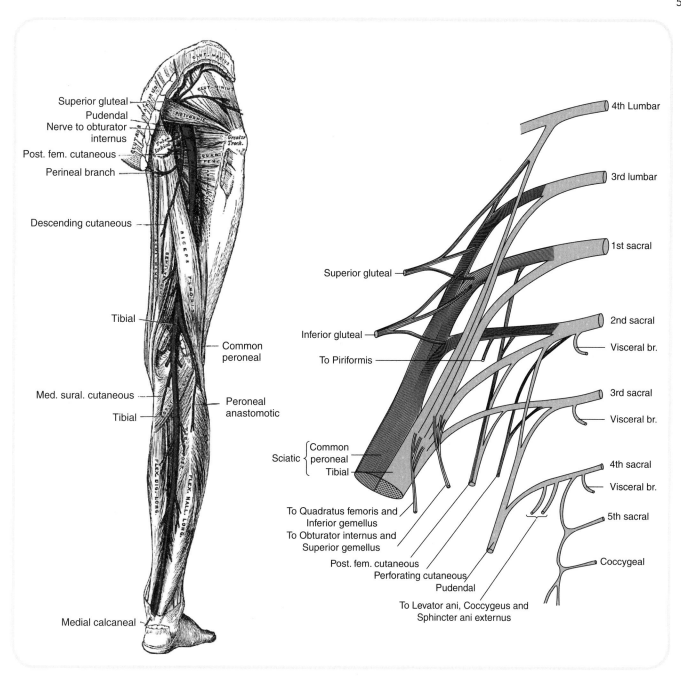

Figure 1. *(Continued)*

SUGGESTED READINGS

Barash P, Cullen BF, Stoelting RK, et al, eds. *Clinical Anesthesia*. 6th ed. Philadelphia, PA: Lippincott Williams & Wilkins; 2009:1384–1385.

Brown DL. *Atlas of Regional Anesthesia*: *Expert Consult—Online and Print*. Philadelphia, PA: Saunders/Elsevier; 2010:90–120.

Gray H. *Anatomy of the Human Body*. 20th ed. Philadelphia, PA: Lea & Febiger; 1918.

TPN Discontinuation: Hypoglycemia and Cx
Subspecialties: Critical Care

Jammie Ferrara and Kevan Stanton
Edited by Hossam Tantawy

KEY POINTS

1. Total parenteral nutrition (TPN) provides nutritional support in patients in whom enteric feeding is contraindicated or absorption via the gastrointestinal (GI) tract is inadequate.
2. TPN formulas are hyperosmolar solutions of amino acids, glucose, and lipids and generally require administration by central venous catheters.
3. The abrupt cessation of TPN can result in hypoglycemia secondary to increased circulating endogenous concentrations of insulin.
4. When discontinuing or tapering TPN, blood glucose levels should be measured frequently until they stabilize and should be maintained at 100 to 150 mg per dL.
5. If TPN is continued during an anesthetic, hyperglycemia can result because the neuroendocrine stress response to surgery typically worsens glucose intolerance and can lead to hyperosmolar nonketotic acidosis.

DISCUSSION

TPN is used when the GI tract is a contraindicated or inadequate route for nutritional support. TPN is a hyperosmolar solution that consists of amino acids, glucose, and lipids, typically administered centrally; peripheral administration can irritate the veins and produce thrombophlebitis.

Adverse effects of TPN include hyperglycemia, hypoglycemia, fluid overload, increased carbon dioxide production, catheter-related sepsis, electrolyte abnormalities, hepatic dysfunction, renal dysfunction, and thrombosis of central veins (see Table 1). Patients on TPN should undergo a careful preoperative evaluation, since electrolyte imbalances and other metabolic abnormalities are common and may necessitate correction before going to the OR. For example, hypophosphatemia is often noted in patients on TPN and can worsen postoperative muscle weakness and respiratory failure. Furthermore, the plan regarding discontinuation versus tapering versus intra-operative continuation of parenteral nutrition (or replacement with 10% dextrose) must be noted. The abrupt cessation of TPN can result in hypoglycemia secondary to increased circulating endogenous concentrations of insulin. Blood glucose levels should be measured frequently intraoperatively until they stabilize and should be maintained at 100 to 150 mg per dL.

Table 1. Adverse Effects of TPN

Hyperglycemia
Hypoglycemia
Fluid overload
Increased carbon dioxide production
Catheter-related sepsis
Electrolyte abnormalities
    Hypokalemia
    Hypocalcemia
    Hypophosphatemia
    Hypomagnesemia
Hepatic dysfunction
Renal dysfunction
Thrombosis of central veins

In contrast, in patients with baseline glucose intolerance, the neuroendocrine response to surgical stress can further exacerbate insulin resistance. In such patients, continuation of TPN intraoperatively can cause significant hyperglycemia. To prevent hyperglycemia-induced hyperosmolar nonketotic acidosis, it is recommended to decrease the infusion rate of TPN before induction. It is also appropriate to decrease the infusion rate of intravenous maintenance fluids to minimize the risk of congestive heart failure secondary to fluid overload.

The following are the strategies to reduce the risk of hypoglycemia due to cessation of TPN:

1. Avoid overfeeding. Do not exceed daily caloric needs with TPN administration.
2. Use of TPN formulations containing lower glucose: lipid ratios (70:30 to 50:50) reduces the incidence of hypoglycemia after abrupt discontinuation of TPN.
3. A conservative strategy for TPN cessation is to decrease the TPN administration rate the night prior to surgery if it is planned to discontinue the infusion on the day of surgery.
4. TPN may also be substituted with 10% glucose and gradually decreased while monitoring blood glucose levels closely.
5. When stopping TPN, any insulin infusion must also be stopped.
6. Ideally, the TPN formulation should be continued at the original rate during the surgery and blood glucose closely monitored.

SUGGESTED READINGS

Barash PG, Cullen BF, Stoelting RK, et al, eds. *Clinical Anesthesia*. 6th ed. Philadelphia, PA: Lippincott Williams & Wilkins; 2009:1462.

Miller RD, Eriksson LI, Fleisher LA, et al. *Miller's Anesthesia*. 7th ed. Philadelphia, PA: Churchill Livingstone; 2010:1078, 2949.

Morgan GE, Mikhail MS, Murray MJ. *Clinical Anesthesiology*. 4th ed. New York, NY: McGraw Hill; 2006:1060–1062.

Stoelting RK, Miller RD. *Basics of Anesthesia*. 5th ed. Philadelphia, PA: Elsevier; 2007:450.

T

TPN: Metabolic Effects

Subspecialties: Critical Care

Alexander Timchenko

Edited by Ala Haddadin

KEY POINTS

1. The effects of total parenteral nutrition (TPN) as well as its complications can be divided into mechanical, infectious, and metabolic.
2. Metabolic effects refer to high or low serum level of any component of TPN solution, liver disease, and bone disease.
3. Days after initiating TPN, hyperglycemia is common because of underproduction of endogenous insulin in the face of carbohydrate load.
4. Hypoglycemia may occur after discontinuation of TPN because of upregulation of endogenous insulin production seen with TPN administration.
5. Exceeding caloric requirements with TPN may result in hypercapnia and respiratory acidosis, leading to difficulty with ventilator weaning.

DISCUSSION

Clinical manifestations of nutrient deficiencies are summarized in Table 1 below:

Most common metabolic problems associated with TPN are described as follows:

Hyperglycemia. Most common cause is excessive dextrose infusion. After the start of TPN, transient elevation of serum glucose develops. Later, endogenous insulin production adjusts to TPN dextrose content and infusion rate. Factors that trigger tolerance to dextrose are inability of insulin synthesis to catch up with TPN infusion rate and underlying conditions. Risk factors include sepsis, diabetes, acute pancreatitis, and corticosteroid use. Hyperglycemia results in immune system dysfunction and increased susceptibility to infection. Excessive caloric load stimulates glucose conversion to fat, leading to hypertriglyceridemia and hepatic steatosis. *Prevention:* The blood glucose is to be maintained 80 to 110 mg per dL, dextrose should be infused at a rate of 4 to 5 mg/kg/min, and dextrose in TPN should be increased slowly to meet caloric goal.

Table 1. Nutrient Deficiencies

Sign or Symptom	Potentially Depleted Nutrient
Muscle and fat wasting	Calories, protein, or both
Peripheral edema	Thiamine (heart failure), protein (low oncotic pressure)
Glossitis	Folate, vitamin B_{12}, niacin, riboflavin, thiamine, iron
Cheilosis, angular stomatitis	Riboflavin, niacin, folate, vitamin B_{12}
Loss of vibratory or position sense, fatigue	Vitamin B_{12}
Dermatitis (sun-exposed skin), dementia, diarrhea	Niacin (pellagra)
Symmetric motor or sensory dysfunction, ataxia, nystagmus, heart failure, altered mental status	Thiamine (beriberi)
Bleeding gums, petechiae, ecchymosis	Vitamin C, vitamin K
Poor wound healing	Calories, protein, or both; vitamin C; vitamin A; zinc
Bone pain	Vitamin D (osteomalacia)
Follicular hyperkeratosis, night blindness	Vitamin A
Flaky, whitish dermatitis	Essential fatty acids (linoleic, linolenic)
Sparse hair, easily pluckable hair	Zinc, protein
Pale skin, nail spooning	Iron
Loss of taste; reddish dermatitis around nose, mouth, groin; hair loss	Zinc
Peripheral neuropathies, gait abnormalities, weakness, fatigue	Copper
Muscle pain, heart failure	Selenium
Paresthesias, carpal pedal spasm	Calcium, magnesium, phosphorus, or potassium

T

Hypoglycemia. Most common reason is sudden interruption of TPN (e.g., before surgery). After cessation of TPN, the endogenous insulin is being secreted in response to caloric load. Reactive hypoglycemia usually occurs 15 to 60 minutes after TPN cessation. To prevent this complication, gradual tapering of TPN over 1 to 2 hours before complete cessation should be performed.

Hyperlipidemia (HLD). Most common cause is excess of lipids in the TPN or impaired lipid clearance. Risk factors for decreased lipid clearance obesity, diabetes, sepsis, pancreatitis, and liver disease. HLD can precipitate acute pancreatitis if serum triglyceride levels are above 1,000 mg per dL. If HLD develops, dextrose load should be reconsidered and reduced, and then lipid infusion rate should be decreased. Lipid infusion should not exceed 0.12 g/kg/h. Continuous lipid infusion has better lipid clearance characteristics as compared with cyclic lipid infusion. Propofol precautions should be taken into account, as propofol represents a source of extra lipid calories, 1.1 kcal per mL. Daily lipid infusion should be stopped if serum triglyceride concentration exceeds 400 mg per dL.

Hypercapnia. Overfeeding of total calories and dextrose can result in excess of carbon dioxide production, which results in respiratory acidosis—increased respiratory muscle work to compensate for acidosis, and therefore difficulty weaning from mechanical ventilation. Reduction of caloric load helps to prevent hypercapnia.

Refeeding syndrome. The cause is rapid nutritional repletion in severely malnourished persons—infusion of dextrose stimulates insulin secretion, which is responsible for shifting of phosphorus and potassium intracellularly. Refeeding syndrome presents as combination of following metabolic derangements:

- Hypernatremia
- Hypophosphatemia—weakness, convulsions, respiratory failure (unable to wean off ventilator), cardiac failure. In the red blood cells, hypophosphatemia prevents formation of 2,3-DPG, which leads to decreased O_2 delivery to tissues
- Hypokalemia
- Hypomagnesemia
- Increased blood volume—may trigger preexisting heart failure

To prevent refeeding syndrome, TPN should be advanced gradually to achieve nutritional goals over 3 to 5 days in patients with severe malnutrition.

Hepatobiliary disorders. Most common cause is caloric overfeeding that leads to increased lipogenesis in the liver. In turn, impaired fat mobilization leads to steatosis. Acalculous cholecystitis was reported to be present in approximately 4% of patients on TPN for more than 3 months. Biliary sludge was reported in 50% of the patients after 4 to 6 weeks, and in almost 100% after 6 weeks.

SUGGESTED READINGS

Powell-Tuck J. Nutritional interventions in critical illness. *Proc Nutr Soc.* 2007;66:16–24.
Ukleja A, Romano MM. Complications of parenteral nutrition. *Gastroenterol Clin North Am.* 2007;36:23–46.
Ziegler TR. Parenteral nutrition in the critically ill patient. *N Engl J Med.* 2009;361(11):1088–1097.

TRALI: Treatment
Organ-based Clinical: Hematologic

Gabriel Jacobs

Edited by Hossam Tantawy

1. Transfusion-related acute lung injury (TRALI) is a form of noncardiogenic pulmonary edema associated with transfusion of blood products, most frequently platelets, fresh frozen plasma (FFP), and other plasma-containing components.
2. The pathophysiology of TRALI involves donor anti-human leukocyte antigen (anti-HLA) mediators or antigranulocyte antibodies that activate host leukocytes, which then become sequestered in the lung and create local capillary damage.
3. Treatment of TRALI is mostly supportive, with cessation of transfusion if symptoms occur while blood product infusion is ongoing and supplemental O_2 and/or low-tidal volume ventilation is similar to that recommended in acute respiratory distress syndrome (ARDS) protocols.

TRALI is a form of noncardiogenic pulmonary edema that is associated with the transfusion of blood products, especially plasma-containing products. Although TRALI can occur with transfusion of many types of blood components, it occurs most frequently with platelet or FFP transfusions. Incidence is estimated at 1/1,200 to 1/5,000 units transfused, and the mortality rate reaches 5%. Symptoms of dyspnea, fever, chills, and the characteristic bilateral infiltrate pattern on chest X-ray typically appear within 6 hours of transfusion.

Mechanism of Pathophysiology

Over 90% of incidences of TRALI are thought to occur when donor plasma mediators (usually anti-HLA, class I or class II) cause recipient leukocytes to become activated and to express surface adhesion markers that lead to their sequestration in the lungs. These activated leukocytes sequestered in the recipient's lungs can secrete inflammation products that promote capillary damage and leakage. The resulting increase in capillary permeability leads to bilateral pulmonary edema. In contrast, in the remaining minority of TRALI cases, the opposite pathologic phenomenon occurs: donor leukocytes, which are present in the transfused donor plasma, get recognized by recipient-preformed antibodies and aggregate in the recipient's lungs, leading to the same type of capillary injury.

The donor plasma mediators that activate host leukocytes are typically biologically active lipids, termed *biologic response modifiers* (BRMs). BRMs accumulate in donor plasma because of membrane breakdown over time. Consequently, older blood products are more likely to be implicated in cases of TRALI than fresh plasma products. Furthermore, donors that have been previously transfused or exposed to foreign antigens (e.g., by pregnancy) are most likely to have antileukocyte antibodies in their plasma. Multiparous female donors are the most likely to contribute blood products containing antileukocyte antibodies, which may later trigger TRALI.

A two-hit theory has been proposed to explain leukocyte activation and pulmonary sequestration central to the development of TRALI. The first "hit" is typically a physiologic insult (trauma, sepsis, shock, surgery), which "primes" the recipient's granulocytes to express surface adhesion molecules and is sequestered in the lung parenchyma. The second "hit," the transfusion itself, then delivers BRMs (mostly in the form of lysophosphatidylcholines). The BRMs activate the sequestered recipient leukocytes and cause them to release substances that damage the capillary endothelial lining, leading to the rapid development of noncardiogenic pulmonary edema.

Diagnosis of TRALI

1. Acute hypoxemia → Usually within 6 hours of transfusion.
2. Bilateral lung field infiltrates appreciated on chest X-ray consistent with acute lung injury.
3. No evidence of left atrial hypertension (noncardiogenic).
4. Absence of other causes of acute lung injury.

Treatment

Treatment of TRALI is mostly supportive, with immediate cessation of transfusion, if the symptoms present while the transfusion is ongoing. Supplemental oxygenation—either by noninvasive means or via mechanical ventilation with low tidal volumes—is instituted. Glucocorticoids can be considered, but no definitive evidence supports this intervention. Diuretics generally do not help, as the clinical picture is of acute lung capillary damage and not cardiogenic edema. Symptoms generally improve after 12 to 48 hours. In terms of preventing repeat episodes of injury in patients with history of TRALI and ongoing anemia necessitating further transfusions, no clear guidelines have been provided. The use of washed RBCs is preferred, but supportive studies are lacking. Universal leukoreduction and restrictions on the use of plasma products from alloimmunized donors (multiparous women and those with prior transfusions) are ways to reduce the incidence of this significant complication.

SUGGESTED READINGS

Drummond JC, Petrovitch CT, Lane TA. Hemostasis and transfusion medicine. In: Barash PG, Cullen BF, Stoelting RK, et al, eds. *Clinical Anesthesia.* 6th ed. Philadelphia, PA: Lippincott Williams & Wilkins; 2009:374–375.

Marino P. Anemia and red blood cell transfusions in the ICU. In: *The ICU Book.* 3rd ed. Philadelphia, PA: Lippincott Williams & Wilkins; 2007:675–676.

Morgan E, Mikhail M. Fluid management and transfusion. In: *Clinical Anesthesiology.* 4th ed. New York, NY: McGraw-Hill Co; 2006:701.

T

Transdermal Fentanyl Indications
Subspecialties: Pain

Ira Whitten

Edited by Jodi Sherman

1. Transdermal fentanyl is indicated for the treatment of moderate-to-severe chronic pain states such as chronic neuropathic pain or cancer-related pain.
2. It should be avoided in opioid-naïve patients because of the drugs respiratory depressant effects.
3. It is not appropriate for acute pain or unstable pain states requiring rapid dose titration.

Transdermal fentanyl is indicated for the management of chronic pain such as neuropathic pain or cancer-related pain. It provides a basal rate of fentanyl administration over 48 to 72 hours, with maximal plasma concentrations reached within 17 to 48 hours. This method of drug delivery may offer certain advantages over oral or parenteral opioid formulations, such as ease of administration and more consistent plasma drug concentrations. Transdermal fentanyl may also be used to transition from oral morphine, as it has a better side-effect profile, including lower incidence of constipation, nausea, and daytime drowsiness. Dose adjustments to the patch must be made slowly to avoid respiratory depressant effects.

Transdermal fentanyl patches alone are not sufficient to control acute exacerbations of chronic pain, and in these cases, short-acting opioids or alternative pharmacologic therapies should be added. The transdermal fentanyl system should not be used in acute or unstable pain states because this delivery system does not allow for rapid titration and because drug remains in the subcutaneous tissue depot dose for several hours after removing the patch.

Loeser JD, Butler SH, Chapman CR, et al. *Bonica's Management of Pain*. Philadelphia, PA: Lippincott Williams & Wilkins; 2001:1701.
Miller RD. *Miller's Anesthesia*. 7th ed. Philadelphia, PA: Elsevier; 2009:769–824.
Walsh D. *Palliative Medicine*. 1st ed. Philadelphia, PA: Saunders; 2008:554–570.
Warfield CA. *Principles and Practice of Pain Medicine*. 2nd ed. New York, NY: McGraw-Hill; 2004:583–601.

T

Transfusion Mortality: Causes

Organ-based Clinical: Hematologic

Ervin Jakab

Edited by Ala Haddadin

KEY POINTS

1. Acute transfusion reactions present within 24 hours of a blood transfusion and may include severe, but uncommon, events such as transfusion-related acute lung injury (TRALI), sepsis, anaphylaxis, or immune-mediated acute hemolytic reactions (nonimmune mediated being generally benign).
2. The most frequent events are allergic or nonhemolytic febrile reactions, which typically resolve promptly without specific treatment or complications.

DISCUSSION

1. *Transfusion-related acute lung injury (TRALI)*
   a. Manifests as noncardiogenic pulmonary edema.
   b. The most frequently reported fatal complication of blood transfusion in the United States.
   c. Most commonly associated with plasma-containing blood components such as platelets or fresh frozen plasma.
   d. Estimated to occur in 0.014% to 0.08% of blood component transfusions or in 0.04% to 0.16% of patients transfused.
   e. Proposed pathophysiologic mechanisms: (a) the *antibody hypothesis* (a human leukocyte antigen [HLA class I, HLA class II] or human neutrophil antigen [HNA] antibody in the transfused component reacts with neutrophil antigens in the recipient; the recipient's neutrophils lodge in the pulmonary capillaries and release mediators that cause pulmonary capillary leakage); and (b) *the neutrophil priming hypothesis* (certain clinical conditions, such as infection, surgery, or inflammation, predispose to neutrophil priming and endothelial activation; bioactive substances in the transfused component activate the primed, sequestered neutrophils, and pulmonary endothelial damage ensues).
2. *Bacterial contamination/endotoxemia*
   a. Septic reactions: approximately 1/700 pooled random donor platelet concentrates; approximately 1/4,000 single-donor (apheresis) platelet products; approximately 1/250,000 RBCs.
   b. Mortality rate: approximately 1/50,000 platelet units.
   c. Caused by inadequate sterile preparation of the phlebotomy site, opening the blood container in a nonsterile environment, or the presence of bacteria in the donor's circulation at the time of blood collection.
3. *Acute hemolytic, immune mediated*
   a. Mortality rate: approximately 1/250,000 to 600,000 population.
   b. Caused by immunoglobulin M (IgM) anti-A, anti-B, or anti-A/B, resulting in severe complement-mediated intravascular hemolysis; most severe reactions result from inadvertent transfusion of group AB or group A red cells to a group O recipient.
   c. Renal failure and disseminated intravascular coagulation are potential complications for patients who survive the initial acute reaction; mortality increases directly with the volume of incompatible blood that was transfused.
   d. Immune-mediated hemolytic reactions caused by IgG, Rh, Kell, Duffy, or other non-ABO antibodies typically result in extravascular sequestration and shortened survival of transfused red cells and produce relatively mild clinical reactions.

4. *Anaphylaxis*
   a. Estimated at approximately 1 in 20,000 to 1 in 47,000 blood components transfused.
   b. Mortality rate for anaphylaxis is estimated to be approximately 1 per year.
   c. Often associated with anti-IgA in recipients who are IgA deficient or in patients with congenital haptoglobin deficiency.

SUGGESTED READINGS

Davenport RD. Pathophysiology of hemolytic transfusion reactions. *Semin Hematol.* 2005;42(3):165–168.

Hillyer CD, Josephson CD, Blajchman MA, et al. Bacterial contamination of blood components: risks, strategies, and regulation: joint ASH and AABB educational session in transfusion medicine. *Hematology Am Soc Hematol Educ Program.* 2003;575–589.

Sazama K, DeChristopher PJ, Dodd R, et al. Practice parameter for the recognition, management, and prevention of adverse consequences of blood transfusion. College of American Pathologists. *Arch Pathol Lab Med.* 2000;124(1):61–70.

Silliman CC, Boshkov LK, Mehdizadehkashi Z, et al. Transfusion-related acute lung injury: epidemiology and a prospective analysis of etiologic factors. *Blood.* 2003;101(2):454–462.

Toy P, Popovsky MA, Abraham E, et al. Transfusion-related acute lung injury: definition and review. *Crit Care Med.* 2005;33(4):721–726.

T

Traumatic Brain Injury: CPP
Organ-based Clinical: Neurologic and Neuromuscular

Rongjie Jiang

Edited by Ramachandran Ramani

KEY POINTS

1. Cerebral perfusion pressure (CPP) = MAP (mean arterial pressure) – ICP (intracranial pressure) or CVP (central venous pressure), whichever is higher.
2. The goal of CPP is 50 to 70 mm Hg in severe traumatic brain injury (TBI).
3. Hyperventilation therapy to $PaCO_2$ of 25 mm Hg is no longer recommended as a prophylactic treatment. The recommended target $PaCO_2$ is between 30 and 35 mm Hg.

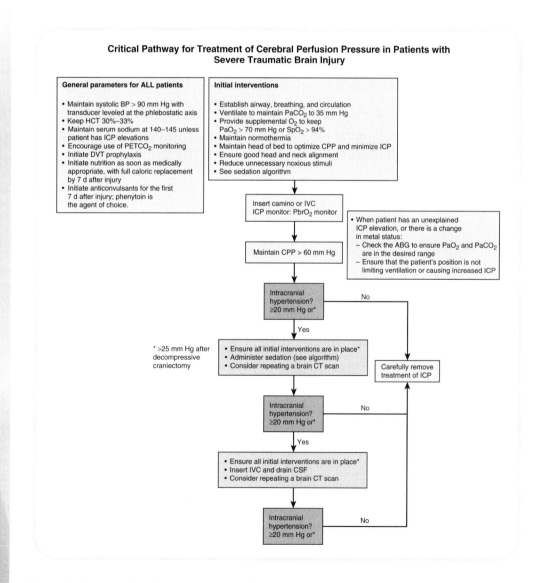

Figure 1. Clinical pathway for the management of severe traumatic brain injury part 1.

576

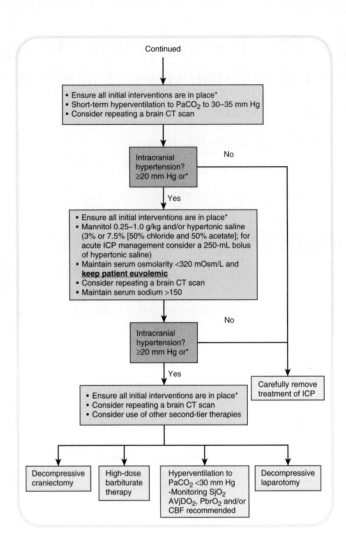

Figure 2. Clinical pathway for the management of severe traumatic brain injury part 2.

DISCUSSION

Severe TBI is classified as a Glasgow Coma Score (GCS) less than or equal to 8 on admission. Patients with TBI are very sensitive to hypotension (systolic BP <90 mm Hg) and hypoxia (PaO_2 <60 mm Hg). Elevated ICP is very common from acute brain injury; however, hypotension due to bleeding from other injuries also frequently accompanies trauma to brain and other areas. In fact, hypotension is the most common cause of death in head-injured patients. Hypotension and hypovolemia lead to decreased CPP, resulting in tissue hypoxia and neuronal cell death. A CPP of 50 to 70 mm Hg is needed to ensure adequate cerebral blood flow (CBF). It has been shown that hypotension less than 90 mm Hg even for a brief duration increases mortality by up to 50%. Therefore, CPP must be maintained in the range of 50 to 70 mm Hg by resuscitation with intravenous fluids and pressors (e.g., phenylephrine), maintaining optimal MAP, and ICP must be maintained below 20 Hg.

$$CPP = MAP \text{ (mean arterial pressure)} - ICP \text{ (intracranial pressure)}$$
$$\text{or CVP (central venous pressure).}$$

Early targeted CPP management (Figs. 1 and 2) is critical to improve the outcome in TBI patients. The goal of CPP should be normal or high normal, given that CBF is low in brain regions with acute insults. It is currently recommended that a CPP of 50 to 70 mm Hg be maintained. Previously, a higher CPP target (>70 mm Hg) was recommended, but studies have shown an increased incidence of acute respiratory distress syndrome (ARDS) with higher CPP pressure goal. In the absence of ICP monitoring, mean blood pressure should be kept above 80 mm Hg. Maintaining a euvolemic, normoxic (PaO_2 >95) state and keeping the hematocrit greater than 30% are important initial management goals as well.

577

Hyperventilation therapy to a $PaCO_2$ of 25 mm Hg is no longer recommended as a prophylactic treatment in TBI. Brain ischemia from hypoperfusion may be worsened with this more aggressive regimen, even when the CPP is maintained within the target range. Interestingly, hyperventilation in patients with severe TBI may also be associated with acute lung injury as a result of increased vascular resistance. Current guidelines recommend no hyperventilation in the first 24 hours after TBI and mild hyperventilation targeting a $PaCO_2$ between 30 and 35 mm Hg for episodes of elevated ICP that cannot be controlled with other standard treatment measures.

SUGGESTED READINGS

Barash P, Cullen BF, Stoelting RK, et al, eds. Anesthesia for trauma and burn patients. In: *Clinical Anesthesia*. 6th ed. Philadelphia, PA: Lippincott Williams & Wilkins; 2009:899–901.

Miller RD, Eriksson LI, Fleisher LA, et al, eds. *Miller's Anesthesia*. 7th ed. Philadelphia, PA: Elsevier, Churchill and Livingstone; 2009:2070, 2296–2298.

T

Trigeminal Neuralgia: Rx

Subspecialties: Pain

Emilio Andrade

Edited by Thomas Halaszynski

1. Trigeminal neuralgia, also known as *tic douloureux*, is a disorder of the trigeminal nerve that can be characterized by abrupt "shock-like" pain limited to the distribution of one or more divisions of the trigeminal nerve.
2. Trigeminal neuralgia is usually treated effectively with medications such as carbamazepine.
3. Clonazepam and gabapentin with baclofen have also been used in the treatment of trigeminal neuralgia.
4. For immediate relief of trigeminal neuralgia, intravenous (IV) lidocaine or phenytoin can be used until patients are able to tolerate oral medications.
5. Cases refractory to medical treatment may benefit from surgical procedures such as glycerol rhizolysis, radiofrequency rhizotomy, or gamma knife therapy.

Trigeminal neuralgia is characterized by brief electrical shock-like pain that follows the distribution of one or more branches of the trigeminal nerve. It is more commonly unilateral and rarely bilateral. The duration of symptoms can be from a few seconds to 2 minutes. Exacerbating factors associated with trigeminal neuralgia can be chewing, talking, brushing teeth, cold air, or smiling. Trigger zones may also be present, and the majority of cases begin in middle and old age.

Initial treatment is medical, and the first-line choice is carbamazepine. Starting dose is 50 mg twice a day. If this is not enough, baclofen can be added. In situations where immediate pain relief is needed, IV phenytoin is effective. Other medications used to treat this disorder are oxcarbazepine, valproate, clonazepam, pimozide, gabapentin, lamotrigine, topiramate, perphenazine, olanzapine, and tizanidine.

Additional treatment modalities include behavioral modifications and lifestyle changes to avoid known triggers, such as certain facial motions, cold breezes, aggressive chewing, and other actions, and these may help reduce exacerbation of symptoms. Alternative therapies such as biofeedback, relaxation therapy, and acupuncture are some additional techniques to utilize before implementation of interventional therapies.

When medical therapy fails, surgical treatment can be performed. Ablation of the trigeminal nerve can be performed by glycerol injection of the nerve. The success rate of ablation treatment is near 90% and has very few side effects. During the following 18 months, approximately 20% of patients will return for a second injection. An alternative to glycerol injection is radiofrequency gangliolysis (RFL) or thermocoagulation of the trigeminal ganglion. RFL relieves symptoms in 80% to 85% of cases, but glycerol injection is better tolerated and has less complications than RFL for most patients. Other interventional alternatives include microvascular decompression surgery, stereotactic thalamic stimulation, and trigeminal nerve or gasserian ganglion block performed using a combination of local anesthetic and corticosteroid.

Warfield C, Bajwa Z, eds. *Principles and Practice of Pain Medicine.* 2nd ed. New York, NY: McGraw-Hill Professional; 2004:650, 1420.

Longnecker D, Brown D, Newman M, et al, eds. *Longnecker's Anesthesiology.* New York, NY: McGraw-Hill Professional; 2007:1521–1530.

Trigger Point Injection Indications
Subspecialties: Pain

Trevor Banack

Edited by Jodi Sherman

KEY POINTS

1. A trigger point is a hyperirritable focal area located within a taut band of skeletal muscle.
2. Trigger point injections are used to aid in the treatment of many conditions including chronic pain, low back pain, myofascial pain syndrome, temporomandibular joint pain, tension headaches, and whiplash injuries.
3. The indications for a trigger point injection include musculoskeletal pain and subsequent impaired range of motion.
4. Contraindications to trigger point injections should include local or systemic infection, patient refusal, and altered mental status.

DISCUSSION

A trigger point is a hyperirritable focal area located within a taut band of skeletal muscle. The area is painful on compression and can produce referred pain, referred tenderness, motor dysfunction, and autonomic phenomena. A trigger point injection consists of inserting a needle into the trigger point and injecting a solution that may contain local anesthetic, saline, or botulin toxin. It is believed that the mechanisms of action of a trigger point injection are mechanical, with the needle disrupting the pathologic contractile elements in the muscle as well as the solution diluting the accumulated toxins felt to precipitate the trigger point response. Local anesthetic can cause local vasodilatation, which improves the abnormally reduced blood flow and further helps eliminate toxins in the sensitized area.

Trigger point injections are used to aid in the treatment of many conditions including chronic pain, low back pain, myofascial pain syndrome, temporomandibular joint pain, tension headaches, and whiplash injuries. The indications for a trigger point injection include musculoskeletal pain and subsequent impaired range of motion. Contraindications to trigger point injections should include local or systemic infection, patient refusal, and altered mental status.

SUGGESTED READINGS

Alvarez DJ, Rockwell PG. Trigger points diagnosis and management. *Am Fam Physician.* 2002;65:653–660.

Ashburn MA, Rice LJ, eds. *The Management of Pain.* New York, NY: Churchill Livingstone Inc; 1998:685.

Simons DG, Travell JG, Simons LS. *Travell & Simons' Myofascial Pain and Dysfunction: The Trigger Point Manual.* 2nd ed. Baltimore, MD: Williams & Wilkins; 1999:5.

Tumescent Liposuction: Lidocaine Dose

Generic, Clinical Sciences: Anesthesia Procedures, Methods, Techniques

Holly Barth

Edited by Lars Helgeson

KEY POINTS

1. Lidocaine with epinephrine is used as part of an infiltrate solution during fat removal.
2. The large amounts of local anesthetic used could result in lidocaine toxicity.
3. Although lidocaine toxicity is thought of as 7 mg per kg, 35 to 55 mg per kg of lidocaine has been used safely in liposuction.
4. Lidocaine administered in this manner behaves similar to sustained-release medications, and thus peak serum levels may not take place for 12 to 14 hours after injection.

DISCUSSION

Liposuction is the second most common cosmetic operation performed by plastic surgeons and dermatologists. Tumescent liposuction is a popular surgery that requires the use of inserting hollow rods into small incisions in the skin and suctioning out subcutaneous fat. Large volumes (1 to 4 mL) of infiltrate solution for each 1 cm³ of fat removed.

This infiltrate solution may be composed of normal saline or lactated Ringer with lidocaine 0.025% to 0.1% with 1:100,000 of epinephrine. It is placed under the skin where the fat is to be removed. The more fat that is to be removed requires larger amounts of infiltrate solution. Therefore, the large volume of local anesthetic is a potential risk for lidocaine toxicity.

Local anesthetic toxicity may manifest itself with mental status changes such as confusion, delirium, or seizures. Cardiovascular toxicity includes hypotension, bradycardia, or arrhythmias such as ventricular fibrillation.

The toxic dose of lidocaine is 7 mg per kg. However, doses of 35 to 55 mg per kg have been used safely because the tumescent technique allows for a single compartment clearance similar to that of a sustained-release medication. The peak serum levels of lidocaine occur 12 to 14 hours after injection.

SUGGESTED READING

Barash PG, Cullen BF, Stoelting RK, et al, eds. *Clinical Anesthesia*. 6th ed. Philadelphia, PA: Lippincott Williams & Wilkins; 2009:854.

Tumescent Liposuction Complications

Generic Clinical Sciences: Anesthesia Procedures, Methods, Techniques

Ashley Kelley

Edited by Lars Helgeson

KEY POINTS

1. Liposuction is a common cosmetic surgical procedure, often performed on an outpatient basis.
2. Tumescent liposuction uses a large volume of isotonic solution (normal saline or lactated Ringer) to which lidocaine and epinephrine have been added.
3. Complications include local anesthetic toxicity, pulmonary embolism, fat embolism, abdominal cavity/viscus perforation, and fluid and electrolyte derangements.

DISCUSSION

Liposuction is often performed as an outpatient procedure, and ranks second only to breast augmentation in terms of most sought after cosmetic procedures. It can be performed under general anesthesia or Monitored Anesthesia Care (MAC) with sedation. Liposuction is typically performed using hollow rods through which large amounts of subcutaneous fat can be aspirated. These rods are inserted through small skin incisions. Large volumes of isotonic solution (normal saline or lactated Ringer) containing lidocaine 0.025% to 0.1% and epinephrine 1/1,000,000 are used to wash away the removed adipose tissue. Epinephrine is included in the infiltrate solution in an effort to cause vasoconstriction and decrease the amount of blood loss for the procedure.

During liposuction, the volume of wetting solution used is based on the amount of fat to be removed. The traditional safe upper limit for lidocaine with epinephrine is 7 mg per kg; however, during liposuction, much higher amounts (up to 35 or even 55 mg per kg) have been used without apparent ill effects. Peak lidocaine serum levels do not occur until 11 to 15 hours after injection because the distribution and pharmacokinetics of the drug are different with tumescent liposuction than during intravenous administration. This is thought to be because lidocaine clearance follows single compartment kinetics in this instance, as would be seen with sustained release medications.

Complications of tumescent liposuction are numerous. The large volume of tumescent solution can cause electrolyte abnormalities, and aspiration of large volumes may cause third spacing of fluid. Absorption of the wetting solution containing local anesthetic and epinephrine may cause local anesthetic toxicity, resulting in seizures, cardiac arrhythmias, and hypertension. Blood loss is generally 1% of the aspirate, but can still be significant depending on the extent of the procedure. Other surgical risks include perforation of the abdominal cavity and injury to abdominal viscera, hematoma/seroma formation, and sensory nerve impairment.

The most common cause of morbidity and mortality associated with liposuction, however, is pulmonary embolism, with fat embolism also being a risk of the procedure. Risks associated with sedation and anesthesia include excessive sedation leading to hypoventilation and airway obstruction, and worsening of hypotension and tumescent fluid absorption due to vasodilation/decreased systemic vascular resistance.

SUGGESTED READINGS

Barash PG, Cullen BF, Stoelting RK, et al, eds. *Clinical Anesthesia*. 6th ed. Philadelphia, PA: Lippincott Williams & Wilkins; 2009:854.

Jaffe RA, Samuels SI, eds. *Anesthesiologist's Manual of Surgical Procedures*. 5th ed. Philadelphia, PA: Lippincott Williams & Wilkins; 2009:1098–1101.

TURP Syndrome: Rx

Organ-based Clinical: Renal/ Urinary/ Electrolytes

Dallen Mill

Edited by Ala Haddadin

1. Transurethral resection of the prostate (TURP) syndrome results from excessive absorption of irrigation solution, which typically consists of a slightly hypotonic, nonelectrolyte solution containing glycine, sorbitol, or mannitol.
2. Therapy is supportive, focusing mainly on appropriate restoration of extracellular tonicity.
3. Specific treatments include free water restriction and loop diuretics for mild cases of TURP syndrome, and hypertonic saline (3% sodium chloride) for severe toxicity.
4. To minimize the theoretical risk of osmotic demyelination syndrome (ODS), aggressive therapy is recommended for severe TURP syndrome only while patients remain symptomatic and serum sodium is less than 120 mEq per L.

TURP syndrome describes a constellation of symptoms resulting from the excessive absorption of irrigation solution used during urologic procedures. During TURP, tissue is excised through a resectoscope using electrocautery. Consequently, electrolyte solutions such as normal saline or lactated Ringer cannot be used to wash away the resected tissue or to improve surgical visualization, as they would disperse the electrical current and place the patient and surgeon at risk. Instead, hypotonic solutions are typically used, containing glycine 1.5% (230 mOsm per L), mixed sorbitol 2.7%, and mannitol 0.54% (195 mOsm per L), or more rarely dextrose (2.5% to 4%) or urea (1%). Distilled water can provide an excellent optical view, but causes water intoxication as well as intravascular hemolysis, and the precipitation of hemoglobin in the renal tubules can lead to renal failure. Because all the commonly used irrigation solutions are hypotonic, a significant amount of water can be absorbed over the course of the procedure. In addition, the surgical procedure itself predisposes to increased systemic fluid absorption by opening up the prostatic venous sinuses.

TURP syndrome generally manifests as altered mental status, visual disturbances, nausea, bradycardia, and hypertension or hypotension. Pulmonary edema and congestive heart failure can result. In addition, each irrigating solution has unique risks resulting from the metabolism or toxicity of the main component, for example, central nervous system toxicity and transient blindness resulting from hyperglycinemia, fluid overload with mannitol-containing solutions, and hyperglycemia with sorbitol or dextrose-containing irrigants.

Supportive therapy, including the maintenance of adequate oxygenation and circulatory support, constitute the mainstay of treatment while efforts are made to restore extracellular tonicity (see Table 1). Cessation of the surgery and electrocautery use allows for irrigation of the bladder with normal saline. Avoidance of hypotension prevents further irrigant absorption. For the symptomatic patient with a serum sodium concentration greater than 120 mEq per L, correction can be achieved by free water restriction. The addition of a loop diuretic, such as furosemide, may also be beneficial. For patients with a serum sodium concentration less than 120 mEq per L, the administration of hypertonic saline (3% sodium chloride) intravenously (IV) may be considered.

Table 1. Treatment of the Transurethral Resection Syndrome

- Ensure oxygenation and circulatory support.
- Notify surgeon and terminate procedure as soon as possible.
- Consider insertion of invasive monitors if cardiovascular instability occurs.
- Send blood to laboratory for evaluation of electrolytes, creatinine, glucose, and arterial blood gases.
- Obtain 12-lead ECG.
- Treat mild symptoms (with serum Na^+ concentration >120 mEq/L) with fluid restriction and loop diuretic (furosemide).
- Cautious treatment of severe symptoms (if serum Na^+ <120 mEq/L) with 3% sodium chloride IV at a rate <100 mL/h.
- Discontinue 3% sodium chloride when serum Na^+ >120 mEq/L.

Reproduced from Stafford-Smith M, Shaw A, George R, et al. The renal system and anesthesia for urologic surgery. In: *Clinical Anesthesia*. 6th ed. Philadelphia, PA: Lippincott Williams & Wilkins; 2009:1367, with permission.

Controversy exists concerning the rate of correction of hyponatremia associated with TURP syndrome. To decrease the risk of ODS, a serum sodium correction rate no greater than 0.5 mEq/L/h has traditionally been recommended. However, evidence exists that correcting sodium levels too slowly may be associated with higher rates of morbidity and mortality. ODS, which is typically associated with the correction of chronic hyponatremia, has not been reported with the correction of the acute hyponatremia associated with TURP syndrome. If symptoms are severe, serum sodium may be corrected aggressively at rates higher than 0.5 mEq/L/h, but only until symptoms resolve and a serum sodium concentration greater than 120 mEq per L is achieved.

SUGGESTED READINGS

Gravenstein D, Hahn RG. TURP syndrome. In: *Complications in Anesthesiology*. Philadelphia, PA: Lippincott Williams & Wilkins; 2008:483.

Miller RD. Anesthesia and the renal and genitourinary systems. In: *Miller's Anesthesia*. 7th ed. Philadelphia, PA: Elsevier; 2008:2121–2122.

Stafford-Smith M, Shaw A, George RB, et al. The renal system and anesthesia for urologic surgery. In: *Clinical Anesthesia*. 6th ed. Philadelphia, PA: Lippincott Williams & Wilkins; 2009:1367–1368.

Ultrasound Structures: Echogenicity
Anatomy

Meredith Brown and Margaret Rose
Edited by Jodi Sherman

KEY POINTS

1. Hypoechoic tissues, such as blood, have a high water content and reflect very little beam. The resultant image is very dark.
2. Tissues with low water content (bone, tendon) reflect a large portion of the beam, and the strong signal creates a bright white (hyperechoic) signal.
3. The echogenicity of solid organs similarly varies by the water content, which may further vary by disease states (e.g., cirrhotic liver).
4. Ultrasound wave penetrance of air is poor. Air bubbles or poor transducer contact may cast "shadows" on deeper structures.

DISCUSSION

In ultrasound imaging, high-frequency sound waves are projected into tissues, a portion of which is reflected, while another portion is absorbed, depending on their water content. The beam passes easily through tissues with high water content, such as blood, effusions, or cysts, and a very dark image is created. These tissues are considered to have low echogenicity. Tissues with high echogenicity reflect a very high percentage of the beam, and the strong signal creates a bright white image. These highly echogenic tissues (bone, tendon, fat) have very little water content. The echogenicity of solid organs similarly varies by the water content, which may further vary by disease states (e.g., cirrhotic liver). The ultrasound machine has difficulty delineating between adjacent tissues of similar echogenicity, which thus may appear as a single structure.

Ultrasound waves are not transmitted through air well. A large air bubble, or poor contact of the transducer, will obscure deeper structures by reflecting much of the beam. These bubbles may appear to cast "shadows." Because of these properties, ultrasound has great utility in imaging solid organs, the heart, and the gravid uterus with fetus. Abdominal structures deep to the bowel cannot adequately be imaged.

The wavelength of the projected sound waves determines resolution, which increases with a shorter wavelength. These higher-frequency sound waves are quickly attenuated, however, limiting the depth of penetration.

SUGGESTED READINGS

Hadzic A, ed. *The New York School of Regional Anesthesia Textbook of Regional Anesthesia and Pain Management.* New York, NY: McGraw-Hill Medical; 2007:657–664.

Magee P, Tooley M. *The Physics, Clinical Measurement, and Equipment of Anaesthetic Practice.* New York, NY: Oxford University Press; 2005:56–61.

Ultrasound Visualization: IJ Compression
Anatomy

Kellie Park

Edited by Qingbing Zhu

KEY POINTS

1. A wide anatomic variation exists in the location of the internal jugular vein (IJ) with respect to the carotid artery.
2. Ultrasound visualization and guidance decreases the complication rates of central line placement in the IJ.
3. To confirm the identity of the IJ, one must at least demonstrate both the compressibility and the distensibility of the vessel on two-dimensional (2D) ultrasound visualization.

DISCUSSION

The location of the carotid artery in relation to the IJ demonstrates wide anatomic variation. This results in not infrequent puncture and occasional cannulation of the carotid artery during attempted central line placement by anatomic landmarks only. Furthermore, blind attempts to find the IJ occasionally lead to deep and inferior needle probing that can result in lung puncture and pneumothorax. Data suggest that the use of ultrasound visualization and guidance of central line placement in the IJ can greatly decrease these complications.

In 2D Doppler imaging, a cross-section through the short axis of the vessels traditionally shows the IJ superficial and lateral to the carotid artery. However, an immediately anterior or even medial IJ location with respect to the artery may also be seen. The IJ generally appears oblong and thin walled in cross-section, as compared with the round, thick-walled, and pulsatile conformation of the carotid artery. To confirm the correct identification of the vessel by ultrasound, two essential criteria must be met: (1) the IJ must be compressible when external pressure is applied with the ultrasound probe, and (2) the IJ must be distensible with Valsalva maneuver or Trendelenburg positioning by color Doppler when probe head tilts toward patient head, artery fills with red color, but IJ fills with blue color. When probe head tilts away from patient head, artery fills with blue color, but IJ fills with red color.

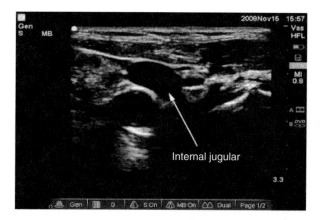

Figure 1. Ultrasound image of internal jugular vein. (Modified from Kumar A, Chuan A. Ultrasound guided vascular access: efficacy and safety. *Best Pract Res Clin Anaesthesiol.* 2009;23(3):299–311, with permission).

SUGGESTED READINGS

Barash PG, Cullen BF, Stoelting RK, et al, eds. *Clinical Anesthesia*. 6th ed. Philadelphia, PA: Lippincott Williams & Wilkins; 2009:746–747.

Denys BG, Uretsky BF. Anatomical variations of internal jugular vein location: impact on central venous access. *Crit Care Med*. 1991;19(12):1516–1519.

Karakitsos D, Labropoulos N, De Groot E, et al. Real-time ultrasound-guided catheterization of the internal jugular vein: a prospective comparison with the landmark technique in critical care patients. *Crit Care*. 2006;10(6):R162.

Kumar A, Chuan A. Ultrasound guided vascular access: efficacy and safety. *Best Pract Res Clin Anaesthesiol*. 2009;23(3):299–311.

U

Uncuffed ETT: Max Leak Pressure

Subspecialties: Pediatric Anesthesia

Bijal Patel

Edited by Mamatha Punjala

KEY POINTS

1. The narrowest portion of the airway in the pediatric patient population is the cricoid cartilage.
2. The correct size of endotracheal tube (ETT) to be used in children can be approximated by the formula: 4 + (age/4).
3. The maximum leak pressure around the ETT should be approximately 25 to 30 cm H_2O. Values higher than this can result in subglottic edema and postextubation croup.

DISCUSSION

In the pediatric patient population, the narrowest portion of the airway is the cricoid cartilage. This is in contrast to adults, in whom the vocal folds create the narrowest diameter. Meticulous care with ETT size selection, tube position, and stabilization must be taken to avoid upper airway injury or airway edema in children. With this in mind, uncuffed ETT are often selected in infants and children less than 6 to 8 years of age. Arguments for uncuffed ETTs in children include (1) the presence of a leak, which ensures that the tube is not compressing the tracheal mucosa against the nondistensible cricoid ring; (2) presumed extra care required for correct placement of an uncuffed tube; (3) cuffs can cause trauma to the trachea via pressure, and cuff pressure must be monitored, (4) using an uncuffed tube allows placement of a larger ETT and improves the ability to suction and ventilate. One formula used to approximate the size of ETT in children is 4 + (age/4).

Once the ETT is in place, the pressure leak around the ETT should be assessed. If a leak is found at a low pressure (<10 cm H_2O), then one cannot ensure adequate ventilation. A maximum leak pressure is around 25 to 30 cm H_2O. If the leak is greater than this value, a smaller-sized ETT should be placed. At high leak pressures, the child is at risk for subglottic edema and postextubation stridor/croup (up to 4.4%). Furthermore, long-term intubation with a tightly fitting tube has been shown to increase the risk of subglottic stenosis.

Other considerations need to be kept in mind when selecting, placing, and testing ETT for leaks in very young children. The anatomy of the cricoid lumen in children is important: it is typically not circular, but rather ellipsoid. Round uncuffed tracheal tubes inserted into the noncircular cricoid lumen therefore have to be sufficiently large to adequately seal the airway without creating excessive leaks. Uncuffed tubes, then, can create considerable (uneven) pressure on the posteriolateral walls of the cricoid. Thus, the air leak at an inspiratory pressure of 25 cm H_2O, thought to prevent excessive mucosal pressure, may actually arise only from the anterior part of the cricoid lumen. This phenomenon is termed *cricoidal sealing*. In contrast, cuffed ETTs are usually selected with a smaller diameter and do not wedge against parts of the cricoid ring. With a cuffed ETT, the cuff creates a potentially more even pressure sealing the airway. This in turn is termed *tracheal sealing*. Tracheal sealing with a high volume, low-pressure cuff (HVLP) allows for more precise estimation and easier adjustment of the cuff pressure, potentially lessening the risk of mucosal damage. In conclusion, although traditionally uncuffed tubes have been preferred over cuffed ETT in the management of very young children, recent data suggest that cuffed ETT may not be any less effective and may not be associated with increased rates of postextubation complications over uncuffed tubes.

SUGGESTED READINGS

Barash PG, Cullen BF, Stoelting RK, et al, eds. *Clinical Anesthesia*. 6th ed. Philadelphia, PA: Lippincott Williams & Wilkins; 2009:752, 1215.

Lerman J, Coté CJ, Steward DJ. *Manual of Pediatric Anesthesia*. 6th ed. Philadelphia, PA: Churchill Livingstone Elsevier; 2010:15, 95.

Stoelting RK, Miller RD, eds. *Basics of Anesthesia*. 5th ed. Philadelphia, PA: Churchill Livingstone Elsevier; 2007:507.

Unilateral Blindness: Etiology

Organ-based Clinical: Neurologic and Neuromuscular and Generic, Clinical Sciences: Anesthesia Procedures, Methods, Techniques

Anna Clebone

Edited by Ramachandran Ramani

KEY POINTS

1. Incidence of blindness after surgery is higher, especially in cases of spine surgery in the prone position or procedures involving cardiopulmonary bypass.
2. Unilateral blindness is more common with anterior ischemic optic neuropathy (AION) than with posterior ischemic optic neuropathy (PION).
3. Postoperative vision loss may not manifest for several days.
4. Suspected mechanisms involve decreases in perfusion pressure to the optic nerve and retina by decreased arterial blood pressure or increased intraocular pressure (direct mechanical pressure on the eyes or decreased venous drainage).

DISCUSSION

Partial or complete loss of vision after surgery occurs infrequently, but is a known complication. Surgeries involving cardiopulmonary bypass or prone positioning, in particular, carry an increased risk. Postoperative vision loss may not become apparent for several days.

The most common mechanism of injury is ischemic damage to the optic nerve (anterior or posterior). Vision loss may be bilateral or unilateral. Unilateral blindness is more common with AION than with PION. The greater association with bilateral injury in PION could be due to involvement of the optic chiasm. Other possible etiologies include retinal artery thrombosis, retinal ischemia, damage to the vision centers in the cerebral cortex or visual pathways, hemorrhagic retinopathy, and acute glaucoma.

Common occurrences during surgery such as hypotension and blood loss have been associated with postoperative blindness. The proposed mechanism is decreased perfusion of the optic nerve, leading to injury. The prone position is a known risk factor for eye injury, possibly related to pressure on the optic globe, mechanically decreasing blood flow to the optic nerve. Positioning may also interfere with venous drainage, leading to increased intraoptic pressure and decreased perfusion pressure.

Potential risks should be minimized in an effort to prevent injury, although postoperative vision loss can occur despite precautions. Some authors advocate the use of Mayfield pins to suspend the head, thus avoiding any direct pressure on the face. Specially designed cushions may be used to support the head and protect the face, but care must be taken to ensure that the cushion is clear of the eyes as well as other facial features. The eyes and face should be checked immediately after turning prone as well as many times throughout the procedure. However, according to the ASA Visual Loss Registry, only 10% of the visual loss is related to direct trauma to the eyeball.

It is essential that anesthesiologists are aware of factors placing patients at risk for this complication, so that preventive measures can be taken. Although overall incidence is low, patients do suffer eye injuries, and even blindness, despite preventative measures.

Anesthesiologists should consider discussing this risk preoperatively with patients deemed to be at risk. Furthermore, should any visual changes be noted by patients postoperatively, an urgent ophthalmology consult is imperative.

SUGGESTED READINGS

Barash PG, Cullen BF, Stoelting RK, et al, eds. *Clinical Anesthesia.* 6th ed. Philadelphia, PA: Lippincott Williams & Wilkins; 2009:1337–1345.

Lee LA, Lam AM. Unilateral blindness after prone lumbar spine surgery. *Anesthesiology.* 2001;95(3):793–795.

Nakra D, Bala I, Pratap M. Unilateral postoperative visual loss due to central retinal artery occlusion following cervical spine surgery in prone position. *Paediatr Anesth.* 2007;17(8):805–808.

U

Upper Extremity Nerve Blocks: Indications
Regional Anesthesia

Frederick Conlin

Edited by Jodi Sherman

1. Blocking branches of C5–T1 nerve roots as they travel from the brachial plexus to more distal locations can produce surgical anesthesia for surgeries on the upper extremity.
2. The four most commonly applied techniques achieve anesthesia by injecting local anesthetic via an interscalene, supraclavicular, infraclavicular, or axillary approach.
3. Performing blocks at each of the four anatomic locations will produce either more proximal or distal coverage. The surgical site, whether the block is for anesthesia or analgesia, and whether a tourniquet will be utilized by the surgeon, all dictate the appropriate block approach.
4. Bier blocks and isolated nerve blocks of the ulnar, median, and radial nerves as they cross the elbow or wrist are viable methods of providing anesthesia or analgesia for procedures on the distal upper extremity.

DISCUSSION

Regional anesthesia can provide patients with surgical anesthesia or postoperative analgesia, while decreasing or even eliminating the need for systemic medication. When selecting a regional technique, the anesthesiologist must consider surgical site, personal experience with placing the block, patient's ability to tolerate positioning and procedure, surgeon's preference, and other patient factors (i.e., underlying comorbidities). There is always a potential need to induce general anesthesia because of block failure, block complications, or patient intolerance, and emergency airway equipment must always be available.

For upper extremity surgery, regional anesthesia entails blocking the brachial plexus or its distal nerves. The four most common approaches are the interscalene, supraclavicular, infraclavicular, and axillary blocks. The orientation of the nerves changes as they travel distally, and with patient positioning. Knowing the anatomic course of the nerves and the distribution that they supply allows the anesthesiologist to select the most appropriate block for surgical anesthesia or analgesia.

Interscalene block. The interscalene is the most proximal approach to the brachial plexus block and is performed at the level of the C6 vertebra. It therefore has the most proximal coverage of the four approaches, and is most often placed for shoulder or proximal humerus surgeries. Blocking the plexus at this level often misses some C8 and T1 fibers, and therefore, incomplete blocks typically fail to cover the distribution of the ulnar nerve. The most common complication is anesthesia of the phrenic nerve, and therefore, patients who are unlikely to tolerate temporary hemidiaphragmatic paralysis are poor candidates for this block. Other potential complications include Horner syndrome, pneumothorax, and epidural or intrathecal injection.

Supraclavicular block. The supraclavicular approach to the brachial plexus block is performed just above the clavicle at the level of the first rib. This block is used for surgeries involving the distal humerus, elbow, forearm, wrist, and hand. Potential complications include phrenic nerve anesthesia (although less so than the interscalene block), as well as Horner syndrome, or pneumothorax.

Infraclavicular block. Like the supraclavicular block, the infraclavicular provides coverage of the distal humerus, elbow, forearm, wrist, and hand. This approach also carries the chance of pneumothorax, although its greatest advantage over the supraclavicular block is the lack of risk of phrenic nerve anesthesia.

U

Axillary block. The axillary approach is performed in the axilla and also covers the distal humerus, elbow, forearm, wrist, and hand. The musculocutaneous nerve is often missed with this approach because it exits the brachial plexus early and courses separately within the coracobrachialis muscle. Furthermore, as the medial arm and axilla are supplied by the lateral cutaneous branch of the T2 intercostal nerve, a supplemental block is helpful if a tourniquet is planned. The axillary block has a higher safety profile than the more proximal approaches because there is no risk of pulmonary complications, but provides incomplete coverage of the upper extremity.

For surgical anesthesia of the wrist and hand without postoperative analgesia, the intravenous Bier block may be performed. The greatest limitation of this block is the potential for systemic toxicity, so a tourniquet must be utilized for an appropriate duration. The advantage of this block is that once the tourniquet is released, the anesthesia is ended, and it is well suited for small procedures. Alternatively, it is also possible to block the median, radial, and ulnar nerve individually, at the level of the elbow or wrist.

All nerve blocks carry a risk of local anesthesia toxicity, intravascular injection, hematoma, nerve injury, infection, and failed or incomplete coverage. When selecting a block, the benefits must be weighed against these and the risks particular to the approach.

SUGGESTED READINGS

Barash PG, Cullen BF, Stoelting RK, et al, eds. *Clinical Anesthesia.* 6th ed. Philadelphia, PA: Lippincott, Williams & Wilkins; 2006:726–732.

Miller RD, ed. *Miller's Anesthesia.* 7th ed. Philadelphia, PA: Churchill Livingstone; 2009:1640–1649.

U

KEYWORD

Upper Extremity Tourniquet Pain Prevention

SECTION

Generic Clinical Sciences: Anesthesia Procedures, Methods, Techniques

Kristin Richards

Edited by Thomas Halaszynski

KEY POINTS

1. Definitive treatment for tourniquet pain is to release the tourniquet from the extremity.
2. In patients with extremity tourniquets inflated, patient discomfort usually occurs after the tourniquet time approaches 45 minutes. This phenomenon can be seen in patients under either general or regional anesthesia.
3. Intraoperatively, opioids and hypnotics can usually prove somewhat effective at treating or mitigating the tourniquet pain.
4. Etiology of tourniquet inflation induced pain is believed to be from ischemic pain.

DISCUSSION

Tourniquets are used to minimize blood loss and optimize the operating field for a host of surgical procedures (usually orthopedic) on the extremities. It remains important to be aware of tourniquet inflation pressures that are being used, as well as of the distribution of the pressure applied. Controversy exists with regard to the tourniquet pressures needed to prevent bleeding. In general, a cuff pressure of 100 mm Hg above a patient's systolic pressure proves adequate for a thigh cuff and 50 mm Hg above systolic pressure is appropriate for an arm cuff.

In addition, cuff size and cuff diameter are important to provide uniform distribution of pressure so as to minimize injury to neurovascular bundles and skeletal muscle. The cuff should be large enough to comfortably circle the limb, and it is recommended that the width of the cuff be more than half of the limb diameter. The duration of tourniquet inflation is an area of controversy. Some have recommended a time frame as short as 30 minutes, and others claim that up to 4 hours in duration should be fine. It has been argued that deflation/reperfusion for 5 minutes after every 1 to 2 hours of planned tourniquet inflation use may help minimize complications such as nerve compression injury, arterial spasms, and venous thrombosis.

When a tourniquet is used with a regional anesthetic, patients may complain of dull, aching pain, or simply become restless. Patient discomfort usually appears approximately 45 minutes after the tourniquet is inflated and becomes more intense over additional time. Even if the patient is under general anesthesia, a similar phenomenon can occur at approximately 45 minutes after the tourniquet is inflated. Evidence of lightening anesthesia, observed increases in patient blood pressure and heart rate, can be noted even though the level of anesthesia being delivered is unchanged.

The pathophysiology of tourniquet pain has not been clearly elucidated. It is currently thought that tourniquet pain is transmitted through both A-delta and C fibers and is modulated in the dorsal horn. The definitive treatment for tourniquet pain is release of the tourniquet; however, during surgery, opioids and hypnotics may often, and usually, prove to be effective.

SUGGESTED
READINGS

Barash PB, Cullen BF, Stoelting RK, et al, eds. *Clinical Anesthesia*. 6th ed. Philadelphia, PA: Lippincott Williams & Wilkins; 2009:1387–1388.

Hagenouw RP, Bridenbaugh PO, van Egmond J, et al. Tourniquet pain: a volunteer study. *Anesth Analg.* 1986;65:1175–1180.

Valli H, Rosenberg PH. Effects of three anesthetic methods on haemodynamic responses connected with the use of thigh tourniquets in orthopaedic patients. *Acta Anaesthesiol Scand.* 1985;29:142–147.

U

Uptake of Inhaled Anesthetics: V/Q Mismatch

Pharmacology

Thomas Gallen

Edited by Raj K. Modak

1. There are three factors that determine anesthetic uptake of volatile anesthetic from alveoli to blood: cardiac output (pulmonary blood flow), agent solubility, and alveolar-to-venous partial pressure difference.
2. Ventilation:perfusion (V/Q) mismatch raises alveolar partial pressure of volatile anesthetics but decreases arterial partial pressure, decreasing rate of induction.
3. Highly soluble anesthetics are affected by V/Q mismatch less than poorly soluble anesthetics.

To appreciate the effect of V/Q mismatch on the induction of anesthesia using volatile anesthetics, it is critical to understand the factors governing their uptake. Of primary importance in the induction of anesthesia with volatiles is their partial pressure within the alveoli. Therefore, increasing the alveolar partial pressure more rapidly speeds the induction of anesthesia. The transfer of volatile anesthetics from the alveoli to blood is governed by three factors: cardiac output (pulmonary blood flow), agent solubility, and the alveolar-to-venous partial pressure difference.

The combined effect of these factors is not additive, but rather is a product of the three. Thus, if any of the three factors approaches zero, the remaining two cannot compensate.

- *Cardiac output* is generally equal to pulmonary blood flow, presuming normal physiology. When cardiac output increases (and therefore pulmonary blood flow), the rise in the alveolar partial pressure of the anesthetic slows, resulting in a slower inhalational induction. With a high cardiac output, the blood passes quickly through the lungs, and the absorbed anesthetic is carried out of the lungs before its partial pressure between the alveoli and blood can be reached, thereby slowing induction.
- *Agent solubility* is represented by its blood–gas partition coefficient (the relative capacity of the two phases for the anesthetic). As solubility increases, the gas diffuses from the alveoli into the blood more readily, leaving a decreased alveolar partial pressure of the gas and prolonging induction.
- *Alveolar-to-venous partial pressure difference* is determined by the degree of anesthetic uptake by tissues, a process governed by similar factors (regional blood flow, agent solubility, and partial pressure differences). Less tissue uptake will increase the venous partial pressure of the anesthetic, and thus allow the alveolar partial pressure to increase as less anesthetic diffuses into the blood.

V/Q Mismatch

With V/Q mismatch, portions of lung tissue are not contributing to gas exchange, whether from dead space or shunt. The effect on the volatile anesthetics is a decrease in the arterial partial pressure while increasing the alveolar partial pressure. Overall, the rate of uptake and induction is slowed despite an increasing alveolar partial pressure. The degree of this effect is affected by the agent solubility: The arterial partial pressure of a highly soluble agent will be less reduced than that of a poorly soluble agent.

The blood from the underventilated lung tissue dilutes the anesthetic partial pressure of the blood from the ventilated lung tissue. With highly soluble anesthetics, the alveolar partial pressure of the agent will rise higher than typical in hyperventilated lung tissue, causing a higher arterial partial pressure from that tissue, potentially compensating for underventilated tissues. However, less soluble agents do not demonstrate the same compensation.

SUGGESTED READINGS

Longnecker DE, Brown DL, Newman MF, et, eds. *Anesthesiology.* New York, NY: McGraw-Hill; 2008:745–775.

Miller RD, ed. *Miller's Anesthesia.* 6th ed. Philadelphia, PA: Lippincott Williams & Wilkins; 2005:539–548.

U

Uterine Rupture: Dx
Subspecialties: Obstetric Anesthesia
Kimberly Slininger and Ervin Jakab
Edited by Lars Helgeson

1. Uterine rupture is a rare but potentially devastating obstetrical occurrence. It is more likely to occur in women with a previous hysterotomy scar (prior C-section).
2. Uterine rupture carries up to a 5% maternal mortality and a 50% fetal mortality.
3. Signs and symptoms of uterine rupture are nonspecific, which include vaginal bleeding, abdominal pain, fetal distress, and maternal hypotension progressing to shock. More specific signs are loss of uterine tone and loss of fetal station.
4. Diagnosis begins with a high index of suspicion in women at higher risk for this complication. Definitive diagnosis is made by manual examination of the uterus and laparotomy.

Uterine rupture is a rare but potentially catastrophic obstetric complication. The incidence is 0.1% to 0.5% of all pregnancies and less than 1% of pregnancies with a scarred uterus. The major risk factor is having a hysterotomy scar, as from a previous caesarean delivery or prior extensive myomectomy. Scar dehiscence involves the breakdown of a previous scar within the muscle without disruption of the overlying visceral peritoneum (uterine serosa). Uterine rupture, in contrast, involves extrusion of the fetus and/or placenta into the abdominal cavity, and carries a much higher risk of bleeding and fetal/maternal demise if not immediately surgically addressed.

The risk of uterine rupture depends on the type of uterine scar: a classical C-section or inverted T-shaped scar confers the highest risk. A low transverse scar confers a lower risk. Other well-established risk factors include history of uterine rupture, abnormal fetal presentation, and excessive use of oxytocin. Uterine distention from multiple gestations, polyhydramnios, or fetal macrosomia also significantly increases risk of rupture during labor. When uterine rupture does occur, it carries up to a 5% maternal mortality rate and up to 50% fetal mortality rate.

Diagnosis of uterine rupture begins with a high index of suspicion in women who are at risk for rupture. There are no heralding signs of impending uterine rupture. Signs and symptoms are nonspecific and include vaginal bleeding, which can be attributed to placental abruption; abdominal pain, which can be masked by epidural anesthesia; fetal distress (decreased heart rate); and maternal hypotension progressing to shock. More specific signs are loss of uterine tone and loss of fetal station. The most common signs are fetal distress (50% to 70%) or loss of fetal heart sounds.

Because of the very short time frame (10 to 30 minutes) before definitive treatment is required, complex diagnostic studies (MRI, CT) generally have no role in the acute management of patients with suspected uterine rupture. A definitive diagnosis is made by manual exploration of the uterus and laparotomy.

Of note, ultrasound (transabdominal, transvaginal, or sonohysterographic [saline ultrasound] that distends the uterine cavity and allows better sonographic evaluation of the uterine walls) may be useful for detecting uterine-scar defects before labor onset. In particular, a decreased thickness of the lower uterine segment measured at 36 to 38 weeks of gestation (<3.5 mm) may have a greater than 85% sensitivity, greater than 70% specificity, 12% positive predictive value, and 99% negative predictive value for subsequent uterine rupture.

SUGGESTED READINGS

Chestnut DH, Polley LS, Tsen LC, et al, eds. *Chestnut's Obstetric Anesthesia: Principles and Practice.* 4th ed. Philadelphia, PA: Mosby Elsevier; 2009:817.

DeCherney AH, Nathan L.*Current Obstetric & Gynecological Diagnosis & Treatment.* 9th ed. New York, NY: McGraw-Hill Medical; 2002:365–367.

Gibbs RS, Karlan BY, Haney AF, et al, eds. *Danforth's Obstetrics and Gynecology.* 10th ed. Philadelphia, PA: Lippincott Williams & Wilkins; 2008:500–501.

Lydon-Rochelle M, Holt VL, Easterling TR, et al. Risk of uterine rupture during labor among women with prior cesarean delivery. *N Engl J Med.* 2001;345:3–8.

Miller RD, ed. *Miller's Anesthesia.* 7th ed. Philadelphia, PA: Churchill Livingstone Elsevier; 2010:2233.

Morgan GE Jr, Mikhail MS, Murray MJ. *Clinical Anesthesiology.* 4th ed. New York, NY: McGraw Hill/Lange Medical Books; 2006:908–909.

Rozenberg P, Goffinet F, Philippe HJ, et al. Thickness of the lower uterine segment: its influence in the management of patients with previous cesarean sections. *Eur J Obstet Gynecol Reprod Biol.* 1999;87(1):39–45.

Ruskin KJ, Rosenbaum S. *Anesthesia Emergencies.* 1st ed. New York, NY: Oxford University Press; 2011:199–201.

Stoelting RK, Miller RD. *Basics of Anesthesia.* 5th ed. Philadelphia, PA: Churchill Livingstone Elsevier; 2007:496.

U

Vaporizer Output Calculation
Physics, Monitoring, and Anesthesia Delivery

Kevan Stanton

Edited by Raj K. Modak

KEY POINTS

1. The three main determinants of vaporizer output are the saturated vapor pressure of the anesthetic, the carrier gas flow rate, and the barometric pressure.
2. Temperature can affect the vaporizer output, though modern vaporizers have a relatively linear output over a significant range of temperatures.
3. Intermittent backpressure as a result of positive pressure ventilation, known as the pumping effect, can lead to higher vaporizer output than expected.
4. Properties of the carrier gas such as viscosity, density, and solubility in the volatile anesthetic can cause vaporizer output to be higher or lower than expected.

DISCUSSION

Multiple factors influence vaporizer output, though only three variables are used directly in calculating output. These are (1) the vapor pressure of the volatile anesthetic, (2) the carrier gas flow rate, and (3) the barometric pressure.

The following equation is used to calculate vaporizer output:

$$VO = \frac{CG \times SVP_{anes}}{P_b - SVP_{anes}}$$

where VO is the vaporizer output in mL per minute, CG is the carrier gas flow in mL per minute, SVP_{anes} is the (saturated) vapor pressure of the anesthetic, and P_b is the barometric pressure.

The first variable is the vapor pressure of the volatile anesthetic. It determines how readily anesthetic molecules escape from the liquid phase into the gaseous phase (by evaporation) to become available for pickup by the carrier gas. Vapor pressure is independent of the barometric pressure, but it does vary with temperature.

The second variable affecting vaporizer output is the carrier gas flow rate through the vaporizer. Carrier flow rate most obviously influences vaporizer output at the extremes of flow: maximal and minimal flow rates. At both extremes, the vaporizer output is less than stated on the dial. At low flow rates, this is because insufficient turbulence is generated in the vaporizer chamber to pick up vapor molecules. At high flow rates, it is due to incomplete mixing and inability to fully saturate the carrier gas.

The third variable affecting vaporizer output is the barometric pressure. Because the vapor pressure is independent of the barometric pressure, as the barometric pressure falls, vaporizer output becomes primarily dependent on the vapor pressure of the volatile anesthetic. As barometric pressure falls, then, the vaporizer output increases (greater volume of evaporated anesthetic gas is carried away per unit time).

Temperature can also affect vaporizer output. Because vapor pressure is dependent on temperature, and because vapor pressure is a main determinant of vaporizer output, temperature thus affects output. Modern vaporizers have a relatively linear output over a range of temperatures. This is accomplished both by altering the amount of carrier gas directed into the vaporizing chamber, depending on the temperature, and by constructing vaporizers out of materials that minimize the effect of cooling that results from vaporization.

Another factor that can influence vaporizer output is the intermittent backpressure resulting from positive pressure ventilation or from the use of the oxygen flush valve. Both of these can lead to a higher vaporizer output than expected. This effect, called the pumping effect, is more prominent with low dial settings, low flows, and a low level of liquid anesthetic in the vaporizer. High respiratory rates, high peak pressures, and rapid pressure decreases also augment this effect.

The final major factor affecting vaporizer output is the carrier gas composition. Depending on the viscosity, density, and solubility of the carrier gas in the anesthetic liquid, the output can be greater or less than expected when switching between carrier gasses.

SUGGESTED READINGS

Barash PG, Cullen BF, Stoelting RK, et al, eds. *Clinical Anesthesia*. 6th ed. Philadelphia, PA: Lippincott Williams & Wilkins; 2009:663–664.

Ehrenwerth J, Eisenkraft JB. *Anesthesia Equipment: Principles and Applications*. St Louis, MO: Mosby-Year Book; 1993: 61.

Miller RD, Eriksson LI, Fleisher LA, et al. *Miller's Anesthesia*. 7th ed. Philadelphia, PA: Churchill Livingstone; 2010:685–687.

V

Vasodilators: Pharmacodynamics and Renal Blood Flow

Pharmacology

Jinlei Li and Archer Martin

Edited by Benjamin Sherman

1. There are many classes of vasodilators that are used widely in clinical practice.
2. The vasodilators covered are sodium nitroprusside, nitroglycerin, hydralazine, adenosine, and fenoldopam.
3. The use of various vasodilators should be tailored to the specific clinical situation. Side effects and toxicity should be monitored accordingly.
4. The effects on renal blood flow vary among the vasodilators.

Classes of Vasodilators

1. Direct vasodilators: nitroglycerin, nitroprusside, hydralazine
2. Calcium channel blockers: amlodipine, bepridil, diltiazem, felodipine
3. Beta-blockers: metoprolol, esmolol
4. Alpha- and beta-adrenergic blockers: labetalol
5. Alpha-adrenergic blockers: phentolamine, prazosin, tolazoline
6. Angiotensin-converting enzyme (ACE) inhibitors: lisinopril, captopril
7. Angiotensin II receptor blockers (ARBs): losartan, irbesartan
8. Central alpha-2-agonist: clonidine
9. Dopamine agonist/antagonist: fenoldopam
10. Natriuretic peptide receptor agonist: nesiritide
11. Prostaglandin (PG) agonist: alprostadil, epoprostenol

Common Vasodilators

- *Sodium nitroprusside.* It relaxes venous smooth muscle via the release of nitric oxide (NO) status post metabolism of the parent compound. After administration, the lowering of the arterial blood pressure (BP) leads to subsequent release of renin and catecholamines. Renal function is well maintained despite drops in arterial BP and overall renal perfusion.
- *Nitroglycerin.* It relaxes venous smooth muscle via NO, as discussed above with sodium nitroprusside. According to Elkayam et al., nitroglycerin causes "a selective vasodilatory effect on renal conductance but not on resistance of blood vessels, and fails to increase renal blood flow."
- *Hydralazine.* Its mechanism of action may be through vasodilatation via interference of calcium utilization and activation of guanylyl cyclase. The renal blood flow is maintained or even increased, and thus it is used for patients with renal impairment.
- *Adenosine.* It is a vasodilator that selectively affects vessels responsible for afterload, with a minor effect on preload, working on specific adenosine receptors located in vascular beds. "Adenosine causes renal vasoconstriction with a drop in renal blood flow, GFR, and urinary output" according to Elkayam et al.
- *Fenoldopam.* It is a vasodilator that works via the D1-dopamine receptors, with the R-isomer predominately being the biologically active compound. It increases renal blood flow via the D1-receptor activation, even in the face of a decreased arterial BP.

Common Indications for the use of Vasodilators

1. Hypertension (HTN) secondary to increased systemic vascular resistance (SVR)
2. Congestive heart failure (CHF): acute and chronic CHF when preload and afterload need to be decreased
3. Pulmonary HTN: nitroglycerin, nitroprusside, NO, epoprostenol
4. Cardiovascular surgery: controlled hypotension
5. Acute coronary syndrome: nitroglycerin
6. Cerebral vasospasm: nimodipine

Common Side Effects

1. By decreasing SVR and BP, vasodilators can induce reflex sympathetic stimulation (baroreceptor mediated) manifested by tachycardia and increased contractility. This can be detrimental in situations as acute cardiac ischemia.
2. Some vasodilators such as clonidine or beta-blockers can cause rebound HTN if discontinued abruptly. This can be attenuated by coadministration of beta-blocker and ACE inhibitor or ARB.
3. Nitroprusside needs to be monitored closely for cyanide toxicity.

Example Site of Actions

Exclusive Arterial Dilatation	Arterial and Venous Dilatation
Calcium channel blockers	ACE inhibitors: angiotensin-converting enzyme inhibitor
Hydralazine: direct vasodilator	ARB: angiotensin receptor antagonist
Phentolamine: alpha-adrenergic blockers	Nitroglycerin: direct vasodilator
	Nitroprusside: direct vasodilator
	Prazosin: alpha-adrenergic blockers
	Alprostadil: PGE1 agonist
	Trimethaphan: ganglionic blocker and direct vasodilator
	Nesiritide: natriuretic factor receptor agonist

SUGGESTED READINGS

Elkayam U, Cohen G, Gogia H, et al. Renal vasodilatory effect of endothelial stimulation in patients with chronic congestive heart failure. *J Am Coll Cardiol.* 1996;28(1):176–182.

Hensley FA Jr, Martin DE, Gravlee GP, eds. *A Practical Approach to Cardiac Anesthesia.* 4th ed. Philadelphia, PA: Lippincott Williams & Wilkins; 2008:64–83.

Morgan GE Jr, Mikhail MS, Murray MJ. *Clinical Anesthesiology.* 4th ed. New York, NY: McGraw Hill/Lange Medical Books; 2006:256–261.

Vasopressin Rx: Diabetes Insipidus
Organ-based Clinical: Endocrine/Metabolic

Roberto Rappa

Edited by Ala Haddadin

KEY POINTS

1. Diabetes insipidus is a clinical condition characterized by an inability to concentrate urine.
2. Diabetes insipidus may be central (inadequate secretion of antidiuretic hormone [ADH]) or nephrogenic (decreased renal tubule responsiveness to ADH).
3. The treatment of choice for central diabetes insipidus is vasopressin or its synthetic derivative, desmopressin.
4. Perioperative vasopressin therapy is not indicated until plasma osmolality rises above 290 mOsm per L.

DISCUSSION

Diabetes insipidus is a clinical condition characterized by an inability to concentrate urine. It can result from either the inadequate secretion of ADH (central diabetes insipidus), or failure of the renal tubules to respond appropriately to circulating ADH (nephrogenic diabetes insipidus). Signs and symptoms include the production of copious amounts of dilute urine, often greater than 6 L per day, and polydipsia. Without an intact thirst mechanism, patients can quickly become severely dehydrated and demonstrate signs/symptoms of severe hypovolemia (dizziness, tachycardia, orthostatic hypotension, dry mucous membranes, etc.). Patients often develop hypovolemic hypernatremia, as free water losses often exceed daily intake.

Vasopressin, also known as arginine vasopressin (AVP), argipressin, or ADH, is the treatment of choice for acute central diabetes insipidus. It is an endogenous peptide hormone that is initially synthesized as a preprohormone precursor in the hypothalamus, and stored in vesicles in the posterior pituitary gland. It is secreted directly into the blood stream in response to reduced circulating plasma volume and to increased plasma osmolality. It is also commercially available (trade name Pitressin) as a sterile, aqueous solution of synthetic vasopressin. It is standardized to contain 20 pressor units per mL.

The treatment of central diabetes insipidus includes the administration of vasopressin or its long-acting synthetic analogue, desmopressin. Vasopressin can be administered as an aqueous preparation with an intravenous bolus of 100 mU, followed by a constant infusion of 100 to 200 mU per hour along with an isotonic crystalloid solution. Alternatively, it can be administered as a tannate in oil intramuscularly.

The synthetic derivative, desmopressin (DDAVP), can be administered intranasally, orally, or parenterally. It has a prolonged duration of antidiuretic activity (12 to 24 hours) and is associated with markedly reduced pressor activity. It demonstrates 2,000-fold more specific antidiuretic activity than its naturally occurring cousin, L-AVP.

When treating patients with vasopressin or desmopressin, plasma osmolality should be measured routinely. It is advisable to measure plasma osmolality every hour intraoperatively and immediately after surgery. Dosages require careful titration, as there is considerable interpatient variability. Useful titration parameters include urine output and routine plasma osmolality assessment.

Vasopressin replacement therapy should only be considered for those patients with complete diabetes insipidus. In patients with a partial deficiency of ADH production, nonosmotic triggers (i.e., volume depletion) in conjunction with surgical stimulation are sufficient enough to promote adequate release of endogenous ADH in the perioperative period. In fact, perioperative vasopressin therapy is not indicated until plasma osmolality rises above 290 mOsm per L.

V

SUGGESTED READINGS

Barash PG, Cullen BF, Stoelting RK, et al, eds. *Clinical Anesthesia*, 6th ed. Philadelphia, PA: Lippincott Williams & Wilkins; 2009:1019–1020.

Roizen MF, Fleisher LA. Anesthetic implications of concurrent diseases. In: Miller RD, Eriksson LI, Fleisher LA, et al, eds. *Miller's Anesthesia*. 7th ed. Philadelphia, PA: Churchill Livingstone; 2009.

Kronenberg HM, Melmed S, Polonsky KS, et al, eds. *Williams Textbook of Endocrinology*. 11th ed. Philadelphia, PA: Saunders Elsevier; 2008.

Vasopressors: Risk of Myocardial Ischemia
Organ-based Clinical: Cardiovascular

Veronica Matei

Edited by Benjamin Sherman

KEY POINTS

1. Vasopressors belong to a larger family of agents, called vasoactive agents.
2. Vasoactive drugs are used to treat the hemodynamic changes associated with different types of shock.
3. Many of the vasopressors in use have varied clinical effects because of their mixed receptor activity. Some of these effects are undesirable, which include myocardial ischemia.
4. Risks of myocardial ischemia are mostly related to exaggerated effects on afterload, which include decreased cardiac output, reflex bradycardia, and increased myocardial oxygen consumption.
5. It is possible for vasoconstrictors, including alpha-mediated and vasopressin, to cause direct coronary vasoconstriction severe enough to cause myocardial ischemia.

DISCUSSION

Vasoactive agents are classically subdivided on the basis of their pharmacologic activity into two separate class types: vasopressors and inotropes. Vasoactive drugs are used to treat the hemodynamic changes associated with different types of shock. Vasoactive drug therapy is used to manipulate the relative distribution of blood flow and restore tissue perfusion. The proper selection of one or more agents greatly depends on a basic understanding of the physiologic mechanisms driving a particular shock state.

Vasopressors improve perfusion pressure and preserve regional distribution of cardiac output through an increase in mean arterial pressure (MAP) above autoregulatory thresholds. Vasopressors may also improve cardiac preload by decreasing venous compliance and augmenting venous return.

Vasopressors function primarily through stimulation of adrenergic or nonadrenergic receptors. Many of the drugs in use have varied effects because of their mixed receptor activity, and some of these effects can be undesirable.

The desired responses (i.e., vasoconstriction) can stimulate feedback responses that might counter the intended effect (increased perfusion). For example, vasoconstriction leads to an increase in systemic vascular resistance (SVR) and a resultant increase in MAP. Elevated MAPs can trigger reflex bradycardia, causing a decrease in CO (decreased perfusion). In addition, increases in SVR (afterload) can also negatively impact CO, particularly in patients with weakened or ischemic myocardium. Elevated afterload also increases myocardial oxygen consumption with possible manifestations of ischemia in patients with severe coronary artery disease. It is possible for vasoconstrictors, including alpha-mediated and vasopressin, to cause direct coronary vasoconstriction severe enough to cause myocardial ischemia. Common complications associated with vasopressors and inotropic agents include dysrhythmias, myocardial ischemia, hyperglycemia, and hypoperfusion.

SUGGESTED READINGS

Barash PG, Cullen BF, Stoelting RK, et al, eds. *Clinical Anesthesia*. 6th ed. Philadelphia, PA: Lippincott Williams & Wilkins; 2009.

Heusch G. Alpha-adrenergic mechanisms in myocardial ischemia. *Circulation*. 1990;81:1–13.

Maturi MF, Martin SE, Markle D, et al. Coronary vasoconstriction induced by vasopressin. Production of myocardial ischemia in dogs by constriction of nondiseased small vessels. *Circulation*. 1991;83(6):2111–2121.

V

Venous Air Embolism: Diagnosis

Organ-based Clinical: Neurologic and Neuromuscular and Physics, Monitoring, and Anesthesia Delivery Devices

Ashley Kelley, Dallen Mill, Marianne Saleeb,

and Ira Whitten

Edited by Ramachandran Ramani

KEY POINTS

1. Venous air embolism is the entrapment of air into the pulmonary circulation.
   a. Occurs when there is subatmospheric pressure within an open vein.
   b. Patient is at risk when the wound is above the level of the heart.
2. Highest incidence occurs in sitting craniotomies.
3. Diagnosis of air embolism should be suspected with a sudden decrease in measured end-tidal CO_2 ($ETCO_2$), a sudden increase in measured end-tidal nitrogen (ETN_2), and sudden attempts to self-ventilate by patients who are being mechanically ventilated.
4. Later signs of venous air embolism include cardiac arrhythmias, hypotension, tachycardia, a "mill wheel" murmur, and cyanosis.
5. Diagnosis can be confirmed with transesophageal echocardiography (TEE; most sensitive), precordial Doppler, or air aspiration from a central venous catheter.
6. TEE is the most sensitive modality for the detection of venous air embolism, but its use is limited.
7. Treatment:
   - Flood surgical field with saline
   - Deliver 100% oxygen
   - Aspirate central venous catheter
   - Give volume to increase central venous pressure (CVP)
   - Treat hemodynamic changes appropriately

DISCUSSION

Venous air embolism is the entrapment of air into the pulmonary circulation. Air embolism is a complication of the head-elevated surgical position and with any surgical position where the surgical field is located more than 10 to 15 cm above the right heart (when CVP becomes negative). The pathophysiology of venous air embolism involves increased dead-space ventilation from occlusion of small pulmonary vessels. Air may pass into the right ventricle and compromise right ventricular output as well as into the cerebral and coronary circulation via a patent foramen ovale. This can lead to shock, pulmonary edema, myocardial infarction, or cerebrovascular accident.

Venous air embolism should be suspected with a sudden decrease in measured $ETCO_2$ or sudden attempts at spontaneous ventilation by patients who are being mechanically ventilated. Later signs of venous air embolism include cardiac arrhythmias, hypotension, auscultation of a "mill wheel" murmur, and cyanosis. Other signs include increased CVP, hypoxemia, and increased ETN_2 (measured with mass spectrometry).

The most sensitive method of diagnosing venous air embolism is TEE; however, this may be inconvenient and not readily available to the anesthesiologist in all settings. The next most sensitive method is a precordial Doppler ultrasound that can detect as little as 0.25 mL of entrapped air. In comparison with $ETCO_2$, ETN_2 is of comparable or greater sensitivity, and changes associated with venous air embolism (VAE) can be detected

30 to 90 seconds earlier. ETN_2 is not widely available, and its utility in the detection of VAE is compromised in the presence of hypotension or nitrous oxide use. Pulse oximetry, ECG, and the use of an esophageal stethoscope are additional methods of detection, which are limited by low sensitivity. The diagnosis can also be made by aspiration of air from a central venous catheter (Table 1).

Table 1. Comparison of Methods of Detection of Vascular Air Embolism

Method of Detection	Sensitivity (mL/kg)	Availability	Invasiveness	Limitations
TEE	High (0.02)	Low	High	Expertise required, expensive, invasive
Precordial Doppler	High (0.05)	Moderate	None	Obese patients
PA catheter	High (0.25)	Moderate	High	Fixed distance, small orifice
TCD	High	Moderate	None	Expertise required
ETN_2	Moderate (0.5)	Low	None	N_2O, hypotension
$ETCO_2$	Moderate (0.5)	Moderate	None	Pulmonary disease
Oxygen saturation	Low	High	None	Late changes
Direct visualization	Low	High	None	No physiologic data
Esophageal stethoscope	Low (1.5)	High	Low	Late changes
ECG	Low (1.25)	High	Low	Late changes

N_2O, nitrous oxide; PA, pulmonary artery; TCD, transcranial Doppler.

The treatment of VAE includes the following:

- Flooding the surgical field with saline.
- Discontinuing nitrous oxide and delivering 100% oxygen.
- Aspirating the venous embolism via a central venous catheter that is placed high in the right atrium.
- Increasing CVP with intravascular volume.
- Treating hypotension with vasopressors.
- Attempting to create back bleeding, with bilateral jugular vein compression, to help the surgeon identify the source of the embolism.
- Choosing positive end-expiratory pressure (PEEP) to increase cerebral venous pressure, but this is controversial.
- Trendelenburg position and wound closure, which may be needed.
- Resuscitation, if circulatory arrest ensues.

SUGGESTED READINGS

Barash PG, Cullen BF, Stoelting RK, et al, eds. *Clinical Anesthesia.* 6th ed. Philadelphia, PA: Lippincott Williams & Wilkins; 2009:811.

Miller RD, Eriksson LI, Fleisher LA, et al, eds. Neurosurgical anesthesia. In: *Miller's Anesthesia.* 7th ed. Philadelphia, PA: Churchill Livingstone; 2009:2054–2057.

Mirski MA, Lele AV, Fitzsimmons L, et al. Diagnosis and treatment of vascular air embolism. *Anesthesiology.* 2007;106:164–177.

Morgan GE, Mikhail MS, Murray MJ. *Clinical Anesthesiology.* 4th ed. New York, NY: McGraw-Hill Companies; 2006:638–639.

Shaikh N, Ummunisa F. Acute management of vascular air embolism. *J Emerg Trauma Shock.* 2009;2:180–185.

Stoelting RK, Miller RD, eds. *Basics of Anesthesia.* 5th ed. Philadelphia, PA: Churchill Livingstone; 2007:298, 459–460.

Vent Modes: Pressure Waveform
Organ-based Clinical: Respiratory

Brooke Albright

Edited by Veronica Matei

1. Various modes of ventilation are in current clinical use, and each has a distinct pressure waveform pattern.
2. Pressure waveform analysis provides valuable information regarding lung mechanics, specifically airways resistance.
3. Triggered ventilation modes result in a negative deflection of the pressure waveform prior to the delivered breath.
4. Synchronized intermittent mandatory ventilation uses an observation window to deliver a mandatory breath at the beginning or the end of a breath interval to avoid breath stacking.

1. Controlled Mechanical Ventilation (CMV) versus Pressure Control Ventilation (PCV)

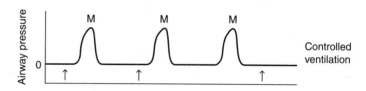

In CMV, all breaths are volume-fixed mandatory breaths. The patient cannot trigger a breath. PCV is similar to CMV in that the rate is fixed and the breaths are controlled; however, in PCV, a peak inspiratory pressure is set rather than a tidal volume so that both tidal volume and minute ventilation can vary if the patient's lung-thorax compliance or airway resistance changes. Note that in the pressure waveforms seen above, airway pressure is at 0 until the ventilator initiates a breath, which is signified by the sharp increase in airway pressure. Once the breath is completed, the airway pressure returns back to 0.

2. Pressure Support Ventilation (PSV)

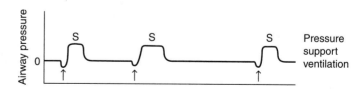

PSV helps augment each breath during spontaneous ventilation by maintaining a preset positive pressure during inspiration. It is essentially spontaneous breathing with a boost at each inspiration. Advantages of PSV include decreased work of breathing, improved synchronization between the patient and the ventilator, reduced inspiratory pressures, and facilitation of weaning. The disadvantage is if apnea occurs, then the patient receives no ventilation. PSV is considered at a minimum when the level of support is <8 cm H_2O. In Figure 2, notice the negative deflection of the airway pressure tracing signifying the patient

V

triggering a breath, followed by the steep and rapid rise in the flow tracing, representing machine-delivered positive pressure support.

3. Spontaneous Intermittent Mandatory Ventilation (SIMV)

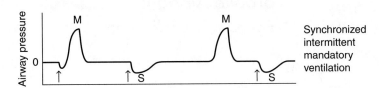

In SIMV, the ventilator synchronizes mandatory scheduled breaths of a fixed tidal volume and rate around the patient's own spontaneous ventilation. The additional minute ventilation is determined by the patient's own respiratory efforts. If no inspiratory effort is detected within a set time frame, then the ventilator delivers a mandatory breath at the scheduled time. Depending on the patient's own respiratory efforts, the ventilator is able to vary the machine cycle times slightly. PSV can be set in conjunction with SIMV to decrease the work of breathing when the patient initiates the breath. IMV is considered at a minimum when the rate is no more than 4 to 6 breaths per minute.

4. Assist Control Ventilation (ACV)

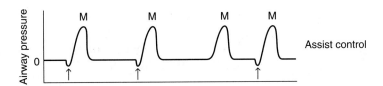

In ACV, the patient may trigger the set-volume ventilator breaths at a more rapid rate than the controlled mandatory respiratory rate. In Figure 5 to the left, notice the slight negative deflection of the airway pressure tracing as the patient triggers the breath.

5. High-Frequency Ventilation (HFV)

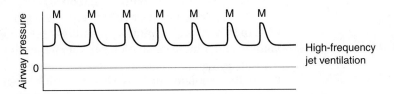

HFV is a generic term describing mechanical ventilation that operates at a frequency at least four times higher than the natural breathing frequency of the patient. HFV most often uses a small cannula to deliver a jet stream of flow to the lungs during inspiration. Expiration is usually passive, except in high-frequency oscillatory ventilation (HFOV), where the ventilator actively drives expiratory flows by a rotary driven piston that produces to-and-fro movement of gas in the airway. HFV is characterized by low peak and mean airway pressures.

HFV is indicated in the following situations:

- In special procedures requiring adequate visualization for surgeons to operate such as bronchoscopy, laryngoscopy and tracheal reconstruction.
- Respiratory failure in patients with bronchopleural fistulas, tracheoesophageal fistulas, barotraumas, pulmonary fibrosis, acute respiratory distress syndrome, pulmonary hemorrhage, and persistent fetal circulation in the neonate to enhance CO_2 elimination.

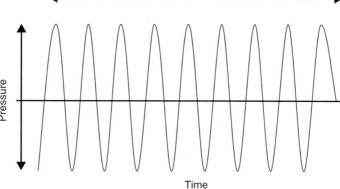

Frequency:
Increasing frequency may paradoxically lead to decreased CO_2 removal by increasing lung impedence and airway resistance, decreasing tidal volume to alveoli.

Amplitude:
Increasing amplitude will increase tidal volume and improve CO_2. Care needs to be taken to avoid over-inflation, which would compromise systemic circulation.

Pressure

Time

A type of HFV, high-frequency jet ventilation, displays an intrinsic PEEP effect at inspiratory times greater than 40% and high drive pressures. Of note on the pressure waveform, the airway pressure is always greater than 0.

Precautions to HFV use include the following:

- Adequate expiratory time should always be considered to prevent barotrauma.
- Adequate humidification should always be used to prevent tracheal injury.
- Automatic shutoff mechanisms should be functioning properly to allow termination of ventilation in overpressure situations.

SUGGESTED READINGS

Froese AB. *High Frequency Ventilation: Uses and Abuses* (ASA refresher courses in anesthesiology). Park Ridge, IL: American Society of Anesthesiologists; 1986:127–138.

Morgan GE, Mikhail MS, Murray MJ. *Clinical Anesthesiology*. 4th ed. New York, NY: McGraw Hill; 2006:1032–1035.

Pierson D. *A Primer on Mechanical Ventilation* (Clinical Respiratory Diseases & Critical Care Medicine). Seattle, WA: University of Washington School of Medicine 4th year Curriculum Guide; 2008: 1–12.

Robertson K, Lubarsky D, Sudharma R. *Anesthesiology Board Review*. 2nd ed. New York, NY: McGraw Hill; 2006:202, 372.

Yao F, Fontes M, Malhotra V. *Anesthesiology Problem-Oriented Patient Management*. 6th ed. Philadelphia, PA: Lippincott Williams & Wilkins; 2008:77–80.

V

Ventilator: Low Tidal Volume and Protect Effects

Generic, Clinical Sciences: Anesthesia Procedures, Methods, Techniques and Organ-based Clinical: Respiratory

Svetlana Sapozhnikova and Neil Sinha
Edited by Raj K. Modak

1. The ARDSnet protocol describes a low tidal volume strategy, and incremental increases in positive end-expiratory pressure (PEEP) and FiO_2 to maintain appropriate oxygenation.
2. Low tidal volumes of less than or equal to 6 mL/kg in combination with plateau airway pressures of less than or equal to 30 cm H_2O have been shown to reduce mortality by 22% in patients with acute lung injury (ALI)/acute respiratory distress syndrome (ARDS).
3. Tidal volumes have to be based on predicted ideal body weight and not on actual patient's weight.
4. Respiratory acidosis from low volume ventilation can be treated with increase in respiratory rate.
5. Classically, tidal volumes of 10 to 15 mL/kg have been used to ensure appropriate oxygenation and provide respiratory compensation for metabolic acidosis.
6. ALI is characterized by capillary leakage, a decrease in lung compliance, noncardiogenic pulmonary edema, and hypoxemia.

ALI is characterized by capillary leakage, a decrease in lung compliance, noncardiogenic pulmonary edema, and hypoxemia caused by local and systemic inflammation. There are two forms of ALI. Primary ALI results from direct injury to the lung (e.g., pneumonia), and secondary ALI results from indirect insult (e.g., sepsis). There are two phases to ALI. The acute phase results from the destruction of the alveolar–capillary interface causing leakage of fluid into the alveolar and interstitial space. The reparative phase is characterized by fibrotic changes and reorganization of the lung.

ALI is characterized by the following: (1) bilateral pulmonary infiltrates on chest X-ray, (2) pulmonary capillary wedge pressure (PCWP) less than 18 mm Hg, and (3) PaO_2/FiO_2 less than 300 mm Hg. More severe lung injury with PaO_2/FiO_2 less than 200 mm Hg is defined as ARDS.

Classically, tidal volumes of 10 to 15 mL/kg of body weight have been used for patients with acute lung injury (compared with normal rest tidal volumes of 7 to 8 mL/kg) to ensure appropriate oxygenation and to help provide respiratory compensation for metabolic acidosis. However, these tidal volumes may result in excessive distension and "stretch" of the ventilated lung causing a release of inflammatory markers and ultimately, the further exacerbation of ALI.

The ARDSnet trial was a prospective study comparing classical ventilatory strategies to low tidal volume ventilation in patients with ALI. The study was stopped after the fourth interim analysis as the use of lower tidal volumes caused a reduction in mortality by 22% and significant reduction in the number of ventilator-free days. The ARDSnet protocol for ventilation in patients with ALI involves initial Vt of 8 mL/kg; the tidal volumes should be reduced by 1 mL/kg at intervals of 1 to 2 hours until low tidal volume ventilation is achieved (Vt = 6 mL/kg). The respiratory rate should be increased to maintain minute ventilation. Oxygenation should be maintained (PaO_2 of 55 to 80 mm Hg or SpO_2 88% to 95%) by using a minimum PEEP of 5 cm H_2O and incremental and alternative increases in FiO_2 and PEEP. The plateau pressures should be maintained at less than 30 cm H_2O, and further decreases in tidal volume or changes in ventilator modes should be taken to achieve this.

In patients whose plateau pressure remains greater than or equal to 30 cm H_2O tidal volumes need to be decreased gradually to a minimum tidal volume of 4 mL/kg. If patients develop respiratory acidosis, respiratory rate can be increased. Respiratory rates up to 35 breaths per minute can be used as a compensation for low tidal volumes.

SUGGESTED READINGS

Barash PG, Cullen BF, Stoelting RK, et al, eds. *Clinical Anesthesia*. 6th ed. Philadelphia, PA: Lippincott Williams & Wilkins; 2009:1458–1459.

Fink EL, et al. *Textbook of Critical Care*. 5th ed. Philadelphia, PA: Saunders; 2005:193, 576–578.

Miller RD, et al. *Miller's Anesthesia*. 7th ed. Philadelphia, PA: Churchill Livingstone; 2010:2854–2857.

Papadakos PJ, et al. *Mechanical Ventilation*. 1st ed. Philadelphia, PA: Saunders; 2007:503–504.

The Acute Respiratory Distress Syndrome Network. Ventilation with lower tidal volumes as compared with traditional tidal volumes for acute lung injury and the acute respiratory distress syndrome. *N Engl J Med*. 2000;342:1301–1308.

V

Ventilator Disconnect: Detection

Physics, Monitoring, and Anesthesia Delivery

Emilio Andrade

Edited by Raj K. Modak

KEY POINTS

1. One hazard associated with ventilator use in the operating room is ventilator disconnection resulting in inadequate ventilation of the patient.
2. The most common site of anesthesia delivery system disconnect is the breathing circuit, specifically at the Y-piece.
3. The three most common types of disconnection monitors are pressure, volume, and end-tidal carbon dioxide monitors.
4. Utilization of one or all of these alarms will not guarantee detection. Ultimately, the anesthesiologist should remain vigilant and monitor for breath sounds and chest rise to detect ventilator disconnection.

DISCUSSION

Multiple hazards are associated with ventilator use in the operating room. One such problem is ventilator disconnection resulting in inadequate ventilation of the patient. The disconnection can be partial or complete. The most common site of anesthesia delivery system disconnect is the breathing circuit, specifically at the Y-piece. Preexisting leaks may also occur in the disposable circuits that are commonly used. Important detection devices/alarms have been established to alert the anesthesiologist when disconnection occurs.

The three most common types of disconnection monitors are pressure, volume, and end-tidal carbon dioxide monitors. Pressure monitors (pneumatic or electronic) measure the amplitude of ventilator-generated pressure in the breathing circuit. The effectiveness of these monitors depends on sensor location, site of disconnection, inspiratory flow rates, pressure alarm limits, and the resistance of the circuit. Some of these factors depend on the type of ventilator being used, such as the location of the sensor. Alarm values may be preset or adjustable. If the peak inspiratory pressure of the circuit falls below the set limit, then the alarm will go off. If the alarm limit is adjustable, it should be set within 5 cm H_2O of the peak inspiratory pressure. If it is set less than this value, then a disconnection may go unnoticed.

Respiratory volume monitors may also prove valuable in the detection of ventilator disconnections. These types of monitors may sense exhaled or inhaled tidal volume, minute volume, or a combination of the three. Again, the type of machine will dictate where these sensors are placed and the type of volume being monitored. Appropriate upper and lower volume limits should be set based on what is expected to be delivered to the patient.

End-tidal carbon dioxide monitors are extremely effective and rapid at detecting ventilator disconnections. Carbon dioxide analyzers use infrared analysis to detect changes in every breath. These analyzers measure CO_2 near the Y-piece. A disconnection may have occurred if there is an acute absence of end-tidal CO_2 or acute changes in the difference between end-tidal and inspiratory carbon dioxide concentrations.

However, utilization of one or all of these alarms will not guarantee detection. Ultimately, the anesthesiologist should remain vigilant and monitor for breath sounds and chest rise to detect ventilator disconnection.

SUGGESTED READINGS

Barash PG, Cullen BF, Stoelting RK, et al. *Clinical Anesthesia.* 6th ed. Philadelphia, PA: Lippincott Williams & Wilkins; 2009:676–679.

Lobato E, Gravenstein N, Kirby R. Anesthesia machine malfunction. In: *Complications in Anesthesiology.* 1st ed. Philadelphia, PA: Lippincott Williams & Wilkins; 2008:811.

Petty C. Safety features of the anesthesia machine. In: *The Anesthesia Machine.* Philadelphia, PA: Churchill Livingstone; 1987:187–192.

V

Ventricular PV Loops
Organ-based Clinical: Cardiovascular, Physiology

Neil Sinha
Edited by Qingbing Zhu

1. The left ventricular pressure–volume (LVPV) loop is a graphic depiction of the left ventricular (LV) pressure plotted against the LV volume during the various stages of the cardiac cycle.
2. The width of the ventricular PV loop reflects the stroke volume (EDV–ESV), and the area within the loop is the stroke work.

The LVPV loop is a graphic depiction of the LV pressure (*y*-axis) plotted against the LV volume (*x*-axis) during the various stages of the cardiac cycle (see Fig. 1). Point 1 reflects the state of the LV at the end of diastole, which is the end-diastolic volume (EDV). Phase "b" is isovolumetric contraction, which occurs with the closure of the mitral valve and ends with the opening of the aortic valve. During this phase, the LV pressure begins to increase (without a change in the LV volume) until the LV pressure exceeds the aortic diastolic pressure (point 2) and the aortic valve opens. Phase "c" reflects the ejection of the blood from the LV to the systemic circulation. During this phase, the LV pressure increases upto a maximum value (peak systolic pressure) and then slowly starts to decline as ventricular relaxation begins. The LV volume declines as the blood volume is ejected through the aortic valve into the systemic circulation.

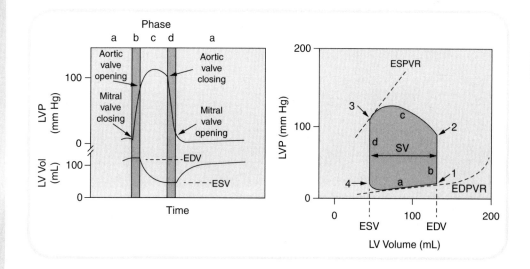

Figure 1. Ventricular PV loops. (From Klabunde RE. *Cardiovascular Physiology Concepts*. Philadelphia, PA: Lippincott Williams & Wilkins; 2005:67, with permission.)

Point 3 refers to the closure of the aortic valve, at which point ejection stops and the LV begins isovolumetric relaxation (phase "d"). Both the mitral and the aortic valve are closed during this phase, resulting in a decline in the LV pressure in the absence of change to the LV volume. The LV volume during phase "d" is also known as end-systolic volume (ESV).

614

Point 4 occurs when the LV pressure falls below the left atrial pressure, resulting in the opening of the mitral valve. Phase "a" reflects diastole and the filling of the LV. Initially, the LV pressure declines as LV volume increases because the ventricle is still relaxing. Slowly, however, the LV pressure increases in response to the LV volume increasing. The width of the ventricular PV loop reflects the stroke volume (EDV – ESV), and the area within the loop is the stroke work.

The ventricular PV loops can be used to further analyze different cardiac disease states. Systolic dysfunction results in the loss of intrinsic inotropy of the LV, causing a decrease in the slope of the end-systolic PV curve and ultimately an increase in the ESV with a compensatory increase in EDV. The PV loop in systolic dysfunction is typically depicted with a global right shift of the loop. Diastolic dysfunction results from a reduction of ventricular compliance. The PV loop will demonstrate a decrease in ventricular filling and a decrease of EDV, and ultimately a drop in the stroke volume.

The ventricular PV loop helps depict changes in the LV volume and pressure during various phases of the cardiac cycle and is a useful tool to analyze changes in systolic and/or diastolic function of the heart.

SUGGESTED READINGS

Klabunde RE. *Cardiovascular Physiology Concepts*. Philadelphia, PA: Lippincott Williams & Wilkins; 2005:67.
Kono A, Maughan WL, Sunagawa K, et al. The use of left ventricular end-ejection pressure and peak pressure in the estimation of the end-systolic pressure–volume relationship. *Circulation*. 1984;70:1057–1065.

V

VE/PaCO$_2$ Relationship: Hypoxia
Physiology

Alexander Timchenko

Edited by Shamsuddin Akhtar

KEY POINTS

1. Under normoxic conditions, central chemoreceptors in the brainstem as well as peripheral chemoreceptors in the carotid body detect changes in PaCO$_2$. Together they generate a linear ventilatory response curve.
2. Peripheral chemoreceptors are primarily responsible for an exponentially increasing respiratory stimulus in response to decreasing levels of PaO$_2$ (less than 70 mm Hg).
3. Synergistic output from peripheral and central chemoreceptors generates increasing respiratory responses under conditions of hypoxia and hypercapnia.

DISCUSSION

At normal or near-normal levels of oxygen, CO$_2$ levels in the blood are the primary driver of ventilation. Approximately 80% to 85% of the ventilatory response to CO$_2$ results from stimulation of central chemoreceptors in the medulla. The rest results from effects of PaCO$_2$ on the carotid bodies. Some of these central receptors, which are located in the inferolateral aspect of the ventral medulla, are exquisitely responsive to cerebrospinal fluid (CSF) pH. CO$_2$ easily crosses the blood–brain barrier into the minimally buffered CSF, leading to carbonic acid formation and a decrease in the CSF pH. Other central chemoreceptors respond to a more delayed increase in interstitial fluid pH. In combination, this process leads to an initial rapid increase in ventilation, with a peak central chemoreceptor response in 1 to 2 minutes after an acute change in PaCO$_2$.

As PaCO$_2$ increases 2 to 3 mm Hg above normal, there is a linear relationship between PaCO$_2$ and minute ventilation, although at extremely high levels this response begins to flatten. On average, the hypercapneic ventilatory response in the awake patient ranges between 1 and 4 L/min/mm Hg. This response is not sustained chronically due to bicarbonate buffering by the kidneys, which in large part compensates for the change in pH detected by central chemoreceptors.

Under hypoxic conditions, changes in respiration come about through the activation of the peripheral chemoreceptors. Little additional contribution to respiration occurs via the central receptors under hypoxic conditions. Instead, the level of ventilation is altered primarily by the action of peripheral chemoreceptors located in the carotid bodies. This is important because under normoxic conditions, peripheral chemoreceptors contribute only 15% to 20% to the linear hypercapneic response. Under normocapneic conditions, the peripheral chemoreceptors respond to levels of PaO$_2$ less than 70 mm Hg with an exponentially increasing stimulus to the respiratory system. Interestingly, peripheral receptors are insensitive to conditions such as anemia or carbon monoxide poisoning that lower blood oxygen content without affecting the PaO$_2$. When both oxygen and CO$_2$ levels change, however, peripheral chemoreceptors respond in a highly synergistic manner. Under low O$_2$ and high CO$_2$ conditions, they therefore generate an exaggerated arterial response to the hypercapneic hypoxic conditions. For example, the normal hypercapneic response is doubled when measured during hypoxia at a PaO$_2$ of 55 mm Hg.

Chronically, there is a central response to prolonged hypoxia that dampens the heightened respiratory drive mediated by peripheral chemoreceptors. This phenomenon is known as hypoxic ventilatory decline. Hypoxic ventilatory decline, a centrally mediated response, usually occurs 15 to 20 minutes after the initial increase in minute ventilation.

V

**SUGGESTED
READINGS**

Caruano-Montaldo B, Gleeson K, Zwillich CW. The control of breathing in clinical practice. *Chest.* 2000;117(1):205–225.

Hemmings HC, Hopkins PM. *Foundations of Anesthesia: Basic Sciences for Clinical Practice.* Philadelphia, PA; Elsevier; 2006:565–566.

Stoelting Rk, Miller RD. *Basics of Anesthesia.* 5th ed. Philadelphia, PA; Churchill Livingstone; 2007:61–63.

VF: Epinephrine Mechanism
Organ-based Clinical: Cardiovascular

Trevor Banack

Edited by Benjamin Sherman

KEY POINTS

1. The cardiovascular effects of epinephrine result from the direct stimulation of alpha- and beta-adrenergic receptors.
2. Numerous studies discuss the effect of epinephrine on hemodynamics by the increase in systemic vascular resistance (SVR).
3. Epinephrine has been thought to play a role in the treatment of ventricular fibrillation, because it has been reported to narrow dispersion and improve synchronization of repolarization, resulting in a more homogenous recovery of the myocardium.
4. The improvement in synchronization of repolarization with epinephrine use may also facilitate defibrillation.

DISCUSSION

Epinephrine is secreted from the adrenal medulla with effects on bronchial and vascular smooth muscle tone, glandular secretions, glycogenolysis, heart rate, lipolysis, and myocardial contractility. The cardiovascular effects of epinephrine result from the direct stimulation of alpha- and beta-adrenergic receptors. The dose of epinephrine determines which type of receptor is stimulated more than the other. For example, beta-2 receptors are predominantly stimulated at intravenous epinephrine doses of 1 to 2 μg per minute, whereas beta-1 receptor activation predominates at doses of 4 μg per minute. Larger doses (10 to 20 μg per minute) stimulate both alpha and beta receptors, with alpha receptor stimulation predominating in most vascular beds.

Epinephrine is listed as one of the integral drugs for treating ventricular fibrillation in the advanced cardiovascular life support protocol. Numerous studies discuss the effect of epinephrine on hemodynamics by the increase in SVR. It is believed that the increase in SVR results in improved coronary blood flow, leading to improvement in the electrical properties of the heart, and may facilitate resuscitation. Also, epinephrine has been thought to play a role in ventricular fibrillation because it has been reported to narrow dispersion and improve synchronization of repolarization, resulting in a more homogenous recovery of the myocardium. The improvement in synchronization of repolarization may also facilitate defibrillation. On the basis of these different studies, epinephrine has multiple roles in the treatment of ventricular fibrillation.

SUGGESTED READINGS

Michael JR, Guerci AD, Koehler RC, et al. Mechanisms by which epinephrine augments cerebral and myocardial perfusions during cardiopulmonary bypass in dogs. *Circulation.* 1984;69:822–835.

Stoetling RK, Hiller SC. *Pharmacology and Physiology in Anesthetic Practice.* 4th ed. Philadelphia, PA: Lippincott Williams & Wilkins; 2006:259–277.

Suddath WO, Deychak Y, Varghese PJ. Electrophysiologic basis by which epinephrine facilitates defibrillation after prolonged episodes of ventricular fibrillation. *Ann Emerg Med.* 2001;38(3):201–206.

V

V/Q Mismatch—Emphysema
Organ-based Clinical: Respiratory

Nehal Gatha
Edited by Shamsuddin Akhtar

KEY POINTS

1. Emphysema is defined by destruction of airways distal to the terminal bronchioles.
2. Loss of the pulmonary capillary bed results in impaired gas exchange and pulmonary hypertension.
3. Emphysema is characterized by increased dead space ventilation. Ventilation/perfusion (V/Q) mismatch occurs due to ventilation of large bullae and increased alveolar pressure compressing capillaries in adjacent tissue.

DISCUSSION

Emphysema is one of the two major causes of chronic obstructive pulmonary disease (COPD), the other being chronic bronchitis. Emphysema leads to the gradual destruction of lung tissue, specifically the airways distal to the terminal bronchioles. The destruction of elastic tissue results in permanent enlargement and increased compliance of alveolar sacs with destruction of the pulmonary capillary bed. The loss of surface area limits gas exchange, decreasing ability for oxygenation of blood. The loss of the capillary bed also causes pulmonary hypertension. With disease progression, hypercapnia and hypoxia occur, with hypoxic pulmonary vasoconstriction exacerbating pulmonary hypertension and causing potential right heart failure.

V/Q mismatch in emphysema is primarily a defect of increased dead space. Ventilation occurs in large bullae that do not contribute to gas exchange. Moreover, increased pressure within these enlarging alveoli can exceed capillary and arteriole pressure, further limiting gas exchange that may occur in adjacent intact tissues.

SUGGESTED READINGS

Barash PG, Cullen BF, Stoelting RK, eds. *Clinical Anesthesia.* Philadelphia, PA: Lippincott Williams & Wilkins; 2006:800–810.

Wall O$_2$ Failure: Signs
Physics, Monitoring, and Anesthesia Delivery

Holly Barth
Edited by Raj K. Modak

KEY POINTS

1. The pipeline (from a central supply source) is the primary source of oxygen to the anesthesia machine, while the cylinder provides a backup if the pipeline fails.
2. Anesthesia machines have a low pressure sensor that will trigger an electric alarm or gas whistle if the oxygen pressure falls below a set value, generally ranging from 20 to 35 psig.
3. If the cylinder is left open, the anesthesia machine will preferentially choose the cylinder supply when the central supply falls below 45 psig.
4. In the event that oxygen supply pressure decreases, oxygen failure cutoff valves (fail-safe valves) for other gases will proportionally decrease or shut off to limit their delivery.
5. There can be the accidental mixing of nitrous oxide and oxygen from central supply. In this case, the oxygen cylinder located on the back of the anesthesia machine must be turned on and the central pipeline of oxygen must be disconnected.

DISCUSSION

Oxygen, nitrous oxide, and often air have two supply sources: pipeline and cylinder. The pipeline (from a central supply source) is the primary source of gas to the anesthesia machine, whereas the cylinder provides a backup if the pipeline fails. Generally, most machines have two pressure gauges for each gas supplied (for pipeline and cylinder). Oxygen from the pipeline is generally delivered at a constant pressure of 50 psig. It is possible for there to be a failure in the delivery of central supply oxygen. Anesthesia machines have a low pressure sensor that will trigger an electric alarm or gas whistle if the oxygen pressure falls below a set value, generally ranging from 20 to 35 psig. The cylinder source is governed by a pressure regulator that reduces the gas pressure to about 45 psig. Usually, the cylinder source is closed off and needs to be opened in the event of central gas supply failure. However, if the cylinder is left often, the anesthesia machine will preferentially choose the cylinder supply when the central supply falls below 45 psig. Therefore, in the event the cylinder is open and is being used, it may be a sign of a central oxygen delivery problem.

A safety device known as the oxygen failure cutoff valve (also referred to as fail-safe valve) is located downstream from each of the gas sources supplying flowmeters, except for oxygen. In the event that oxygen supply pressure decreases, the valves for these gases will proportionally decrease or shut off to limit their delivery. However, this does not necessarily prevent against delivery of hypoxic mixtures, which is further controlled by a flow-proportioning system.

There are different types of fail-safe valves. Some anesthesia machines have a pressure-sensor shutoff valve. If the oxygen supply pressure falls below a certain threshold value, the valve closes and prevents delivery of other gases. Other machines use a proportioning system rather than a set threshold value, which will allow for gas pressures to decrease in accordance with oxygen pressures.

Gas from the central supply enters through specific inlet fittings known as Diameter Index Safety System. It provides noninterchangeable connections, which minimizes error. However, there can be the accidental mixing of nitrous oxide and oxygen. If the anesthesiologist suspects a crossover, two actions must be done. The oxygen cylinder located on

620

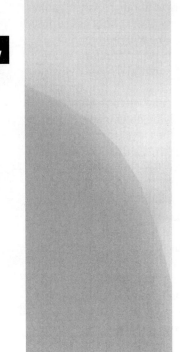

SUGGESTED
READINGS

the back of the anesthesia machine must be turned on, and the central pipeline of oxygen must be disconnected. This second step is mandatory because the machine preferentially uses the pipeline due to its lower pressure, as discussed above.

Barash PG, Cullen BF, Stoelting RK, et al, eds. *Clinical Anesthesia*. 6th ed. Philadelphia, PA: Lippincott Williams and Wilkins; 2009:653–655.

Morgan GE, Mikhail MS, Murray MJ. *Clinical Anesthesiology*. 4th ed. New York, NY: McGraw-Hill; 2006:47–54.

W

WHO Analgesic Ladder
Subspecialties: Pain

Meredith Brown

Edited by Thomas Halaszynski

KEY POINTS

1. The WHO analgesic ladder was originally created as a method for treatment of cancer pain.
2. WHO analgesic ladder consists of a three-step framework and involves the administration of both nonopioid and opioid medications as well as several other adjunct therapies.
3. Step 1 of the ladder includes administration of nonopioids (e.g., acetaminophen and nonsteroidal anti-inflammatory drugs [NSAIDs]), step 2 includes administration of weak opioids (codeine), and step 3 involves administration of stronger opioids.
4. Adjuvant therapy should also be used when appropriate, and includes corticosteroids, antidepressants, anxiolytics, gabapentin, pregabalin, and carbamazepine.

DISCUSSION

The WHO analgesic ladder was originally created in 1986 as a method for treatment of cancer pain. The WHO ladder consists of a three-step framework and involves the administration of both nonopioid and opioid medications as well as adjuvant medication therapy (Fig. 1). Effective pain control has been noted with this method in 75% to 90% of cancer-related pain patients.

The first step involves the administration of nonopioids, which includes medications such as acetaminophen and NSAIDs. If pain relief is not achieved with these classes of medications, advancement to the second step of the ladder should occur. The second step includes mild opioids, such as codeine, for the treatment of mild-to-moderate pain. If pain relief is still not provided or deemed inadequate, progression to stage 3 of the ladder occurs, which includes administration of stronger opioids such as morphine for the treatment of moderate-to-severe pain.

W

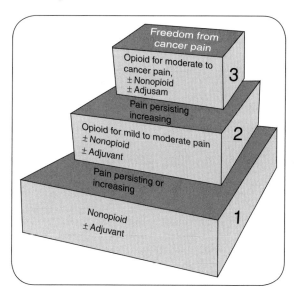

Figure 1. WHO's pain relief ladder. (Courtesy of http://www.who.int/cancer/palliative/painladder/en)

Throughout all stages of the WHO analgesic ladder, adjuvant therapy should always be considered, to complement the medications within each of the steps described above. Potential adjuvant therapy includes corticosteroids, antidepressants, anxiolytics, gabapentin, pregabalin, and carbamazepine. Furthermore, adverse effects of analgesic medications should be managed appropriately (e.g., use of antiemetics and stool softeners) to avoid potential failure of treatment resulting from side-effect profiles from the drugs highlighted within each step of the ladder.

Oral formulations of the medications are preferred over other routes of administration. However, in the case of refractory vomiting, dysphagia, and obstruction of the gastrointestinal tract, other routes may be considered (including rectal, transdermal, parenteral, and sublingual). Analgesic medications should be administered along a regimented schedule or on an around-the-clock basis, following adequate medication titration success to control continuous pain. In addition, breakthrough pain medication should also be established. Most importantly, treatment plans should be individualized on the basis of evidence of clinical needs and the response(s) of each patient.

SUGGESTED READINGS

Barash PG, Cullen BF, Stoelting RK, et al, eds. *Clinical Anesthesia*. 6th ed. Philadelphia, PA: Lippincott Williams & Wilkins; 2009:1518.

Fishman SM, Ballantyne JC, Rathmell JP, eds. *Bonica's Management of Pain*. 4th ed. Philadelphia, PA: Lippincott Williams & Wilkins; 2009:586–588.

W

Work of Breathing: Neonate vs. Adult
Subspecialties: Pediatric Anesthesia

Anna Clebone

Edited by Mamatha Punjala

KEY POINTS

1. Tidal volume and functional residual capacity (FRC) on a per-weight basis are similar in neonates and adults, approximately 7 and 30 cc per kg, respectively.
2. Oxygen consumption, respiratory rate, and minute ventilation are all higher in neonates when compared with adults.
3. The work of breathing is higher in neonates secondary to low lung compliance and high airway resistance due to a decreased number of small airways.
4. Neonates have pliable rib cages that attenuate mechanical support. Increased work of breathing is seen, as this lack of support results in functional airway closure and less efficient gas exchange.

DISCUSSION

There are several similarities and differences when comparing the respiratory system of a neonate with an adult. Tidal volume and FRC on a per-weight basis are similar, approximately 7 and 30 cc per kg, respectively, in both neonates and adults. Oxygen consumption is higher in neonates, 7 to 9 cc/kg/min compared with 3 cc/kg/min in adults. To account for this higher value, neonates have a higher baseline respiratory rate (30 to 50 breaths per minute) and thus also a higher minute ventilation (100 to 150 cc/kg/min) compared with adults (60 cc/kg/min).

The work of breathing is higher in neonates when compared with older children and adults. It is increased by high airway resistance and low lung compliance. Neonates have relatively low lung compliance while having high chest wall compliance. They also have pliable rib cages that attenuate mechanical support. Increased work of breathing is seen, as this lack of support results in functional airway closure and less efficient gas exchange. Furthermore, neonates have poorly developed intercostal muscles and a relatively weak diaphragm secondary to a lack of type one muscle fibers. Also, there is increase in airway resistance secondary to decreased numbers of small airways, and the complete maturation of alveoli does not occur until approximately 8 years of age. Lung resistance is six times greater in awake neonates compared with adults.

The problems of resistance are compounded for the neonate undergoing anesthesia when a breathing tube and circuit are introduced. The much smaller radius of a neonatal endotracheal tube leads to a large increase in resistance, explained by Poiseuille law ($R = 8\,nl/\pi r^4$). Anesthesia circuits that involve a one-way valve (e.g., circle systems) require additional inspiratory force from the spontaneously breathing neonate for opening, further increasing resistance.

W

SUGGESTED READINGS

Barash PG, Cullen BF, Stoelting RK, et al., eds. *Clinical Anesthesia*. 6th ed. Philadelphia, PA: Lippincott Williams & Wilkins; 2009:1174, 1428–1430.

Cote CJ, Lerman J, Todres ID, eds. *A Practice of Anesthesia for Infants and Children*. 4th ed. Philadelphia, PA: Saunders Elsevier; 2009:747–766.

Morgan GE, Mikhail MS, Murray MJ. *Clinical Anesthesiology*. 4th ed. New York, NY: McGraw Hill; 2006:923.